ENVIRONMENTAL CHEMISTRY AND TOXICOLOGY OF MERCURY

ENVIRONMENTAL CHEMISTRY AND TOXICOLOGY OF MERCURY

Edited by

GUANGLIANG LIU
YONG CAI
NELSON O'DRISCOLL

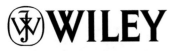

A JOHN WILEY & SONS, INC., PUBLICATION

Published by John Wiley & Sons, Inc., Hoboken, New Jersey
Published simultaneously in Canada

For general information on our other products and services or for technical support, please contact our Customer Care Department within the United States at (800) 762-2974, outside the United States at (317) 572-3993 or fax (317) 572-4002.

Wiley also publishes its books in a variety of electronic formats. Some content that appears in print may not be available in electronic formats. For more information about Wiley products, visit our web site at www.wiley.com.

Library of Congress Cataloging-in-Publication Data:

Advances in environmental chemistry and toxicology of mercury / edited by Guangliang Liu, Yong Cai, Nelson O'Driscoll.
   p. cm.
  Includes index.
  ISBN 978-0-470-57872-8 (hardback)
  1. Mercury–Toxicology. 2. Mercury–Environmental aspects. 3. Mercury–Metabolism. I. Liu, Guangliang, 1972– II. Cai, Yong, 1961– III. O'Driscoll, Nelson J., 1973–
  RA1231.M5335 2012
  615.9′25663–dc23

                                          2011021001

Printed in the United States of America

10 9 8 7 6 5 4 3 2 1

CONTENTS

PREFACE

Mercury is a global contaminant posing severe risks to the health of ecosystems and humans worldwide. The biogeochemical cycling of mercury is rather complicated, involving various transformations and transport processes of mercury species in the environment. A comprehensive review of all the various aspects of mercury transformation and transport is essential for better understanding the mercury cycle and assessing the risks of mercury contamination. Substantial progress has been made in the area of mercury biogeochemistry over the past years; however, there are currently few places where researchers and students can obtain a complete review of the state of the science in this field. This book brings together many of the foremost experts in the field of environmental chemistry and toxicology of mercury and provides a comprehensive overview of the current mercury science. We believe that this book will serve as an excellent resource for researchers, graduate students, environmental regulators, and others.

This book is organized as follows. The first chapter of the book provides a brief overview of mercury in the environment, followed by two chapters discussing environmental analytical chemistry of mercury species and measurement of industrial gas phase mercury emissions. The main part of the book is then devoted to addressing the important transformation and transport processes of mercury in the environment. The following topics are covered under mercury transformation: atmospheric chemical processes, microbial transformations, and aquatic photochemical reactions of mercury species, mercury speciation in soils/sediments, interaction of mercury with organic matter, and isotopic fractionation. For mercury transport, the following topics are examined: atmospheric transport, partition between water and solids, and exchange between the atmosphere and the earth surface (including oceans and terrestrial systems) of mercury. The last part of the book covers bioaccumulation, toxicity, metallomics, and human health risks of mercury. Author's name in boldface on the chapter opening pages indicates the lead author of that chapter.

GUANGLIANG LIU
YONG CAI
NELSON O'DRISCOLL

ACKNOWLEDGMENTS

We thank all the authors for their contribution to this book. We are grateful to the peer reviewers of the chapters for their expertise and efforts. We acknowledge Michael Leventhal at John Wiley & Sons Inc. for devoting great efforts in coordinating the book.

CONTRIBUTORS

GEORGE R. AIKEN, US Geological Survey, 3215 Marine St., Suite E127, Boulder, CO

MARC AMYOT, GRIL, Département de sciences biologiques. Université de Montréal, Montréal, Quebec, Canada

TAMAR BARKAY, Department of Biochemistry and Microbiology, Rutgers University, New Brunswick, NJ and National Environmental Research Institute (NERI), Aahus University, Roskilde, Denmark

SURESH K. BHARGAVA, Advanced Materials and Industrial Chemistry Group, School of Applied Sciences, RMIT University, Melbourne, Victoria, Australia

YONG CAI, Department of Chemistry and Biochemistry and Southeast Environmental Research Center, Florida International University, Miami, FL

ANNA L. CHOI, Department of Environmental Health, Harvard School of Public Health, Boston, MA

MEREDITH CLAYDEN, Canadian Rivers Institute and Biology Department, University of New Brunswick, Saint John, New Brunswick, Canada

XINBIN FENG, State Key Laboratory of Environmental Geochemistry, Institute of Geochemistry, Chinese Academy of Sciences, Guiyang, China

CHASE A. GERBIG, Department of Civil, Environmental, and Architectural Engineering, University of Colorado, Boulder, CO

PHILIPPE GRANDJEAN, Department of Environmental Health, Harvard School of Public Health, Boston, MA Department of Environmental Medicine, University of Southern Denmark, Odense, Denmark

MAE SEXAUER GUSTIN, Department of Natural Resources and Environmental Sciences, University of Nevada-Reno, Reno, NV

HOLGER HINTELMANN, Department of Chemistry, Trent University, Peterborough, Ontario, Canada

KONRAD HUNGERBÜHLER, Safety and Environmental Technology Group, Swiss Federal Institute of Technology (ETH Zürich), Zürich, Switzerland

SAMUEL J. IPPOLITO, Advanced Materials and Industrial Chemistry Group, School of Applied Sciences, RMIT University, Melbourne, Victoria, Australia

TIM JARDINE, Australian Rivers Institute, Griffith University, Brisbane, Queensland, Australia

GUIBIN JIANG, State Key Laboratory of Environmental Chemistry and Ecotoxicology, Research Center for Eco-Environmental Sciences, Chinese Academy of Sciences, Beijing, China

AKIYOSHI KAKITA, Department of Pathological Neuroscience, Resource Branch for Brain Disease Research CBBR, Brain Research Institute, Niigata University, Niigata, Japan

MOHAMMAD A. K. KHAN, Department of Chemistry, University of Manitoba, Winnipeg, Manitoba, Canada

KAREN KIDD, Canadian Rivers Institute and Biology Department, University of New Brunswick, Saint John, New Brunswick, Canada

MARCOS LEMES, Department of Environment and Geography and Department of Chemistry, University of Manitoba, Winnipeg, Manitoba, Canada

YANBIN LI, Department of Chemistry and Biochemistry and Southeast Environmental Research Center, Florida International University, Miami, FL

CHE-JEN LIN, Department of Civil Engineering, Lamar University, Beaumont, TX

CHU-CHING LIN, Department of Biochemistry and Microbiology, Rutgers University, New Brunswick, NJ

GUANGLIANG LIU, Department of Chemistry and Biochemistry and Southeast Environmental Research Center, Florida International University, Miami, FL

MATTHEW MACLEOD, Department of Applied Environmental Science, Stockholm University, Stockholm, Sweden

KATSUYUKI MURATA, Department of Environmental Health Sciences, Akita University School of Medicine, Akita, Japan

NELSON J. O'DRISCOLL, Department of Earth and Environmental Sciences, K.C. Irving Environmental Science Center, Acadia University, Wolfville, Nova Scotia, Canada

SIMO O. PEHKONEN, Department of Chemical Engineering, Masdar Institute, Abu Dhabi, United Arab Emirates

ASIF QURESHI, Safety and Environmental Technology Group, Swiss Federal Institute of Technology (ETH Zürich), Zürich, Switzerland

JOSEPH N. RYAN, Department of Civil, Environmental, and Architectural Engineering, University of Colorado, Boulder, CO

YLIAS M. SABRI, Advanced Materials and Industrial Chemistry Group, School of Applied Sciences, RMIT University, Melbourne, Victoria, Australia

MINESHI SAKAMOTO, Department of International Affairs and Environmental Sciences, National Institute for Minamata Disease, Minamata, Japan

MASANORI SASAKI, Department of Basic Medical Science, National Institute for Minamata Disease, Minamata, Japan

PATTARAPORN SINGHASUK, Department of Industrial Engineering, Lamar University, Beaumont, TX

ULF SKYLLBERG, Department of Forest Ecology and Management, Swedish University of Agricultural Sciences, Umeå, Sweden

ELSIE SUNDERLAND, School of Public Health, Harvard University, Boston, MA

OLEG TRAVNIKOV, Meteorological Synthesizing Centre-East, EMEP, Moscow, Russia

EMMA E. VOST, Department of Earth and Environmental Science, K. C. Irving Environmental Science Center, Acadia University, Wolfville, Nova Scotia, Canada

FEIYUE WANG, Department of Environment and Geography and Department of Chemistry, University of Manitoba, Winnipeg, Manitoba, Canada

NATHAN YEE, Department of Environmental Sciences, Rutgers University, New Brunswick, NJ

YONGGUANG YIN, State Key Laboratory of Environmental Chemistry and Ecotoxicology, Research Center for Eco-Environmental Sciences, Chinese Academy of Sciences, Beijing, China

WANG ZHENG, Environmental Sciences Division, Oak Ridge National Laboratory, Oak Ridge, TN

CHAPTER 1

OVERVIEW OF MERCURY IN THE ENVIRONMENT

GUANGLIANG LIU, YONG CAI, NELSON O'DRISCOLL, XINBIN FENG, and GUIBIN JIANG

1.1 INTRODUCTION

Mercury (Hg) is a naturally occurring element that is present throughout the environment. Mercury is recognized as a global contaminant because it can undergo long-range transport in the atmosphere, be persistent in the environment, be accumulated in the food web, and pose severe adverse effects on the human and ecosystem health (Nriagu, 1979; Fitzgerald et al., 2007b). The environmental contamination of land, air, water, and wildlife in various ecosystems with mercury around the world due to the natural release and extensive anthropogenic use of Hg has been a global concern for decades (Lindberg and Turner, 1977; Ebinghaus et al., 1999; Fitzgerald et al., 2005; Mason et al., 2009). This being the first chapter of the book, it will briefly discuss the health risks associated with mercury exposure and the natural and anthropogenic sources of mercury emissions, and then provide a very brief overview of the biogeochemical cycling of mercury.

In the environment and in biological systems, mercury can exist in three oxidation states, namely, Hg(0) (metallic), Hg(II) (mercuric), and Hg(I) (mercurous), with the monovalent form being rare owing to its instability (Ullrich et al., 2001; Fitzgerald et al., 2007a,b). In general, the dominant form of mercury in water, soil, and sediment is the inorganic Hg(II) form while methylmercury (MeHg) is dominant in biota, and in the atmosphere Hg(0) is the primary species (USEPA, 1997; Ullrich et al., 2001).

Environmental Chemistry and Toxicology of Mercury, First Edition.
Edited by Guangliang Liu, Yong Cai, and Nelson O'Driscoll.
© 2012 John Wiley & Sons, Inc. Published 2012 by John Wiley & Sons, Inc.

1.2 TOXICITY AND HEALTH RISKS OF MERCURY EXPOSURE

All forms of mercury are toxic, but particularly problematic are the organic forms such as MeHg, which is a neurotoxin (Committee on the Toxicological Effects of Methylmercury, 2000; Clarkson and Magos, 2006). Acute mercury exposure can produce permanent damage to the nervous system, resulting in a variety of symptoms such as paresthesia, ataxia, sensory disturbances, tremors, blurred vision, slurred speech, hearing difficulties, blindness, deafness, and death (USEPA, 1997; Committee on the Toxicological Effects of Methylmercury, 2000; Clarkson and Magos, 2006). In addition to neurotoxicity, mercury, in inorganic and/or organic forms, can affect other systems and sequentially cause adverse effects including renal toxicity, myocardial infarction, immune malfunction, and irregular blood pressure (USEPA, 1997; Committee on the Toxicological Effects of Methylmercury, 2000).

Human exposure to Hg can pose a variety of health risks, with the severity depending largely on the magnitude of the dose. Historically, there were two notorious poisoning episodes associated with the extremely high MeHg exposures, that is, in Minamata where individuals were poisoned by MeHg through consumption of contaminated fish and in Iraq where the consumption of MeHg-treated (as a fungicide) grain led to poisoning (Committee on the Toxicological Effects of Methylmercury, 2000). Nowadays, acute poisoning incidents from high Hg exposure are rare and the health risks mercury poses to human population are mainly from chronic MeHg exposure through consumption of contaminated fish and other aquatic organisms, particularly large predatory fish species (USEPA, 1997). A major concern related to the health risks of chronic MeHg exposure is the possibility of developmental toxicity in the fetal brain, since MeHg can readily cross the placenta and the blood–brain barrier (Clarkson and Magos, 2006). Prenatal Hg exposure interferes with the growth and migration of neurons and has the potential to cause irreversible damage to the developing central nervous system (Committee on the Toxicological Effects of Methylmercury, 2000). For instance, because of prenatal MeHg exposure from maternal fish consumption, infants might display deficits in subtle neurological endpoints such as IQ deficits, abnormal muscle tone, and decrements in motor function (Committee on the Toxicological Effects of Methylmercury, 2000).

1.3 SOURCES OF MERCURY

Both naturally occurring and anthropogenic processes can release mercury into air, water, and soil, and emission into the atmosphere is usually the primary pathway for mercury entering the environment (Camargo, 1993; Berg et al., 2006; Jiang et al., 2006; Bone et al., 2007; Bookman et al., 2008; Streets et al., 2009; Cheng and Hu, 2010). It is estimated that the total annual global input to the atmosphere from all sources (i.e., from natural and anthropogenic emissions) is around 5000–6000 t (Mason et al., 1994; Lamborg et al., 2002; Gray and Hines,

2006). The relative importance of natural versus anthropogenic sources of mercury has not been accurately determined, with the ratio of natural to anthropogenic mercury emissions being reported to be within a wide range (e.g., from 0.8 to 1.8) (Nriagu and Pacyna, 1988; Nriagu, 1989, 1994; Bergan et al., 1999; Gustin et al., 2000; Lin and Tao, 2003; Nriagu and Becker, 2003; Seigneur et al., 2003, 2004; Gbor et al., 2007; Shetty et al., 2008).

1.3.1   Natural Sources of Mercury

There are a number of natural processes that can emit Hg into the atmosphere. These processes may include geologic activities (in particular volcanic and geothermal emissions), volatilization of Hg in marine environments, and emission of Hg from terrestrial environments (including substrates with elevated Hg concentrations and background soils) (Nriagu, 1989, 1993, 1994; Gustin et al., 2000, 2008; Gustin, 2003; Nriagu and Becker, 2003; Gray and Hines, 2006). Owing to the lack of data and the complexity of geological processes (e.g., vast variability spatially and temporally) (Gustin et al., 2000, 2008), it is rather difficult to accurately estimate natural Hg emissions, resulting in high degrees of uncertainties being associated with the reported Hg emissions from natural sources. The annual global Hg emissions from natural sources are estimated to range from 800 to 5800 t, with a middle range from 1800 to 3000 t (Lindberg and Turner, 1977; Nriagu, 1989; Lindberg et al., 1998; Bergan et al., 1999; Pirrone et al., 2001; Seigneur et al., 2001, 2004; Lamborg et al., 2002; Mason and Sheu, 2002; Pacyna and Pacyna, 2002; Pirrone and Mahaffey, 2005; Pacyna et al., 2006; Shetty et al., 2008). Among different natural processes, the global volcanic, geothermal, oceanic, and terrestrial Hg emissions are estimated to be 1–700, ~60, 800–2600, and 1000–3200 t per year, respectively (Nriagu, 1989; Lindberg et al., 1998, 1999; Bergan et al., 1999; Ferrara et al., 2000; Lamborg et al., 2002; Mason and Sheu, 2002; Nriagu and Becker, 2003; Pyle and Mather, 2003; Seigneur et al., 2004; Fitzgerald et al., 2007b). Gaseous elemental mercury (GEM) is the predominant form (>99%) of Hg from natural emissions, which is different than anthropogenic emissions that may also contain reactive gaseous mercury (RGM) and particulate Hg (PHg) (Stein et al., 1996; Streets et al., 2005; Pacyna et al., 2006). It should be noted that some processes of natural Hg emissions include reemission of Hg previously deposited from the atmosphere by wet and dry processes derived from both anthropogenic and natural sources. For instance, emission from low Hg-containing substrates and background soils is assumed to be predominantly reemission of Hg previously deposited (Gustin et al., 2000; Seigneur et al., 2004; Gustin et al., 2008; Shetty et al., 2008).

1.3.2   Anthropogenic Sources of Mercury

Extensive anthropogenic emission and use of Hg have caused worldwide mercury contamination in many aquatic and terrestrial ecosystems (Lee et al., 2001; Streets

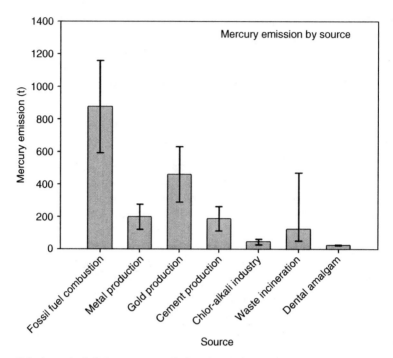

Figure 1.1 Annual global mercury emission (tons) from major anthropogenic sources. *Source*: Data are extracted from the UNEP reports (AMAP/UNEP, 2008; UNEP Chemicals Branch, 2008). Fossil fuel combustion refers to burning of coal and other fossil fuels in power plants and commercial and residential heating units. Metal production includes mercury production, but does not include gold mining and production, which is listed separately.

et al., 2005, 2009; Hope, 2006; Wu et al., 2006; Zhang and Wong, 2007; Sunderland et al., 2009). Comparisons of contemporary (within the past 20–30 years) measurements and historical records indicate that the total global atmospheric mercury burden has increased by a factor of between 2 and 5 since the beginning of the industrialized period (USEPA, 1997). Although anthropogenic emission of Hg has been reduced in the past three decades, anthropogenic processes are still responsible for a significant proportion of global Hg input to the environment. It has been suggested that, among the 5000–6000 t of Hg that is estimated to be released into the atmosphere each year, about 50% may be from anthropogenic sources (Mason et al., 1994; Lamborg et al., 2002; Gray and Hines, 2006), which agrees with some other studies where the annual global anthropogenic emissions of mercury are estimated to be in the range of 2000–2600 t (Pacyna et al., 2001, 2006; Pirrone et al., 2001; Pacyna and Pacyna, 2002; Pirrone and Mahaffey, 2005). Unlike natural sources, anthropogenic sources can emit different species of Hg including GEM, RGM, and PHg with a distribution of about 50–60% GEM, 30% RGM, and 10% PHg (Streets et al., 2005; Pacyna et al., 2006).

Anthropogenic emissions of mercury can be from point (e.g., incinerators and coal-fired power plants) as well as diffuse (e.g., landfills, sewage sludge amended fields, and mine waste) sources (Nriagu, 1989; Sigel and Sigel, 2005; Malm, 1998; Schroeder and Munthe, 1998; Quemerais et al., 1999; Lee et al., 2001; Horvat, 2002; Gustin, 2003; Nelson, 2007; Feng et al., 2010; Pacyna et al., 2010). Point sources, including combustion, manufacturing, and miscellaneous sources (e.g., dental amalgam), are thought to be the main anthropogenic sources of mercury, accounting for approximately more than 95% of anthropogenic mercury emissions (USEPA, 1997). Combustion sources include burning of fossil fuels (e.g., coal and oil), medical waste incinerators, municipal waste combustors, and sewage sludge incinerators. Fossil fuel combustion can be associated with power generation, industrial and residential heating, and various industrial processes. Combustion processes emit divalent mercury and elemental mercury, in gaseous as well as particulate form, depending on the fuels and materials burned (e.g., coal, oil, municipal waste) and fuel gas cleaning and operating temperature, into the atmosphere (USEPA, 1997; UNEP Chemicals Branch, 2008). Manufacturing sources refer to extensive use (especially in the past and in some undeveloped areas) of mercury compounds in many industrial processes such as gold mining, chlor-alkali production, and paper and pulp manufacturing. Unlike combustion sources, manufacturing processes can release mercurial compounds directly into aquatic and terrestrial environments, in addition to the atmosphere (Lindberg and Turner, 1977; Nriagu et al., 1992; Nriagu, 1994; USEPA, 1997; AMAP/UNEP, 2008; UNEP Chemicals Branch, 2008).

Of the three anthropogenic point sources, combustion generally contributes more than 80% of anthropogenic mercury emissions, although varying from region to region (USEPA, 1997; UNEP Chemicals Branch, 2008). Figure 1.1 illustrates the global inventory of mercury emissions from major anthropogenic sources, as estimated by the United Nations Environmental Programme (UNEP) (AMAP/UNEP, 2008; UNEP Chemicals Branch, 2008). Fossil fuel combustion for power generation and industrial and residential heating contributes about 45% of total global emission (880 t out of 1930 t) (Fig. 1.1). Owing to the enormous amount of coal that is burned, coal burning is the largest single source of anthropogenic emissions of Hg to the atmosphere (AMAP/UNEP, 2008). Waste incineration contributes another significant proportion (about 120 t) of mercury emission, but with a wide range between 50 and 470 t due to lack of reliable estimation data, in particular in countries outside Europe and North America. In addition, fuel combustion in industrial processes, including cement and metal production, can release mercury into the atmosphere. Meanwhile, these industrial processes, in particular, the production of iron and nonferrous metals, can release mercury as it can be present as impurity in ores (AMAP/UNEP, 2008). The data illustrated in Fig. 1.1 for these industrial processes include mercury from fuel combustion and from impurities in ores.

Manufacturing sources mainly include gold mining and chlor-alkali industry. Globally, gold mining and production, primarily artisanal and small-scale gold mining using mercury to extract gold, contribute about 20% of anthropogenic mercury emission, while the fraction for chlor-alkali production is about 3% (Fig. 1.1) (AMAP/UNEP, 2008; UNEP Chemicals Branch, 2008). Although industrial use of mercury has been largely reduced in developed countries, it may still contribute to a significant portion of Hg emission in developing countries (e.g., in Asia and South America). As seen from Fig. 1.2, there are significant geological disparities in anthropogenic mercury emissions, with Asia alone accounting for about 65% of total global emission (1280 t out of 1930 t). It should be borne in mind that the data in Fig. 1.2 refer merely to the current emission inventory by region estimated by UNEP, with historical contributions being unaccounted for. Moreover, the relative contributions of different sources to total anthropogenic mercury emission vary with geological region (Fig. 1.3). The most striking characteristic in geological variability of anthropogenic mercury emissions is the dominant contribution of gold mining to overall anthropogenic mercury emission in South America. On the global scale, fossil fuel combustion for power and heating is the primary source of mercury emission, but in South America, gold mining contributes over 60% of total anthropogenic mercury emission (Fig. 1.3).

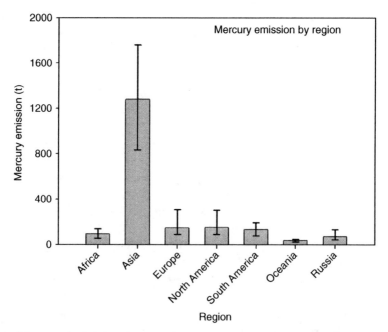

Figure 1.2 Annual global anthropogenic mercury emission (tons) in different regions of the world. *Source*: Data are extracted from the UNEP reports (AMAP/UNEP, 2008; UNEP Chemicals Branch, 2008). Fossil fuel combustion refers to burning of coal and other fossil fuels in power plants and commercial and residential heating units. Metal production includes mercury production, but does not include gold mining and production, which is listed separately.

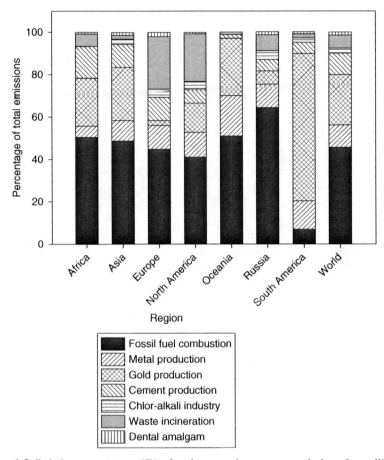

Figure 1.3 Relative percentages (%) of anthropogenic mercury emissions from different sources worldwide and in different regions of the world. *Source*: Data are extracted from the UNEP reports (AMAP/UNEP, 2008; UNEP Chemicals Branch, 2008). Fossil fuel combustion refers to burning of coal and other fossil fuels in power plants and commercial and residential heating units. Metal production includes mercury production, but does not include gold mining and production, which is listed separately.

1.4 OVERVIEW OF MERCURY BIOGEOCHEMICAL CYCLING

After entering the environment, mercury undergoes a series of complicated transport and transformation processes during its biogeochemical cycling. The biogeochemical cycling of mercury is closely associated with the chemical forms of mercury present in different phases of the environment.

In the atmosphere, elemental mercury (Hg(0)) constitutes the majority of Hg (>90%) and is the predominant form in the gaseous phase, which facilitates the long-range transport of Hg at a global scale (USEPA, 1997; Ebinghaus et al.,

1999; Pirrone and Mahaffey, 2005). On the other hand, Hg(II) species present in atmospheric waters, either dissolved or adsorbed onto particles in droplets, has a tendency to readily deposit on the earth's surface through wet and dry deposition, which is important to the local and regional cycle of Hg (Nriagu, 1979; Schroeder and Munthe, 1998).

In water, sediment, and soil environments, mercury is present primarily as various Hg(II) compounds, including inorganic (e.g., mercuric hydroxide) and organic (e.g., MeHg) mercuric compounds, and secondarily as Hg(0), which plays an important role in the exchange of mercury between the atmosphere and aquatic and terrestrial surfaces (Stein et al., 1996; Ullrich et al., 2001; Fitzgerald et al., 2007a,b). These Hg(II) compounds (including inorganic and organic) are present in a variety of physical and chemical forms through complexing with various inorganic (e.g., chloride and sulfide) and organic (e.g., organic matter) ligands (Ullrich et al., 2001). Although in aquatic and soil environments MeHg may constitute a minor fraction of total mercury present (typically less than 10% and 3% in water and soil/sediment, respectively), the formation of MeHg is an important step in mercury cycling (USEPA, 1997; Ullrich et al., 2001). This is because MeHg can be bioaccumulated along the food web and reach high concentrations in organisms, in particular, in aquatic environments. In fishes and wildlife that prey on fish, MeHg can be the dominant form of mercury species owing to bioaccumulation and biomagnification (Stein et al., 1996; Fitzgerald et al., 2007a).

Associated with transformation between different mercury species and transport of mercury between different environmental phases, there are a number of processes that are important in the biogeochemical cycling of mercury. These processes include oxidation of Hg(0) and reduction of Hg(II) (including photochemical and microbial processes), methylation of inorganic mercury (primarily mediated by microbes), distribution of mercury between water and sediment, deposition of mercury from the atmosphere, long-range transport of mercury in the atmosphere, exchange of mercury between the earth surface (oceans and terrestrial ecosystems) and the atmosphere, and bioaccumulation of mercury through food webs (Nriagu, 1979; Ebinghaus et al., 1999; Pirrone and Mahaffey, 2005; Fitzgerald et al., 2007b).

1.5 STRUCTURE OF THE BOOK

The biogeochemical cycling of mercury is rather complicated, involving various transport and transformation processes that determine the fate of mercury and the health risks on ecosystem and humans. A comprehensive summary of the various aspects regarding transformation and transport of mercury is essential for better assessing the risks of mercury contamination. In the past years, a great deal of research has been done to advance the understanding of important aspects of mercury biogeochemical cycling and has produced a wealth of material. This book is aimed to develop a comprehensive review of the state of environmental mercury research by summarizing all the key aspects of the mercury cycle.

Following this opening chapter, environmental analytical chemistry of mercury species and measurement of industrial gas phase mercury emissions are discussed. The main body of the book is devoted to address the important transformation and transport processes of mercury in the environment (as mentioned in Section 1.4), which includes the interaction of mercury with organic matter and the isotope fractionation of mercury. In addition, the toxicity, metallomics, and health risks associated with mercury (in particular MeHg) exposure are discussed in Part IV of the book.

1.6 CONCLUDING REMARKS

Both naturally occurring and anthropogenic processes can release mercury into the environment, and the latter has led to a current total global atmospheric mercury burden two- to fivefold higher than before the industrialized period. There are significant geological disparities not only in the amounts of anthropogenic mercury emissions but also in the relative importance of different anthropogenic sources for each region.

After entering the environment, mercury undergoes a series of complicated transport and transformation processes during its biogeochemical cycling. Through formation of MeHg in the (particularly aquatic) environment and bioaccumulation of MeHg (particularly in fishes) through food webs, human populations can be exposed to mercury (especially MeHg) through consumption of mercury-contaminated fishes. Human exposure to mercury can pose a variety of health risks, mainly as neurological damages, especially in the fetal brain. This book covers environmental analysis of mercury, important transformation and transport processes of mercury in the environment, and toxicological aspects of mercury.

REFERENCES

AMAP/UNEP. Technical Background Report to the Global Atmospheric Mercury Assessment. Arctic Monitoring and Assessment Programme/UNEP Chemicals Branch; 2008. p 159.

Berg T, Fjeld E, Steinnes E. Atmospheric mercury in Norway: contributions from different sources. Sci Total Environ 2006;368:3–9.

Bergan T, Gallardo L, Rodhe H. Mercury in the global troposphere: a three-dimensional model study. Atmos Environ 1999;33:1575–1585.

Bone SE, Charette MA, Lamborg CH, Gonneea ME. Has submarine groundwater discharge been overlooked as a source of mercury to coastal waters. Environ Sci Technol 2007;41:3090–3095.

Bookman R, Driscoll CT, Engstrom DR, Effler SW. Local to regional emission sources affecting mercury fluxes to New York lakes. Atmos Environ 2008;42:6088–6097.

Camargo JA. Which source of mercury pollution. Nature 1993;365:302–302.

Cheng H, Hu Y. China needs to control mercury emissions from municipal solid waste (MSW) incineration. Environ Sci Technol 2010;44:7994–7995.

Clarkson TW, Magos L. The toxicology of mercury and its chemical compounds. Crit Rev Toxicol 2006;36:609–662.

Committee on the Toxicological Effects of Methylmercury. Toxicological effect of methylmercury. Washington (DC): Board on Environmental Studies and Toxicology Commission on Life Sciences National Research Council, National Academy Press; 2000.

Ebinghaus R, Turner RR, Lacerda D, Vasiliev O, Salomons W. Mercury contaminated sites-characterization, risk assessment and remediation. Berlin, Heidelberg, New York: Springer Environmental Science, Springer Verlag; 1999. p 538.

Feng X, Foucher D, Hintelmann H, Yan H, He T, Qiu G. Tracing mercury contamination sources in sediments using mercury isotope compositions. Environ Sci Technol 2010;44:3363–3368.

Ferrara R, Mazzolai B, Lanzillotta E, Nucaro E, Pirrone N. Volcanoes as emission sources of atmospheric mercury in the Mediterranean basin. Sci Total Environ 2000;259:115–121.

Fitzgerald WF, Engstrom DR, Lamborg CH, Tseng CM, Balcom PH, Hammerschmidt CR. Modern and historic atmospheric mercury fluxes in northern Alaska: global sources and arctic depletion. Environ Sci Technol 2005;39:557–568.

Fitzgerald WF, Lamborg CH, Hammerschmidt CR. Marine biogeochemical cycling of mercury. Chem Rev 2007a;107:641–662.

Fitzgerald WF, Lamborg CH, Heinrich DH, Karl KT. Geochemistry of mercury in the environment. Treatise on geochemistry. Oxford: Pergamon; 2007b. p 1–47.

Gbor PK, Wen D, Meng F, Yang F, Sloan JJ. Modeling of mercury emission, transport and deposition in North America. Atmos Environ 2007;41:1135–1149.

Gray JE, Hines ME. Mercury: distribution, transport, and geochemical and microbial transformations from natural and anthropogenic sources. Appl Geochem 2006;21:1819–1820.

Gustin MS. Are mercury emissions from geologic sources significant? A status report. Sci Total Environ 2003;304:153–167.

Gustin MS, Lindberg SE, Austin K, Coolbaugh M, Vette A, Zhang H. Assessing the contribution of natural sources to regional atmospheric mercury budgets. Sci Total Environ 2000;259:61–71.

Gustin MS, Lindberg SE, Weisberg PJ. An update on the natural sources and sinks of atmospheric mercury. Appl Geochem 2008;23:482–493.

Hope BK. An assessment of anthropogenic source impacts on mercury cycling in the Willamette Basin, Oregon, USA. Sci Total Environ 2006;356:165–191.

Horvat M. Mercury as a global pollutant. Anal Bioanal Chem 2002;374:981–982.

Jiang G-B, Shi J-B, Feng X-B. Mercury pollution in China. Environ Sci Technol 2006;40:3672–3678.

Lamborg CH, Fitzgerald WF, O'Donnell J, Torgersen T. A non-steady-state compartmental model of global-scale mercury biogeochemistry with interhemispheric atmospheric gradients. Geochim Cosmochim Acta 2002;66:1105–1118.

Lee X, Bullock OR Jr, Andres RJ. Anthropogenic emission of mercury to the atmosphere in the northeast United States. Geophys Res Lett 2001;28:1231–1234.

Lin X, Tao Y. A numerical modelling study on regional mercury budget for eastern North America. Atmos Chem Phys 2003;3:535–548.

Lindberg SE, Hanson PJ, Meyers TP, Kim KH. Air/surface exchange of mercury vapor over forests–the need for a reassessment of continental biogenic emissions. Atmos Environ 1998;32:895–908.

Lindberg SE, Turner RR. Mercury emissions from chlorine-production solid waste deposits. Nature 1977;268:133–136.

Lindberg SE, Zhang H, Gustin M, Vette A, Marsik F, Owens J, Casimir A, Ebinghaus R, Edwards G, Fitzgerald C, Kemp J, Kock HH, London J, Majewski M, Poissant L, Pilote M, Rasmussen P, Schaedlich F, Schneeberger D, Sommar J, Turner R, Wallschläger D, Xiao Z. Increases in mercury emissions from desert soils in response to rainfall and irrigation. J Geophys Res 1999;104:21879–21888.

Malm O. Gold mining as a source of mercury exposure in the Brazilian Amazon. Environ Res 1998;77:73–78.

Mason RP, Fitzgerald WF, Morel FMM. The biogeochemical cycling of elemental mercury: anthropogenic influences. Geochim Cosmochim Acta 1994;58:3191–3198.

Mason R, Pirrone N, Pirrone N, Cinnirella S, Feng X, Finkelman RB, Friedli HR, Leaner J, Mason R, Mukherjee AB, Stracher G, Streets DG, Telmer K. Global mercury emissions to the atmosphere from natural and anthropogenic sources. Mercury fate and transport in the global atmosphere. New York (NY): Springer; 2009. p 1–47.

Mason RP, Sheu GR. Role of the ocean in the global mercury cycle. Global Biogeochem Cycles 2002;16:1093.

Nelson PF. Atmospheric emissions of mercury from Australian point sources. Atmos Environ 2007;41:1717–1724.

Nriagu JO. The biogeochemistry of mercury in the environment. New York: Elsevier/North Holland Biomedical Press; 1979. p 696.

Nriagu JO. A global assessment of natural sources of atmospheric trace metals. Nature 1989;338:47–49.

Nriagu JO. Legacy of mercury pollution. Nature 1993;363:589.

Nriagu JO. Mercury pollution from the past mining of gold and silver in the Americas. Sci Total Environ 1994;149:167–181.

Nriagu JO, Becker C. Volcanic emissions of mercury to the atmosphere: global and regional inventories. Sci Total Environ 2003;304:3–12.

Nriagu JO, Pacyna JM. Quantitative assessment of worldwide contamination of air, water and soils by trace metals. Nature 1988;333:134–139.

Nriagu JO, Pfeiffer WC, Malm O, Souza CMM, Mierle G. Mercury pollution in Brazil. Nature 1992;356:389–389.

Pacyna EG, Pacyna JM. Global emission of mercury from anthropogenic sources in 1995. Water Air Soil Pollut 2002;137:149–165.

Pacyna EG, Pacyna JM, Fudala J, Strzelecka-Jastrzab E, Hlawiczka S, Panasiuk D. Mercury emissions to the atmosphere from anthropogenic sources in Europe in 2000 and their scenarios until 2020. Sci Total Environ 2006;370:147–156.

Pacyna EG, Pacyna JM, Pirrone N. European emissions of atmospheric mercury from anthropogenic sources in 1995. Atmos Environ 2001;35:2987–2996.

Pacyna EG, Pacyna JM, Sundseth K, Munthe J, Kindbom K, Wilson S, Steenhuisen F, Maxson P. Global emission of mercury to the atmosphere from anthropogenic sources in 2005 and projections to 2020. Atmos Environ 2010;44:2487–2499.

Pirrone N, Costa P, Pacyna JM, Ferrara R. Mercury emissions to the atmosphere from natural and anthropogenic sources in the Mediterranean region. Atmos Environ 2001;35:2997–3006.

Pirrone N, Mahaffey KR. Dynamics of mercury pollution on regional and global scales: atmospheric processes and human exposures around the world. New York: Springer; 2005. p 744.

Pyle DM, Mather TA. The importance of volcanic emissions for the global atmospheric mercury cycle. Atmos Environ 2003;37:5115–5124.

Quemerais B, Cossa D, Rondeau B, Pham TT, Gagnon P, Fortin B. Sources and fluxes of mercury in the St Lawrence River. Environ Sci Technol 1999;33:840–849.

Schroeder WH, Munthe J. Atmospheric mercury—An overview. Atmos Environ 1998;32:809–822.

Seigneur C, Karamchandani P, Lohman K, Vijayaraghavan K, Shia R-L. Multi-scale modeling of the atmospheric fate and transport of mercury. J Geophys Res 2001;106:27795–27809.

Seigneur C, Lohman K, Vijayaraghavan K, Shia R-L. Contributions of global and regional sources to mercury deposition in New York State. Environ Pollut 2003;123:365–373.

Seigneur C, Vijayaraghavan K, Lohman K, Karamchandani P, Scott C. Global source attribution for mercury deposition in the United States. Environ Sci Technol 2004;38:555–569.

Shetty SK, Lin CJ, Streets DG, Jang C. Model estimate of mercury emission from natural sources in East Asia. Atmos Environ 2008;42:8674–8685.

Sigel A, Sigel H. Mercury and its effects on environment and biology. Volume 34, Metal ions in biological systems. New York: Marcel Dekker, Inc; 1997. p 604.

Stein ED, Cohen Y, Winer AM. Environmental distribution and transformation of mercury compounds. Crit Rev Environ Sci Technol 1996;26:1–43.

Streets DG, Hao J, Wu Y, Jiang J, Chan M, Tian H, Feng X. Anthropogenic mercury emissions in china. Atmos Environ 2005;39:7789–7806.

Streets DG, Zhang Q, Wu Y. Projections of global mercury emissions in 2050. Environ Sci Technol 2009;43:2983–2988.

Sunderland EM, Krabbenhoft DP, Moreau JW, Strode SA, Landing WM. Mercury sources, distribution, and bioavailability in the North Pacific Ocean: insights from data and models. Global Biogeochem Cycles 2009;23:GB2010.

Ullrich SM, Tanton TW, Abdrashitova SA. Mercury in the aquatic environment: a review of factors affecting methylation. Crit Rev Environ Sci Technol 2001;31:241–293.

UNEP Chemicals Branch. The global atmospheric mercury assessment: sources, emissions and transport. Geneva: UNEP-Chemicals Branch; 2008. p 44.

USEPA. EPA Mercury Study Report to Congress. Washington (DC): Office of Air Quality and Standards and Office of Research and Development, U.S. Environmental Protection Agency; 1997. EPA-452/R-97-009.

Wu Y, Wang S, Streets DG, Hao J, Chan M, Jiang J. Trends in anthropogenic mercury emissions in china from 1995 to 2003. Environ Sci Technol 2006;40:5312–5318.

Zhang L, Wong MH. Environmental mercury contamination in china: sources and impacts. Environ Int 2007;33:108–121.

PART I

ANALYTICAL DEVELOPMENTS

CHAPTER 2

ADVANCES IN SPECIATION ANALYSIS OF MERCURY IN THE ENVIRONMENT

YANBIN LI, YONGGUANG YIN, GUANGLIANG LIU, and **YONG CAI**

2.1 INTRODUCTION

Mercury (Hg) has recently emerged as a highly pervasive global pollutant, which occurs widely in the environment (sediment, water, and atmosphere) in various chemical species. The existing chemical forms in which Hg is present inevitably affect the biogeochemical transformation, transport, toxicity, bioaccumulation, and fate of Hg in the environment. Therefore, there is a clear need for developing sensitive and cost-effective methods for Hg speciation analysis. There are five important chemical forms of mercury in the environment, including elemental Hg (Hg^0), divalent inorganic mercury (Hg^{2+}), monomethylmercury (MeHg), dimethylmercury (DMeHg), and monoethylmercury (EtHg). Hg^0 is the predominant species of mercury in the atmosphere, and it can undergo long-range transport from source regions via atmospheric circulation. Divalent inorganic mercury represents the largest fraction of this element in the terrestrial and aquatic environment, while MeHg is the species of concern owing to its prevalent existence, high toxicity, accumulation through food chain, and big threats posed to human and wildlife. Although EtHg is not as prevalent as MeHg in nature, its occurrence has been reported in some wetland systems (Cai et al., 1997; Siciliano et al., 2003; Mao et al., 2010).

The speciation analysis of Hg mainly involves three steps, extraction of Hg from matrix, separation of different Hg species, and detection. High performance liquid chromatography (HPLC) and gas chromatography (GC) are the most commonly used separation techniques for Hg speciation analysis. The application of HPLC-based techniques is limited by their poor limit of detection (LOD). Therefore, it is hard to apply these methods for the mercury speciation analysis of environmental samples with low concentration of mercury (e.g., natural water

Environmental Chemistry and Toxicology of Mercury, First Edition.
Edited by Guangliang Liu, Yong Cai, and Nelson O'Driscoll.
© 2012 John Wiley & Sons, Inc. Published 2012 by John Wiley & Sons, Inc.

samples). It is very easy to couple GC with highly effective preconcentration methods, such as purge and trap, which can significantly improve the sensitivity and makes GC the first choice for analyzing ultra-low concentrations of Hg species in environmental samples. A third technique, capillary electrophoresis (CE), has been extensively studied and demonstrated to be a complementary tool to GC and HPLC in analyzing mercury species, especially in studying the interaction of alkylated mercury with biomolecules (Trumpler et al., 2009). Various element-specific detectors, such as atomic absorption spectrometry (AAS), inductively coupled plasma mass spectrometry (ICP-MS), atomic fluorescence spectrometry (AFS), and atomic emission spectrometry (AES), have been coupled on-line to GC, HPLC, or CE for Hg speciation analysis. The AFS detector is sensitive, selective, and cost-effective, which make it one of the most popular detectors for mercury detection (Cai, 2000; Leermakers et al., 2005). ICP-MS is another popularly used detector owing to its high sensitivity, selectivity, and the opportunity to perform isotope dilution (ID) analysis of mercury species (Leermakers et al., 2005).

This chapter reviews recent analytical developments on the Hg speciation analysis. The bulk of the review is organized on the basis of different separation techniques (GC, HPLC, and CE). In addition, a fourth section is provided to describe the application of ID technique in Hg speciation analysis. ID analysis provides a powerful and unique tool for elemental speciation owing to its high accuracy and precision (Monperrus et al., 2004; Rodriguez-Gonzalez et al., 2005; Bjorn et al., 2007). Lastly, X-ray absorption spectroscopy (XAS) in mercury speciation is also briefly reviewed, considering its importance in the *in situ* probing of the chemical microenvironment of Hg, including structure and bonding.

2.2   SAMPLE PREPARATION FOR Hg SPECIATION IN ENVIRONMENTAL SAMPLES

Extraction of mercury species from matrix is usually required before analysis when solid samples are analyzed. Acid (e.g., concentrated HCl) and alkaline (e.g., KOH in methanol) leaching are among the most popular methods for Hg species extraction from soil, sediment, and biological samples (Tables 2.1 and 2.2). In the past decade, various mild leaching methods using mercaptoethanol (Lin et al., 2008), L-cysteine (Hight and Cheng, 2006), or thiourea (Shade, 2008) as complexation reagent have also been developed for extracting Hg species from biological samples, including hair, fish, mussel, bovine liver, blood, zooplankton, rice, and flour. The virtue of leaching using thiol reagents is that the extracted solution can be directly injected into the HPLC column without the requirement of pH adjustment (Wang et al., 2007). Microwave and ultrasound have been widely used to accelerate the solid–liquid leaching procedure. Compared to conventional leaching procedures, these techniques can reduce the sample preparation time and solvent consumption and improve the leaching efficiency (Rio-Segade and Bendicho, 1999). Aqueous samples can be directly

TABLE 2.1 Summary of the GC Methods for Mercury Speciation

Hg Species	Sample Matrix	Leaching Protocol	Pre-concentration	Derivatization	Detector	LOD (ng/L for Water and ng/g for Solid Matrices)				References
						Hg^{2+}	MeHg	EtHg	Others	
Hg^{2+}	River water	—	SDME	Ph	FID	20,000	—	—	—	Yazdi et al. (2010)
MeHg	Fish sediment	Dithizone distillation	PT	Eth	MS	—	0.1 (Fish) 0.05 (Sediment)	—	—	Park et al. (2010)
Hg^{2+}, MeHg	Fish	TMAH (microwave)	SE	Eth	EI-MS	10	10	—	—	Castillo et al. (2010)
MeHg	Sediment	TSE	PT	Eth	ICP-MS	—	—	—	—	Avramescu et al. (2010)
Hg^{2+}, MeHg	Water	—	SE	Eth	MS ICP-MS	—	—	—	—	Nsengimana et al. (2009)
MeHg	Medicine	HCl	SE	—	ECD	—	2	—	—	Jung et al. (2009)
MeHg	Water	—	PT	Eth	ICP-MS	—	0.003	—	—	Jackson et al. (2009)
Hg^{2+}, MeHg, EtHg	Drinking water	—	SBSE	Pr	MS	200	20	10	—	Ito et al. (2009)
MeHg, EtHg	Biota	Aqueous KOH	HS-SPME	Pr	AFS	—	0.04	0.04	—	Carrasco et al. (2009)
Hg^{2+}, MeHg	Human urine, saliva, serum	—	HS-SPME	Eth	MS	10–61	15–81	—	—	Zachariadis and Kapsimali (2008)

(continued)

TABLE 2.1 (*Continued*)

Hg Species	Sample Matrix	Leaching Protocol	Pre-concentration	Derivatization	Detector	LOD (ng/L for Water and ng/g for Solid Matrices)				References
						Hg^{2+}	MeHg	EtHg	Others	
MeHg, EtHg	Water, soil, fish	KBr/H_2SO_4 and $CuSO_4$ for soil 18% NaOH–methanol for fish	PT	Ph	AFS ICP-MS	—	0.03 (AFS) 0.02 (ICP-MS)	0.03 (AFS) 0.01 (ICP-MS)	—	Mao et al. (2008)
MeHg	Biological samples	KOH-ethanol	PT	Eth	MS	—	0.9	—	—	Lee et al. (2007)
MeHg, EtHg	Biological samples, vaccine	KBr/H_2SO_4 and $CuSO_4$	PT	Pr	CV-AFS	—	0.01 (Blood) 0.01 (Saliva) 0.01 (Vaccine) 5 (Hair)	0.01 (Blood) 0.01 (Saliva) 0.01 (Vaccine) 5 (Hair)	—	Gibicar et al. (2007)
MeHg	Standard solution	—	HS-SPME	Pr	AED	—	0.016	—	—	Geerdink et al. (2007)
MeHg	Plant	$HBr/CuSO_4$ (microwave)	—	—	ECD	—	0.35	—	—	Canario et al. (2006)
Hg^{2+}, MeHg	Sediment, biota, seawater	$HCl–CH_3OH$ for sediment 25%KOH for biota (sonication)	SPME	Ph	MS	0.1 (Sediment) 12.5 (Biota) 2.0 (Seawater)	0.04 (Sediment) 0.5 (Biota) 0.8 (Seawater)	—	—	Mishra et al. (2005)

Analyte	Sample	Digestion/Extraction	Technique	Derivatization	Detection				LOD	Reference
Hg²⁺, MeHg	Fish	TMAH or HNO₃ (microwave)	SE	Eth	ICP-MS AFS	—	—	—	—	Krystek and Ritsema (2005)
MeHg	Fish	25% KOH–methanol or 18% NaOH–methanol	SPME	Ph	AFS	—	—	—	—	Jokai et al. (2005)
$(CH_3)_2Hg$	Air	—	Carbotrap™	—	CV-AFS	—	—	—	0.01 ng/m³	Bloom et al. (2005)
MeHg	Hair	Acid digest	SPME	Eth	CV-AFS	—	40	—	—	Montuori et al. (2004)
Hg²⁺, MeHg	Fish	TMAH	SE	Eth	ICP-MS	—	—	—	—	Krystek and Ritsema (2004)
MeHg	Biological samples	Acetic acid (microwave)	HS-SPME	Eth or Ph	ICP-MS	—	0.004	—	—	Davis et al. (2004)
MeHg	Fish	TMAH (microwave)	SE	Pr	EI-MS	—	40	—	—	Chen et al. (2004)

(continued)

TABLE 2.1 (*Continued*)

Hg Species	Sample Matrix	Leaching Protocol	Pre-concentration	Derivati-zation	Detector	LOD (ng/L for Water and ng/g for Solid Matrices)				References
						Hg^{2+}	MeHg	EtHg	Others	
Hg^{2+}, MeHg	Sea water	—	SPME	Pr	ICP-MS	0.35	0.17	—	—	Bravo-Sanchez et al. (2004)
Hg^{2+}, MeHg	Water	—	CT	HG	AFS	—	—	—	—	Stoichev et al. (2002)
Hg^{2+}, MeHg	Water	—	PT	Eth	AFS	0.06	0.006	—	—	Logar et al. (2002)
Hg^{2+}, MeHg	Standard solution	—	PT	Eth	ICP-TOF-MS	0.15	0.002	—	—	Leenaers et al. (2002)
MeHg	Food samples	KOH–methanol or TMAH or enzymolysis	SE	—	AFS	—	200 ng/L	—	—	Ebdon et al. (2002)
MeHg, Hg^{2+}	Hair	HCl	HS-SPME	Eth	CV-AFS	80	50	—	—	Diez and Bayona (2002)
MeHg, EtHg, Hg^{2+}	Seawater	—	HS-SPME	Ph	AED	300	100	100	—	Carro et al. (2002)
MeHg, EtHg, Hg^{2+}	Standard solution	—	SE	Grignard	RF- HC-GD- AES	0.2 pg	0.2 pg	0.2 pg	—	Velado et al. (2000)
MeHg	Biological samples	NaCl–HCl	SE	Eth	MIP-AES ICP-MS	—	4.4 (MIP-AES) 2.6 (ICP-MS)	—	—	Tu et al. (2000)

MeHg	Fish	KOH–methanol	SE	Ph	MIP-AED	—	100	—	Palmieri and Leonel (2000)
MeHg	Blood	KOH–methanol	SE	Eth	CV-AFS	—	0.02	—	Liang et al. (2000)
MeHg	Soil	Subcritical water extraction	HS-SPME	Eth	MS	—	5.0	—	Beichert et al. (2000)
MeHg	Rain	—	PT	Eth	AFS ICP-MS	—	0.05 (AFS) 0.02 (ICP-MS)	—	Holz et al. (1999)
DMeHg, MeHg	Ocean water	—	PT	Eth	AFD	—	0.005	0.005 (DMeHg)	Pongratz and Heumann (1998)
MeHg, EtHg, Hg^{2+}	Standard solution	—	—	Grignard	GD-AES	3000	1300	1300	Orellana-Velado et al. (1998)
MeHg, EtHg	Standard solution	—	SE	Pr	ICP-MS	—	210	210	De Smaele et al. (1998)
MeHg	Fish, water	Aqueous KOH for fish	SPME	Eth	AFS	—	3.0 (Water) 6.6 (Fish)	—	Cai et al. (1998)

(continued)

TABLE 2.1 (*Continued*)

Hg Species	Sample Matrix	Leaching Protocol	Pre-concentration	Derivati-zation	Detector	LOD (ng/L for Water and ng/g for Solid Matrices)				References
						Hg^{2+}	MeHg	EtHg	Others	
MeHg	Water	—	Steam distillation	Eth	CV-AFS	—	0.024	—	—	Bowles and Apte (1998)
MeHg, Hg^{2+}	Biological samples	TMAH	PT	Eth	AES	0.2	1.4	—	—	Jimenez and Sturgeon (1997)
MeHg	Sediment	KOH–methanol (sonication)	SE	—	ECD	—	—	—	—	Caricchia et al. (1997)
MeHg, EtHg	Water	—	SPE	—	AFS	—	0.01	—	—	Cai et al. (1996)
MeHg	Water, biological samples	KOH–methanol for biota	PT	Eth	CV-AFS	—	0.05 (Water) 1.4 (Biota)	—	—	Saouter and Blattmann (1994)
MeHg	Hair	Alkaline digest	SE	—	ECD	—	50	—	—	Chiavarini et al. (1994)

TMAH, tetramethylammonium hydroxide; PT, purge and trap; CT, cryogenic trapping; Eth, ethylation; HG, hydride generation; TSE, thiosulfate extraction.

TABLE 2.2 Summary of the HPLC Methods for Mercury Speciation

Hg Species	Sample Matrix	Leaching Protocol	Pre-concentration	Detector	Interface	LOD (µg/L)				References
						Hg(II)	MeHg	EtHg	PhHg	
Hg^{2+}, MeHg, EtHg, PhHg	Standard	—	—	UV	—	110	79	108	50	dos Santos et al. (2006)
Hg^{2+}, MeHg, PhHg	Standard	—	—	UV	—	4	8.5	—	11.5	Shaw et al. (2003)
MeHg, EtHg, PhHg	Water, fish	HCl (sonication)	HF-LLLME	UV	—	—	3.8	0.7	0.3	Xia et al. (2007)
Hg^{2+}, MeHg, EtHg, PhHg	Fish, seafood	HCl (sonication)	FI displacement sorption	UV	—	—	—	—	—	Dong et al. (2004)
Hg^{2+}, MeHg, PhHg	Water	—	Dithizone-modified C18 SPE	UV	—	0.14	0.14	—	0.16	Sanchez et al. (2000)
Hg^{2+}, MeHg, PhHg	Water	—	Triazenide-modified C18 extraction disks	UV	—	0.0013	0.0010	—	0.0008	Hashempur et al. (2008)
Hg^{2+}, MeHg, EtHg, PhHg	Water	—	SDME	UV	—	22.8	1.0	1.6	7.1	Pena-Pereira et al. (2009)
Hg^{2+}, MeHg	Water	—	—	PED	—	0.23	0.21	—	—	Palenzuela et al. (2004)

(continued)

TABLE 2.2 (*Continued*)

Hg Species	Sample Matrix	Leaching Protocol	Pre-concentration	Detector	Interface	LOD (μg/L) Hg(II)	MeHg	EtHg	PhHg	References
Hg^{2+}, MeHg, EtHg, PhHg	River water	—	APDC-modified C18 SPE	APCI-ion-trap MS	—	0.090	0.370	0.280	0.250	Houserova et al. (2007)
Hg^{2+}, MeHg, PhHg	Standard	—	—	PB-EI-MS	—	1.55	15.0	—	1.03	Krishna et al. (2007)
Hg^{2+}, MeHg	Water, fish	—	APDC-modified C18 SPE	AAS	CVG	0.000068	0.000034	—	—	Qvarnstrom et al. (2000)
Hg^{2+}, MeHg	Sediment	25% KOH–methanol (sonication)	—	AAS	Photo-oxidation—CVG	0.05	0.05	—	—	Campos et al. (2009)
Hg^{2+}, MeHg	Fish	HCl and NaCl	—	RGD-AES	$K_2S_2O_8$ oxidation (microwave)—CVG	1.2	1.8	—	—	Martinez et al. (2001)
Hg^{2+}, MeHg	Human urine	—	—	ICP-AES	—	1000	2000	—	—	Percy et al. (2007)
Hg^{2+}, MeHg	Zooplankton, fish	Thiourea, HCl, and HAc	Online SPE by thiol or iodide-complex poly divinyl-benzene resin	AFS	$KBrO_3$ oxidation—CVG	0.00014	0.00008	—	—	Shade (2008)

Analyte	Matrix									Reference
Hg^{2+}, MeHg, EtHg, PhHg	Fish	CPE	HCl (sonication)	AFS	K$_2$S$_2$O$_8$ oxidation (knotted reactor)—CVG	0.002	0.009	0.004	0.004	Yu (2005)
Hg^{2+}, MeHg	Fish	Thiol trapping	KBr–KBr$_2$SO$_4$ and CuSO$_4$	AFS	H$_2$O$_2$ oxidation (UV)—CVG	0.0002	0.0002	—	—	Shade and Hudson (2005)
Hg^{2+}, MeHg, EtHg, PhHg	Fish, seafood	—	HCl (sonication)	AFS	K$_2$S$_2$O$_8$ oxidation (knotted reactor)—CVG	0.19	0.27	0.26	0.21	Li et al. (2005b)
Hg^{2+}, MeHg, EtHg, PhHg	Fish	—	HCl and NaCl (microwave)	AFS	KBr–KBrO$_3$ oxidation—CVG	0.07	0.2	0.12	0.06	Houserova et al. (2006)
Hg^{2+}, MeHg, EtHg, PhHg	Fish	—	HCl (100°C)	AFS	KBr–KBrO$_3$ oxidation (knotted reactor)—CVG	0.46	0.51	0.51	0.57	Bramanti et al. (2005)

(continued)

25

TABLE 2.2 *(Continued)*

Hg Species	Sample Matrix	Leaching Protocol	Pre-concentration	Detector	Interface	LOD (µg/L)				References
						Hg(II)	MeHg	EtHg	PhHg	
Hg^{2+}, MeHg	Fish, lobster	KOH–methanol (microwave)	—	AFS	Photo-oxidation—CVG	0.051	0.051	—	—	Ramalhosa et al. (2001b)
Hg^{2+}, MeHg	Sediment	KOH–methanol (microwave)	—	AFS	Photo-oxidation—CVG	0.051	0.051	—	—	Ramalhosa et al. (2001a)
Hg^{2+}, MeHg	Sediment	KOH–methanol (sonication)	—	AFS	KBr–$KBrO_3$ oxidation—CVG	0.05	0.05	—	—	Ramalhosa et al. (2001c)
Hg^{2+}, MeHg	Freshwater	—	—	AFS	$K_2S_2O_8$ photooxidation—CVG	11	8	—	—	Gomez-Ariza et al. (2004)
Hg^{2+}, MeHg, EtHg, PhHg	Fish, oyster	KOH–methanol	—	AFS	$K_2S_2O_8$ oxidation (microwave)—CVG	15	10	8.5	7	Liang et al. (2003)
Hg^{2+}, MeHg, EtHg, PhHg	Sediment, zoobenthos, river water	HCl, 50% aqueous methanol, and citric acid	2-Mercaptophenol-modified C18 SPE	AFS	$KBr/KBrO_3$ photooxidation—CVG	0.8	4.3	1.4	0.8	Margetinova et al. (2008)

Hg^{2+}, MeHg, EtHg, PhHg	Fish, mollusk	KOH–methanol	—	AFS	Photo-CVG with formic acid	1.01	0.81	0.20	0.87	Yin et al. (2007b)
Hg^{2+}, MeHg, EtHg, PhHg	Fish, mollusk	KOH–methanol	—	AFS	Photo-CVG with formic acid in mobile phase	0.085	0.033	0.029	0.038	Yin et al. (2008)
Hg^{2+}, MeHg, EtHg, PhHg	Fish, mollusk	KOH–methanol	—	AFS	Photo-CVG with reaction agent in mobile phase	0.53	0.22	0.18	0.25	Yin et al. (2009a)
Hg^{2+}, MeHg, EtHg, PhHg	Fish, mollusk, sediment	HCl for biological sample and KOH–methanol for sediment	—	AFS	Photo-CVG with formic acid and TiO_2 catalyst	—	—	—	—	Yin et al. (2007a)

(continued)

TABLE 2.2 (*Continued*)

Hg Species	Sample Matrix	Leaching Protocol	Pre-concentration	Detector	Interface	LOD (µg/L)				References
						Hg(II)	MeHg	EtHg	PhHg	
Hg²⁺, MeHg, EtHg	Fish, lobster	KOH–methanol	—	AFS	L-cysteine—CVG	0.10	0.05	0.07	—	Yin et al. (2007c)
Hg²⁺, MeHg, EtHg	Fish, hair	KOH–methanol	—	AFS	Direct CVG-flame atomization	0.4	0.2	0.4	—	Yin et al. (2009b)
Hg²⁺, MeHg, EtHg	Coal	TMAH (microwave)	—	AFS	$K_2S_2O_8$ photooxidation—CVG	—	—	—	—	Gao et al. (2008)
Hg²⁺, MeHg	Freshwater	—	—	AFS, ICP-MS	$K_2S_2O_8$ photooxidation—CVG	12(AFS), 0.9(ICP-MS)	8(AFS), 1.1(ICP-MS)	—	—	Gomez-Ariza et al. (2005)
Hg²⁺, MeHg, EtHg	Hair	Mercaptoethanol, L-cysteine, and HCl (sonication)	—	ICP-MS	—	—	—	—	—	(de Souza et al. (2010)
Hg²⁺, MeHg	Fish	Perchloric acid, L-cysteine, and toluene: methanol (1:1) (sonication)	—	ICP-MS	—	0.9	0.7	—	—	Santoyo et al. (2009)

Species	Matrix	Extraction	Preconcentration	Detection					Reference
Hg^{2+}, MeHg	Human hair	HNO$_3$ (100°C, microwave)	—	ICP-MS	—	—	—	—	Rahman et al. (2009)
Hg^{2+}, MeHg	Tuna fish	Alkaline extraction (microwave or sonication)	—	ICP-MS	—	0.46	0.78	—	Reyes et al. (2008)
Hg^{2+}, MeHg, EtHg	Seafood	L-cysteine, HCl, H$_2$O (60°C)	—	ICP-MS	—	0.02	0.03	—	Hight and Cheng (2006)
Hg^{2+}, MeHg, EtHg, PhHg	Sediment	NH$_4$Ac in n-butanol	DDTC-modified polyurethane foam	ICP-MS	—	0.0046	0.0052	—	dos Santos et al. (2009)
Hg^{2+}, MeHg	Water, human hair	Nitric acid (sonication)	CPE	ICP-MS	—	0.004	0.010	—	Chen et al. (2009a)
Hg^{2+}, MeHg, EtHg, PhHg	Water, human hair, fish	HCl (sonication)	CPE	ICP-MS	—	0.006	0.013	0.008	Chen et al. (2009b)
Hg^{2+}, MeHg	Fish	HCl (sonication)	—	ICP-MS	—	0.05	0.08	—	Vallant et al. (2007)
Hg^{2+}, MeHg	River water	—	DDTC-modified C18 SPE	ICP-MS	—	0.0052	0.0056	—	Blanco et al. (2000)

(continued)

TABLE 2.2 (Continued)

Hg Species	Sample Matrix	Leaching Protocol	Pre-concentration	Detector	Interface	LOD (µg/L)				References
						Hg(II)	MeHg	EtHg	PhHg	
Hg^{2+}, MeHg	Fish	Enzymatic hydrolysis	—	ICP-MS	—	0.5	0.5	—	—	Rai et al. (2002)
Hg^{2+}, MeHg,	Fish, oyster	TMAH (sonication)	—	ICP-MS	—	—	—	—	—	Qvarnstrom and Frech (2002)
Hg^{2+}, MeHg, EtHg, PhHg	Water	—	—	ICP-MS	—	0.011	0.023	0.008	0.032	Castillo et al. (2006)
Hg^{2+}, MeHg, EtHg	Blood	HCl, L-cysteine, and 2-mercaptoethanol (sonication)	—	ICP-MS	—	0.25	0.1	—	—	Rodrigues et al. (2010)
Hg^{2+}, MeHg	Fish	HCl and NaCl (microwave)	—	ICP-MS	—	—	—	—	—	Reyes et al. (2009)
Hg^{2+}, MeHg	Human urine	—	—	ICP-MS	—	2.5	2.0	—	—	Li et al. (2007a)
Hg^{2+}, MeHg, EtHg	Fish	ETDA and 2-mercaptoethanol (microwave)	—	ICP-MS	—	0.2	0.2	0.3	—	Chang et al. (2007)

Analytes	Sample	Sample preparation	Separation	Detection	Derivatization					Reference
Hg²⁺, MeHg	Seawater	—	Opti-LynxTM trap cartridge	ICP-MS	—	0.00007	0.00002	—	—	Cairns et al. (2008)
Hg²⁺, MeHg	Fish, hair	TMAH (microwave)	—	ICP-MS	—	—	—	—	—	Vidler et al. (2007)
Hg²⁺, MeHg	Human hair	HNO₃ and H₂O₂ (microwave)	—	ICP-MS	—	—	—	—	—	Morton et al. (2002)
Hg²⁺, MeHg	Fish, mussel, bovine liver	HCl, KCl and mercaptoethanol	—	ICP-MS	—	0.2	0.2	—	—	Wang et al. (2007)
Hg²⁺, MeHg, EtHg	Water	Dithizone-modified C18 SPE	—	ICP-MS	—	0.003	0.003	0.003	—	Yin et al. (2010)
Hg²⁺, MeHg	Human urine	—	—	ICP-MS	Photo-CVG with formic acid and TiO₂ catalyst	0.10	0.03	—	—	Chen et al. (2009c)
Hg²⁺, MeHg, EtHg	Fish	L-cysteine and mercaptoethanol (microwave)	—	ICP-MS	CVG	0.06	0.05	0.09	—	Chiou et al. (2001)
Hg²⁺, MeHg, EtHg	Rice, wheat flour, fish	2-Mercaptoethanol in methanol (microwave)	—	ICP-MS	CVG	0.004	0.003	0.006	—	Lin et al. (2008)
Hg²⁺, MeHg	Soil	Methanol and HCl (microwave)	—	ICP-MS	CVG	0.035	0.073	—	—	Tu et al. (2003)

Fl, flow injection; RGD, radiofrequency glow discharge.

injected into HPLC or CE without the need for leaching or derivatization. For GC technique, ionic mercury species need to be converted to nonpolar mercury species by various precolumn derivatization methods, which is detailed in Section 2.3.

After leaching Hg species from the sample matrix, various cleanup, preconcentration, and derivatization strategies are required before GC, HPLC, or CE separation.

2.3   APPLICATION OF GC TECHNIQUE IN Hg SPECIATION ANALYSIS

Gas chromatography is the most commonly used technique for separation of Hg species owing to its high separation efficiency and the capability to easily couple with highly effective preconcentration methods. Table 2.1 summarizes the reported applications of GC in Hg speciation analysis in various environmental or biological matrices, including water (Ito et al., 2009; Jackson et al., 2009; Nsengimana et al., 2009; Yazdi et al., 2010), sediment (Stoichev et al., 2004; Avramescu et al., 2010), plant (Canario et al., 2006), fish (Jokai et al., 2005; Krystek and Ritsema, 2005; Castillo et al., 2010), and blood (Liang et al., 2000). As direct injection of ionic mercury can result in loss of column efficiency, deterioration of column performance, and damage of the detector, ionic mercury species are usually converted to nonpolar mercury species by precolumn derivatization before injection into the GC column. Hydride generation (He and Jiang, 1999; Stoichev et al., 2002, 2004), Grignard derivatization (Cai et al., 1997), ethylation (Jackson et al., 2009; Nsengimana et al., 2009; Avramescu et al., 2010; Castillo et al., 2010; Park et al., 2010), propylation (Geerdink et al., 2007; Gibicar et al., 2007; Ito et al., 2008; Carrasco et al., 2009), and phenylation (Jokai et al., 2005; Mishra et al., 2005; Mao et al., 2008) are the most frequently used derivatization methods in mercury speciation.

In most uncontaminated water samples, concentrations of Hg species are at low part per trillion (ppt) levels. Hence, preconcentration procedures are necessary before these derivatives can be analyzed by GC coupled with element-specific detectors. Preconcentration procedures commonly utilized for the speciation analysis of Hg include solvent extraction (SE) (Krystek and Ritsema, 2005; Jung et al., 2009; Nsengimana et al., 2009), solid-phase microextraction (SPME) (Mishra et al., 2005; Geerdink et al., 2007; Zachariadis and Kapsimali, 2008; Carrasco et al., 2009), stir bar sorptive extraction (SBSE) (Ito et al., 2008, 2009), single-drop microextraction (SDME) (Yazdi et al., 2010), and purge and trap (Lee et al., 2007; Mao et al., 2008; Jackson et al., 2009; Avramescu et al., 2010; Castillo et al., 2010; Park et al., 2010). Among these preconcentration techniques, purge and trap, with an almost infinite enrichment factor, is the most effective and commonly used preconcentration technique in Hg speciation analysis.

2.3.1 Derivatization

2.3.1.1 *Grignard Derivatization.* Grignard derivatization, a traditional technique for mercury speciation analysis, can convert ionic inorganic or organic Hg to volatile alkylated Hg species. For example, during the derivatization with butylmagnesium chloride, Hg^{2+} is transformed to $Hg(Bu)_2$ and MeHg is converted to MeHgBu, while EtHg forms EtHgBu. These nonpolar dialkyl derivatives are then separated by GC and detected by AFS (Cai et al., 1997), glow discharge atomic emission spectrometry (GD-AES) (Orellana-Velado et al., 1998), or microwave-induced plasma atomic emission spectrometry (MIP-AES) (Bulska et al., 1991). This technique has been applied in the determination of EtHg in sediment (Cai et al., 1997) and the detection of MeHg in fish tissue (Orellana-Velado et al., 1998). The major drawback of this method is that sample preparation is tedious and time consuming. In addition, the derivatization must be carried out in nonaqueous environments. These issues limit the usage of this technique in the speciation analysis of Hg in environmental and biological samples.

2.3.1.2 *Hydride Generation (HG).* Organomercuric species are converted to their hydrides with KBH_4 or $NaBH_4$ as derivatization reagent, while Hg^{2+} is converted to Hg^0. These hydride species, for example, MeHgH, are then separated by GC and then detected by various detectors, such as Fourier transform infrared (FTIR) spectrometer (Filippelli et al., 1992) and AFS (Stoichev et al., 2004). For example, simultaneous detection of Hg^{2+} and MeHg by hydride generation, cryofocusing, GC separation, and AFS detection has been recently reported (Stoichev et al., 2004). Low detection limit was achieved by using this reported method, with an LOD of 0.13 ng/L for Hg^{2+} and 0.01 ng/L for MeHg. Separation of organomercuric chlorides (MeHg, EtHg, phenylmercury (PhHg)) by GC is also possible after derivatization with KBH_4 (He and Jiang, 1999). A drawback of hydride generation is that the presence of metal ions in matrix strongly decreases the sensitivity in the determination of mercury species (de Diego et al., 1998), consequently limiting the application of hydride generation in analyzing metal-rich samples (de Diego et al., 1998) (e.g., sediments, waste effluents, and sediment pore waters). Another drawback is that ambient temperature traps (carbon or Tenax) cannot be used to preconcentrate the derivatized mercury species because of the instability of the hydride species of organic mercury.

2.3.1.3 *Aqueous Alkylation.* Aqueous alkylation, especially ethylation, is the most commonly used technique in MeHg analysis. Rapsomanikis et al. first reported the ethylation of MeHg with tetraethylborate ($NaBEt_4$) (Rapsomanikis et al., 1986). Although other reagents (e.g., bromomagnesium tetraethylborate ($BrMgEt_4B$) (Nsengimana et al., 2009)) can also produce ethylation, $NaBEt_4$ is most commonly used (Bowles and Apte, 1998; Pereiro et al., 1998; Pongratz and Heumann, 1998; Holz et al., 1999; Jackson et al., 2009; Avramescu et al., 2010; Castillo et al., 2010; Park et al., 2010). This method has been widely utilized in the speciation analysis of Hg in various matrices, for example, water (Ito et al., 2009; Jackson et al., 2009), sediment (Avramescu et al., 2010; Park et al., 2010), biota (Krystek and Ritsema, 2005; Lee et al., 2007; Zachariadis and Kapsimali, 2008; Castillo et al., 2010; Park et al., 2010), blood (Liang et al., 2000), and hair (Diez and Bayona, 2002). The major advantage of this derivatization method is that the reaction is performed in aqueous solution and thus can be coupled with an on-line purge-and-trap preconcentration system and a sensitive element-specific detector (e.g., AFS or ICP-MS). Low LOD (pg/L level) can be achieved with such arrangement (Slaets et al., 1999; Leenaers et al., 2002; Jackson et al., 2009). Unfortunately, this method should be used with caution in certain circumstances because several significant interferences can result from the sample matrix. Chloride ion and dissolved organic matter (DOM) strongly decrease the sensitivity and reproducibility of the method (Bloom, 1989; de Diego et al., 1998; Demuth and Heumann, 2001). To eliminate these matrix effects, extraction/back-extraction or sample distillation is often necessary before aqueous ethylation when salty or organic-rich water samples are analyzed. In addition, $NaBEt_4$ dissolved in water is unstable and needs to be freshly made and handled under protective gas (Mao et al., 2008). These steps make the analysis of mercury more tedious, time consuming, and expensive. Moreover, artifactual MeHg could be formed during the process of distillation (Bloom et al., 1997). The presence of this artifact may be significant particularly in the analysis of sediments and Hg-contaminated water samples, where the measured fraction of MeHg is <1% of the total (Bloom et al., 1997). One approach to reduce these interferences is to use the ID technique by GC-ICP-MS (Demuth and Heumann, 2001). Another drawback of aqueous ethylation is that it cannot distinguish Hg^{2+} from EtHg because these two species form the same derivative, $Hg(Et)_2$. This disadvantage limits the application of ethylation in the environment where EtHg coexists with Hg^{2+}.

Aqueous propylation with sodium tetrapropylborate ($NaBPr_4$) is another alkylation technique used in Hg speciation. This method was first proposed by De Smaele et al. (1998), and it has been frequently used for mercury speciation since then (Geerdink et al., 2007; Gibicar et al., 2007; Ito et al., 2008; Carrasco et al., 2009). During propylation with $NaBPr_4$, Hg^{2+} is converted to $Hg(Pr)_2$, MeHg is transformed to MeHgPr, and EtHg forms EtHgPr. The advantages of propylation include its ability to distinguish Hg^{2+} from EtHg, and its resistance to interferences from chlorides (Demuth and Heumann, 2001). Coupled with purge and trap or head space solid-phase microextraction (HS-SPME), this technique has been applied to determine low concentrations of mercury species in biota (Gibicar et al., 2007) (LOD, 10 pg/g) and water samples (Geerdink et al., 2007) (LOD, 0.016 ng/L). However, this method should also be used with caution because of the formation of artifactual organomercury compounds during $NaBPr_4$ derivatization (Huang, 2005). The purity of the derivatization agent is also a factor. Artifactual monoethylmercury accounted for 0.99% to 2.9% of the Hg^{2+} present depending on the quality of the reagent (Huang, 2005). This issue may limit its application in the determination of EtHg in environmental samples. Similar to $NaBEt_4$, $NaBPr_4$ dissolved in water is unstable and needs to be freshly made and handled under protective gas, which increases the time and cost of analysis.

2.3.1.4 Aqueous Phenylation. Application of aqueous phenylation with sodium tetraphenylborate (NaBPh$_4$) in Hg analysis was first proposed in 1978 (Luckow and Rüssel, 1978). This technique has several advantages: aqueous solutions of NaBPh$_4$ are very stable, phenylation is not affected by interferences from chloride ions and decomposed tissues (Luckow and Rüssel, 1978), and it can distinguish Hg^{2+} from EtHg. Combined with SE or SPME, aqueous-phase phenylation has been widely used for the Hg speciation analysis in biota (Pereiro et al., 1998; Abuin et al., 2000; Mishra et al., 2005), soil/sediment (Mishra et al., 2005), and water (Carro et al., 2002; Mishra et al., 2005). However, when SE or SPME-aqueous phenylation is applied, the detection limit is relatively high for the analysis of trace level organomercury in environmental samples, especially in water samples. In order to overcome this problem, coupling of a more effective preconcentration technique, for example, purge and trap, with the phenylation is necessary. Nevertheless, initial studies indicate that it is difficult to purge the phenylation products from the aqueous phase owing to their poor volatilities. In a recent study, a method was successfully developed using aqueous-phase phenylation-purge-and-trap preconcentration-GC separation followed by AFS or ICP-MS detection for organomercury speciation analysis (Mao et al., 2008). During the development of this method, the problem of purge efficiency was resolved by adding NaCl and increasing the purge temperature. This new method can simultaneously detect MeHg and EtHg in environmental samples, with low detection limit and less interference than alkylation. In this method, detection limits were determined to be 0.03 ng/L for both MeHg and EtHg when AFS was used as detector. Because the phenylation reaction is not affected by the presence of chloride ion and DOM (Mao et al., 2008), this new method is particularly useful for direct analysis of freshwater samples without extraction or distillation. One drawback of this method is the interference of K$^+$. A depression of $\sim 50\%$ in the system response was observed when artificial seawater (K$^+$, 0.38%) was analyzed (Mao et al., 2008). Another drawback of this method is that the phenylation derivative of Hg^{2+} cannot be efficiently purged; thus this method cannot be used to quantify Hg^{2+} in samples.

2.3.2 Detection

GC coupled with electron capture detector (ECD) (Chiavarini et al., 1994) is the traditional technique for Hg speciation analysis in the environment. The application of ECD is limited by its nonspecificity and the resulting potential for co-elution of mercury species with interfering compounds. Therefore, this detector has been replaced by other element-specific detection methods. GC has been coupled to MS, AAS, MIP-AES, AFS, ICP-MS, and electron ionization mass spectrometry (EI-MS) (Table 2.1) for mercury speciation. Among these detectors, AFS and ICP-MS are the most commonly used. AFS is sensitive, selective, and relatively inexpensive, which make it one of the most popular detectors for mercury detection (Cai, 2000; Leermakers et al., 2005). The use of ICP-MS has also increased tremendously as a result of its high sensitivity, selectivity, and capability in applying the ID technique in mercury speciation analysis (Leermakers et al., 2005).

2.4   APPLICATION OF HPLC TECHNIQUE IN Hg SPECIATION ANALYSIS

Although GC is still the most popular method for Hg speciation analysis, HPLC-based separation coupled with various detectors, including ultraviolet (UV), AAS, AES, AFS, atomic MS (ICP-MS), and molecular MS, has been widely used for Hg speciation analysis in various environmental and biological matrices. Unlike GC-based methods, derivatization of the ionic mercury species to produce volatile compounds is not required for HPLC, which makes the analytical procedure much simpler. Table 2.2 summarizes the reported applications of HPLC in Hg speciation analysis.

2.4.1   Preconcentration Techniques for HPLC

HPLC coupled with atomic spectrometry techniques permits the determination of Hg species at sub-ppb levels. Generally, this method can be used to directly determine Hg species in biological samples without preconcentration. However, for samples with low Hg concentration, especially in pristine natural water, analysis using HPLC is a great challenge (Leopold et al., 2009). In recent years, various solid-phase and liquid-phase preconcentration strategies, including solid-phase extraction (SPE) (Dong et al., 2004; Margetinova et al., 2008; Shade, 2008), cloud point extraction (CPE) (Yu, 2005; Chen et al., 2009a), hollow fiber-based liquid–liquid–liquid microextraction (HF-LLLME) (Xia et al., 2007), and SDME (Pena-Pereira et al., 2009), have been developed for the determination of Hg.

2.4.2   Coupling HPLC with Atomic Spectrometer

The main advantage of HPLC is the possibility of simultaneously separating a great variety of organomercury compounds (Leermakers et al., 2005). Although cation exchange (Vallant et al., 2007; Shade, 2008; Chen et al., 2009c) and multiphase (Tu et al., 2003) separations have also been reported in recent years, reversed phase (RP) (C18 and C8 column) separation is the most commonly used procedure for mercury speciation (Sanchez et al., 2000; Shaw et al., 2003; Xia et al., 2007). Various chelating or ion pair reagents are used as mobile phase additives to improve the chromatographic separation of Hg species. The commonly used reagents include mercaptoethanol (de Souza et al., 2010), L-cysteine (Rahman et al., 2009), thiourea (Shade, 2008), diethyldithiocarbamate (DDTC) (Chen et al., 2009a), pyrrolidinedithiocarbamate (APDC) (Li et al., 2005b), ethylenediaminetetraacetic acid (EDTA) (Sanchez et al., 2000), tetrabutylammonium bromide (Gomez-Ariza et al., 2004), heptafluorobutanoic acid (Li et al., 2007a), and pentanesulfonic acid (Chang et al., 2007).

Direct coupling of HPLC with an atomic spectrometric detector (e.g., ICP-MS and AAS) can be easily realized using a nebulizer to transport the HPLC eluent as aerosol into a plasma or AAS. The main drawbacks of this direct hyphenation of HPLC to atomic spectrometric detectors are poor sensitivity and matrix interferences. Therefore, post-column derivatization using chemical vapor generation (CVG) is commonly used to convert Hg^{2+} to Hg^0 to improve sensitivity and minimize interferences. When organomercury species are present, it is usually necessary to convert them to Hg^{2+} or to hydrides before cold vapor generation. Usually, borohydride is used to convert organomercury species to their hydrides, which can then be determined by ICP-MS (Wan et al., 1997). When AAS or AFS serves as the detector, organomercury is usually decomposed to Hg^{2+} before generating cold vapor by reacting with oxidation reagents, such as $K_2S_2O_8$ or $KBr-KBrO_3$, and with the assistance of heating, UV, or microwave to improve the efficiency.

In the past few years, some new techniques have been developed to simplify the post-column degradation procedure, such as the addition of L-cysteine to the mobile phase (Wang et al., 2010) and the application of photoinduced chemical vapor generation (photo-CVG) (Yin et al., 2007a,b, 2008, 2009a; Chen et al., 2009c). An efficient post-column oxidation system without an external heat source was recently developed for HPLC-CV-AFS (Li et al., 2005b). Oxidation of organomercury species under ambient temperature using this on-line system was achieved by mixing the HPLC effluent with a $K_2S_2O_8$ solution (Li et al., 2005b). L-cysteine was recently found to be able to induce degradation of MeHg and EtHg in the presence of KBH_4 and HCl. By using a mobile phase consisting of L-cysteine, a simple on-line HPLC-CV-AFS method that did not require oxidation reagents or external heat sources was developed for Hg speciation analysis (Wang et al., 2010). Compared with the conventional HPLC-CV-AFS systems, this system is simpler and cheaper. Photo-CVG has recently been applied in Hg speciation using HPLC-AFS (Yin et al., 2007a,b, 2008, 2009a) and HPLC-ICP-MS (Chen et al., 2009c). By mixing the organomercury compounds separated by HPLC with formic acid, the decomposition of organomercury species and the reduction of Hg^{2+} to elemental mercury can be completed in one step with a photo-CVG system (Yin et al., 2007b). In another example, a simple HPLC–AFS interface was developed using formic acid in mobile phase as the reaction reagent for photo-CVG (Yin et al., 2008). In this system, post-column derivatization of organomercury with borohydride is avoided, thus reducing the possibility of contamination. In addition, the flow injection system required in the traditional CVG procedure can be omitted.

2.4.3 Identification of Hg-Binding Forms in Biota

Mercury can be taken up by plants and animals, and it can be further translocated and accumulated in different tissues. Hg^{2+} and organomercury in the intracellular environment are believed to predominantly bind to thiol-containing biomolecules (Harris et al., 2003). The interaction of mercury with biomolecules in biota plays a very important role in the transport and detoxification of Hg. However, the identities of these target biomolecules and their interactions with mercury are yet to be determined (Lemes and Wang, 2009). Liquid-phase-based separation techniques coupled to UV, elemental MS (ICP-MS), or molecular MS (electrospray ionization mass spectrometry, ESI-MS) are useful tools in the identification and quantification of the molecular forms of mercury in the tissues of plants and animals.

2.4.3.1 Phytochelatin in Plant.
Hg-bonded phytochelatins (PCs) in plants can be separated and characterized by HPLC coupled with ICP-MS, ESI-MS, or ESI-MS-MS (Iglesia-Turino et al., 2006; Krupp et al., 2009; Chen et al., 2009d). For example, in vivo PCs and their corresponding Hg–PC complexes (oxidized PC_2, PC_3, PC_4, $HgPC_2$, $HgPC_3$, $HgPC_4$, and Hg_2PC_4) were characterized in the roots of *Brassica chinensis* L. using RP-LC-ESI-MS-MS (Chen et al., 2009d). Similarly, RP-HPLC coupled with ICP-MS and ESI-MS permitted the detection of novel Hg–PC complexes, such as $HgPC_2$, $Hg(Ser)PC_2$, $Hg(Glu)PC_2$, and $Hg(des-Gly)PC_2$ (Krupp et al., 2009).

2.4.3.2 Mercury-Containing Proteins and Metallothioneins (MT).
The coupling of size exclusion and RP liquid chromatography with ICP-MS or ESI-MS detection has been widely used to characterize metallothioneins (MT) and other mercury-containing proteins in rats, mice, and carp (Huang et al., 2004, 2007; Kameo et al., 2005; Shen et al., 2005, 2007; Wang et al., 2008). Metal-binding MT isoforms and subisoforms in tissues of rat after oral intake of $HgCl_2$ were purified with size exclusion chromatography (SEC) followed by C8 RP separation and on-line detection by UV, ICP-MS, and ESI-MS (Shen et al., 2005). Using an enriched stable isotopic tracer (^{196}Hg and ^{198}Hg) technique, a method employing SEC coupled with ICP-ID-MS was developed to provide both qualitative and quantitative information on mercury-containing proteins in rats after MeHg exposure (Shi et al., 2007).

HPLC coupled with ICP-MS or ESI-MS has also been applied in the identification of forms of organic mercury in rice, fish, and other biological samples. MeHg-cysteine (the primary form of MeHg in the uncooked rice and fish muscle (Lemes and Wang, 2009)) has been identified in biota by using enzymatic hydrolysis with trypsin followed by HPLC-ICP-MS determination. Studies using HPLC-ICP-MS and HPLC-ESI-MS on the interaction of thimerosal (an EtHg-containing preservative in vaccines) with proteins demonstrated the formation of EtHg-β-lactoglobulin A and EtHg–human serum albumin (HSA) adducts in physiological conditions (Trumpler et al., 2009). After tryptic digestion of β-lactoglobulin A, a free thiol residue in the peptide T13 was identified as the binding site of EtHg. Enzymatic hydrolysis with trypsin followed by the combined application of ICP-MS and ESI-MS provides a promising analytical method for identifying binding sites of mercury species in proteins. Thus, on-line coupling of ESI-MS and ICP-MS to HPLC, which can simultaneously provide both elemental and molecular information, is expected to be a useful tool in identifying forms of mercury species in biota. In addition, HPLC-ICP-MS has been successfully applied in the simultaneous determination of Hg- and Se-containing proteins, which provides new insight into the Hg–Se antagonism (Ikemoto et al., 2004).

2.5 APPLICATION OF CAPILLARY ELECTROPHORESIS TECHNIQUES IN Hg SPECIATION ANALYSIS

CE is a relatively new technique for Hg speciation analysis. It has some advantages over GC and HPLC in terms of separation speed, efficiency, resolution, and sample size. In recent years, it has been extensively studied and demonstrated to be a complementary tool to GC and HPLC (Kubán et al., 2009).

Commercially available UV–visible detection is, by far, the most widely used procedure in CE-based Hg speciation. Cysteine (Pager and Gaspar, 2002), glutathione (Pager and Gaspar, 2002), 2-mercaptonicotinic acid (Pager and Gaspar, 2002), mercaptoacetic acid (Pager and Gaspar, 2002), dithizone sulfonate (Hardy and Jones, 1997), nitrilotriacetic acid, EDTA (Liu and Lee, 1999), and imidazole (Peng et al., 2005) have been commonly used as off-column or on-column derivatization reagents for mercury species to form UV-absorbing complexes in CE analysis. The shortcomings of UV detection include potential interferences from co-migrating species and low sensitivity due to the relatively weak absorbance of the derivatized Hg complexes in the UV–visible region. Off-line and/or on-line preconcentration methods, such as SPE (Manganiello et al., 2002), dual-CPE (Yin, 2007), liquid-phase microextraction (Fan and Liu, 2008), and large-volume sample stacking (Li et al., 2008), can improve detection sensitivity. By combining HF-LLLME with on-line large-volume sample stacking preconcentration, enrichment factors of 2600–4600 were attained for MeHg, EtHg, and PhHg (Li et al., 2008). LODs were in the range of 0.03–0.14 mg/L (Li et al., 2008).

Element-specific and highly sensitive hyphenated techniques, such as CE-ICP-MS, CE-AAS, CE-flame-heated furnace (FHF)-AAS, CE-electrothermal (ET)-AAS, and CE-AFS, are increasingly used in the field of mercury speciation. Although CE can be coupled with ICP-MS directly using a cross-flow or micro-concentric nebulizer, application of chemical vapor generation is commonly suggested in mercury speciation analysis as it can provide higher transport efficiency and better sensitivity for the analyzed mercury species. On-line hyphenation of chip CE or flow injection-miniaturized CE to AFS was recently reported for high throughput analysis of mercury speciation (Li et al., 2005a; Wang et al., 2006). By implementing this technique, about 60 samples can be analyzed within an hour.

CE is becoming a more frequently utilized separation technique for studying the interaction of Hg species and biomolecules (Li et al., 2005c, 2007b). There are several advantages of CE over other separation techniques such as GC and HPLC in this field. The major advantage of CE is that the complete electrophoretic separation can be performed under nearly physiological conditions if proper background electrolyte is employed. In addition, there is no interaction between the analytes and the stationary phase in CE (Kubán et al., 2009). These virtues can minimize the disturbance of the existing Hg–biomolecule equilibrium. In addition to directly demonstrating the formation of mercury-biomolecule complexes, this technique can also provide the thermodynamic and kinetic information on the interaction of mercury species with biomolecules. For instance, a CE-ET-AAS hyphenated system was recently developed and applied to study the interaction of Hg^{2+} and salmon sperm DNA (Li et al., 2005c), and the interaction of Hg^{2+}, MeHg, EtHg, and PhHg with HSA (Li et al., 2007b).

2.6 APPLICATION OF X-RAY ABSORPTION SPECTROSCOPY IN PROBING CHEMICAL MICROENVIRONMENT OF Hg

X-ray absorption spectroscopy is increasingly being applied to probe the chemical microenvironment of Hg including structure and bonding. Although a relatively high concentration of Hg is generally required, this technique has the benefit of being element specific and nondestructive to the chemical environment, and its sample preparation is simple. X-ray absorption near-edge structure (XANES) can provide information on the oxidation state and geometry of Hg. Extended X-ray absorption fine structure (EXAFS) can probe the number, type, and proximity of neighboring atoms to Hg (Andrews, 2006). Both techniques are widely applied in various aspects of mercury study, such as mercury speciation analysis in various environmental samples and the interaction of Hg^{2+} and MeHg with thiols and humic substances.

2.6.1 Chemical Identity of Hg in Biological Samples

It was suggested that MeHg may coordinate with cysteine residues of proteins in biological samples many years ago (Westöö, 1967). However, very little has been done to test this assumption because of the lack of proper techniques such as XAS in this field. Hg LIII near-edge spectrometry was implemented to study the chemical identity of mercury in fish with different diets (Harris et al., 2003; George et al., 2008). Cysteine was found to be the most likely thiolate donor for MeHg. By utilizing XANES, MeHg was found to be present in a form similar to MeHg-cysteine in plants (*Eichhornia crassipes*) (Rajan et al., 2008).

Hg–Se antagonism plays a very important role in the detoxification of mercury in organisms (Khan and Wang, 2009). X-ray absorption spectroscopy can simultaneously provide the *in situ* information on the structure and bonding of Hg and Se in biological samples. By implementing EXAFS, mercury and selenium were found to exist in the form of HgSe in the liver of northern fur seal, while Hg(Se, S) granules were suggested as the existing form in the black-footed albatross (Arai et al., 2004). Other researchers found that X-ray absorption spectra of Hg and Se in erythrocytes, plasma, and bile of rabbits exposed to sodium selenite and mercuric chloride were essentially identical to those of synthetic Hg–Se–S species (Gailer et al., 2000).

2.6.2   Hg Species in Ore, Soil, and Their Sorption on Solid Surface

XAS has the ability to identify multiple mercury phases in a heterogeneous sample, such as cinnabar, metacinnabar, $HgCl_2$, $HgSO_4$, and HgO. Thus, it is a proper tool to directly determine Hg species and content in ore, slag, and soil from Hg mines (Bernaus et al., 2005), mine tailings (Lowry et al., 2004; Slowey et al., 2005), mine wastes (Kim et al., 2000), and chlor-alkali plants (Bernaus et al., 2006). By using this technique, mercury was found to occur as a sulfide phase in lake sediment with a local structural environment similar to that in cinnabar (Wolfenden et al., 2005). XAS has also been demonstrated to be a useful tool for studying the sorption of Hg on particle surfaces (Kim et al., 2004), brominated activated carbon (Hutson et al., 2007), and pyrite (Behra et al., 2001).

2.6.3   Interaction of Hg^{2+} and MeHg with Thiol and Organic Matters

Mercury LIII-edge X-ray absorption spectroscopy has recently been used to characterize the interactions of mercuric ions with nonprotein thiols (cysteine (Jalilehvand et al., 2006) and glutathione (Mah and Jalilehvand, 2008), chemical warfare agents (thiodiglycol (Skubal et al., 2005)), and chelation therapy agents (George et al., 2004)). These studies are helpful in understanding cycling of mercury in the environment and designing mercury chelation therapeutic drugs. For example, reduced sulfur functional groups were found to be important in the complexation of Hg^{2+} with humic substances using XAS (Xia et al., 1999; Hesterberg et al., 2001). Disulfide/disulfane S may be involved in the complexation of Hg^{2+} with soil organic matter (Xia et al., 1999). Another study using XANES and EXAFS found that reduced sulfur groups also play an important role in the binding of MeHg to soil and stream organic matter (Qian et al., 2002).

2.7   APPLICATION OF STABLE ISOTOPE DILUTION TECHNIQUE IN MERCURY SPECIATION ANALYSIS

ID analysis has been suggested as the primary method for trace element speciation owing to its high accuracy and precision (Monperrus et al., 2004; Rodriguez-Gonzalez et al., 2005; Bjorn et al., 2007). Application of radio ID in mercury analysis has been reported since the early 1980s (Kanda and Suzuki, 1980). Because this technique utilizes highly radioactive material and requires specific safety measures (Hintelmann and Evans, 1997), it has been adopted in only a few studies (Kanda and Suzuki, 1980; Šmejkal and Teplá, 1983). Over the past decade, stable ID techniques have been increasingly used for mercury speciation by coupling with HPLC (Rahman and Kingston, 2004) or GC (Demuth and Heumann, 2001; Martin-Doimeadios et al., 2002a, 2003; Larsson and Frech, 2003; Monperrus et al., 2003; Qvarnstrom et al., 2003) followed by detection with molecular (i.e., EI-MS) (Barshick et al., 1999; Yang et al., 2003; Castillo et al., 2010) or atomic mass spectrometry (i.e., ICP-MS) (Demuth and Heumann, 2001; Martin-Doimeadios et al., 2002a, 2003; Larsson and Frech, 2003; Monperrus et al., 2003; Qvarnstrom et al., 2003; Rahman and Kingston, 2004).

2.7.1 Species-Unspecific Stable Isotope Dilution

Species-unspecific stable ID is commonly used in mercury speciation analysis using HPLC-ICP-MS, in which a mercury isotope tracer (usually Hg^{2+}) is added to the post-column reagent stream of HPLC, and then the mixture is introduced to the plasma of ICP-MS. As it is not necessary for the isotope tracer to be the same species as the analyte, this technique is especially useful when the structure of the Hg species of interest is not known or the isotope labeled Hg species of interest is not available. It was recently reported in the analysis of mercury in rat (Shi et al., 2007). In that study, an SEC–species-unspecific isotope dilution–ICP-MS method was developed to investigate trace mercury-containing proteins in rats. The major advantage of this technique is that it can correct for random and systematic errors arising from instrumental instabilities or the influence of sample matrix. It is expected to be more widely applied in the mercury speciation in environmental samples and mercury-containing proteins in future.

2.7.2 Species-Specific Stable Isotope Dilution

Species-specific stable ID has been widely applied in mercury speciation analysis since the mid-1990s (Smith, 1993; Hintelmann et al., 1995, 1997; Hintelmann and Evans, 1997). This method allows the generation of accurate and precise results for mercury species even when species transformations and analyte losses occur during analysis. In addition, no external calibration or standard is required for this assay. There are seven stable isotopes of mercury, with ^{202}Hg being the most abundant. Therefore, the mercury species enriched in one (single spike ID) or more (multiple spike ID) stable isotopes can be added to the samples to correct for the analyte losses and artifact effects, providing a valuable tool for accurate detection of mercury species. Isotope-enriched MeHg (Martin-Doimeadios et al., 2002b; Rahman et al., 2003; Bancon-Montigny et al., 2004; Snell et al., 2004), dimethylmercury (Snell et al., 2000), and EtHg (Rahman et al., 2005) can be synthesized in the laboratory from isotope-enriched HgO or Hg^0. Isotope-enriched MeHg is also commercially available (Snell et al., 2004).

2.7.2.1 Single Spike Stable Isotope Dilution. In single spike ID analysis, MeHg and/or the other mercury species enriched in the same isotope are spiked in the samples, and act as internal standards. A few methods utilizing single spike stable ID have been reported recently for mercury speciation analysis (Demuth and Heumann, 2001; Hintelmann and Nguyen, 2005). The main advantage of this method is the ability to correct for the loss of mercury species during sample preparation. For example, halide ions were found to cause the degradation of MeHg to Hg^0 when ethylation was used as the derivatization method (Demuth and Heumann, 2001). This partial transformation of MeHg during this analysis leads to the underestimation of mercury concentration in samples. This loss of MeHg can be amended if ID techniques are adopted (Demuth and Heumann, 2001).

Although the single spike of isotopically enriched MeHg can correct for the loss of MeHg during analysis, it cannot identify and correct for the potential production of MeHg (chemical methylation) in the sample preparation and analytical procedure (Martin-Doimeadios et al., 2003). Thus, double or multiple ID technique is required for simultaneously monitoring losses and interconversion of mercury species during analysis.

2.7.2.2   Multiple Spike Stable Isotope Dilution. In multiple spike ID analysis, MeHg and/or other mercury species (usually MeHg and Hg^{2+}) enriched in two or more isotopes are spiked in the samples. The major advantage of this method over single spike ID is that it can correct for not only the analyte losses but also the interconversion of mercury species during sample analysis. Qvarnstrom and Frech (2002) reported a double ID protocol by spiking $Me^{198}Hg$ and $^{201}Hg^{2+}$ for monitoring the degradation of MeHg and abiotic methylation of Hg^{2+} during extraction using tetramethylammonium hydroxide (TMAH). Up to 11.5% of added $^{201}Hg^{2+}$ was found to be methylated while up to 6.26% of added $Me^{198}Hg$ was demethylated to Hg^{2+}. Partial degradation of EtHg to Hg^{2+} during sample preparation was also detected (Qvarnstrom et al., 2003). By using multiple spike ID, analytical errors derived from these transformations can be amended. Recently, this technique has been used to determine mercury species in various matrices, such as sediment (Monperrus et al., 2008), fish (Castillo et al., 2010), water (Jackson et al., 2009), and gas phase (Larsson and Frech, 2003). In addition, multiple spike ID combined with enriched stable isotope tracer techniques provides a useful tool to study mercury species transformation in natural environments (Lambertsson et al., 2001). Application of this technique can significantly improve the precision and accuracy in mercury transformation rate measurement.

2.8   SUMMARY

Mercury widely exists in the environment in various chemical species. Mercury speciation analysis is important in understanding the cycling of mercury in the environment as well as its toxicity. Various separation tools including HPLC, GC, and CE are commonly used for Hg speciation analysis. The ease of coupling GC with highly effective preconcentration methods, such as purge and trap, makes it the first choice for analyzing ultra-low concentrations of Hg species in environmental samples, especially pristine water. The derivatization of the ionic mercury species into volatile compounds before separation is not required by HPLC, and this makes the analytical procedure for HPLC much simpler than that for GC. However, the use of HPLC-based techniques is limited by its high detection limit; thus, it is mainly applied in analyzing Hg species in soil and biological samples where the concentration of Hg is relatively high—in parts per billion to parts per million levels. CE methods can be useful in studying the interaction of Hg species and biomolecules, although its application in Hg speciation of real environmental samples is limited by its poor sensitivity. Various element-specific detectors are coupled on-line to GC, HPLC, or CE for Hg speciation analysis. Among them, AFS and ICP-MS are the most popular detectors for mercury detection owing to their high sensitivity and selectivity.

Overcoming matrix effects and artifact formation during sample preparation and derivatization is important for identification and quantification of mercury species in various environmental samples. It has been proved that multiple spike stable ID analysis can correct for matrix effects and the interconversion of mercury species during sample analysis; however, this technique is relatively expensive. Aqueous phenylation coupled to purge and trap-GC-AFS provides a potential low cost way to resolve this problem. The presence of chloride ion and DOM do not produce interferences, and it can directly analyze freshwater samples without extraction or distillation. However, it is possible that artifact formation of organomercury compounds occurs during phenylation and this topic needs further investigation.

Although numerous hyphenated techniques have been developed for mercury speciation, the determination of mercury–DOM complexes and mercury species in biota is still a challenging task. Owing to the virtues of being element specific and nondestructive to chemical microenvironment, XAS is expected to be a powerful tool in this field. However, its application is currently constrained by poor detection limit. More work is required to improve the detection power of this technique. Enzymatic hydrolysis followed by simultaneous on-line coupling of ESI-MS and ICP-MS to HPLC is expected to be another promising tool owing to its advantages of providing both elemental and molecular information.

REFERENCES

Abuin M, Carro AM, Lorenzo RA. Experimental design of a microwave-assisted extraction-derivatization method for the analysis of methylmercury. J Chromatogr A 2000;889:185–193.

Andrews, JC. Mercury speciation in the environment using X-ray absorption spectroscopy. In: Mingos DMP, Atwood DA (Eds.), Recent Developments in Mercury Science, Structure and Bonding. Springer, Berlin Heidelberg, 2006;120: p 1–35.

Arai T, Ikemoto T, Hokura A, Terada Y, Kunito T, Tanabe S, Nakai I. Chemical forms of mercury and cadmium accumulated in marine mammals and seabirds as determined by XAFS analysis. Environ Sci Technol 2004;38:6468–6474.

Avramescu ML, Zhu J, Yumvihoze E, Hintelmann H, Fortin D, Lean DRS. Simplified sample preparation procedure for measuring isotope-enriched methylmercury by gas chromatography and inductively coupled plasma mass spectrometry. Environ Toxicol Chem 2010;29:1256–1262.

Bancon-Montigny C, Yang L, Sturgeon RE, Colombini V, Mester Z. High-yield synthesis of milligram amounts of isotopically enriched methylmercury (CH_3[198]$HgCl$). Appl Organomet Chem 2004;18:57–64.

Barshick CM, Barshick SA, Walsh EB, Vance MA, Britt PF. Application of isotope dilution to ion trap gas chromatography mass spectrometry. Anal Chem 1999;71:483–488.

Behra P, Bonnissel-Gissinger P, Alnot M, Revel R, Ehrhardt JJ. XPS and XAS study of the sorption of Hg(II) onto pyrite. Langmuir 2001;17:3970–3979.

Beichert A, Padberg S, Wenclawiak BW. Selective determination of alkylmercury compounds in solid matrices after subcritical water extraction, followed by solid-phase microextraction and GC-MS. Appl Organomet Chem 2000;14:493–498.

Bernaus A, Gaona X, van Ree D, Valiente M. Determination of mercury in polluted soils surrounding a chlor-alkali plant - direct speciation by x-ray absorption spectroscopy techniques and preliminary geochemical characterisation of the area. Anal Chim Acta 2006;565:73–80.

Bernaus A, Gaona X, Valiente M. Characterisation of Almaden mercury mine environment by XAS techniques. J Environ Monit 2005;7:771–777.

Bjorn E, Larsson T, Lambertsson L, Skyllberg U, Frech W. Recent advances in mercury speciation analysis with focus on spectrometric methods and enriched stable isotope applications. Ambio 2007;36:443–451.

Blanco RM, Villanueva MT, Uria JES, Sanz-Medel A. Field sampling, preconcentration and determination of mercury species in river waters. Anal Chim Acta 2000;419: 137–144.

Bloom N. Determination of picogram levels of methylmercury by aqueous phase ethylation, followed by cryogenic gas chromatography with cold vapor atomic fluorescence detection. Can J Fish Aquat Sci 1989;46:1131–1140.

Bloom NS, Colman JA, Barber L. Artifact formation of methyl mercury during aqueous distillation and alternative techniques for the extraction of methyl mercury from environmental samples. Fresenius J Anal Chem 1997;358:371–377.

Bloom NS, Grout AK, Prestbo EM. Development and complete validation of a method for the determination of dimethyl mercury in air and other media. Anal Chim Acta 2005;546:92–101.

Bowles KC, Apte SC. Determination of methylmercury in natural water samples by steam distillation and gas chromatography atomic fluorescence spectrometry. Anal Chem 1998;70:395–399.

Bramanti E, Lomonte C, Onor M, Zamboni R, D'Ulivo A, Raspi G. Mercury speciation by liquid chromatography coupled with on-line chemical vapour generation and atomic fluorescence spectrometric detection (LC-CVGAFS). Talanta 2005;66:762–768.

Bravo-Sanchez LR, Encinar JR, Martinez JIF, Sanz-Medel A. Mercury speciation analysis in sea water by solid phase microextraction-gas chromatography-inductively coupled plasma mass spectrometry using ethyl and propyl derivatization. Matrix effects evaluation. Spectrochim Acta B 2004;59:59–66.

Bulska E, Baxter DC, Frech W. Capillary column gas chromatography for mercury speciation. Anal Chim Acta 1991;249:545–554.

Cai Y. Speciation and analysis of mercury, arsenic, and selenium by atomic fluorescence spectrometry. Trac-Trend Anal Chem 2000;19:62–66.

Cai Y, Jaffe R, Alli A, Jones RD. Determination of organomercury compounds in aqueous samples by capillary gas chromatography atomic fluorescence spectrometry following solid-phase extraction. Anal Chim Acta 1996;334:251–259.

Cai Y, Jaffe R, Jones R. Ethylmercury in the soils and sediments of the Florida Everglades. Environ Sci Technol 1997;31:302–305.

Cai Y, Monsalud S, Furton KG, Jaffe R, Jones RD. Determination of methylmercury in fish and aqueous samples using solid-phase microextraction followed by gas chromatography atomic fluorescence spectrometry. Appl Organomet Chem 1998;12:565–569.

Cairns WRL, Ranaldo M, Hennebelle R, Turetta C, Capodaglio G, Ferrari CF, Dommergue A, Cescon P, Barbante C. Speciation analysis of mercury in seawater from the lagoon of Venice by on-line pre-concentration HPLC-ICP-MS. Anal Chim Acta 2008;622:62–69.

Campos RC, Goncalves RA, Brandao GP, Azevedo MS, Oliveira F, Wasserman J. Methylmercury determination using a hyphenated high performance liquid chromatography ultraviolet cold vapor multipath atomic absorption spectrometry system. Spectrochim Acta B 2009;64:506–512.

Canario J, Caetano M, Vale C. Validation and application of an analytical method for monomethylmercury quantification in aquatic plant tissues. Anal Chim Acta 2006;580:258–262.

Caricchia AM, Minervini G, Soldati P, Chiavarini S, Ubaldi C, Morabito R. GC-ECD determination of methylmercury in sediment samples using a SPB-608 capillary column after alkaline digestion. Microchem J 1997;55:44–55.

Carrasco L, Diez S, Bayona JM. Simultaneous determination of methyl- and ethyl-mercury by solid-phase microextraction followed by gas chromatography atomic fluorescence detection. J Chromatogr A 2009;1216:8828–8834.

Carro AM, Neira I, Rodil R, Lorenzo RA. Speciation of mercury compounds by gas chromatography with atomic emission detection. Simultaneous optimization of a headspace solid-phase microextraction and derivatization procedure by use of chemometric techniques. Chromatographia 2002;56:733–738.

Castillo A, Rodriguez-Gonzalez P, Centineo G, Roig-Navarro AF, Alonso JIG. Multiple spiking species-specific isotope dilution analysis by molecular mass spectrometry: simultaneous determination of inorganic mercury and methylmercury in fish tissues. Anal Chem 2010;82:2773–2783.

Castillo A, Roig-Navarro AF, Pozo OJ. Method optimization for the determination of four mercury species by micro-liquid chromatography-inductively coupled plasma mass spectrometry coupling in environmental water samples. Anal Chim Acta 2006;577:18–25.

Chang LF, Jiang SJ, Sahayam AC. Speciation analysis of mercury and lead in fish samples using liquid chromatography-inductively coupled plasma mass spectrometry. J Chromatogr A 2007;1176:143–148.

Chen SS, Chou SS, Hwang DF. Determination of methylmercury in fish using focused microwave digestion following by Cu^{2+} addition, sodium tetrapropylborate derivatization, n-heptane extraction, and gas chromatography-mass spectrometry. J Chromatogr A 2004;1024:209–215.

Chen HT, Chen JG, Jin XZ, Wei DY. Determination of trace mercury species by high performance liquid chromatography-inductively coupled plasma mass spectrometry after cloud point extraction. J Hazard Mater 2009a;172:1282–1287.

Chen JG, Chen HW, Jin XZ, Chen HT. Determination of ultra-trace amount methyl-, phenyl- and inorganic mercury in environmental and biological samples by liquid chromatography with inductively coupled plasma mass spectrometry after cloud point extraction preconcentration. Talanta 2009b;77:1381–1387.

Chen KJ, Hsu IH, Sun YC. Determination of methylmercury and inorganic mercury by coupling short-column ion chromatographic separation, on-line photocatalyst-assisted vapor generation, and inductively coupled plasma mass spectrometry. J Chromatogr A 2009c;1216:8933–8938.

Chen LQ, Yang LM, Wang QQ. In vivo phytochelatins and Hg-phytochelatin complexes in Hg-stressed *Brassica chinensis* L. Metallomics 2009d;1:101–106.

Chiavarini S, Cremisini C, Ingrao G, Morabito R. Determination of methylmercury in human hair by capillary GC with electron capture detection. Appl Organomet Chem 1994;8:563–570.

Chiou CS, Jiang SJ, Danadurai KSK. Determination of mercury compounds in fish by microwave-assisted extraction and liquid chromatography-vapor generation-inductively coupled plasma mass spectrometry. Spectrochim Acta B 2001;56:1133–1142.

Davis WC, Vander Pol SS, Schantz MM, Long SE, Day RD, Christopher SJ. An accurate and sensitive method for the determination of methylmercury in biological specimens using GC-ICP-MS with solid phase microextraction. J Anal At Spectrom 2004;19:1546–1551.

De Smaele T, Moens L, Dams R, Sandra P, Van der Eycken J, Vandyck J. Sodium tetra(n-propyl)borate: a novel aqueous in situ derivatization reagent for the simultaneous determination of organomercury, -lead and -tin compounds with capillary gas chromatography inductively coupled plasma mass spectrometry. J Chromatogr A 1998;793:99–106.

Demuth N, Heumann KG. Validation of methylmercury determinations in aquatic systems by alkyl derivatization methods for GC analysis using ICP-IDMS. Anal Chem 2001;73:4020–4027.

de Diego A, Tseng CM, Stoichev T, Amouroux D, Donard OFX. Interferences during mercury speciation determination by volatilization, cryofocusing, gas chromatography and atomic absorption spectroscopy: comparative study between hydride generation and ethylation techniques. J Anal At Spectrom 1998;13:623–629.

Diez S, Bayona JM. Determination of methylmercury in human hair by ethylation followed by headspace solid-phase microextraction-gas chromatography-cold-vapour atomic fluorescence spectrometry. J Chromatogr A 2002;963:345–351.

Dong LM, Yan XP, Li Y, Jiang Y, Wang SW, Jiang DQ. On-line coupling of flow injection displacement sorption preconcentration to high-performance liquid chromatography for speciation analysis of mercury in seafood. J Chromatogr A 2004;1036:119–125.

Ebdon L, Foulkes ME, Le Roux S, Muñoz-Olivas R. Cold vapour atomic fluorescence spectrometry and gas chromatography-pyrolysis-atomic fluorescence spectrometry for routine determination of total and organometallic mercury in food samples. Analyst 2002;127:1108–1114.

Fan Z, Liu X. Determination of methylmercury and phenylmercury in water samples by liquid-liquid-liquid microextraction coupled with capillary electrophoresis. J Chromatogr A 2008;1180:187–192.

Filippelli M, Baldi F, Brinckman FE, Olson GJ. Methylmercury determination as volatile methylmercury hydride by purge and trap gas chromatography in line with Fourier transform infrared spectroscopy. Environ Sci Technol 1992;26:1457–1460.

Gailer J, George GN, Pickering IJ, Madden S, Prince RC, Yu EY, Denton MB, Younis HS, Aposhian HV. Structural basis of the antagonism between inorganic mercury and selenium in mammals. Chem Res Toxicol 2000;13:1135–1142.

Gao EL, Jiang GB, He B, Yin YG, Shi JB. Speciation of mercury in coal using HPLC-CV-AFS system: comparison of different extraction methods. J Anal At Spectrom 2008;23:1397–1400.

Geerdink RB, Breidenbach R, Epema OJ. Optimization of headspace solid-phase microextraction gas chromatography-atomic emission detection analysis of monomethylmercury. J Chromatogr A 2007;1174:7–12.

George GN, Prince RC, Gailer J, Buttigieg GA, Denton MB, Harris HH, Pickering IJ. Mercury binding to the chelation therapy agents DMSA and DMPS and the rational design of custom chelators for mercury. Chem Res Toxicol 2004;17:999–1006.

George GN, Singh SP, Prince RC, Pickering IJ. Chemical forms of mercury and selenium in fish following digestion with simulated gastric fluid. Chem Res Toxicol 2008;21:2106–2110.

Gibicar D, Logar M, Horvat N, Marn-Pernat A, Ponikvar R, Horvat M. Simultaneous determination of trace levels of ethylmercury and methylmercury in biological samples and vaccines using sodium tetra(n-propyl)borate as derivatizing agent. Anal Bioanal Chem 2007;388:329–340.

Gomez-Ariza JL, Lorenzo F, Garcia-Barrera T. Simultaneous determination of mercury and arsenic species in natural freshwater by liquid chromatography with on-line UV irradiation, generation of hydrides and cold vapor and tandem atomic fluorescence detection. J Chromatogr A 2004;1056:139–144.

Gomez-Ariza JL, Lorenzo F, Garcia-Barrera T. Comparative study of atomic fluorescence spectroscopy and inductively coupled plasma mass spectrometry for mercury and arsenic multispeciation. Anal Bioanal Chem 2005;382:485–492.

Hardy S, Jones P. Capillary electrophoresis determination of methylmercury in fish and crab meat after extraction as the dithizone sulphonate complex. J Chromatogr A 1997;791:333–338.

Harris HH, Pickering IJ, George GN. The chemical form of mercury in fish. Science 2003;301:1203–1203.

Hashempur T, Rofouei MK, Khorrami AR. Speciation analysis of mercury contaminants in water samples by RP-HPLC after solid phase extraction on modified C-18 extraction disks with 1,3-bis(2-cyanobenzene)triazene. Microchem J 2008;89:131–136.

He B, Jiang GB. Analysis of organomercuric species in soils from orchards and wheat fields by capillary gas chromatography on-line coupled with atomic absorption spectrometry after in situ hydride generation and headspace solid phase microextraction. Fresenius J Anal Chem 1999;365:615–618.

Hesterberg D, Chou JW, Hutchison KJ, Sayers DE. Bonding of Hg(II) to reduced organic, sulfur in humic acid as affected by S/Hg ratio. Environ Sci Technol 2001;35:2741–2745.

Hight SC, Cheng J. Determination of methylmercury and estimation of total mercury in seafood using high performance liquid chromatography (HPLC) and inductively coupled plasma-mass spectrometry (ICP-MS): Method development and validation. Anal Chim Acta 2006;567:160–172.

Hintelmann H, Evans RD. Application of stable isotopes in environmental tracer studies-Measurement of monomethylmercury (CH_3Hg^+) by isotope dilution ICP-MS and detection of species transformation. Fresenius J Anal Chem 1997;358:378–385.

Hintelmann H, Evans RD, Villeneuve JY. Measurement of mercury methylation in sediments by using enriched stable mercury isotopes combined with methylmercury determination by gas chromatography-inductively coupled plasma mass spectrometry. J Anal At Spectrom 1995;10:619–624.

Hintelmann H, Falter R, Ilgen G, Evans RD. Determination of artifactual formation of monomethylmercury (CH_3Hg^+) in environmental samples using stable Hg^{2+} isotopes with ICP-MS detection: calculation of contents applying species specific isotope addition. Fresenius J Anal Chem 1997;358:363–370.

Hintelmann H, Nguyen HT. Extraction of methylmercury from tissue and plant samples by acid leaching. Anal Bioanal Chem 2005;381:360–365.

Holz J, Kreutzmann J, Wilken RD, Falter R. Methylmercury monitoring in rainwater samples using in situ ethylation in combination with GC-AFS and GC-ICP-MS techniques. Appl Organomet Chem 1999;13:789–794.

Houserova P, Matejicek D, Kuban V. High-performance liquid chromatographic/ion-trap mass spectrometric speciation of aquatic mercury as its pyrrolidinedithiocarbamate complexes. Anal Chim Acta 2007;596:242–250.

Houserova P, Matejicek D, Kuban V, Pavlickova J, Komarek J. Liquid chromatographic-cold vapour atomic fluorescence spectrometric determination of mercury species. J Sep Sci 2006;29:248–255.

Huang JH. Artifact formation of methyl- and ethyl-mercury compounds from inorganic mercury during derivatization using sodium tetra(n-propyl)borate. Anal Chim Acta 2005;532:113–120.

Huang ZY, Shen JC, Zhuang ZX, Wang XR, Lee FSC. Investigation of metal-binding metallothioneins in the tissues of rats after oral intake of cinnabar. Anal Bioanal Chem 2004;379:427–432.

Huang ZY, Zhang Q, Chen J, Zhuang ZX, Wang XR. Bioaccumulation of metals and induction of metallothioneins in selected tissues of common carp (*Cyprinus carpio L.*) co-exposed to cadmium, mercury and lead. Appl Organomet Chem 2007;21:101–107.

Hutson ND, Attwood BC, Scheckel KG. XAS and XPS characterization of mercury binding on brominated activated carbon. Environ Sci Technol 2007;41:1747–1752.

Iglesia-Turino S, Febrero A, Jauregui O, Caldelas C, Araus JL, Bort J. Detection and quantification of unbound phytochelatin 2 in plant extracts of *Brassica napus* grown with different levels of mercury. Plant Physiol 2006;142:742–749.

Ikemoto T, Kunito T, Anan Y, Tanaka H, Baba N, Miyazaki N, Tanabe S. Association of heavy metals with metallothionein and other proteins in hepatic cytosol of marine mammals and seabirds. Environ Toxicol Chem 2004;23:2008–2016.

Ito R, Kawaguchi M, Sakui N, Honda H, Okanouchi N, Saito K, Nakazawa H. Mercury speciation and analysis in drinking water by stir bar sorptive extraction with in situ propyl derivatization and thermal desorption-gas chromatography-mass spectrometry. J Chromatogr A 2008;1209:267–270.

Ito R, Kawaguchi M, Sakui N, Okanouchi N, Saito K, Seto Y, Nakazawa H. Stir bar sorptive extraction with in situ derivatization and thermal desorption-gas chromatography-mass spectrometry for trace analysis of methylmercury and mercury(II) in water sample. Talanta 2009;77:1295–1298.

Jackson B, Taylor V, Baker RA, Miller E. Low-level mercury speciation in freshwaters by isotope dilution GC-ICP-MS. Environ Sci Technol 2009;43:2463–2469.

Jalilehvand F, Leung BO, Izadifard M, Damian E. Mercury(II) cysteine complexes in alkaline aqueous solution. Inorg Chem 2006;45:66–73.

Jimenez MS, Sturgeon RE. Speciation of methyl- and inorganic mercury in biological tissues using ethylation and gas chromatography with furnace atomization plasma emission spectrometric detection. J Anal At Spectrom 1997;12:597–601.

Jokai Z, Abranko L, Fodor P. SPME-GC-pyrolysis-AFS determination of methylmercury in marine fish products by alkaline sample preparation and aqueous phase phenylation derivatization. J Agric Food Chem 2005;53:5499–5505.

Jung MJ, Yang DH, Sung YK, Kim MJ, Kang SJ, Kwon DY, Kwon Y. Rapid determination of trace methylmercury in natural crude medicine of animal origin. Microchim Acta 2009;164:345–349.

Kameo S, Nakai K, Kurokawa N, Kanehisa T, Naganuma A, Satoh H. Metal components analysis of metallothionein-III in the brain sections of metallothionein-I and metallothionein-II null mice exposed to mercury vapor with HPLC/ICP-MS. Anal Bioanal Chem 2005;381:1514–1519.

Kanda Y, Suzuki N. Substoichiometric isotope dilution analysis of inorganic mercury and methylmercury with thionalide. Anal Chem 1980;52:1672–1675.

Khan MAK, Wang FY. Mercury-selenium compounds and their toxicological significance: toward a molecular understanding of the mercury-selenium antagonism. Environ Toxicol Chem 2009;28:1567–1577.

Kim CS, Brown GE, Rytuba JJ. Characterization and speciation of mercury-bearing mine wastes using X-ray absorption spectroscopy. Sci Total Environ 2000;261:157–168.

Kim CS, Rytuba JJ, Brown GE. EXAFS study of mercury(II) sorption to Fe- and Al-(hydr)oxides-II. Effects of chloride and sulfate. J Colloid Interface Sci 2004;270:9–20.

Krishna MVB, Castro J, Brewer TM, Marcus RK. Online mercury speciation through liquid chromatography with particle beam/electron ionization mass spectrometry detection. J Anal At Spectrom 2007;22:283–291.

Krupp EM, Mestrot A, Wielgus J, Meharg AA, Feldmann J. The molecular form of mercury in biota: identification of novel mercury peptide complexes in plants. Chem Commun 2009;28:4257–4259.

Krystek P, Ritsema R. Determination of methylmercury and inorganic mercury in shark fillets. Appl Organomet Chem 2004;18:640–645.

Krystek P, Ritsema R. Mercury speciation in thawed out and refrozen fish samples by gas chromatography coupled to inductively coupled plasma mass spectrometry and atomic fluorescence spectroscopy. Anal Bioanal Chem 2005;381:354–359.

Kubán P, Pelcová P, Margetínová J, Kubán V. Mercury speciation by CE: an update. Electrophoresis 2009;30:92–99.

Lambertsson L, Lundberg E, Nilsson M, Frech W. Applications of enriched stable isotope tracers in combination with isotope dilution GC-ICP-MS to study mercury species transformation in sea sediments during in situ ethylation and determination. J Anal At Spectrom 2001;16:1296–1301.

Larsson T, Frech W. Species-specific isotope dilution with permeation tubes for determination of gaseous mercury species. Anal Chem 2003;75:5584–5591.

Lee JS, Ryu YJ, Park JS, Jeon SH, Kim SC, Kim YH. Determination of methylmercury in biological samples using dithizone extraction method followed by purge & trap GC-MS. B Kor Chem Soc 2007;28:2293–2298.

Leenaers J, Van Mol W, Infante HG, Adams FC. Gas chromatography-inductively coupled plasma-time-of-flight mass spectrometry as a tool for speciation analysis of organomercury compounds in environmental and biological samples. J Anal At Spectrom 2002;17:1492–1497.

Leermakers M, Baeyens W, Quevauviller P, Horvat M. Mercury in environmental samples: speciation, artifacts and validation. Trac-Trend Anal Chem 2005;24:383–393.

Lemes M, Wang FY. Methylmercury speciation in fish muscle by HPLC-ICP-MS following enzymatic hydrolysis. J Anal At Spectrom 2009;24:663–668.

Leopold K, Foulkes M, Worsfold PJ. Preconcentration techniques for the determination of mercury species in natural waters. Trac-Trend Anal Chem 2009;28:426–435.

Li PJ, Duan JK, Hu B. High-sensitivity capillary electrophoresis for speciation of organomercury in biological samples using hollow fiber-based liquid-liquid-liquid microextraction combined with on-line preconcentration by large-volume sample stacking. Electrophoresis 2008;29:3081–3089.

Li F, Wang DD, Yan XP, Lin JM, Su RG. Development of a new hybrid technique for rapid speciation analysis by directly interfacing a microfluidic chip-based capillary electrophoresis system to atomic fluorescence spectrometry. Electrophoresis 2005a;26:2261–2268.

Li Y, Yan XP, Dong LM, Wang SW, Jiang Y, Jiang DQ. Development of an ambient temperature post-column oxidation system for high-performance liquid chromatography on-line coupled with cold vapor atomic fluorescence spectrometry for mercury speciation in seafood. J Anal At Spectrom 2005b;20:467–472.

Li YF, Chen CY, Li B, Wang Q, Wang JX, Gao YX, Zhao YL, Chai ZF. Simultaneous speciation of selenium and mercury in human urine samples from long-term mercury-exposed populations with supplementation of selenium-enriched yeast by HPLC-ICP-MS. J Anal At Spectrom 2007a;22:925–930.

Li Y, Yan XP, Chen C, Xia YL, Jiang Y. Human serum albumin-mercurial species interactions. J Proteome Res 2007b;6:2277–2286.

Li Y, Yan XP, Jiang Y. Interfacing capillary electrophoresis and electrothermal atomic absorption spectroscopy to study metal speciation and metal–biomolecule interactions. Angew Chem Int Ed 2005c;44:6387–6391.

Liang L, Evens C, Lazoff S, Woods JS, Cernichiari E, Horvat M, Martin MD, DeRouen T. Determination of methyl mercury in whole blood by ethylation-GC-CVAFS after alkaline digestion-solvent extraction. J Anal Toxicol 2000;24:328–332.

Liang LN, Jiang GB, Liu JF, Hu JT. Speciation analysis of mercury in seafood by using high-performance liquid chromatography on-line coupled with cold-vapor atomic fluorescence spectrometry via a post column microwave digestion. Anal Chim Acta 2003;477:131–137.

Lin LY, Chang LF, Jiang SJ. Speciation analysis of mercury in cereals by liquid chromatography chemical vapor generation inductively coupled plasma-mass spectrometry. J Agric Food Chem 2008;56:6868–6872.

Liu WP, Lee HK. Simultaneous analysis of lead, mercury and selenium species by capillary electrophoresis with combined ethylenediaminetetraacetic acid complexation and field-amplified stacking injection. Electrophoresis 1999;20:2475–2483.

Logar M, Horvat M, Akagi H, Pihlar B. Simultaneous determination of inorganic mercury and methylmercury compounds in natural waters. Anal Bioanal Chem 2002;374:1015–1021.

Lowry GV, Shaw S, Kim CS, Rytuba JJ, Brown GE. Macroscopic and microscopic observations of particle-facilitated mercury transport from new idria and sulphur bank mercury mine tailings. Environ Sci Technol 2004;38:5101–5111.

Luckow V, Rüssel HA. Gas chromatographic determination of trace amounts of inorganic mercury. J Chromatogr A 1978;150:187–194.

Mah V, Jalilehvand F. Mercury(II) complex formation with glutathione in alkaline aqueous solution. J Biol Inorg Chem 2008;13:541–553.

Manganiello L, Arce L, Rios A, Valcarcel M. Piezoelectric screening coupled on line to capillary electrophoresis for detection and speciation of mercury. J Sep Sci 2002;25:319–327.

Mao YX, Liu GL, Meichel G, Cai Y, Jiang GB. Simultaneous speciation of monomethylmercury and monoethylmercury by aqueous phenylation and purge-and-trap preconcentration followed by atomic spectrometry detection. Anal Chem 2008;80:7163–7168.

Mao YX, Yin YG, Li YB, Liu GL, Feng XB, Jiang GB, Cai Y. Occurrence of monoethylmercury in the Florida Everglades: identification and verification. Environ Pollut 2010;158:3378–3384.

Margetinova J, Houserova-Pelcova P, Kuban V. Speciation analysis of mercury in sediments, zoobenthos and river water samples by high-performance liquid chromatography hyphenated to atomic fluorescence spectrometry following preconcentration by solid phase extraction. Anal Chim Acta 2008;615:115–123.

Martin-Doimeadios RCR, Krupp E, Amouroux D, Donard OFX. Application of isotopically labeled methylmercury for isotope dilution analysis of biological samples using gas chromatography/ICPMS. Anal Chem 2002a;74:2505–2512.

Martin-Doimeadios RCR, Stoichev T, Krupp E, Amouroux D, Holeman M, Donard OFX. Micro-scale preparation and characterization of isotopically enriched monomethylmercury. Appl Organomet Chem 2002b;16:610–615.

Martin-Doimeadios RCR, Monperrus M, Krupp E, Amouroux D, Donard OFX. Using speciated isotope dilution with GC-inductively coupled plasma MS to determine and unravel the artificial formation of monomethylmercury in certified reference sediments. Anal Chem 2003;75:3202–3211.

Martinez R, Pereiro R, Sanz-Medel A, Bordel N. Mercury speciation by HPLC-cold-vapour radiofrequency glow-discharge optical-emission spectrometry with on-line microwave oxidation. Fresenius J Anal Chem 2001;371:746–752.

Mishra S, Tripathi RM, Bhalke S, Shukla VK, Puranik VD. Determination of methylmercury and mercury(II) in a marine ecosystem using solid-phase microextraction gas chromatography-mass spectrometry. Anal Chim Acta 2005;551:192–198.

Monperrus M, Gonzalez PR, Amouroux D, Alonso JIG, Donard OFX. Evaluating the potential and limitations of double-spiking species-specific isotope dilution analysis for the accurate quantification of mercury species in different environmental matrices. Anal Bioanal Chem 2008;390:655–666.

Monperrus M, Krupp E, Amouroux D, Donard OFX, Martin-Doimeadios RCR. Potential and limits of speciated isotope-dilution analysis for metrology and assessing environmental reactivity. Trac-Trend Anal Chem 2004;23:261–272.

Monperrus M, Martin-Doimeadios RCR, Scancar J, Amouroux D, Donard OFX. Simultaneous sample preparation and species-specific isotope dilution mass spectrometry analysis of monomethylmercury and tributyltin in a certified oyster tissue. Anal Chem 2003;75:4095–4102.

Montuori P, Jover E, Alzaga R, Diez S, Bayona JM. Improvements in the methylmercury extraction from human hair by headspace solid-phase microextraction followed by gas-chromatography cold-vapour atomic fluorescence spectrometry. J Chromatogr A 2004;1025:71–75.

Morton J, Carolan VA, Gardiner PHE. The speciation of inorganic and methylmercury in human hair by high-performance liquid chromatography coupled with inductively coupled plasma mass spectrometry. J Anal At Spectrom 2002;17:377–381.

Nsengimana H, Cukrowska EM, Dinsmore A, Tessier E, Amouroux D. In situ ethylation of organolead, organotin and organomercury species by bromomagnesium tetraethylborate prior to GC-ICP MS analysis. J Sep Sci 2009;32:2426–2433.

Orellana-Velado NG, Pereiro R, Sanz-Medel A. Glow discharge atomic emission spectrometry as a detector in gas chromatography for mercury speciation. J Anal At Spectrom 1998;13:905–909.

Pager C, Gaspar A. Possibilities of determination of mercury compounds using capillary zone electrophoresis. Microchem J 2002;73:53–58.

Palenzuela B, Manganiello L, Rios A, Valcarcel M. Monitoring inorganic mercury and methylmercury species with liquid chromatography-piezoelectric detection. Anal Chim Acta 2004;511:289–294.

Palmieri HE, Leonel LV. Determination of methylmercury in fish tissue by gas chromatography with microwave-induced plasma atomic emission spectrometry after derivatization with sodium tetraphenylborate. Fresenius J Anal Chem 2000;366:466–469.

Park JS, Lee JS, Kim GB, Cha JS, Shin SK, Kang HG, Hong EJ, Chung GT, Kim YH. Mercury and methylmercury in freshwater fish and sediments in South Korea using newly adopted purge and trap GC-MS detection method. Water Air Soil Pollut 2010;207:391–401.

Pena-Pereira F, Lavilla I, Bendicho C, Vidal L, Canals A. Speciation of mercury by ionic liquid-based single-drop microextraction combined with high-performance liquid chromatography-photodiode array detection. Talanta 2009;78:537–541.

Peng ZL, Qu F, Song G, Lin JM. Simultaneous separation of organomercury species by nonaqueous capillary electrophoresis using methanol containing acetic acid and imidazole. Electrophoresis 2005;26:3333–3340.

Percy AJ, Korbas M, George GN, Gailer J. Reversed-phase high-performance liquid chromatographic separation of inorganic mercury and methylmercury driven by their different coordination chemistry towards thiols. J Chromatogr A 2007;1156:331–339.

Pereiro IR, Wasik A, Lobinski R. Determination of mercury species in fish reference materials by isothermal multicapillary gas chromatography with atomic emission detection after microwave-assisted solubilization and solvent extraction. J Anal At Spectrom 1998;13:743–747.

Pongratz R, Heumann KG. Determination of concentration profiles of methyl mercury compounds in surface waters of polar and other remote oceans by GC-AFD. Int J Environ Anal Chem 1998;71:41–56.

Qian J, Skyllberg U, Frech W, Bleam WF, Bloom PR, Petit PE. Bonding of methyl mercury to reduced sulfur groups in soil and stream organic matter as determined by x-ray absorption spectroscopy and binding affinity studies. Geochim Cosmochim Acta 2002;66:3873–3885.

Qvarnstrom J, Frech W. Mercury species transformations during sample pre-treatment of biological tissues studied by HPLC-ICP-MS. J Anal At Spectrom 2002;17:1486–1491.

Qvarnstrom J, Lambertsson L, Havarinasab S, Hultman P, Frech W. Determination of methylmercury, ethylmercury, and inorganic mercury in mouse tissues, following administration of thimerosal, by species-specific isotope dilution GC-inductively coupled plasma-MS. Anal Chem 2003;75:4120–4124.

Qvarnstrom J, Tu Q, Frech W, Ludke C. Flow injection-liquid chromatography-cold vapour atomic absorption spectrometry for rapid determination of methyl and inorganic mercury. Analyst 2000;125:1193–1197.

Rahman GMM, Fahrenholz T, Kingston HM. Application of speciated isotope dilution mass spectrometry to evaluate methods for efficiencies, recoveries, and quantification of mercury species transformations in human hair. J Anal At Spectrom 2009;24:83–92.

Rahman GMM, Kingston HMS. Application of speciated isotope dilution mass spectrometry to evaluate extraction methods for determining mercury speciation in soils and sediments. Anal Chem 2004;76:3548–3555.

Rahman GMM, Kingston HMS, Bhandari S. Synthesis and characterization of isotopically enriched methylmercury ($CH_3{}^{201}Hg^+$). Appl Organomet Chem 2003;17:913–920.

Rahman GMM, Kingston HMS, Pamukcu M. High yield synthesis and characterization of isotopically enriched monoethylmercury chloride ($C_2H_5{}^{201}HgCl$). Appl Organomet Chem 2005;19:1215–1219.

Rai R, Maher W, Kirkowa F. Measurement of inorganic and methylmercury in fish tissues by enzymatic hydrolysis and HPLC-ICP-MS. J Anal At Spectrom 2002;17:1560–1563.

Rajan M, Darrow J, Hua M, Barnett B, Mendoza M, Greenfield BK, Andrews JC. Hg L-3 XANES study of mercury methylation in shredded *Eichhornia crassipes*. Environ Sci Technol 2008;42:5568–5573.

Ramalhosa E, Segade SR, Pereira E, Vale C, Duarte A. Microwave-assisted extraction for methylmercury determination in sediments by high performance liquid chromatography-cold vapour-atomic fluorescence spectrometry. J Anal At Spectrom 2001a;16:643–647.

Ramalhosa E, Segade SR, Pereira E, Vale C, Duarte A. Microwave treatment of biological samples for methylmercury determination by high performance liquid chromatography-cold vapour atomic fluorescence spectrometry. Analyst 2001b;126:1583–1587.

Ramalhosa E, Segade SR, Pereira E, Vale C, Duarte A. Simple methodology for methylmercury and inorganic mercury determinations by high-performance liquid chromatography-cold vapour atomic fluorescence spectrometry. Anal Chim Acta 2001c;448:135–143.

Rapsomanikis S, Donard OFX, Weber JH. Speciation of lead and methyllead ions in water by chromatography/atomic absorption spectrometry after ethylation with sodium tetraethylborate. Anal Chem 1986;58:35–38.

Reyes LH, Rahman GMM, Fahrenholz T, Kingston HMS. Comparison of methods with respect to efficiencies, recoveries, and quantitation of mercury species interconversions in food demonstrated using tuna fish. Anal Bioanal Chem 2008;390:2123–2132.

Reyes LH, Rahman GMM, Kingston HMS. Robust microwave-assisted extraction protocol for determination of total mercury and methylmercury in fish tissues. Anal Chim Acta 2009;631:121–128.

Rio-Segade S, Bendicho C. Ultrasound-assisted extraction for mercury speciation by the flow injection cold vapor technique. J Anal At Spectrom 1999;14:263–268.

Rodrigues JL, de Souza SS, de Oliveira Souza VC, Barbosa F. Methylmercury and inorganic mercury determination in blood by using liquid chromatography with inductively coupled plasma mass spectrometry and a fast sample preparation procedure. Talanta 2010;80:1158–1163.

Rodriguez-Gonzalez P, Marchante-Gayon JM, Alonso JIG, Sanz-Medel A. Isotope dilution analysis for elemental speciation: a tutorial review. Spectrochim Acta B 2005;60:151–207.

Sanchez DM, Martin R, Morante R, Marin J, Munuera ML. Preconcentration speciation method for mercury compounds in water samples using solid phase extraction followed by reversed phase high performance liquid chromatography. Talanta 2000;52:671–679.

dos Santos JS, de la Guardia M, Pastor A. A multinjection strategy for mercury speciation. Talanta 2006;69:534–537.

dos Santos JS, de la Guardia M, Pastor A, dos Santos MLP. Determination of organic and inorganic mercury species in water and sediment samples by HPLC on-line coupled with ICP-MS. Talanta 2009;80:207–211.

Santoyo MM, Figueroa JAL, Wrobel K, Wrobel K. Analytical speciation of mercury in fish tissues by reversed phase liquid chromatography-inductively coupled plasma mass spectrometry with Bi^{3+} as internal standard. Talanta 2009;79:706–711.

Saouter E, Blattmann B. Analyses of organic and inorganic mercury by atomic fluorescence spectrometry using a semiautomatic analytical system. Anal Chem 1994;66:2031–2037.

Shade CW. Automated simultaneous analysis of monomethyl and mercuric Hg in biotic samples by Hg-thiourea complex liquid chromatography following acidic thiourea leaching. Environ Sci Technol 2008;42:6604–6610.

Shade CW, Hudson RJM. Determination of MeHg in environmental sample matrices using Hg-thiourea complex ion chromatography with on-line cold vapor generation and atomic fluorescence spectrometric detection. Environ Sci Technol 2005;39:4974–4982.

Shaw MJ, Jones P, Haddad PR. Dithizone derivatives as sensitive water soluble chromogenic reagents for the ion chromatographic determination of inorganic and organomercury in aqueous matrices. Analyst 2003;128:1209–1212.

Shen JC, Huang ZY, Zhuang ZX, Wang XR, Lee FSC. Investigation of mercury metallothionein complexes in tissues of rat after oral intake of $HgCl_2$. Appl Organomet Chem 2005;19:140–146.

Shi JW, Feng WY, Wang M, Zhang F, Li B, Wang B, Zhu MT, Chai ZF. Investigation of mercury-containing proteins by enriched stable isotopic tracer and size-exclusion chromatography hyphenated to inductively coupled plasma-isotope dilution mass spectrometry. Anal Chim Acta 2007;583:84–91.

Siciliano SD, Sangster A, Daughney CJ, Loseto L, Germida JJ, Rencz AN, O'Driscoll NJ, Lean DRS. Are methylmercury concentrations in the wetlands of Kejimkujik National Park, Nova Scotia, Canada, dependent on geology? J Environ Qual 2003;32:2085–2094.

Skubal LR, Biedron SG, Newville M, Schneider JF, Milton SV, Pianetta P, O'Neill HJ. Mercury transformations in chemical agent simulant as characterized by x-ray absorption fine spectroscopy. Talanta 2005;67:730–735.

Slaets S, Adams F, Pereiro IR, Lobinski R. Optimization of the coupling of multicapillary GC with ICP-MS for mercury speciation analysis in biological materials. J Anal At Spectrom 1999;14:851–857.

Slowey AJ, Rytuba JJ, Brown GE. Speciation of mercury and mode of transport from placer gold mine tailings. Environ Sci Technol 2005;39:1547–1554.

Šmejkal Z, Teplá Z. Exchange extraction equilibrium of mercury(II) and bis(diethyldithiocarbamato)copper in sub-and superequivalent method of isotope dilution analysis. J Radioanal Chem 1983;77:49–56.

Smith RG. Determination of mercury in environmental samples by isotope dilution/ICPMS. Anal Chem 1993;65:2485–2488.

Snell JP, Quetel CR, Lambertsson L, Qvarnstrom J. Preparation and certification of ERM-AE670, a ^{202}Hg enriched methylmercury isotopic reference material. J Anal At Spectrom 2004;19:1315–1324.

Snell JP, Stewart II, Sturgeon, RE, Frech, W. Species specific isotope dilution calibration for determination of mercury species by gas chromatography coupled to inductively coupled plasma- or furnace atomisation plasma ionisation-mass spectrometry. J Anal At Spectrom 2000;15:1540–1545.

de Souza SS, Rodrigues JL, de Oliveira Souza VC, Barbosa F. A fast sample preparation procedure for mercury speciation in hair samples by high-performance liquid chromatography coupled to ICP-MS. J Anal At Spectrom 2010;25:79–83.

Stoichev T, Martin-Doimeadios RCR, Amouroux D, Molenat N, Donard OFX. Application of cryofocusing hydride generation and atomic fluorescence detection for dissolved mercury species determination in natural water samples. J Environ Monit 2002;4:517–521.

Stoichev T, Martin-Doimeadios RCR, Tessier E, Amouroux D, Donard OFX. Improvement of analytical performances for mercury speciation by on-line derivatization, cryofocussing and atomic fluorescence spectrometry. Talanta 2004;62:433–438.

Trumpler S, Lohmann W, Meermann B, Buscher W, Sperling M, Karst U. Interaction of thimerosal with proteins-ethylmercury adduct formation of human serum albumin and beta-lactoglobulin A. Metallomics 2009;1:87–91.

Tu Q, Johnson W, Buckley B. Mercury speciation analysis in soil samples by ion chromatography, post-column cold vapor generation and inductively coupled plasma mass spectrometry. J Anal At Spectrom 2003;18:696–701.

Tu Q, Qian J, Frech W. Rapid determination of methylmercury in biological materials by GC-MIP-AES or GC-ICP-MS following simultaneous ultrasonic-assisted in situ ethylation and solvent extraction. J Anal At Spectrom 2000;15:1583–1588.

Vallant B, Kadnar R, Goessler W. Development of a new HPLC method for the determination of inorganic and methylmercury in biological samples with ICP-MS detection. J Anal At Spectrom 2007;22:322–325.

Velado NGO, Pereiro R, Sanz-Medel A. Mercury speciation by capillary gas chromatography with radiofrequency hollow cathode glow discharge atomic emission detection. J Anal At Spectrom 2000;15:49–53.

Vidler DS, Jenkins RO, Hall JF, Harrington CF. The determination of methylmercury in biological samples by HPLC coupled to ICP-MS detection. Appl Organomet Chem 2007;21:303–310.

Wan CC, Chen CS, Jiang SJ. Determination of mercury compounds in water samples by liquid chromatography inductively coupled plasma mass spectrometry with an in situ nebulizer/vapor generator. J Anal At Spectrom 1997;12:683–687.

Wang M, Feng WY, Shi JW, Zhang F, Wang B, Zhu MT, Li B, Zhao YL, Chai ZF. Development of a mild mercaptoethanol extraction method for determination of mercury species in biological samples by HPLC-ICP-MS. Talanta 2007;71:2034–2039.

Wang M, Feng WY, Wang HJ, Zhang Y, Li J, Li B, Zhao YL, Chai ZF. Analysis of mercury-containing protein fractions in brain cytosol of the maternal and infant rats after exposure to a low-dose of methylmercury by SEC coupled to isotope dilution ICP-MS. J Anal At Spectrom 2008;23:1112–1116.

Wang D-D, Li F, Yan X-P. On-line hyphenation of flow injection, miniaturized capillary electrophoresis and atomic fluorescence spectrometry for high-throughput speciation analysis. J Chromatogr A 2006;1117:246–249.

Wang ZH, Yin YG, He B, Shi JB, Liu JF, Jiang GB. L-cysteine-induced degradation of organic mercury as a novel interface in the HPLC-CV-AFS hyphenated system for speciation of mercury. J Anal At Spectrom 2010;25:810–814.

Westöö G. Determination of methylmercury compounds in foodstuffs. II. Determination of methylmercury in fish, egg, meat, and liver. Acta Chem Scand 1967;21:1790–1800.

Wolfenden S, Charnock JM, Hilton J, Livens FR, Vaughan DJ. Sulfide species as a sink for mercury in lake sediments. Environ Sci Technol 2005;39:6644–6648.

Xia LB, Hu B, Wu YL. Hollow fiber-based liquid-liquid-liquid microextraction combined with high-performance liquid chromatography for the speciation of organomercury. J Chromatogr A 2007;1173:44–51.

Xia K, Skyllberg UL, Bleam WF, Bloom PR, Nater EA, Helmke PA. X-ray absorption spectroscopic evidence for the complexation of Hg(II) by reduced sulfur in soil humic substances. Environ Sci Technol 1999;33:257–261.

Yang L, Colombini V, Maxwell P, Mester Z, Sturgeon RE. Application of isotope dilution to the determination of methylmercury in fish tissue by solid-phase microextraction gas chromatography-mass spectrometry. J Chromatogr A 2003;1011:135–142.

Yazdi AS, Banihashemi S, Es'haghi Z. Determination of Hg(II) in natural waters by diphenylation by single-drop microextraction: GC. Chromatographia 2010;71:1049–1054.

Yin XB. Dual-cloud point extraction as a preconcentration and clean-up technique for capillary electrophoresis speciation analysis of mercury. J Chromatogr A 2007;1154:437–443.

Yin YG, Chen M, Peng JF, Liu JF, Jiang GB. Dithizone-functionalized solid phase extraction-displacement elution-high performance liquid chromatography-inductively coupled plasma mass spectrometry for mercury speciation in water samples. Talanta 2010;81:1788–1792.

Yin YG, Liu JF, He B, Shi JB, Jiang GB. Simple interface of high-performance liquid chromatography-atomic fluorescence spectrometry hyphenated system for speciation of mercury based on photo-induced chemical vapour generation with formic acid in mobile phase as reaction reagent. J Chromatogr A 2008;1181:77–82.

Yin YG, Liu JF, He B, Shi JB, Jiang GB. Mercury speciation by a high performance liquid chromatography-atomic fluorescence spectrometry hyphenated system with photo-induced chemical vapour generation reagent in the mobile phase. Microchim Acta 2009a;167:289–295.

Yin YG, Wang ZH, Peng JF, Liu JF, He B, Jiang GB. Direct chemical vapour generation-flame atomization as interface of high performance liquid chromatography-atomic fluorescence spectrometry for speciation of mercury without using post-column digestion. J Anal At Spectrom 2009b;24:1575–1578.

Yin YM, Liang J, Yang LM, Wang QQ. Vapour generation at a UV/TiO$_2$ photocatalysis reaction device for determination and speciation of mercury by AFS and HPLC-AFS. J Anal At Spectrom 2007a;22:330–334.

Yin YG, Liu JF, He B, Gao EL, Jiang GB. Photo-induced chemical vapour generation with formic acid: novel interface for high performance liquid chromatography-atomic fluorescence spectrometry hyphenated system and application in speciation of mercury. J Anal At Spectrom 2007b;22:822–826.

Yin YM, Qiu JH, Yang LM, Wang QQ. A new vapor generation system for mercury species based on the UV irradiation of mercaptoethanol used in the determination of total and methyl mercury in environmental and biological samples by atomic fluorescence spectrometry. Anal Bioanal Chem 2007c;388:831–836.

Yu LP. Cloud point extraction preconcentration prior to high-performance liquid chromatography coupled with cold vapor generation atomic fluorescence spectrometry for speciation analysis of mercury in fish samples. J Agric Food Chem 2005;53:9656–9662.

Zachariadis GA, Kapsimali DC. Effect of sample matrix on sensitivity of mercury and methylmercury quantitation in human urine, saliva, and serum using GC-MS. J Sep Sci 2008;31:3884–3893.

CHAPTER 3

MEASURING GAS PHASE MERCURY EMISSIONS FROM INDUSTRIAL EFFLUENTS

SAMUEL J. IPPOLITO, YLIAS M. SABRI, and **SURESH K. BHARGAVA**

3.1   INTRODUCTION

A number of hazardous and toxic gaseous species are emitted into the atmosphere from a large variety of industrial-scale processes. Of the trace metal species that have been identified in industrial gaseous emissions, mercury and its compounds (expressed as mercury or Hg) have received the most attention because of the perceived health and environmental risks associated with its release into the atmosphere. Hg emitted from the industrial sources is therefore now recognized as a major concern by governments and environmental bodies worldwide.

Anthropogenic emissions have resulted in global atmospheric Hg deposition rates $\sim$3 times higher than in preindustrial times, with increases of 2 to 10 times in and around the most industrialized regions (Hylander and Meili, 2003). The United States Environmental Protection Agency (US-EPA), in its *Mercury Study Report to Congress* (US-EPA, 1997) in 1997, reported that the amount of mercury released into the atmosphere from human activities in 1995 was between 50% and 75% of the total yearly release (including natural, anthropogenic, and oceanic emissions) of 5500 Mg. The most common estimates for anthropogenic Hg emissions into the atmosphere range between 2000 and 2900 Mg/year. China is widely cited as the largest anthropogenic emitter, being responsible for approximately a quarter of global emissions with $\sim$690 Mg in 2003 (Wu et al., 2006). While there are comprehensive Hg emission inventories regarding industrial processes for many countries, significant gaps still remain within the data. Additional uncertainties remain about how far mercury may travel from its respective emission sources, and thus its impacts on the surrounding environment cannot be fully quantified.

Environmental Chemistry and Toxicology of Mercury, First Edition.
Edited by Guangliang Liu, Yong Cai, and Nelson O'Driscoll.
© 2012 John Wiley & Sons, Inc. Published 2012 by John Wiley & Sons, Inc.

The continuous monitoring and controlling of these emissions are important factors in increasing the sustainability of many industrial processes worldwide. Globally, Hg emissions have been decreasing; more than 11% reduction in the levels has been observed between the year 2000 (2190 Mg) and 2005 (1930 Mg) (Pacyna et al., 2006b; UNEP, 2008b). Although it is expected that Hg emissions from industrial sources in the year 2020 will be reduced to ±20% of the year 2000 levels (Pacyna et al., 2006b), others (Sundseth et al., 2010) estimate that an increase of ~25% on 2005 levels will occur if no further action is taken to reduce emissions globally. Such increases, when based merely on the loss of IQ (intelligence quotient), are expected to have an annual cost of ~US$3.7 billion dollar values of year 2005 in 2020 (Sundseth et al., 2010). The ability to rapidly detect Hg emissions over a range of industrial processes will significantly assist various industries in complying with new and future Hg emission guidelines. Furthermore, it will provide a better understanding of the causes and effects of how different process-operating conditions influence Hg emission rates from the many different types of industrial sources worldwide.

3.1.1   Mercury Emissions from Industry

Historically, mercury has been used for a variety of diverse applications that range from batteries, thermometers, and electrical switches to liquid mirrors for telescopes. Currently, mercury is primarily used in some specialized electrical, lighting, and electronic devices and in the manufacture of some industrial chemicals, and thus is a valuable commercial commodity. In industrial situations, mercury can enter into the environment through its improper disposal (e.g., land-fill or incineration) or via its direct release into the atmosphere from stationary industrial sources that use combustion and high temperature processes, such as those found in coal-fire combustion processes for power generation and within the mining and mineral refining sectors.

Given the efforts of the US-EPA to regulate Hg emissions from industrial sources over the past few decades (Stokstad, 2004; Metcalfe, 2010; S.1630 US Library of Congress S.1630; US Library of Congress S.2995), it is foreseeable that new air emission standards for coal- and oil-fired power utilities operating in the United States will force the utilities to comply with tougher monitoring and emission regulations (Neville, 2010). Thereafter, it is anticipated that other industries contributing to the total amount of mercury emitted into the atmosphere are also likely to be subjected to similar regulations, in much the same way as the cement industries in European countries (Baier, 2009). Since the year 2000, for example, continuous monitoring of Hg emission in cement kilns in Germany has become mandatory (Renzoni et al., 2010) with Hg emission limits of 50 and 30 $\mu g/m^3$ for half-hourly and daily averages, respectively (Baier, 2009).

In order to understand the significance of the issue, much effort has been dedicated to identifying which industries are the predominant emitters, as well as trying to understand the mercury cycle within each industrial process, so as to limit Hg emissions into the atmosphere. Typically, the main industrial processes that emit Hg into the atmosphere can be broken down into the following categories:

- Combustion of coal, oil, municipal waste, and natural gas
- Mining and refining processes (e.g., smelting, refining of minerals, and hydrocarbons)
- Some chemical and manufacturing processes (e.g., caustic soda and cement production).

Apart from the industries that fall into the categories discussed above, environmental contamination occurring from the dental/medical community and landfill are also the known causes. However, in comparison, the associated Hg emissions are much lower than those of large industrial sources. Similarly, it should be noted that open biomass burning, which is not always considered anthropogenic, can also be an important source of Hg emissions in certain parts of the world (Brunke et al., 2001a, 2010; Weiss-Penzias et al., 2007; Friedli et al., 2009).

The first global emission inventories were compiled by Pacyna et al. (Pacyna and Pacyna, 2002; Pacyna et al., 2003), and Pirrone et al. (1996), with more recent mercury emission inventories compiled in Pacyna et al. (2006b), Pirrone et al. (2010), and Wilson et al. (2006). It has been estimated that 7527 Mg of Hg was emitted worldwide in the year 2010, which includes the primary emissions and re-emissions of the already deposited mercury and natural sources (Pirrone et al., 2009, 2010). Approximately, 2320 Mg is said to be emitted from anthropogenic sources where the major global sources are from fossil-fuel-fired utilities (810 Mg), gold mining (400 Mg), manufacturing of nonferrous metals (310 Mg), cement production (236 Mg), and caustic soda production (163 Mg) (Pirrone et al., 2010). Future estimates of Hg emissions until the year 2020 in Europe and 2050 globally have been projected by Pacyna et al. (2006a) and Streets et al. (2009) (and references therein), respectively. Streets et al. (2009) also list a number of studies covering Hg emissions from particular regions and countries as well as a breakdown of emissions for each industry.

Figure 3.1 shows some of the major Hg emission contributions from different regions of the world. It may be deduced that most of the regional emission rates are decreasing with time, with the exception of China, Australia, and the United States. Although there is a lack of data available for developing countries and countries with economies in transition (such as India and China), it can be observed that China experienced an increase in Hg emissions until the year 2003. This was partially because of the coal combustion and nonferrous metals smelting sectors increasing from 3% to 4.2% every year (up to 2003), which comprises ~80% of China's total Hg emission sources (Wu et al., 2006). This is of major concern as it is estimated that China represented over 26% of global anthropogenic Hg emissions in the same year (Pirrone et al., 2010). Unfortunately, there is a lack of data for the four years before 2010 (data for 2005 was taken from an United Nations Environmental Program (UNEP) report (UNEP, 2008b) and can be identified by the marked arrows). Similarly, India lacks anthropogenic Hg emissions data; however, it is estimated that India's anthropogenic emissions decreased from 321 Mg in the year 2000 to 253 Mg in 2004 (Pirrone et al., 2010). The main sources are reported to be coal combustion (52%) and

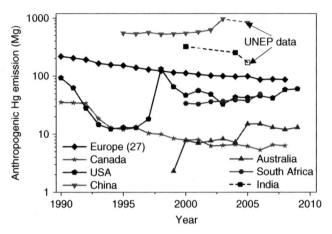

Figure 3.1 Hg emission contributors around the world. Extracted from various sources for each region: Europe, Canada, USA, China 1995–2003 (Wu et al., 2006), India 2000 and 2004 (Mukherjee et al., 2009), China and India 2005 (UNEP, 2008b), Australia, and South Africa (Masekoameng et al., 2010).

waste disposal via incineration (32%). The reduction in India's Hg emission is attributed to the conversion of over 86% of its chlor-alkali caustic soda processes to mercury-free membrane cell technology; however, emissions from coal-fired power plants and municipal solid incineration increased by ~20% and 40% over the same period, respectively.

In comparison to developing and economically transitioning countries, it is easier to predict the major Hg emission sources for countries such as the United States, Canada, Australia, and most of Europe, where emission inventories are well developed and readily available to the general public from national pollutant inventory websites. The increased emissions in Australia observed in Fig. 3.1 are due to mining comprising one of the most significant sectors that contributed to Australia's gross domestic product, increasing from 4.5% in 1994 to 8% in 2007 (www.abs.gov.au). Subsequently, over 40.6% of the total Hg emitted from Australia in the year 2009 originated from the nonferrous metal sector. Similar information is also available for European countries, with the average Hg emission for Europe-27 (excluding Iceland, Liechtenstein, Greece, Luxembourg, and Turkey because of a lack of data) representing 3% of the total emissions in 2004 (97.9 Mg). Further decreases, spurred by regulations restricting the use of mercury and the progressive closure of mercury-emitting industries, have lead to 2% reductions in 2008 in Europe (87.4 Mg). The overall reduction in Hg emissions in the past decade is more evident when comparing the detailed technical background report presented to UNEP, which covers Hg emissions and sources from each country around the globe for the year 2005 (UNEP, 2008b), with other studies reporting Hg emissions for years before 2005. For example, comparing the data from UNEP report with that of Mukherjee et al. (2009), it is observed that India cut its total Hg emissions in 2005 to nearly half of its 2000 emission levels.

In order to improve Hg inventory data, the US-EPA is pursuing bilateral programs with China and India on air quality, promoting best management practices to reduce environmental Hg releases and to encourage Hg emission monitoring and data management/inventory collections (Mital and MacDonald, 2006; Metcalfe, 2010). Limited information is also available for anthropogenic Hg emissions from African countries. However, it is widely regarded that most of the Hg emissions originates from mining and small-scale artisanal gold mining activities (Pirrone et al., 2010). South Africa is of particular interest (Leaner et al., 2009) because of its rapid industrial growth, resulting in ferrous metal production and power generation accounting for ~81% of its emission sources (Pirrone et al., 2010) at an estimated 40.2 Mg in 2004 (Pirrone et al., 2009). Interestingly, out of the top 10 anthropogenic emitting countries, the first three (China, India, and United States) are responsible for nearly 60% of the total Hg emissions globally in 2005, while the bottom three (Australia, Republic of Korea, and Columbia) emitted <5% of the total global emissions (UNEP, 2008b). In addition, new data available on the Hg content of Australian coal has reduced Hg emission estimates by 240 Mg (~10% of global emissions) from Australian anthropogenic sources (UNEP, 2008a), placing it below Brazil on the 2005 top 10 list of countries having the highest anthropogenic Hg emissions (UNEP, 2008b). Brazil, the sixth highest emitter for 2005, is estimated to emit over 45% of its mercury from gold production (UNEP, 2008b); although it has the second largest coal reserve in South America (Mukherjee et al., 2008), it only emits 5.7 Mg of Hg from coal-fired power plant sources annually (Mukherjee et al., 2009). Sources of data regarding natural emissions, which are omitted from Fig. 3.1, can be found in Mason (2009), Pirrone et al. (2009, 2010), UNEP (2008b), and references therein.

3.1.1.1 Thermal Power and Industrial Boilers.
The largest contributing category of Hg emissions from stationary industrial sources into the atmosphere is widely recognized to be fossil-fuel-fired thermal power plants and large industrial boilers. Although relatively large volumes of oil and natural gas are burned each year for power or steam generation, Hg emission from oil and natural gas combustion represents a minor contribution compared to that emitted from coal combustion (Pirrone et al., 2010). Thus, in comparison to other fossil fuels, mercury emission into the atmosphere from coal-fired combustion is found to be significantly higher (Pudasainee et al., 2010). Depending on the grade and origin of coal, trace amounts of mercury can vary substantially from 0.02 to 0.25 ppm, with an average content of 0.09 ppm (Change and Offen, 1995). Although coal does not contain a high concentration of mercury, owing to the large quantity of coal consumed and large number of coal-fired power stations worldwide, it is estimated that ~878 Mg of Hg was emitted into the atmosphere from fossil-fuel combustion for power and heating purposes in 2005 (UNEP, 2008b), which represents ~45% of all anthropogenic mercury emissions worldwide for that year. In addition, mercury is released from coal gasification processes and when coal is burned for heating and cooking purposes, which is prevalent in rural areas

in countries such as China (Wang et al., 2000) and South Africa (Leaner et al., 2009).

Mercury is vaporized during coal combustion processes, where some of the mercury condenses on the ash and the rest passes into the stack gas. It is widely recognized that there has been a substantial reduction in Hg emissions from coal burning facilities over the last few decades because of the industry's continued adoption of air pollution control devices (APCD) and other associated mercury removal technologies, which has been shown to remove upward of 90% of Hg in an economically sustainable manner. A bill presented to the US senate in 2010 for the Clean Air Act Amendments (CAAAs) introduces further legislation requiring coal-fired power plants to cut mercury emissions by 90% across the United States by the year 2015 by utilizing the maximum available control technology (MACT). The total mercury (Hg^T) in the coal-derived flue gas can be broken down into three forms: elemental ($Hg(0)$), oxidized (Hg^{2+}), and particle-bound mercury (Hg^P) (Presto and Granite, 2006). Electrostatic precipitators (ESPs), fabric filters (FFs), baghouses, and flue gas desulfurization (FGD) processes are efficient in removing Hg^{2+} and Hg^P species; however, they are not suitable for removing $Hg(0)$. The most widely used process for removing $Hg(0)$ is based on activated carbon injection. Owing to the high complexity and the large composition variability of streams in plants located in different regions of the world, there has been a strong push to understand how different chemicals affect the removal efficiencies for each of the different removal technologies. The lifetime of the three different forms of Hg is also significantly different. In the case of $Hg(0)$, a lifetime of between six months and two years in the atmosphere has been reported (Galbreath and Zygarlicke, 1996; Pavlish et al., 2003), whereas Hg^{2+} and Hg^P species are reported to have an atmospheric lifetime of only a few days and tend to be deposited on nearby land and vegetation. However, the overall environmental impact of Hg^{2+} and Hg^P is marginal in comparison to $Hg(0)$ emissions, since Hg^{2+} and Hg^P are relatively easy to remove from flue gases by FGD equipment and FF/ESPs, respectively (Presto and Granite, 2006).

Given that $Hg(0)$ vapor has a low affinity for oxygen, is chemically inert, has very low water solubility (49.4×10^{-6} g/L at $20°C$), high volatility (vapor pressure of 0.180 Pa at $20°C$), and is extremely mobile, it is thought to be the most abundant form of mercury, representing 90–99% of the total mercury in the atmosphere. Galbreath et al. (2005) reported that the Hg^T concentration in coal combustion flue gas ranges from 5 to 50 $\mu g/m^3$, with variations in the concentrations of $Hg(0)$, Hg^{2+}, and Hg^P being dependent on combustion conditions, coal composition, and flue gas quench rate. Hg^T concentrations as high as 10 mg/m^3 have been reported (Laudal and French, 2000); however, this could be due to the use of low quality coal or an untreated stream. During combustion, mercury is liberated from coal as $Hg(0)$. However, as the flue gas cools, some of the $Hg(0)$ is oxidized, presumably to Hg(II) chloride ($HgCl_2$) (Presto and Granite, 2006) because of the large excess of chlorine present in some coal ores. Other compounds within the stream such as SO_2, NO_x, CO, O_2, oxidized calcium, chlorine, and fly ash particles are also known to significantly influence the transformation of mercury between its elemental, ionic, and particulate forms within various stages throughout a coal-fired combustion process. For instance, the concentration of Hg(0) is generally much higher than that of Hg^{2+}; however, when Cl_2, NO_x, and SO_2 concentrations increase within the stream, it has been shown that the percentage of Hg^{2+} typically increases proportionally (Duan et al., 2010). Similar findings from other studies have found that Hg reacts with Cl_2, HCl, NO_2, and O_2 but not with NH_3, N_2O, or H_2S, which indicates that Hg could be oxidized by a number of different routes (Hall et al., 1991, 1995), thus demonstrating the complex chemistry of Hg within coal-fired combustion processes. In addition, it has also been shown that 100 ppm of SO_2 in flue gas at 150°C can reduce the capture rate of mercury from 90% to 40%. This effect was largely reversed when this gas mixture also contained 100 ppm of HCl (Krivanek, 1996). It should be noted that gas desulfurization equipment, which is based on the same technology that is used to remove other pollutants such as NH_3, NO_x, and SO_2 via selective catalytic reactors (SCRs) and wet scrubbers, can be adapted to efficiently remove Hg^{2+} from coal-fire combustion streams. However, adsorption-based collection processes (typically carbon based) are still needed because of the higher quantities of Hg(0) in the flue gas, which is substantially harder to collect (Pudasainee et al., 2010).

3.1.1.2 Waste Incineration.
Waste incinerators (municipal, industrial, hazardous, medical, sewage sludge, etc.) and human crematoria are also recognized as major sources that emit Hg into the atmosphere. Similarly, combustion processes that use either natural gas or oil are also known sources of mercury emissions, however, to a far lower extent. In the case of municipal waste combustors (MWCs), the levels of mercury can be 10 to 100 times higher than those of coal-fired combustion processes. In addition, as the flue gases typically also have far higher chlorine content, ESP, FF, and FGD systems can be used more effectively (Senior et al., 2003).

Although incineration is a very efficient means of reducing municipal and hazardous waste, if not properly treated, emissions of particulate matter and other heavy metals besides Hg can have adverse effects on human health and the ecosystem (Yuan et al., 2005). In many countries, including China, incineration is increasingly replacing landfill as the preferred waste management strategy (Cheng and Hu, 2010a,b). As atmospheric Hg emissions from incinerators are highly dependent on the original mercury content of the waste being incinerated, it is possible to effectively limit or prevent Hg emissions by removing mercury-loaded waste from the source feed. In addition, emission regulations requiring incineration facilities to undergo air pollution control processes have been implemented. However, owing to the different national regulations and technology implementations, Hg emission standards vary unsurprisingly from 0.05 to 0.08 mg/m^3 for Europe and the United States to up to 0.2 mg/m^3 for China (Cheng and Hu, 2010b). Overall, medical waste incineration is reported to be the fourth largest contributor of Hg to the global environment (Zimmer and McKinley, 2008).

Recently, Kim et al. (2010) compiled a list of anthropogenic Hg emission sources in Korea for the year 2007. Although the list is limited to Korean emissions, it highlights the high contribution of anthropogenic Hg emissions due to incineration in comparison to coal-fired power stations and various other sources. It was estimated that 17% of Hg emissions came from various types of incineration compared to 26% being released from the coal-fired power plants (Kim et al., 2010). In general, emissions from incinerators have decreased because of the use of efficient Hg removal systems and the progressive decommissioning of high polluting facilities governed by better environmental management practices. Such practices were presumably spurred by the US-EPA ruling between 1995 and 1997 that all municipal and medical incinerators cut their emissions by 90% to 94% in the United States (Stokstad, 2004). Mercury reductions have been achieved by the implementation of direct injection of activated carbon or sodium sulfide, wet or dry scrubbing, and the use of activated carbon beds (Change and Offen, 1995). The effectiveness of these techniques is due to mercury being present primarily in the soluble Hg^{2+} form. In contrast, thermal power plant flue gas contains lower concentrations of total mercury; however, they have larger proportions of Hg(0) (nonsoluble) than Hg^{2+} species. In addition, thermal power plants have significantly larger volumes of stack gas than municipal or hazardous waste incineration plants.

3.1.1.3 Cement Manufacturing. In the case of cement manufacturing, Hg emissions emanate from the cement kiln exhaust gas, which is generated from a combination of the pyroprocessing of the raw materials and the fuel combustion process used to raise part of the kiln to temperatures of $\sim 1480°C$ (Jones et al., 2008). Hg emissions from the latter are the major contributing source for the cement manufacturing process. It is estimated that to produce each ton of clinker (cement), 3–6 GJ of fuel is required, depending on the raw materials and the process used. Primarily, cement is manufactured by heating mixtures of limestone, shale, clay, or sand with other materials in a long rotary kiln to produce a powdered mixture of calcium, silicon, alumina, ferric, and magnesium oxides, which is then suitable for mixing with water to form a hydrated solid. Most cement kilns consume large quantities of coal and petroleum coke as the primary fuel feed, and to a lesser extent natural gas, oil and/or alternative fuels, such as solid waste and tire-derived fuels (Jones et al., 2008; Mlakar et al., 2010). Mercury emission issues from cement plants arise mostly from those plants that burn hazardous waste in their cement kilns (Senior et al., 2003). Although the majority of cement plants do not use waste as their primary source of fuel, there is a large number of facilities that consider burning waste to be a viable alternative fuel and thus may choose to change their fuel feeds in the future. In addition, selected waste and by-products containing useful minerals such as calcium, silica, alumina, and iron can be used as raw materials in the kiln, replacing raw materials such as clay, shale, and limestone. For example, sewage sludge has a low but significant calorific value, though it burns to give ash-containing minerals useful in the clinker matrix. This sometimes leads to confusion when categorizing waste materials either as an alternative fuel or as raw materials. Both dry and wet process kilns can be designed to utilize waste fuel, which in effect can subsidize their running costs not by only reducing raw material needs but also by providing additional waste disposal service to other industries. Apart from raw material changes, other common methods for Hg reduction processes used by the cement industry are dust removal, wet scrubbing, mercury roasting systems, dry sorbent injection, and dry and semidry scrubbing. These processes have been covered in detail in Paone (2010).

The high temperature calcination process of the raw materials (limestone, clay minerals, and potentially waste by-products) can lead to the release of gas, dust, and fly ash that is rich in volatile heavy metals (i.e., thallium, cadmium, etc.) other than mercury. These elements are often found in trace quantities in minerals such as pyrite, galena, and zinc blends, and also need to be captured before the gas escaping through the kiln exhaust. In addition, owing to the inherent recycling of Hg between the hot and cold end of a kiln, and also from the reinjection of Hg-containing cement kiln dust into the kiln, it is difficult to quantitatively measure the distribution of Hg within a kiln (Senior et al., 2003). It has been shown that the process can comprise of many mercury cycles that are strongly dependent on the operating conditions and kiln processes used. In a recent study (Mlakar et al., 2010), it was not only found that the cycling process causes a significant enrichment of Hg inside the kiln but also observed that the efficiency of Hg removal was strongly related to the dust removal efficiency. This is one of the reasons that dust control devices such as ESPs and bag filters are used in many industries (Park et al., 2008), with bag filters being shown to be very efficient at removing all mercury species (Mlakar et al., 2010). However, in a dry kiln process, the cycling of Hg tends to occur at the point between the preheater and the exhaust exit, where it can condense and partially readsorb on the raw materials entering the kiln. In the case of a wet kiln process, the gases cool to $\sim 200°C$ or less at the kiln exhaust, where Hg can oxidize and/or recondense back on the raw materials only to be revaporized in the middle of the kiln after the solids dry and begin calcining. Therefore the recycling loop is potentially larger than what would occur in dry kiln process.

It can take a long time for mercury to reach a steady state within the kiln because of large temperature gradients and the actual recycling of Hg species, making it difficult to accurately mass balance the mercury entering the kiln and that being removed by APCDs. Attempts to model the Hg cycle within a cement kiln have been used to predict its distribution within the kiln, with the intent that the models might be used in conjunction with control technologies to minimize Hg emissions (Senior et al., 2003). A better understanding of the Hg cycle in individual parts of the process, especially in the coal mill, the preheater (cyclones), the cooling tower, and filters would also promote better design of Hg control technologies as well as increase production yields (Mlakar et al., 2010). Such improvements are especially encouraged by the National Emission Standards for Hazardous Air Pollutants (NESHAP) implemented by the US-EPA in 2010 to regulate Hg emissions from cement manufacturing industries (Laudal et al.,

2010; Tracy, 2010; Weise, 2010). The standard requires the installation of Hg emissions control technology on $\sim$163 kilns in 35 states, requiring each kiln to control its Hg emission concentration to <12 $\mu g/m^3$ for existing facilities and 4 $\mu g/m^3$ for new facilities (Renzoni et al., 2010). These rules are estimated by the US-EPA to cost the industry up to \$950 million annually in 2013, with an estimated 10% of the plants in the United States being shut down as they will not be able to meet the Hg control costs to comply with the regulations (Tracy, 2010; Weise, 2010).

3.1.1.4 Mining and Refining Processes. The process of mining and refining minerals, metals, and fossil fuels contributes significantly to anthropogenic Hg emissions into both the atmosphere and the localized surrounding environment. The production of zinc, copper, lead, iron, alumina, gold, silver, and mercury are the major causes. Although there are uncertainties between the emission data provided by different countries, it is estimated that China followed by Australia are the largest emitters of Hg from industrial ore processing activities. Other regions of interest are South America and Africa. In 2003, China's emissions from zinc, copper, and lead smelters alone were estimated to be between 203 and 275 Mg (Wu et al., 2006; Feng et al., 2009), which is equivalent to $\sim$39% of China's total emission for that year. Typically, processes that require ore roasting can release significant Hg emissions. Such processes are used for the extraction of Hg from cinnabar ore or other sulfide-containing minerals, such as corderoite and livingstonite. The Hg is extracted by heating the ore and condensing the vapor to liquid mercury, which is then sold for use in other industrial processes or products. Roughly half of all Hg mined globally in history has been used to mine gold and silver, although the annual production of Hg peaked during the twentieth century as a result of increased industrial use (Hylander and Meili, 2003). Interestingly, the increase in demand for compact fluorescent bulbs has encouraged the reopening of some old cinnabar mines to obtain the Hg required for compact fluorescent bulb manufacture in China. Unfortunately, such sites, as well as other abandoned Hg mine processing sites, often contain hazardous waste piles of roasted cinnabar calcines, which are recognized sources of ecological damage.

Ore roasting, which is generally the first step in refining iron, zinc, or lead, is another significant process that can result in Hg emissions into the atmosphere. The purpose of the roasting process at high temperatures ($>1000°C$) is to remove moisture and volatile impurities such as Hg from the ore before the roasted ore is coke-fired (smelted) and refined by one of a number of electrolysis techniques. In the case of iron and steel manufacturing, the ore is generally roasted before being chemically reduced in blast furnaces to form pig iron. The addition of coal to the blast furnace during the coking process also contributes to Hg emissions, where the mercury from the coal mixes with the additional Hg impurities in the ore. Mercury emission inventories indicate that a significant quantity of mercury (45.4 Mg) was emitted globally in 2005 by pig iron and steel production (UNEP, 2008b). Zinc and lead refining make up an even more significant portion of the emissions resulting from nonferrous metal smelting activities worldwide. In China alone, 115–187.6 and 70.7 Mg out of the total 320 Mg for nonferrous metal smelting activities were emitted for zinc- and lead-refining activities, respectively, in 2003 (Wu et al., 2006). In fact, over 100 mg/m^3 of Hg has been estimated to escape in the flue gas generated from smelting processes owing to sulfide-rich ores that can contain between 100 and 300 mg of Hg for every kilogram of ore (Li et al., 2010). This clearly indicates that the environment surrounding a zinc plant would contain significantly higher levels of Hg deposits when compared to a large thermal power plant. Emissions for ore-roasting copper pyrites to extract copper are also known to release significant quantities of Hg; however, these quantities are much lower when compared to emissions from zinc- and lead-refining processes. Reductions in emissions from copper processes are also partly due to advances in smelter technologies that now limit ore-roasting requirements.

In the context of alumina refineries, trace quantities of Hg have been found in emissions from various sources, in particular oxalate kilns, digestion, calciners, and other minor sources such as liquor burners and boilers. Depending on the origin of the bauxite ore, the mercury content can range between 50 mg/t (Alcoa World Alumina Australia, 2005) and 431 mg/t (Kockman et al., 2005) of bauxite. During the refinery process, much effort is made to capture the Hg before it is emitted into the environment; however, measurable quantities of Hg are still emitted for every metric ton of alumina produced (Dobbs et al., 2005). Often these emissions can be controlled or significantly reduced by using effective gaskets and seals to contain mercury within the process stream; however, Hg buildup within a chemical refining process can occur, which is not dissimilar to the Hg cycling issues that occur within a larger cement kiln process. For instance, during the extraction process of alumina from bauxite (via the Bayer process), the concentration of Hg(0) in the vapor phase reaches a steady state, typically ranging from below 0.1 to 32 mg/m^3 within different stages of the process (Dobbs et al., 2005).This is largely due to the cyclic nature of the Bayer process, which recycles a highly caustic liquor stream through a variety of processes ranging from digestion, evaporation, and calcination that operate at a range of different temperatures between 20°C and 200°C. In contrast to industries such as coal-fired utilities and municipal waste incinerators, which emit all three forms of Hg (i.e., Hg(0), Hg^{2+}, and Hg^P), data collected from the Bayer process shows that Hg emissions are predominantly in the elemental form (Dobbs et al., 2005). Approximately 2.9 Mg of Hg(0) is estimated to have been emitted by Australian alumina refineries in a one-year period spanning 2006–2007. Although these emissions are less significant than those emitted by the zinc- or lead-refining processes, a large alumina refinery would emit higher quantities of mercury into the atmosphere than a comparable stream (flow rate) from a coal-fired power plant.

Emission concerns from both small- and large-scale gold mining operations are also categorized as significant industrial emitters. In the case of small-scale mining operations, gold is extracted using mercury to amalgamate with very small gold particles in the ore, thus separating the gold from the ore. Thereafter, the amalgamated particles are heated to boil off the mercury. This process is very effective in extracting the gold; however, it is hazardous because of the toxicity of Hg vapor that must be reclaimed in an effective and safe manner. Many illegal mining operations dispose of the mercury improperly or allow significant quantities to escape. Unfortunately, owing to its illegal nature, precise data on Hg emissions from small-scale operations employing amalgamation technology are subject to large uncertainties (Wu et al., 2006). In regard to large-scale gold mining operations, amalgamation technology has been gradually phased out. However, it is estimated that artisanal and small-scale gold mining releases between 640 and 1350 Mg of mercury per annum into the environment (rivers, lakes, soil, etc.), with an estimated 300–400 Mg contributing to atmospheric emissions (Telmer and Veiga, 2009). Gold mining conducted in the Amazon region has been reported to contribute to 10% of Brazil's annual Hg emission total (UNEP, 2008b), which mainly results from small-scale gold mining processes (Veiga et al., 2006).

Mining and extraction of fossil fuels such as natural gas, oil, and coal are other major sources from which significant Hg emissions can occur. As one would assume, Hg is only one of a number of harmful substances that are present in small concentrations in these reserves. The natural occurrence of As, Cd, Cr, F, Pb, Se, and Hg within coal leads to their emission into the atmosphere when unwanted solid waste piles undergo spontaneous combustion during the coal mining process. Spontaneous combustion of such piles may be a source of serious environmental pollution in countries such as China, which are credited as the largest coal producer in the world (Zhao et al., 2008). Similarly, in the process of extracting natural gas, the removal of many naturally occurring contaminants such as mercury, CO_2, H_2S, NH_3, thiols, and other sulfide-containing compounds is required. The refining process not only reduces emissions by the end-user but also increases the production and transportation efficiencies of the natural gas. However, the removal of Hg at the extraction/refining site can lead to pollution of the localized surrounding environment; thus, Hg emission control technologies are used by most large facilities. A study conducted in Croatia found that very high Hg concentrations between 0.2 and 2.5 mg/m^3 were measured in extracted natural gas (Spiric and Mashyanov, 2000), which led to the Hg contamination of the soils around gas processing equipment with Hg concentrations of 0.32–40 mg/kg. In the same study, the authors reported that atmospheric testing 54 km away from the processing plant detected an average Hg concentration of 6 ng/m^3. Anomalies of up to 90 ng/m^3 were observed during these measurements, indicating that bursts of Hg vapor also travel vast distances away from the plants. The levels of Hg in the atmosphere were shown to increase with decreasing distance from the process plant, where levels of 120 ng/m^3 were detected at a distance of 6.8 km (Spiric and Mashyanov, 2000).

3.1.1.5 Chemical Manufacture and Other Industrial Processes. The manufacture of chemicals such as chlorine and sodium hydroxide (caustic soda), which utilize mercury within their processes, have historically been the largest Hg emitters from the chemical manufacturing sector. In a chlor-alkali plant using

mercury cell technology, elemental liquid mercury is used to form a cathode electrode in an electrolysis process to produce chlorine and sodium hydroxide from sodium chloride brine. A mercury cell consists of two major parts: an electrolyzer and a decomposer. In the electrolyzer section, sodium chloride is passed along the mercury cathode where the sodium forms an amalgam with the mercury, thus releasing the chloride ions as chlorine gas. In the decomposer, the amalgam is used to produce hydrogen (H_2) gas and sodium hydroxide (NaOH), thus converting the amalgam back into Hg(0) so that the process can be repeated. The process is essentially enclosed and recycles the Hg that is used to amalgamate and provide a transportation mechanism for sodium ions within the mercury cell; however, unintentional losses are unavoidable. Although much of the industry has moved over to mercury-free processes that use mercury-free ion-exchange membranes or diaphragm cell technologies (Bommaraju et al., 2007), it is estimated that $\sim$100 mercury cell plants still operate worldwide, with mercury cell plants accounting for 43% of the capacity in Europe in 2006. Other significant producers of chlorine and caustic soda that use Hg within their processes are based in India and the Middle East (Mukherjee et al., 2009). Interestingly, a study conducted on human exposure to Hg in the vicinity of an Italian chlor-alkali plant concluded that the plant operation posed no health effects above the product of anthropogenic and natural sources of Hg present in the Mediterranean, thereby indicating that the mercury cell chlor-alkali plant itself did not pose an additional risk to human health (Gibicar et al., 2009). However, the authors estimate that 14% of emitted gaseous Hg is deposited within 5 km from its source, with the remaining 86% being dispersed and transported further away where it is supposedly added to the natural atmospheric Hg cycle.

Similarly, it is well known that forest fires are an important pathway for mercury that has previously deposited on soil and vegetation to exchange between the biosphere and atmosphere (Sigler et al., 2003). A study of a mixed vegetation fire in the southern Cape Peninsula in Africa suggests that biomass burning accounts for 12–28% of annual global total gaseous Hg emissions (Brunke et al., 2001b; Sigler et al., 2003). Comparable findings have also been expressed in the United States, where it is estimated that fires emit the equivalent of almost 30% of the total US anthropogenic Hg emissions, which is equivalent to the emissions from coal-fired power plants (Wiedinmyer and Friedli, 2007). Emissions from landfill sites are also known to contribute to atmospheric Hg emissions; however, a lack of data exists for this source. It has been speculated that the entire waste mass of a landfill site can act as a significant Hg emission source and that much of the Hg present is in the elemental form, which is primarily from broken light bulbs and contaminated plumbing (Earle et al., 1999; Kim et al., 2001; Lindberg et al., 2001, 2005; Southworth et al., 2005; de la Rosa et al., 2006).

Although the use of mercury has decreased significantly in the last decade, mercury is still an important material that is used in the manufacturing of products for both commercial and residential use. For example, batteries and fluorescent lamps contribute significantly toward Hg emissions when discarded at the end of their usable lifetime. A survey conducted by Chang et al. (2007) to investigate the fate and management of mercury-containing fluorescent, ultraviolet, and high pressure mercury lamps in Taiwan showed that 886 kg of Hg was used in the year 2004 for these applications. Fortunately, a reduction in the use of mercury with time is partly because of the use of alternative materials used in products that traditionally use mercury in their manufacture (Johnson, 2001). In the case of alkaline batteries, environmental regulations restricting the use of mercury as a corrosion inhibitor for the zinc cathode has significantly reduced Hg emission issues from discarded batteries. Such regulations were passed in the United States and Europe in the 1990s and have also made the recycling of the batteries (which now employ plastic insulators) easier, apart from giving the newer batteries more than twice the capacity of the same size Hg-containing batteries (Powers, 1995). Similarly, the use of alcohols in thermometers and mercury substitutes in other industrial and consumer items has also lead to a reduction of Hg emissions into the environment. However, these reductions have been counterbalanced by the increased demand for fluorescent lamps and PVC, which has resulted in an increase in mercury utilization in China because of import restrictions (Zhang and Wong, 2007; Feng et al., 2009; Li et al., 2009). Other industrial emission sources of mercury and its compounds are glass manufacturing, the wood paper-pulp industry, and the chemical manufacture of chemicals such as acetaldehyde (Dobbs et al., 2005); however, such sources generally result in the release of mercury in its ionic form via aqueous emissions.

3.2   STANDARDIZED METHODS FOR MEASURING MERCURY

Several standardized methods exist for measuring mercury from industrial emission sources or process streams. The first step involves collecting a representative sample of the flue gas either by a sampling train or by a dry sorbent trap technique. Once a representative sample is collected, quantification analyzes of the sample train or sorbent bed/s are performed via a spectroscopic technique, which can be based on either photometry, fluorescence, or mass spectroscopy (Granite, 2003; Abollino et al., 2008). These can include atomic absorption spectroscopy (AAS), atomic fluorescence spectrometry (AFS), UV differential optical absorption spectroscopy (DOAS), inductively coupled plasma atomic emission spectrometry (ICP-AES), and inductively coupled plasma mass spectrometry (ICP-MS) techniques (Clevenger et al., 1997). However, AAS- and AFS-based methods are generally preferred as both have been approved by the US-EPA to perform measurements from industrial point sources (Sánchez Uría and Sanz-Medel, 1998; Blanco et al., 2000; Das et al., 2001; Logar et al., 2002). Although AFS has superior sensitivity and detection limits to AAS, because of the requirements of most industrial applications and the quenching of the fluorescence signal by nitrogen and oxygen being more frequent in the AFS systems, AAS-based systems are more common (Temmerman et al., 1990).

Both AAS and AFS instruments are susceptible to cross-interference by other gases within the many industrial process streams, such as SO_2, NO_2, H_2O, O_3, and carbonyl-containing volatile organic compounds (VOCs) such as benzene, toluene, and acetone. These gas species absorb the same wavelength as mercury (253.7 nm) and can therefore produce misleading results (Weissberg, 1971; Windham, 1972; Logar et al., 2002; Sholupov et al., 2004). In order to overcome the presence of such gases, gold traps or cold vapor (CV) methods are sometimes used in conjunction with the AAS and AFS systems (referred to as *CV AAS* or *CV-AFS*) to determine lower concentrations of Hg. Gold traps involve having a collection material (i.e., gold-coated sand and quartz wool, gold or silver foil, iodized carbon, or other activated carbon) to trap and enrich the Hg before the detection step (Schroeder et al., 1985; Clevenger et al., 1997) and allows direct determination of Hg without an atomizer unit (Clevenger et al., 1997). Mercury vapor is amalgamated with the sorbent material and later released via heating in an argon carrier gas for detection. This allows the ventilation of interfering substances from the gas stream before measurement.

Overall, both the sample train and dry sorbent methods have been shown to provide accurate data when used by experienced operators following strict protocols to collect the flue gas sample. However, the difficulty in measuring mercury arises from issues such as low Hg concentrations, simultaneous existence of speciated forms of Hg (i.e., Hg(0), Hg^{2+}, and Hg^P), complex flue gas chemistry, high temperatures, particulate loading, and mercury reactivity (i.e., interconversion between Hg(0) and Hg^{2+}) within the flue gas samples. Owing to these complexities, a number of standard sampling and measurement protocols have been developed that utilize either sampling train or dry sorbent traps to capture the mercury content for different industrial stream conditions (Holmes and Pavlish, 2004).

3.2.1   Sampling Train Methods

Several sampling train methods exist that are normally used to capture Hg vapor from stationary anthropogenic sources. All the sample train methods described below use isokinetic sampling, with particulate filters attached to the sample nozzle to pass the sample gas through a train of glass impingers containing various chemical agents to collect the mercury. The particulate filters are used to collect the fly ash and Hg^P content in the stream before the sample train, which can be analyzed separately. Each of the methods has its own advantages and limitations depending on conditions such as the flue gas matrix and whether total or speciated mercury needs to be measured in the collected gas sample. Generally, the purpose of the various liquids used in the sample train impingers is to separate and preconcentrate the different species of mercury from the filtered gas sample. The first method that was introduced by the US-EPA for capturing Hg from stationary sources in response to the addition of mercury to the 1990 CAAAs was EPA method 29 (Holmes and Pavlish, 2004).

3.2.1.1   EPA Method 29. EPA method 29 (also known as the multimetals sampling train method) was first introduced as a draft method in 1992 for the determination of metals and/or particulate emissions from stationary sources. It was originally designed to monitor the emission of metals such as Sb, As, Ba, Be, Cd, Cr, Co, Cu, Pb, Mn, Ni, P, Se, Ag, Tl, and Zn; however, its use for Hg speciation analysis was also investigated owing to researchers presuming the physical and chemical properties of Hg (Laudal et al., 2005; Wocken et al., 2006). As a result, the metals Hg, Cd, and Pb were also added in the 1994 proposal before its being approved by the EPA (Holmes and Pavlish, 2004). By 1996, a review of the available mercury measurement methods indicated that the EPA method 29 is the most widely used method for determining Hg in flue gas (Galbreath and Zygarlicke, 1996).

The method comprises seven impingers, the first of which is left empty. The second and third impingers are identical, containing 10% hydrogen peroxide (H_2O_2) and 5% nitric acid (HNO_3) in 100 mL of water. These are followed by another empty impinger and then two identical impingers containing 4% potassium permanganate ($KMNO_4$) and 10% sulfuric acid (H_2SO_4) in water. The final impinger contains silica gel to collect moisture from the sampled gas in order to prevent damage to the dry-gas meter and pump downstream. The stack gas is withdrawn isokinetically and enters the probe/nozzle through a heated filter to collect the particulates, which are used to determine the Hg^P content. In addition, the purpose of the probe is to remove reactive particles that can either oxidize Hg(0) or reduce Hg^{2+} and bias the results. The acidic H_2O_2 solutions are used to capture any Hg^{2+}, while the $KMNO_4$ containing impingers capture Hg(0). For each measurement, the sampling is performed for a continuous 2- to 3-h period in order to obtain a representative sample, as well as to ensure that a detectable concentration of Hg is captured within the solutions. At the end of the capture process, the filters, impingers, and lines are rinsed and all the solutions are sent for analysis. Typically, the Hg content is analyzed using CV-AAS.

Using the same principles as EPA method 29, a comparable European standard (EN 14385, which is also a multielement method) was adapted to measure Hg from stationary emission sources using a side stream sampling technique (EN 13211). Similarly, another European standard for mercury monitoring in industrial gases is the VDI 3868 method (Waltisberg, 2004; Renzoni et al., 2010). However, Laudal et al. (1997) published their research findings concerning the speciation ability of EPA method 29, which were conducted at the North Dakota Energy & Environmental Center (EERC) and were supported by Electric Power Research Institute (EPRI) and the US Department of Energy (DOE). It was found that the EPA method 29 was not able to detect speciated mercury properly in coal combustion flue gas. This shortcoming of the method was due to Hg(0) being captured with Hg^{2+} in the H_2O_2-containing impingers, which resulted in a bias or measurement error.

Ontario Hydro Method. While the Hg speciation issues faced in the EPA method 29 were being investigated, the Ontario Hydro (OH) method was developed in 1994 by Ontario Hydro Technologies (Landis, 1999). Subsequently, in 2005, the US-EPA identified the OH method (also known as the ASTM D6784-02 standard) as the means to measure Hg(0), Hg^{2+}, Hg^P, and Hg^T from coal-fired stationary sources (Laudal et al., 2005; Sarunac, 2007). The method is a modification of EPA method 29 with the only difference being the number and content of the impingers (US-EPA, 1996). In the 8-impinger OH method, the first acidified peroxide solution of EPA method 29 is replaced by three impingers of 1-M potassium chloride (KCl) dissolved in deionized water for a more selective capture of Hg^{2+}. The purpose of these impingers is to eliminate some of the complications that occur during the preparation of the peroxide solution for analysis and to avoid the interference of SO_2 that was shown to exist in the bench-scale studies of EPA method 29 (Laudal et al., 1997). The fourth impinger contains 10% H_2O_2 and 5% HNO_3 solution, while the following three impingers contain 4% $KMNO_4$ and 10% H_2SO_4. The H_2O_2 impinger was specifically added for flue gas containing SO_2, which if not captured in the trap would otherwise react with the $KMNO_4$ and neutralize it, affecting the capture efficiency of Hg(0) and resulting in a measurement error. The final impinger contains silica gel to remove moisture from the sampled gas before the pump and dry-gas meter.

The OH method is able to measure speciated Hg while minimizing the possible interference by SO_2 from the flue gas in CV-AAS measurements (Jun Lee et al., 2004). However, pilot-scale testing undertaken by EERC verified early test results by other researchers showing that mercury is actually lost from some of the solutions in the first three KCl traps. To counter this, acidified permanganate, dichromate, or acidified peroxide solution needs to be added to the KCl solution immediately following sampling. Furthermore, Cl_2 and different ratios of NO/NO_2 (in the presence of fly ash) have also been shown to have a significant effect on Hg speciation as measured by the OH method. This is because Cl_2 reacts with Hg to form $HgCl_2$, while the fly ash can catalyze Hg(0) to Hg^{2+} in the presence of NO/NO_2 (Laudal et al., 2000). In addition, the study showed that HCl appeared to have little influence on Hg speciation at concentrations and temperatures typically found at the outlet of ESPs and baghouses of a coal-fired process stream. This method has also been compared with the European standard reference method for determining Hg in exhaust gases from ducts or chimneys. The average bias between EN 13211 and the OH method was 2.9%, indicating that the bias between the two methods is not statistically significant (Sarunac et al., 2007).

Tris-Buffer Method.   The tris-buffer sampling train method, developed by Radian International (now URS), is another modification of the EPA method 29 designed to measure speciated Hg in industrial flue gas. For this method, the contents of the nitric acid/peroxide impingers in EPA method 29 are replaced with a 1-M tris(hydroxymethyl) aminomethane buffer solution. Ethylene di(tetraamine) or EDTA is added to the tris-buffer solution as a complexing agent to retain $HgCl_2$ (Holmes and Pavlish, 2004). The purpose of the buffer is to remove the SO_2 and Hg^{2+} without removing Hg(0) (US-EPA, 1996); however, a negative aspect of this method is that the solution must be at a pH of 6 or above for it to be effective (Holmes and Pavlish, 2004). Bench-scale experiments conducted at

EERC (Laudal et al., 1997) have shown that sampling and measuring speciated mercury at a baghouse inlet using different Hg sampling methods showed similar results for the tris-buffer and OH methods. Interestingly, it was found that more than 30% of the spiked Hg(0) was measured as Hg^{2+} in the EPA method 29, while nearly 100% was measured using both the OH and tris-buffer methods. Further, bench-scale testing of the different types of coal showed that the difference in speciation between the different sample train methods was affected by the particulate and total Hg concentrations in the flue gas generated by firing different types of coals. Furthermore, mercury recovery from the tris solution has proved to be difficult, as the addition of HNO_3 and H_2O_2 to preserve the mercury in solution results in the evolution of CO_2 and therefore requires great care to be exercised in order to prevent the loss of Hg-containing tris solution. On the basis of the pilot- and bench-scale tests conducted at the EERC, the OH method was shown to better speciate Hg over the tris-buffer method and the EPA method 29 (Laudal et al., 2000).

3.2.1.2   EPA Method 101.

The EPA method 101 was developed for the determination of particulate and gaseous Hg emissions from sources such as chloralkali plants, where the gas sample is mostly comprised of air. Isokinetic sampling is performed to collect the Hg emissions in 0.1-M acidic iodine monochloride (ICl) solution in the first three identical impingers of this 4-impinger method. The final impinger contains 200 g of silica gel and removes moisture from the gas sample. Interference during sample collection is known to occur for gases containing sulfur dioxide (SO_2), which reduces the ICl and prematurely depletes the solution. Following sampling, the ICl needs to be completely removed as concentrations $> 10^{-4}$ M will inhibit the reduction of the Hg (II) ion in the aeration cell of the analytical instrument. This is an extra pretreatment step but necessary to accurately perform the final Hg measurement step.

3.2.1.3   EPA Method 101A.

EPA method 101A is designed for the determination of total gaseous and particulate Hg in the flue gas emissions from sewage sludge incinerators. The method only measures Hg^T but it can be of special interest to sources that need to measure both Hg and Mn emissions. Mercury emissions are withdrawn isokinetically from the source and are collected in the first three identical impingers containing 4% $KMnO_4$ and 10% H_2SO_4 in water. These impingers are designated for Hg(0) capture, whereas the first oxidizing impinger in the OH method is the fourth impinger in this method. The Hg collected (in its mercuric form) is reduced to Hg(0). Thereafter, the solutions are aerated into an optical cell and measured by AAS. In this method, interferences can occur for an industrial gas stream containing excessive oxidizable organic matter, which prematurely depletes the $KMnO_4$ solution and thereby prevents further collection of Hg. Unlike the OH method, interference from SO_2 is possible in this method when analyzing the impinger solutions with AAS (Hedrick et al., 2001; Jun Lee et al., 2004).

3.2.2 Dry Sorbent Methods

Generally speaking, solid sorbent materials are more suitable for flue gas sampling than sample train methods because of their greater stability and ease of handling. For this reason, various solid sorbent methods have also been developed for Hg vapor determination in industrial flue gases over the last two decades (Metzger and Braun, 1987).

3.2.2.1 Certification Procedures. There are two main solid sorbent-based reference methods recognized by the US-EPA that are designed to certify if another method is working properly (Laudal, 2008). These are the Appendix K method and the EPA method 30B.

Appendix K Method. The Code of Federal Regulations (CFR), Title 40, Part 75, Appendix K is a quality assurance and operating procedure that must be met in order for the US-EPA to consider a sorbent type valid for the measurement of mercury from a stack gas. The method encompasses sorbents that are based on iodated charcoal or other suitable reagents and generally refers to a performance-based sorbent trap method; however, Appendix K is not an actual method in itself. Appendix K requires that the flue gas be drawn *in situ* through a pair of traps, each containing a series of three sorbent trap sections. Each section of each sorbent trap is then sent for analysis following a sampling period of approximately three to seven days. In order for any method to be valid, the relative deviation between the two traps must result in $\leq 10\%$ for a Hg concentration of ≥ 1 μg. Furthermore, the first section of a trap must capture the majority of the captured mercury, limiting the second section to contain no more than 5% of the Hg^T being reported. The traps are analyzed either by wet chemistry or thermal desorption/combustion methods that employ absorption or fluorescence spectroscopic analysis, respectively. This method has been reported to suffer from issues with sampling, recovery, and analytical procedures related to both the sampling time and acid gas (e.g., SO_x, NO_x, and HCl) concentrations contained in some flue gases (Jones et al., 2008).

EPA Method 30B. EPA method 30B is a reference method for measuring Hg^T emissions from coal-fired combustion sources using a solid carbon-based sorbent trap that employs sampling and extractive or thermal analytical techniques. This method is only intended for use under relatively low particulate conditions (e.g., sampling after all APCDs). The method is designed to measure Hg^T concentrations in flue gas and is not designed to measure speciated Hg. EPA method 30B differs from Appendix K in that it is a two-section rather than three-section trap and that the sampling time is limited to only 2 h or less. Results from previous studies have shown that the EPA method 30B can produce results similar to the OH method with relative accuracy $\leq 20\%$ (Jones et al., 2008; Cheng et al., 2009).

3.2.2.2   MESA Method. The mercury speciation adsorption (MESA) sampling method employs a series of heated ($90-100°C$) solid phase adsorbent traps to selectively capture and separate mercury species (Prestbo and Bloom, 1995). Flue gas is first withdrawn through heated quartz tubing containing quartz wool to remove particulate matter. Immediately following the quartz wool is the first sorbent containing a mixture of potassium hydroxide, calcium oxide, and potassium chloride, which is designed to capture $HgCl_2$ and methyl mercury (Hg^{2+}). The second sorbent is iodine-impregnated activated carbon, which collects $Hg(0)$. Total Hg is determined by summation of the different species. In the laboratory, CV-AFS is used to measure the collected Hg from the solid sorbents following appropriate sample digestion and preparation processes (Prestbo and Bloom, 1995). The MESA method has been previously evaluated for species stability, matrix effects, breakthrough, artifacts, and precision in coal combustion flue gas at the inlet of pollution control devices. Comparison of the MESA method with other methods (such as EPA method 29 and EPA method 101A) has shown MESA to be precise and in agreement in determining $Hg(0)$, Hg^{2+}, and Hg^T. In addition, the MESA method is capable of mercury speciation for flue gas streams containing Cl_2, which is not always possible with the OH method (Laudal et al., 1996). Compared to EPA method 29, MESA is reported to have a lower detection limit, a much simplified sample collection process and requires less sampling time. However, research conducted at EERC showed that the MESA method did not measure speciated mercury correctly when used in flue gas containing ~600 ppm NO_x and 1500 ppm SO_2 (Laudal et al., 1997). The major limitation of the MESA method is the nonquantitative collection of particulate material (Hg^P). These gas constituents were found to induce an overestimation of Hg^{2+} fraction when using the MESA method and EPA method 29; however, this was not the case with the OH and tris-buffer methods.

3.2.2.3   MIT Method. The MIT method was developed by the Massachusetts Institute of Technology (MIT) for the collection of atmospheric vapor phase Hg using activated charcoal sorbents. Sampling is conducted by passing the flue gas through two activated charcoal-based sorbents connected in series and then analyzing the traps using instrumental neutron activation analysis (INAA) to determine the total Hg collected (Ames, 1995). The sorbent traps are maintained at $100-120°C$ to prevent moisture condensation. The method is used to conduct Hg^T measurements and therefore is of little use for applications of flue gas in coal-fired and cement-type plants where Hg speciation and measurement are necessary as part of the US-EPA regulations. Previous studies that compared the MIT method with EPA method 29, 101A, MESA, and hazardous element sampling train (HEST) (discussed below) showed a reasonably good agreement among the Hg^T measurements for the different methods (Nott, 1995), indicating that the MIT method can be used to confirm Hg^T measurements.

3.2.2.4   HEST Method. The hazardous element sampling train (HEST) method was developed by Chester Environmental and uses an in-stack filter probe to draw gas samples isokinetically through a pack of three filters arranged in series (Cooper, 1994; Nott, 1995). The first filter is made of quartz or Teflon and is used for particulate collection. The second and third filters are carbon-impregnated filters designed to adsorb gas phase Hg(0). Following the sample collection, the filters are analyzed by nondestructive energy dispersive X ray fluorescence (XRF) and result in the determination of total Hg in the gas sample. This method was tested in an industrial coal combustion site along with the EPA method 29 and the dry sorbent MESA method. The correlation between the three methods was found to be excellent, despite the Hg^T concentration within the industrial stream fluctuating by an order of magnitude over the three-day sampling period (Cooper, 1994). The HEST method is able to differentiate between the different speciated forms of Hg and can be used by most Hg-emitting industries where speciation is required, with sampling intervals as short as 10 min. It is claimed that this method can measure Hg and all other elemental hazardous air pollutants (HAPs) in the US-EPA's HAPs list (except beryllium) with a detection limit that is an order of magnitude better than that of the EPA method 29. A comparison of the HEST method and the EPA method 101A at a municipal incinerator showed agreement between the averages (within 4%), proving the method effective in characterizing elemental HAPs emissions (Cooper, 1994).

3.2.2.5 FAMS Method. The flue gas absorption mercury speciation (FAMS) method is based on different solid sorbents that are selective toward the different species of Hg and is therefore able to separate and quantify Hg(0), Hg^{2+}, and Hg^P from emissions in flue gas streams. A 100-mL volume of the flue gas is drawn through the heated ($95 \pm 5°C$) FAMS sorbent train for sampling. The traps are then leak-tested before removing from the sampling train, capping, and shipping to an analytical laboratory. The method requires no exposed glassware, on-site solution preparation, rinses, clogging filters, or hazardous materials. Testing is normally completed within a few days with minimal disruption of plant operations. The US-EPA conducted several comparison tests of the FAMS method with the OH method at the EERC in 2001. It was concluded that the FAMS method was valid for the determination of Hg^T, Hg^P, Hg^{2+}, and Hg(0) concentrations in flue gas matrices and was equivalent to the OH method. Frontier Geosciences (now Frontier Global Sciences), the developer of FAMS as well as Appendix K and EPA method 30B, has compared FAMS with the OH method using over eight years of data collected from emissions in flue gas, where they concluded that the FAMS method is a faster, more reliable, and cost-effective alternative. Others also report the method to be highly precise (repeatable results), sensitive (for low Hg concentrations), and accurate, making it a viable method for measuring speciated Hg in industrial flue gas.

3.2.2.6 FMSS Method. The flue gas mercury sorbent speciation (FMSS) method consists of two lots of dual dry sorbent traps placed in series, which are used to speciate Hg from the flue gas stream. The method relies on a semi-isokinetic sample from a flue gas duct through a particulate filter and a heated solid sorbent sample train. The filter and the sorbent train are analyzed to determine the different species of Hg. The first trap contains dry KCl-coated quartz chips used to capture Hg^{2+} followed by the second trap containing tri-iodine-impregnated activated carbon to capture elemental Hg from the flue gas stream. The entire sample train is sent to a laboratory for analysis using CV-AFS following a vigorous chemical treatment process. The analysis of Hg^P in the fly ash is done by thermal desorption at 800°C using CV-AFS. This method was developed by Frontier Geosciences and validated at the EERC according to a modified EPA method 301 (Wocken et al., 2006). The FMSS showed good agreement with the OH method and its accuracy was better than ±20% for all species for the range of conditions in the validation study tests (Wocken et al., 2006). It is one of the two solid sorbent methods validated by the US-EPA; the second method is the quicksilver emissions monitor (QSEM) method, which does not measure speciated Hg and is used only to determine Hg^T (Laudal et al., 2005).

3.2.2.7 QSEM Method. Following many years of research since 1990 and the development of solid sorbent trap methods for capturing mercury, Frontier Geosciences together with ADA Environmental Solutions and the EPRI developed the QSEM method, otherwise known as the draft EPA method 324 (Laudal et al., 2005). After undergoing various validation tests, the US-EPA published the dry sorbent trap sampling method as draft method 324 in 2004 and the method is now in extensive use for Hg measurements in low dust coal-fired plants and other stationary source applications (Glesmann et al., 2004). QSEM is a nonisokinetic test method that samples flue gas while minimizing particulate capture, and provides Hg^T emission measurements. The sampling and trap analysis methods are similar to the FMSS method except that the solid sorbents used are specially treated forms of activated carbon. The method can be used over periods of time ranging from 30 min to several days with detection limits of an order of magnitude lower than the OH method. The method is relatively simple, can be used for long-term Hg emissions evaluation under various process conditions with minimal effort, and can be conducted in a self-sustained (unmanned) mode with periodic changeover of the sample traps (Glesmann et al., 2004).

3.2.3 Limitations

It is apparent from the existence of well-established analytical instruments that measurement of Hg is not the main issue; the main challenge lies in sampling for speciated Hg from a complex flue gas without manipulating the gas matrix before measurement (IDS-Environment, 2011). In fact, the precision of the method used to sample the different species of Hg is influenced by flue gas concentration and source type as well as procedural and equipment variables. Strict adherence to the chosen method/procedures is therefore necessary to reduce these effects. Several sampling train methods, such as EPA methods 29 and 101A and the tris-buffer and OH methods mentioned above, are approved by the US-EPA; however, results from the OH method (for example) can take several days to turn around if off-site analytic analysis is used. Many of the dry sorbents that use adsorption, amalgamation, diffusion, and/or ion-exchange processes to capture Hg must be transported to a laboratory for preconditioning before analysis is undertaken. As these methods are designed to be used after APCD and particulate control devices, the use of these methods with a filter in a high-dust situation such as the inlet to the ESP or baghouse can bias speciated Hg concentrations. This is particularly true when reactive particulate matter is present, which is known to bias Hg^{2+} and/or Hg^P concentrations (Holmes and Pavlish, 2004). In trying to overcome these limitations, the methods can potentially have the drawbacks of increased expense, lack of real- or long-term data or emission variation data, a requirement for complex sample trains with hazardous chemicals or sorbent processes, and are manual and difficult to apply in practice over the long term (Laudal et al., 1997, 2004; Nelson, 2007). These limitations make the sorbent methods inadequate for use in Hg emissions control loop feedback systems (Holmes and Pavlish, 2004). Hence, there is a need for rapid, on-line continuous emission monitors that are capable of accurately speciating Hg in a variety of different types of industrial flue gas stream environments. Such a system, which would benefit both legislators and plant operators alike, would allow plant operators to make informed decisions concerning their control technology requirements and provide them with feedback for advanced process control technologies (Apogee Scientific, 2010).

3.3   MERCURY CONTINUOUS EMISSION MONITORS (CEMs)

Although the methods described in Section 3.2 are capable of determining total and speciated mercury concentrations in industrial streams, real-time data collection can only be obtained using portable emission analyzers or continuous emission monitoring (CEM) systems. Environmental bodies in the United States, Canada, Europe, and others are working toward the development of regulations requiring industries such as cement, waste incineration, and coal-fired power utilities to monitor their Hg emissions on a continuous basis. Recently, the monitoring and reporting program outlined in the 2010 CAAAs bill submitted to the US Congress requires the operation, reporting, and certification of CEM systems to accurately measure the quantity of mercury that is emitted by electric coal and steam utilities in the United States. This bill, if passed, will be the first clear step in requiring US cement, coal-fired electric, and steam utilities to continuously monitor, verify, and publicly report on their Hg emission levels (Paone, 2010). Some states in the United States and other countries are taking steps to meet the future regulations before such policies are finalized. Massachusetts is incorporating Hg CEMs and sorbent trap protocols into their Hg rule requiring coal-fired utilities to continuously monitor Hg emissions. Similarly, in Germany, it is reported that over 34 cement kilns have Hg CEMs currently installed and that all waste incineration plants are required to continuously monitor total Hg emissions (Renzoni et al., 2010). Although CEM systems are often bulky and costly to purchase and install, they offer a variety of benefits over manual chemical emission measuring techniques, such as (Holmes and Pavlish, 2004).

- real-time measurement capabilities;
- immediate evaluation and feedback for mercury control strategies;
- greater understanding of process variability and identification of "spike" emissions;
- the potential to be less costly than current manual chemical methods;
- availability of significantly larger data sets; and
- greater public assurance that industries are complying with emission reduction targets.

However, on the basis of the current state-of-the-art technologies, mercury CEMs are not without challenges, particularly in terms of ongoing maintenance, the collection of particle-free yet representative gas samples, the presence of interfering gases, and large fluctuations in the low concentrations of Hg to be measured (generally below 10 $\mu g/m^3$) (Laudal, 2001; Nelson, 2007). A detailed report prepared for the US-EPA in 2006 compares several well-known commercially available CEMs for their suitability in a 550-MW coal-fire power utility (Hosenfeld, 2006). It was reported that source characteristics can have a significant effect on a CEM's performance and that the sample transfer and conditioning of the stack gas can be a major issue. Moreover, the challenges with the tested CEMs were found to be more mechanical or physical rather than chemical, and thus the analytical component of the systems were not generally found to contribute to the measurement problems. The report recommended that a CEM system should have a proven track record under the site-specific conditions as well as be customized to the site/source and operated on-site for six months as a requisite to demonstrate its capability to perform reliably and accurately as part of a performance warranty agreement with the manufacturer (Hosenfeld, 2006).

3.3.1 Commercially Available CEMs

Currently, Hg CEMs are primarily based on well-established analytical components such as CV-AAS, CV-AFS, or Zeeman-AAS (ZAAS) (Holmes and Pavlish, 2004). Systems are also being developed on the basis of AES (Narayan, 2006) and laser-based technologies (Magnuson et al., 2008). In addition, in some cases, portable Hg analyzers employ solid-state chemical microsensor technologies that work on mercury amalgamation and/or chemi-adsorption principles (see Section 3.3.2). CEMs come in several forms, each working slightly differently. Apart from the different detector mechanisms, they can be categorized as either extractive or *in situ* (Laudal and French, 2000). Extractive systems are usually located in a central position and may have several switchable gas feeds to sense mercury levels from multiple locations, whereas *in situ* systems are mounted on the duct of a given stack stream. A typical on-line Hg CEM comprises several different key components that integrate to accurately and reliably measure Hg emissions from industrial flue gas. At the heart of the system is the main Hg analyzer (AAS, AFS, etc.), which may or may not employ a preconcentrator based on gold amalgamation. Other important parts can include the isokinetic sampling probe, particulate removal system, and the sample conditioning and sample transfer lines that are required to transfer a representative flue gas sample to the Hg analyzer. In addition, some CEMs require a calibration source for Hg(0) vapor in order to obtain a calibration span. This can be achieved either by an internal permeation device, an external calibrated source, or by introducing a known quantity of mercury. A list of the major commercially available Hg CEM systems and industry used analyzers/monitors is provided in Table 3.1, where the website for each vendor is provided with separate references for research papers that have utilized the analyzer (if applicable). In addition, several of the listed CEMs have been extensively tested in industrial streams, either within the US-EPA Environmental Technology Verification (ETV) program, US-EPA programs (Hosenfeld, 2006), the European-based TüV Rheinland (www.tuv.com) certification program or independent researchers (Laudal and French, 2000; Spiric and Mashyanov, 2000; Laudal et al., 2004).

The US-EPA created the ETV program in 1995, which develops test protocols and verifies the performance of innovative technologies that have the potential to improve the protection of human health and environment. The ETV program is a voluntary program designed to provide credible performance information to purchasers, reducing risk to financial investors in the technology. Similarly, the European-based TüV Rheinland certification provider has also tested and certified some commercially available Hg CEMs by manufactures such as Seefelder, Sick, Durag, Opsis, and Semtech for waste incinerators in Europe (Laudal and French, 2000). The latter has been certified by TüV Rheinland for the determination of compliance with the German legal limit of 50 μg/Nm^3 for total Hg emissions from waste incinerators (Wocken et al., 2006). However, Tekran and Thermo Scientific systems are typically purchased by utilities within the United States (Laudal, 2008). Researchers are also supported by institutes and government environmental bodies (i.e., the US-EPA, DOE, EPRI, etc.) to conduct on-site tests of commercially available and prototype Hg CEMs in order to build confidence in their future usage (Spiric and Mashyanov, 2000; Laudal et al., 2004). Of late, in the absence of a definitive regulatory legislation, the US-EPA has reproposed that newly installed CEMs should at least meet the performance specification 12A (PS-12A), which is a test procedure requiring a CEM to

- be capable of measuring Hg^T (excluding Hg^P);
- include an automatic sampling system and a diluents (CO_2) monitor;
- measure relative accuracy, measurement errors, and drift using specified procedures;
- be installed according to standardized procedures;
- follow measurement and data analysis procedures; and
- follow procedures for comparing the data with a certified reference method.

In order to meet PS-12A, the CEM must contain a filter to remove particulates (e.g., fly ash) and condition any Hg^{2+} content in the flue gas by reducing it to

TABLE 3.1 A List of Commercially Available Gas Phase Hg Analyzers/Equipment and CEMs Predominantly Targeted Toward Industrial Use

Vendor/Product	Analysis Method	Range	Comment/References
Ohio Lumex (www.ohiolumex.com)			
Appendix K—RP-M324[a]	Dry sorbent—ZAAS	1–100,000 ng	Appendix K Trap Mercury Analyzer, RATA approved
RA-915+[a]	ZAAS	2–500 ng/m^3	Hg(0) (Yan et al., 2003; Holmes and Pavlish, 2004; Laudal et al., 2004; Sholupov et al., 2004; Kolesnikov et al., 2010)
RA-915 Light	ZAAS	0.1–100 µg/m^3	Hg(0) (Gochfeld, 2003; Holland, 2005)
IRM-915	ZAAS	0.5–1000 µg/dscm	Hg^T or Hg(0) by TC CEM, RATA approved
RA-915 MiniCEM 2x	ZAAS	0.1–200 µg/m^3	Hg^T by TC CEM, OH replacement
RA-82	AAS	50–99,999 ng/m^3	Portable field-use analyzer
Thermo Electron Corporation (www.thermoscientific.com)			
Model 80i	AFS	0–50 µg/m^3	Used in Freedom System
Mercury Freedom System[a]	AFS	3–9 µg/m^3 verified	Hg^S by TC/SD CEM, meets PS-12A (Hosenfeld, 2006)
Clean Air Engineering (www.cleanair.com/Services/MercuryMonitoring)			
MET-80	Dry sorbent analysis by AAS	—	PS-12A, RATA tested
Nippon Instruments Corporation(www.hg-nic.com/e_index)			
WA-4	AAS	0.01–1000 ng	For use in nonferrous refining
AM-2/3[a]	AAS	5–25 µg/m^3	Hg^S by TC/WC (Laudal et al., 2004)
AM-4	AAS	0.001–1000 ng	
AMG-1	AAS		CEM for use in LNG & LPG
MA-3000	AAS	0.002–25,000 ng	Hg(0) or Hg^T
EMP-1A/B	AAS	0.001–5.0 mg/m^3	Hg(0) portable monitor (Grice et al., 2008)
EM-5	AAS	0.001–2.0 mg/m^3	Hg(0) workplace monitor

84

DM–5[a]	AAS	5–25 µg/m³	Hg^S by WC/TC, CEM (Yan et al., 2003; Holmes and Pavlish, 2004; Laudal et al., 2004)
DM-6/6P[a]	AAS	0.1–1000 µg/m³	Hg^T by TC, CEM for coal (Holmes and Pavlish, 2004)
DM-6B/A/MS1A	AAS	0.1–1000 µg/m³	Hg^S by WC/TC, CEM (Holmes and Pavlish, 2004)
DM-6D	AAS	0.1–50 µg/m³	Hg^S by SD, CEM (Hosenfeld, 2006)
RA series	AAS		Used for liquid-based measurements (ppt–ppm)
PM-2	AAS	0.001–100 ng	Portable workplace monitor
TM-series	AAS	0.01–99.99 mg	For fluorescent tube industry
Tekran, Inc. (www.tekran.com)			
3300[a]	AFS	Up to 0.001 µg/m³ resolution	Hg^S by SD/TC CEM (RATA), for coal-fire, waste (Holmes and Pavlish, 2004; Hosenfeld, 2006)
2537A	AFS	0.0001–10 µg/m³	HgO using SD (Yan et al., 2003; Laudal et al., 2004; Brunke et al., 2010)
1135/1130			Particulate and speciation unit for HgO and Hg^{2+}
Seefelder Messtechnik (www.seefelder-messtechnik.com/english.html)			
HG Monitor 3000	AAS	0.1–2000 µg/m³	Work place monitor
Hg-Mat 2	AAS	0–75 µg/m³	Extractive CEM (Yan et al., 2003)

(continued)

TABLE 3.1 (*Continued*)

Vendor/Product	Analysis Method	Range	Comment/References
PS Analytical (www.psanalytical.com)			
PSA 10.525	AFS	0.001–2500 μg/m³	Hg^S by D/WC CEM for use in LNG and LPG or waste or coal (Kelly et al., 2003; Yan et al., 2003; Holmes and Pavlish, 2004; Kellie et al., 2004; Laudal et al., 2004)
Sir Galahad			
Sir Galahad II[a]			
PSA 10.670	AFS		Hg^S by WC CEM for use in LNG and LPG and petrochemical industry (Webpage)
PSA 10.665			
PSA 10.680			
PSA 10.210	AAS		Hg monitor for chlor-alkali plant
Apogee Scientific (www.apogee-sci.com)			
Quick Silver Inertial Separation System			Sampling probe (Webpage)
Opsis (www.opsis.se)			
AR602/Z/600	DOAS	0–150 μg/m³	Hg(0) (Yan et al. 2003)
HG200[a]	AAS	0.5–1000 μg/m³	Hg^S by SD/TC (Holmes and Pavlish. 2004; Laudal et al., 2004; Hosenfeld, 2006)
Apex Instruments (www.apexinst.com)			
XC-6000EPC[a]			Hg^S sorbent trap system for combustion sources

XC-30B			Hg^T sorbent trap system for coal-fired sources
Arizona Instrument (www.azic.com)			
Jerome 431-X/XE	RGFS	3–999 µg/m³	Portable field-use sensor (Grice et al., 2008)
Jerome J405	RGFS	0.5–999 µg/m³	Portable field-use sensor
Jerome 471	AAS	0.03–250 µg/m³	Portable field-use analyzer (Grice et al., 2008)
Sick UPA GmbH (www.sick.com)			
MERCEM	AAS	0–100 µg/m³	Hg^T by WC CEM (Yan et al., 2003; Holmes and Pavlish, 2004; Laudal et al., 2004)
Semtech Metallurgy AB (www.semtech.se)			
Hg 2010[b]	ZAAS	0.3–160 µg/m³	Hg^T by WC CEM for waste, coal-fire, and refining processes (Yan et al., 2003; Holmes and Pavlish, 2004; Laudal et al., 2004)
Durag Inc. (www.durag.com)			
HM-1400 TR[b]	AAS	0–45 µg/m³	Hg^T by TC CEM (Yan et al., 2003; Holmes and Pavlish, 2004; Laudal et al., 2004; Hosenfeld, 2006)
Aldora/EcoChem Analytics (www.ecochem.biz)			
Hg-MK II	AAS	0–50 µg/m³	Hg^T by TC CEM (Holmes and Pavlish, 2004; Laudal et al., 2004)
Envimetrics (www.envimetrics.com)			
	AES	0–200 µg/m³	Hg^T by TC CEM for coal, cement, waste etc. (Holmes and Pavlish, 2004)
Argus-Hg 1000			
ST2 Technologies			

(continued)

TABLE 3.1 (Continued)

Vendor/Product	Analysis Method	Range	Comment/References
SM–3[b]	AAS	0–500 μg/m³	Hg^S by TC (Holmes and Pavlish, 2004; Laudal et al., 2004)
Mercury Instruments Corporation USA (www.mercury-instrumentsusa.com)			
3000 IP	AAS	0.1–2000 μg/m³	Hg(0) portable monitor (Loredo et al., 2007; Grice et al., 2008)
VM 3000	AAS	0–2000 ug/m³	Hg(0) portable monitor (Choi et al., 2009)
UT 3000	AAS	0.1–10,000 ng/m³	Hg(0) for use in LNG and LPG
MMS	AAS	0.01–2000 μg/m³	Multichannel CEM
MMS-NG	AAS	0.001–2000 μg/m³	Multichannel CEM for LNG
Genesis Laboratory Systems (www.genlabsystems.com/mercury)			
Hg253	AAS	0.001–10 mg/m³	Hg(0) portable monitor (Grice et al., 2008)
Process Sentinel	AAS	0.0001 mg/m³ detection limit	Hg^S by, TC CEM (Laudal et al., 2004; Hosenfeld, 2006)
Sky Sentinel	AAS		Hg^S by TC CEM
MultiMatrix	AAS	< 5 pg to 6 mg/m³	Hg^S by TC CEM
Institute of Physics—Lithuania			
GARDIS 1A	AAS	0–1000 pg	Used in coal-fire (Ferrara and Mazzolai, 1998; Wängberg et al., 2003)

The company websites are provided as well as some references to applicable research papers that have used the analyzer.
Hg^S, reports speciated mercury; D/WC, dry/wet chemistry conversion; Hg^T, reports total mercury; TC, thermal catalytic conversion; Hg(0), reports elemental mercury; SD, sample dilution; DOAS, UV differential optical absorption spectroscopy; RGFS, resistive gold film sensor; LNG, liquefied natural gas; LPG, liquefied petroleum gas.
[a]Evaluated under EPA ETV Program.
[b]Evaluated by TüV Rheinland (www.tuv.com).

Hg(0) before measuring the total Hg content of the stream. It is also proposed that once the CEM has been properly installed, five tests should be conducted to certify the instrument. These five tests are referred to as the *40 CFR Part 75 mercury monitoring provisions, Appendices A and B* and include a seven-day drift test, a cycle time test, a system linearity check, a integrity check, and a relative accuracy test audit (RATA). The basic requirements for a RATA are that a minimum of nine valid paired reference method sorbent traps (either by the OH method, EPA method 29, 30A, or 30B) be taken and compared to the Hg CEM data taken over the same time. The two results should be compared and the relative accuracy calculated (Laudal, 2008, 2009).

3.3.2 Optical and Solid-State Chemical Sensors

A significant amount of work has focused on developing alternative optical and solid-state Hg sensors. Generally, solid-state Hg sensors work on mercury amalgamation or chemi-sorption principles between Hg and a selective layer material that overlays a micro-machined transducer platform. Alternatively, optical-based sensors work on reflectivity or absorption principles. Work spanning the last few decades has seen the use of Au thin-films as a selective material in conjunction with reflectivity, resistivity, or mass-based sensor platforms within the research and development community. However, recently selective layers based on palladium, palladium chloride, nanostructured gold, and polymeric composite-based materials have also been investigated in order to improve both the selectivity and sensitivity characteristics of the developed sensors for Hg sensing applications. The main motivation behind the development of such sensors is their low cost and robust nature in comparison to current analytical techniques (AAS, AFS, etc.). Although much of the developed sensors are initially targeted toward handheld or portable mercury analyzers, there is an ongoing trend of microsensors based on resistive, acoustic, and optical transducer platforms finding their way into commercial products.

3.3.2.1 Chemi-Resistive Sensors. Chemi-resistivity-based sensors, which are also sometimes referred to as conductometric sensors, work by measuring small resistance changes upon the interaction of a chemical (analyte) with the material (sensitive layer) deposited on the transducer. McNerney et al. (1972) was the first to propose Au thin-film-based conductometric sensors for Hg sensing applications in 1972, and one year later, a prototype sensor was developed which claimed to detect 0.05 ng of Hg (McNerney and Buseck, 1973). The sensor determined the concentration of Hg based on the resistivity change of the Au electrode upon the Hg–Au adsorption/amalgamation process. Presently, the commercially available Jerome 431-X mercury analyzer by Arizona Instruments is based on the same principles. The change in resistance of the Au film is thought to be because of an increase in scattering of conduction electrons at the Au film once Hg is adsorbed on the surface. Models have been developed to understand the effect of Au film thickness on the sensitivity of these types of transducers in order to optimize the Hg sensor performance (Raffa et al., 2006). Resistivity-based Hg sensors are typically made by well-established microelectronic fabrication processes; thus they are small sized, have low power consumption, and are highly durable, making them highly suitable for small handheld devices that detect Hg vapor concentrations in indoor Hg spills (e.g., dental clinics) (Ritchie et al., 2004). However, it has been reported that such sensors have a high cross-sensitivity toward ammonia and acetylene along with many other interferant chemicals, thus limiting their use. Furthermore, Arizona Instruments have also commercialized a H_2S sensor (model 631-X) that is based on the same principle. That is, H_2S exposure also induces a measurable resistance change in the Au film, which indicates that H_2S and Hg interactions could be indistinguishable and thus may present significant cross-sensitivity issues (McNerney et al., 1972; McNamara and Wagner, 1996; Cox and Deshusses, 2002). The sensors are also reported to have a minor cross-sensitivity toward other gases such as CH_4, SO_2, and CO that are present in coal-fired and cement plant flue gas.

Materials other than gold have also been studied by NASA to develop an electronic nose (array of conductometric sensors) for Hg detection in air (Ryan et al., 2008). These materials include polymer–carbon black composite films with amines in the polymer structure, gold islands on polymer films, and sintered $PdCl_2$ films (Jet Propulsion Laboratory, 2009). In addition, other work has involved the use of hexadecanethiol self-assembled monolayers (SAMs) that have been successful in repelling some interferant gases such as sulfuric compounds and humidity, yet simultaneously permit the interaction of Hg with the underlining Au film to induce a signal (Mirsky et al., 2002). However, other studies have indicated that Hg adsorption on Au substrates with alkanethiol SAMs induces reorientation and reorganization of the alkanethiols (Thome et al., 1998; Himmelhaus et al., 1999), thus resulting in the formation of Hg nanoparticles at the surface (Aliganga et al., 2004). This is believed to make the sensor unstable when exposed to Hg-containing environments, and thus the development of such surfaces and chemical filter layers is ongoing.

3.3.2.2 Acoustic Sensors.
Acoustic-based sensors, which are also sometimes referred to as resonant or gravimetric sensors, operate by detecting minute changes of mass at the active surface(s) of the device. In addition, some varieties are also sensitive to changes in sheet conductivity of the sensitive layer, and thus can also be used to measure very small changes in conductivity at the surface (Ippolito et al., 2009). Acoustic-based sensors have been widely studied for Hg sensing applications (Yao et al., 1986; Gomes et al., 1999; Ruys et al., 2000; Manganiello et al., 2002; Rogers et al., 2003; Casilli et al., 2004). Bristow (1972) first demonstrated the use of quartz crystal microbalance (QCM) for Hg vapor sensing in 1972, which was based on the adsorption/amalgamation of Hg on the QCM Au thin-film electrodes. Other investigators followed, further demonstrating QCM use for Hg vapor sensing applications (Scheide and Taylor, 1974, 1975; McCammon and Woodfin, 1977; Scheide, 1977; Scheide and Warnar, 1978; Ho et al., 1981; Mogilevski et al., 1991; Spassov et al., 1993). Recent studies by the

authors have also been undertaken to better understand Hg interaction with Au films (Sawant et al., 2009; Sabri et al., 2009b), where modified and nanostructured Au surfaces were studied for potential use as Hg sensors in alumina refinery streams (Sabri et al., 2008, 2009a). Similarly, research conducted by other groups has also demonstrated various other types of gravimetric devices for Hg vapor sensing applications. These devices include surface acoustic wave (SAW) sensors (Caron et al., 1998; Haskell et al., 1999; Haskell, 2003), magnetoelastic sensors (Shao et al., 2007), and piezoelectric microcantilevers (Thundat et al., 1995; Hu et al., 2001; Adams et al., 2005). SAW-based sensors have been identified as possible transducer platforms for Hg CEMs (Laudal, 2001; Yan et al., 2003) owing to their superior sensitivity (they are ~100 times more sensitive than QCM-based sensors). Although SAW sensors have yet to be commercialized, a comparison of SAW sensors with a Semtech Hg 2000 and a PS Analytical Sir Galahad mercury CEM is provided in Laudal (2001). The report shows that the tested SAW sensors have the potential to be made into a relatively low cost portable analyzer even though preconditioning and preconcentration subsystems were needed to deal with interferant gases present in the tested streams. Microcantilever-based sensors, which employ microcantilevers similar to those used in atomic force microscopy (AFM), have also shown promising results, although they suffer the same cross-sensitivity issues because of their use of Au-sensitive layers (Berger et al., 1998; Marie et al., 2002).

3.3.2.3 *Reflective Sensors.*

In 1990, Butler et al. reported that the reflective properties of Au thin films undergo detectable changes following their exposure to Hg (Butler et al., 1990). The group used this property to demonstrate the measurement of various concentrations of mercury vapor in air. The method involved exposing Hg vapor to an optically thin Au film evaporated onto the cleaved end of a multimode optical fiber and simultaneously measuring the amount of light reflected back through the fiber. Similar sensing methods were also demonstrated by Morris et al. (2002). In this case, various Hg vapor concentrations were exposed to Au nanoparticles of 3-, 5-, 12-, or 22-nm size where the resultant blue shift of their surface plasmon resonance (SPR) was monitored, thus demonstrating a novel "litmus" film for Hg vapor. In the same year, the group also demonstrated Hg sensing in air by SPR spectroscopy using Au, Ag, and Au–Ag thin films, showing that a gold-coated Ag film offers greater chemical stability than a pure Ag film and slightly higher sensitivity than a pure Au film (Morris and Szulczewski, 2002a, b). No literature is available on further development of these devices for an industrial-type application, thus presumably it is still in the developmental stage. The simplicity of these devices and the small detection limit in the parts per billion range are quite exceptional. However, other researchers have later demonstrated that Au- (Fontana et al., 1998) and Ag-based surfaces (Butler and Ricco, 1988) are also sensitive to the adsorption of other small gas molecules such as SO_2, CO, H_2S, He, H_2, C_3H_8, and other species commonly found in Hg-emitting industries. Therefore, presumably, such a sensor platform would require a separate filtering step for accurate Hg quantification in industrial gas streams.

3.3.2.4 *Emerging Technologies.*

In addition to the above-mentioned technologies, several new and different competing technologies have also been developed in the last decade to sense Hg within industrial processes. An example is the newly developed differential absorption lidar (DIAL) technique that uses a dye laser system (Weibring et al., 1998). Having been trialed by various chloralkali plants in Europe to measure elemental Hg vapor (Edner et al., 1995), it was found that the system needed frequent servicing because of its fast degrading gain medium (Sjöholm et al., 2004). Similarly, in 2007, Toth et al. (2007) reported the ability to identify and measure Hg by prompt gamma emission, generated by bombardment with neutrons. The method is typically used to sense Hg in ppb concentration ranges in the gaseous phase. Other methods with low detection limits also include laser-induced fluorescence (LIF)-based sensors, which utilize Au thin films to measure gaseous Hg(0) in several gas matrixes (D'ottone, 2006). In this case, Hg is measured by exciting either by 1-photon LIF or 2-photon LIF and subsequently detecting the fluorescent light with an appropriate photomultiplier tube. However, the presence of nitrogen and some other gases can decrease the signal to noise ratio. Similarly, Magnuson et al. (2008) have also reported an *in situ* measurement of Hg vapor from a laboratory-scale coal combustor and flow reactor using a diode-laser-based ultraviolet absorption sensor. The sensor detection limits was reported to be 0.3 ppb and it is said that the method eliminates the need for pretreatment by using a narrow bandwidth source with absorption spectroscopy. However, by using a wide laser-wavelength scan range, the off-resonant baseline was established accurately on both sides of the mercury absorption spectral feature. This is reported to allow for discrimination between Hg absorption and attenuation by other species or particles (Magnuson et al., 2008), thus resulting in the ability to selectively measure Hg in the flue gas. However, the method is not yet validated and needs to be compared with an accepted method for measuring Hg concentrations, such as the OH method.

3.3.3 Limitations

Initially, the majority of CEMs were originally developed for measuring Hg emissions from waste incinerators. However, their application for use in coal-fired combustion processes has not been without significant challenges. This is primarily because of the lower concentrations of Hg present within coal-fired combustion flue gas and the presence of acid gases such as HCl, SO_2, and NO_x that require some form of pretreatment or conversion to avoid interference issues in the analyzer (Laudal and French, 2000). Although several test programs have shown that some systems are capable of measuring mercury from coal-fired combustion streams to within 20% of wet chemistry or dry sorbent methods, several challenges still exist (Hosenfeld, 2006; Wocken et al., 2006).

The main challenge facing Hg CEM manufacturers is providing a "clean" sample gas to the mercury analyzer. This includes the heated sample lines and particulate removal subsystems that filter the stream before the sample is transported to the analyzer (Holmes and Pavlish, 2004). There are now commercially available filters that are being developed to overcome such issues (Webpage). In addition, the majority of the commercially available Hg CEMs are based on CV-AAS or CV-AFS owing to CV attachment making the instrument more selective toward mercury. Furthermore, with the addition of a gold amalgamation trap, it is possible to condition the stream by separating the Hg content from the interferant gas species before the mercury is measured in the AAS or AFS analyzer using the 253.7-nm detection band. This has the added benefit of decreasing the detection limit of the instrument by preconcentrating the mercury on a gold surface and using argon to carry the mercury to an analyzer after being thermally desorbed from the gold trap in an inert carrier gas. However, several challenges are associated with the gold traps technique when applied to industrial streams. Because gold is not sufficiently selective to mercury, its use cannot always guarantee the elimination of interferant gases. Other gases present in industrial streams, such as thiols, sulfides, alcohols, HCl, NO_x, ammonia, and humidity are well known to interact with gold, which results in erroneous mercury measurements (Surplice and Brearley, 1975; Kay et al., 1989; Rocha et al., 1998; Laudal, 2001; de Vooys et al., 2001; Bilic et al., 2002; Mirsky et al., 2002; Richton and Farrow, 2002; Meyer et al., 2004; Nuss and Jansen, 2006). In addition, as conventional traps use Au-coated granulated sand or quartz, during the high temperature heating/release cycle of Hg from the trap, there is the possibility of distillation of the gold. This can lead to condensation of small amounts of Au on the cooler parts of the system, introducing unmonitored collection sites for Hg that can result in systematic error (Schroeder et al., 1985). Moreover, thermodynamic and hydrodynamic problems may occur while releasing Hg from the Au traps for analysis (Caron et al., 1999). Another disadvantage of Au traps is the large pressure drop caused by the densely packed Au-coated adsorbent, making it harder to use high flow rates during sampling procedure. To overcome this limitation, denuder techniques have been proposed, where reactive wall coatings are used to trap the Hg in the flue gas (Larjava et al., 1993; Kvietkus et al., 1995). However, as this procedure is known to work best with laminar flows for optimum adsorption, it may be incompatible with the new mercury monitoring regulations that require isokinetic sampling (using a fixed flow rate and velocity). Furthermore, obstacles with the spectroscopy part of the AAS and AFS measurement techniques present their own issues, including the occurrence of undesired photochemical reactions, collision quenching and spurious scattered incident light, the loss or oxidation of Hg via adsorption or catalysis on solid surfaces, and small temperature fluctuations that cause small changes in the output intensity of the UV source, thus leading to errors (Granite and Pennline, 2002; Tong et al., 2002).

Other methods of sample preconditioning are not without their limitations, such as those that use either wet chemistry or thermal catalytic reduction methods. Typically, these preconditioning systems are used in CEM installations requiring mercury speciation capabilities. Although wet chemistry preconditioning systems are mostly used for research applications, it has been reported that they have worked well in plants burning either lignite or subbituminous coal (Holmes and Pavlish, 2004); however, the large amounts of chemicals generally result in large amounts of waste generation (up to 8 L/day) (Holmes and Pavlish, 2004). Also, wet chemistry preconditioning systems are not always guaranteed to work with streams containing high concentrations of SO_2 or SO_3. Similarly, in the case of thermal catalytic reduction systems, the expense and maintenance of the catalyst materials may become an issue as they need to be frequently regenerated and/or replaced at semi-regular intervals. Another popular method for sample preconditioning involves diluting the sample gas at or near the sample probe and then either using a wet or thermal catalyst preconditioning system. This makes the sample easier to transport and condition within the CEM system; however, because of the dilution process resulting in low mercury concentrations, a CV-AFS analyzer may need to be used over a CV-AAS-based system. Given the fact that each system configuration is subject to a variety of limitations, at this time, there does not appear to be one instrument or measurement technology that will work best in all applications. Several manufactures and bodies such as the EERC have been working on further developing pretreatment systems for Hg CEMs. One such solution is outlined in a report prepared by Laudal for the US DOE (Laudal, 2001), which uses a solid alkali-based sorbent to remove acid gases such as HCl and SO_2, and a stannous chloride solution to convert Hg^{2+} to Hg(0). Therefore speciation data could be provided by the CEM by difference measurements.

There also exists a real need for the development of solid-state transducer platforms if they are to be viable competitors to the already well-established spectroscopic techniques used for Hg vapor measurements in industrial applications. Research and development by various scientific groups is underway into these platforms, as their advantages such as their overall small size, ease of use, ability to be used as continuous on-line sensors, low cost, and low power consumption far outweigh their limitations. In a case similar to most spectroscopic techniques, their most critical disadvantage is the lack of selectivity to Hg in the presence of other interferant gases such as H_2S and SO_2. Similarly, other contaminants present in industrial streams (such as thiols, alcohols, ammonia, and humidity) have also been known to readily provide cross-interference issues (Surplice and Brearley, 1975; Kay et al., 1989; Rocha et al., 1998; de Vooys et al., 2001; Bilic et al., 2002; Mirsky et al., 2002; Richton and Farrow, 2002; Meyer et al., 2004; Nuss and Jansen, 2006). However, developments in nanotechnology and the use of composite materials are being pursued in order to increase both the sensitivity and selectivity of many solid-state transducer platforms. Furthermore, the use of integrated filter layers, surface modifying agents, and Hg sorbent traps could also be potential solutions. Overall, it is generally recognized that the well-established microsensor-based technologies are less sensitive than the currently employed spectroscopic techniques (Dumarey et al., 1985; Clevenger et al., 1997; Mirsky et al., 2002). However, microsensor platforms are cheap predominantly because of their easy fabrication in batch quantities, thus making them thousands of dollars less expensive than competing spectroscopic analyzers (Hughes et al.,

1991; Li and Ma, 2000). Although such sensors are far from reaching the stage of working as an on-line CEM in coal-fired or cement-industry-type flue gases, the race in developing both optical and solid-state Hg sensors for such applications is ongoing.

3.4 FUTURE OUTLOOK

The ill effects of Hg on health and the environment are well documented, yet there is a lack of reliable, robust, cheap, and accurate on-line Hg vapor sensors for monitoring emissions from industrial sources. Although much progress has been achieved in the last few decades, techniques developed so far are not yet mature, signifying that more research and development efforts are required. The current commercially available Hg CEMs and analyzers all have similar drawbacks, centering largely on their lack of a reliable transport method for the sample representing the flue gas stack, Hg selectivity, susceptibility toward interferant gas species, and their ability to deal with particulate matter present within the industrial process streams. In addition, the economic cost associated with installing and maintaining a CEM is another limiting factor. Given that Hg emission control is rapidly moving up the political agenda, it is inevitable that once the technology matures, industries operating in Western counties will be required to install and report their Hg emissions to the public on a regular basis. Recently, 140 countries began to negotiate a UNEP global treaty on mercury that is expected to be signed in 2013 (US Department of State, 2009b). The treaty is aimed at addressing the need to reduce the utilization and trade of mercury-related products, the reduction of atmospheric emissions of mercury, and enhancing national inventories of Hg emissions worldwide (UNEP, 2009). The US-EPA has also approved an Information Collection Request requiring all US power plants with coal- or oil-fired electric generating units to submit their Hg emission data so that it can be used in the development of future air toxics emissions standards (Neville, 2010). In the meantime, it is intended that the new air toxics emissions standard for coal- and oil-fired electric power plants under the Clean Air Act (Section 1.2) will be implemented by March 2011, and finalized by November 2011. Such a ruling would require coal-fired power plants to achieve mercury removal efficiencies of up to 90%; thus there is an urgent need to install mercury control technologies such as wet or dry scrubbers and particulate control devices. It is estimated that by 2013, suppliers of abatement chemicals and catalyst control technologies will service a market of US$500 million a year or more (Reisch, 2008). Although at first the immediate target markets are in the United States, in the coming decade, a McIlvaine on-line article, "Mercury Air Reduction Markets," forecasts a US$2 billion per year market for equipment and consumables to measure and remove mercury from stack gases for the cement, utility boilers, and industrial boiler sectors (Environmental Technology, 2010). Given that Europe and Asia will most likely follow or adapt US regulations and that Chinese cement and power plants emit four times more mercury than US plants, markets outside the United States are predicted to grow substantially in the coming decades. The combination of stringent regulations and industrial growth is prompting the need for Hg CEM developments (Appel et al., 2006; Danet et al., 2009) capable of integrating with Hg removal systems to ensure the environmental sustainability of Hg-emitting industries worldwide.

REFERENCES

Abollino O, Giacomino A, Malandrino M, Piscionieri G, Mentasti E. Determination of mercury by anodic stripping voltammetry with a gold nanoparticle-modified glassy carbon electrode. Electroanalysis 2008;20:75–83.

Adams JD, Rogers B, Manning L, Hu Z, Thundat T, Cavazos H, Minne SC. Piezoelectric self-sensing of adsorption-induced microcantilever bending. Sens Actuators A Phys 2005;121:457–461.

Alcoa World Alumina Australia. 2005. Wagerup refinery unit three environmental review and management program. Available at http://www.alcoa.com/australia/en/infopage/WG3%20Response%20to%20Public%20submissions%20final.pdf. Accessed 2011 Jan 7.

Aliganga AKA, Wang Z, Mittler S. Chemical vapor deposition of mercury on alkanedithiolate self-assembled monolayers. J Phys Chem B 2004;108:10949–10954.

Ames MR. Development and applications of a methodology for measuring atmospheric mercury by instrumental neutron activation analysis PhD [thesis]. Massachusetts Institute of Technology, 1995. Available at http://dspace.mit.edu/bitstream/handle/1721.1/36020/32904702.pdf?sequence=1.

Apogee Scientific, 2010. Quick silver inertial separation system. Available at http://www.apogee-sci.com/QSIS%20Probe%20System.html. Accessed 2011 Jan 12.

Appel D, Grassi JH, Kita D, Socha J. Method and apparatus for detecting the presence of elemental mercury in a gas sample. Patent No: US 2006/0246594 A1, Publication date: Nov. 2, 2006. Available at http://www.freepatentsonline.com/20060246594.pdf. Accessed August 2011.

Baier H. 2009. Legal framework in Germany and EU: The practice of oil shale utilization in power plants and cement production. Available at http://www.medemip.eu/Calc/FM/MED-EMIP/OtherDownloads/Docs_Related_to_the_Region/Oil%20Shale%20-%20Jourdan%20-%20April%202009/Article-ThePracticeOfOilShaleUtilizationIn PowerPlantsAndCementProduction.pdf.

Berger R, Delamarche E, Lang HP, Gerber C, Gimzewski JK, Meyer E, Güntherodt HJ. Surface stress in the self-assembly of alkanethiols on gold probed by a force microscopy technique. Appl Phys A 1998;66: S55–S59.

Bilic A, Reimers JR, Hush NS, Hafner J. Adsorption of ammonia on the gold (111) surface. J Chem Phys 2002;116:8981–8987.

Blanco RM, Villanueva MT, Uría JES, Sanz-Medel A. Field sampling, preconcentration and determination of mercury species in river waters. Anal Chim Acta 2000;419:137–144.

Bommaraju TV, Orosz PJ, Sokol EA. Brine electrolysis. In: Nagy Z, editor. Electrochemistry encyclopedia. Ernest B. Yeager Center for Electrochemical Sciences (YCES); 2007. http://electrochem.cwru.edu/encycl/art-b01-brine.htm.

Bristow Q. An evaluation of the quartz crystal microbalance as a mercury vapour sensor for soil gases. J Geochem Explor 1972;1:55–76.

Brunke EG, Labuschagne C, Ebinghaus R, Kock HH, Slemr F. Gaseous elemental mercury depletion events observed at Cape Point during 2007–2008. Atmos Chem Phys 2010;10:1121–1131.

Brunke EG, Labuschagne C, Scheel HE. Trace gas variations at Cape Point, South Africa, during May 1997 following a regional biomass burning episode. Atmos Environ 2001a;35:777–786.

Brunke EG, Labuschagne C, Slemr F. Gaseous mercury emissions from a fire in the Cape Peninsula, South Africa, during January 2000. Geophys Res Lett 2001b;28:1483–1486.

Butler MA, Ricco AJ. Chemisorption-induced reflectivity changes in optically thin silver films. Appl Phys Lett 1988;53:1471–1473.

Butler MA, Ricco AJ, Baughman RJ. Hg adsorption on optically thin Au films. J Appl Phys 1990;67:4320–4326.

Caron JJ, Haskell RB, Benoit P, Vetelino JF. Surface acoustic wave mercury vapor sensor. IEEE Trans Ultrason Ferroelectr Freq Control 1998;45:1393–1398.

Caron JJ, Haskell RB, Freeman CJ, Vetelino JF. Surface acoustic wave mercury vapor sensors. Orono (ME): Sensor Research and Development Corp. US patent: 5992215 1999.

Casilli S, Malitesta C, Conoci S, Petralia S, Sortino S, Valli L. Piezoelectric sensor functionalised by a self-assembled bipyridinium derivative: characterisation and preliminary applications in the detection of heavy metal ions. Biosens Bioelectron 2004;20:1190–1195.

Chang TC, You SJ, Yu BS, Kong HW. The fate and management of high mercury-containing lamps from high technology industry. J Hazard Mater 2007;141:784–792.

Change R, Offen GR. Mercury emission control technologies: an EPRI synopsis. Power Eng 1995;99:51–57.

Cheng C-M, Chen C-W, Zhu J, Chen C-W, Kuo Y-W, Lin T-H, Wen S-H, Zeng Y-S, Liu J-C, Pan W-P. Measurement of vapor phase mercury emissions at coal-fired power plants using regular and speciating sorbent traps with in-stack and out-of-stack sampling methods. Energy Fuels 2009;23:4831–4839.

Cheng HF, Hu YA. China needs to control mercury emissions from Municipal Solid Waste (MSW) incineration. Environ Sci Technol 2010a;44:7994–7995.

Cheng HF, Hu YN. Municipal Solid Waste (MSW) as a renewable source of energy: current and future practices in China. Bioresour Technol 2010b;101:3816–3824.

Choi HK, Lee SH, Kim SS. The effect of activated carbon injection rate on the removal of elemental mercury in a particulate collector with fabric filters. Fuel Process Technol 2009;90:107–112.

Clevenger WL, Smith BW, Winefordner JD. Trace determination of mercury: a review. Crit Rev Anal Chem 1997;27:1–26.

Cooper JA. Recent advances in sampling and analysis of coal-fired power plant emissions for air toxic compounds. Fuel Process Technol 1994;39:251–258.

Cox HHJ, Deshusses MA. Co-treatment of H2S and toluene in a biotrickling filter. Chem Eng J 2002;87:101–110.

Danet AF, Bratu MC, Radulescu MC, Bratuc A. Portable minianalyzer based on cold vapor atomic absorption spectrometry at 184.9 nm for atmospheric mercury determination. Sens Actuators, B Chem 2009;137:12–16.

Das AK, de la Guardia M, Cervera ML. Literature survey of on-line elemental speciation in aqueous solutions. Talanta 2001;55:1–28.

de la Rosa DA, Velasco A, Rosas A, Volke-Sepulveda T. Total gaseous mercury and volatile organic compounds measurements at five municipal solid waste disposal sites surrounding the Mexico City Metropolitan Area. Atmos Environ 2006;40:2079–2088.

de Vooys ACA, Mrozek MF, Koper MTM, van Santen RA, van Veen JAR, Weaver MJ. The nature of chemisorbates formed from ammonia on gold and palladium electrodes as discerned from surface-enhanced Raman spectroscopy. Electrochem Commun 2001;3:293–298.

Dobbs C, Armanios C, McGuiness L, Bauer G, Ticehurst P, Lochore J, Irons R, Ryan R, Adamek G. Mercury emissions in the bayer process-an overview. 7th International Alumina Quality Workshop; Perth, Western Australia. 2005. p 199–204.

D'ottone LKB. Novel method for the determination of gaseous mercury (0). US patent number: 20060120427, Publication date: Aug 6, 2006. Available at http://www.freepatentsonline.com/y2006/0120427.html. Accessed September 2011.

Duan YF, Zhao CS, Wang YJ, Wu CJ. Mercury emission from co-combustion of coal and sludge in a circulating fluidized-bed incinerator. Energy Fuels 2010;24:220–224.

Dumarey R, Dams R, Hoste J. Comparison of the collection and desorption efficiency of activated charcoal, silver, and gold for the determination of vapor-phase atmospheric mercury. Anal Chem 1985;57:2638–2643.

Earle CDA, Rhue RD, Earle JFK. Mercury in a municipal solid waste landfill. Waste Manage Res 1999;17:305–312.

E-CFR. Quality assurance and operating procedures for sorbent trap monitoring systems. Title 40, Part 75—Continuous Emission Monitoring, Subpart I—Hg Mass Emission Provisions, Electronic Code of Federal Regulations (e-CFR). Available at http://ecfr.gpoaccess.gov or http://rmb-consulting.com/download/Part %2075%20Revisions%20%282010%29.pdf. Accessed September 2011.

Edner H, Ragnarson P, Wallinder E. Industrial emission control using lidar techniques. Environ Sci Technol 1995;29:330–337.

European Environmental Agency. Air pollutant emissions data viewer: Europe. Available at http://www.eea.europa.eu/data-and-maps/. Accessed 2011 Jan 4.

Environmental Technology. US$2 Billion/year market for mercury removal from stack gases. Asian Environ Technol 2010;14:9.

European Environmental Agency. Method implementation document for EN 14385. Available at http://www.s-t-a.org/Files%20Public%20Area/MCERTS-MIDs/ MID14385%20metals.pdf. Accessed 2011 Jan 20.

Feng X, Streets D, Hao J, Wu Y, Li G. Mercury emissions from industrial sources in China. In: Mason, R, Pirrone, N, editors. Mercury fate and transport in the global atmosphere. New York (NY): Springer; 2009. p 67–79.

Ferrara R, Mazzolai B. A dynamic flux chamber to measure mercury emission from aquatic systems. Sci Total Environ 1998;215:51–57.

Fontana E, Dulman HD, Dogeet DE, Pantell RH. Surface plasmon resonance on a single mode optical fiber. IEEE Trans Instrum Meas 1998;47:168–173.

Friedli HR, Arellano AF, Cinnirella S, Pirrone N. Mercury emissions from global biomass burning: spatialand temporal distribution. In: Mason R, Pirrone N, editors. Mercury fate and transport in the global atmosphere. New York (NY): Springer; 2009. p 193–220.

Frontier GeoSciences. Got mercury? Frontier Global Sciences. Available at http://www.frontiergs.com/got-mercury. Accessed 2011 Jan 11.

Galbreath KC, Zygarlicke CJ. Mercury speciation in coal combustion and gasification flue gases. Environ Sci Technol 1996;30:2421–2426.

Galbreath KC, Zygarlicke CJ, Tibbetts JE, Schulz RL, Dunham GE. Effects of NOx, alpha-Fe2O3, gamma-Fe2O3, and HCl on mercury transformations in a 7-kW coal combustion system. Fuel Process Technol 2005;86:429–448.

Gibicar D, Horvat M, Logar M, Fajon V, Falnoga I, Ferrara R, Lanzillotta E, Ceccarini C, Mazzolai B, Denby B, Pacyna J. Human exposure to mercury in the vicinity of chlor-alkali plant. Environ Res 2009;109:355–367.

Glesmann SH, Sjostrom S, Dene C, Prestbo E. Mercury flue gas measurements: understanding draft EPA method 324 and validation results. EPRI-EPA-DOE-AW&MA Power Plant Air Pollutant Control "MEGA" Symposium, Washington, DC 2004. Available at http://www.adaes.com/PDFs/publications/20040830-MercuryFlueGasMeasurements.pdf.

Gochfeld M. Cases of mercury exposure, bioavailability, and absorption. Ecotoxicol Environ Saf 2003;56:174–179.

Gomes MTSR, Oliveira MO, Oliveira JABP. Utilization of a quartz crystal microbalance to obtain Au-Hg phase diagrams. Langmuir 1999;15:8780–8782.

Granite EJ. Obstacles in the development of mercury continuous emissions monitors. Annual International Pittsburgh Coal Conference; Pittsburgh (PA). 2003. p 983–1010.

Granite EJ, Pennline HW. Photochemical removal of mercury from flue gas. Ind Eng Chem Res 2002;41:5470–5476.

Grice KJ, Orman LDV, Young, LA. 2008. Newsletter: Evaluation of portable mercury vapor monitors and their response to a range of simulated oil processing environments. Available at http://www.azic.com/. Accessed 2011 Jan 14.

Hall B, Schager P, Lindqvist O. Chemical-reactions of mercury in combustion flue-gases. Water Air Soil Pollut 1991;56:3–14.

Hall B, Schager P, Weesmaa J. The homogeneous gas-phase reaction of mercury with oxygen, and the corresponding heterogeneous reactions in the presence of activated carbon and fly-ash. Chemosphere 1995;30:611–627.

Haskell RB. A surface acoustic wave mercury vapor sensor [thesis]. Orono (ME): Electrical Engineering, University of Maine; 2003. p 114.

Haskell RLB, Caron JJ, Duptisea MA, Ouellette JJ, Vetelino JF. Effects of film thickness on sensitivity of SAW mercury sensors. Volume 421, 1999 Proceedings of the IEEE Ultrasonics Symposium, Lake Tahoe, NV, USA 1999. p 429–434.

Hedrick E, Lee TG, Biswas P, Zhuang Y. The development of iodine based impinger solutions for the efficient capture of Hg-0 using direct injection nebulization: inductively coupled plasma mass spectrometry analysis. Environ Sci Technol 2001;35:3764–3773.

Himmelhaus M, Buck M, Grunze M. Mercury induced reorientation of alkanethiolates adsorbed on gold. Appl Phys B 1999;68:595–598.

Ho MH, Guilbault GG, Scheide EP. Determination of nanogram quantities of mercury in water with a gold-plated piezoelectric crystal detector. Anal Chim Acta 1981;130:141–147.

Holland K. 2005. Standard operating procedures: Ohio lumex mercury analyzer (RA 915). Available at http://www.renewnyc.com/content/pdfs/130liberty/SeptemberDeconstruction/B_SOP_for_OhioLumex.pdf. Accessed 2009 Apr 7.

Holmes M, Pavlish J. Mercury information clearinghouse, quarterly 2—mercury measurement. Canadian Electricity Association, Springfield, Virginia, USA; 2004. Available at http://mercury.electricity.ca/PDFs/MercuryResearchQuarterly2.pdf.

Holmes MJ, Pavlish JH, Wocken CA, Laudal DL. Mercury Information Clearinghouse, Quarterly 9—Final Report. Canadian Electricity Association, Springfield, Virginia, USA 2005. Available at http://mercury.electricity.ca/PDFs/MercuryClearinghouse_finalreport.pdf. Accessed September 2011.

Hosenfeld J. 2006. Long-term field evaluation of mercury (hg) continuous emission monitoring systems: coal-fired power plant burning eastern bituminous coal. U.S. Environmental Protection Agency. Available at http://www.epa.gov/ttnemc01/cem/hgcemsdemo.pdf.

Hu Z, Thundat T, Warmack RJ. Investigation of adsorption and absorption-induced stresses using microcantilever sensors. J Appl Phys 2001;90:427–431.

Hughes RC, Ricco AJ, Butler MA, Martin SJ. Chemical microsensors. Science 1991;254:74–80.

Hylander LD, Meili M. 500 years of mercury production: global annual inventory by region until 2000 and associated emissions. Sci Total Environ 2003;304:13–27.

IDS-Environment, 2011. Mercury measurements in fossil fuels. Available at http://www.ids-environment.com/Common/Paper/Paper_30/stockwell_mercury_measurments.pdf. Accessed 2011 Jan 12.

Ippolito SJ, Trinchi A, Powell DA, Wlodarski W. Acoustic wave gas and vapor sensors. In: Comini, E, Faglia, G, Sberveglieri, G, editors. Solid state gas sensors. New York (NY): Springer; 2009. p 261–304.

Jet Propulsion Laboratory. 2009. Detecting airborne mercury by use of polymer/carbon films. Available at http://www.techbriefs.com/component/content/article/5891. Accessed 2011 Jan 12.

Jet Propulsion Laboratory. Detecting airborne mercury by use of polymer/carbon films. NASA's Jet Propulsion Laboratory, Pasadena, California. Available at http://www.techbriefs.com/component/content/article/5891. Volume NPO-45003, Accessed 2011 Jan 10.

Johnson J. Power plants to limit mercury. Chem Eng News 2001;79:18–19.

Jones ML, Laudal DL, Pavlish JH. Mercury emission monitoring for the cement industry. 2008 IEEE Cement Industry Technical Conference Record, Miami, FL, USA; 2008. p 161–170.

Jun Lee S, Seo Y-C, Jurng J, Hong J-H, Park J-W, Hyun JE, Gyu Lee T. Mercury emissions from selected stationary combustion sources in Korea. Sci Total Environ 2004;325:155–161.

Kay BD, Lykke KR, Creighton JR, Ward SJ. The influence of adsorbate absorbate hydrogen bonding in molecular chemisorption: NH$_3$, HF, and H$_2$O on Au(111). J Chem Phys 1989; 91: 5120–5121.

Kellie S, Duan Y, Cao Y, Chu P, Mehta A, Carty R, Liu K, Pan W-P, Riley JT. Mercury emissions from a 100-MW wall-fired boiler as measured by semicontinuous mercury monitor and Ontario Hydro Method. Fuel Process Technol 2004;85:487–499.

Kelly T, Willenberg Z, Riggs K, Dunn J, Kinder K, Calcagno J. Environmental technology verification report—Sir Galahad II Mercury continuous emission monitor. PS Analytical Ltd, Columbus, Ohio, USA 2003. Available at http://www.epa.gov/etv/pubs/01_vr_psa_sg11.pdf. Accessed 2011 Jan 14.

Kim KH, Kim MY, Lee G. The soil-air exchange characteristics of total gaseous mercury from a large-scale municipal landfill area. Atmos Environ 2001;35:3475–3493.

Kim JH, Park JM, Lee SB, Pudasainee D, Seo YC. Anthropogenic mercury emission inventory with emission factors and total emission in Korea. Atmos Environ 2010;44:2714–2721.

Kockman D, Horvat M, Jacimovic R, Gibicar D. Determination of total mercury in solid environmental samples. RMZ Mater Geoenviron 2005;52:71–74.

Kolesnikov S, Rubinskaya T, Strel'tsova E, Leonova M, Korshevets I, Zykov A, Anichkov S. Distribution of mercury in the combustion products of coal dust in boilers with liquid slag removal. Solid Fuel Chem 2010;44:50–55.

Krivanek CS. Mercury control technologies for MWC's: The unanswered questions. J Hazard Mater 1996;47:119–136.

Kvietkus K, Xiao Z, Lindqvist O. Denuder-based techniques for sampling, separation and analysis of gaseous and participate mercury in air. Water Air Soil Pollut 1995;80:1209–1216.

Landis SE. 1999. Field validation of the Ontario hydro mercury speciation sampling method at site E-29. Available at http://www.osti.gov. Accessed 2011 Jan 7.

Larjava K, Laitinen T, Kiviranta T, Siemens V, Klockow D. Application of the diffusion screen technique to the determination of gaseous mercury and mercury (II) chloride in flue gases. Int J Environ Anal Chem 1993;52:65–73.

Laudal DL. EM Task 24—Development of an in-situ Instrument for measuring mercury in a gas stream. U.S. Department of Energy; 2001.

Laudal DL. JV Task 125—Mercury measurement in combustion flue gases short course. U.S. Department of Energy; 2008.

Laudal DL. Conducting a RATA of continuous mercury monitors using EPA Method 30B. Fuel Process Technol 2009;90:1343–1347.

Laudal DL, Brown TD, Nott BR. Effects of flue gas constituents on mercury speciation. Fuel Process Technol 2000;65:157–165.

Laudal DL, French NB. State-of-the-art of mercury continuous emission monitors for coal-fired systems. Conference on Air Quality II: Mercury, McLean, Virginia, USA 2000. p 1–16.

Laudal DL, Galbreath KC, Heidt MK, Brown TD, Nott BR, Jones SK. A State-of-the-Art Review of Flue Gas Mercury Speciation Methods. U.S. Department of Energy and EPRI; 1996. TR-107080.

Laudal DL, Kay JP, Jones ML, Pavlish JH. Issues associated with the use of activated carbon for mercury control in cement kilns. 2010 IEEE-IAS/PCA 52nd Cement Industry Technical Conference, Colorado Springs, Colorado, USA 2010. p 1–9.

Laudal D, Nott B, Brown T, Roberson R. Mercury speciation methods for utility flue gas. Fresenius J Anal Chem 1997;358:397–400.

Laudal DL, Thompson JS, Pavlish JH, Brickett LA, Chu P. Use of continuous mercury monitors at coal-fired utilities. Fuel Process Technol 2004;85:501–511.

Leaner JJ, Dabrowski JM, Mason RP, Resane T, Richardson M, Ginster M, Gericke G, Petersen CR, Masekoameng E, Ashton PJ, Murray K. Mercury emissions from point sources in South Africa. In: Mason R, Pirrone N, editors. Mercury fate and transport in the global atmosphere. New York (NY): Springer; 2009. p 113–130.

Li G, Feng X, Li Z, Qiu G, Shang L, Liang P, Wang D, Yang Y. Mercury emission to atmosphere from primary Zn production in China. Sci Total Environ 2010;408:4607–4612.

Li P, Feng XB, Qiu GL, Shang LH, Wang SF, Meng B. Atmospheric mercury emission from artisanal mercury mining in Guizhou Province, Southwestern China. Atmos Environ 2009;43:2247–2251.

Li D, Ma M. Surface acoustic wave microsensors based on cyclodextrin coatings. Sens Actuators B Chem 2000;69:75–84.

Lindberg SE, Southworth GR, Bogle MA, Blasing TJ, Owens J, Roy K, Zhang H, Kuiken T, Price J, Reinhart D, Sfeir H. Airborne emissions of mercury from municipal solid waste. I: new measurements from six operating landfills in Florida. J Air Waste Manage Assoc 2005;55:859–869.

Lindberg SE, Wallschlager D, Prestbo EM, Bloom NS, Price J, Reinhart D. Methylated mercury species in municipal waste landfill gas sampled in Florida, USA. Atmos Environ 2001;35:4011–4015.

Logar M, Horvat M, Akagi H, Pihlar B. Simultaneous determination of inorganic mercury and methylmercury compounds in natural waters. Anal Bioanal Chem 2002;374:1015–1021.

Loredo J, Soto J, Álvarez R, Ordóñez A. Atmospheric monitoring at abandoned mercury mine sites in Asturias (NW Spain). Environ Monit Assess 2007; 130:201–214.

Magnuson JK, Anderson TN, Lucht RP, Vijayasarathy UA, Oh H, Annamalai K, Caton JA. Application of a diode-laser-based ultraviolet absorption sensor for *in situ* measurements of atomic mercury in coal-combustion exhaust. Energy Fuels 2008;22:3029–3036.

Manganiello L, Rios A, Valcarcel M. A method for screening total mercury in water using a flow injection system with piezoelectric detection. Anal Chem 2002;74:921–925.

Marie R, Jensenius H, Thaysen J, Christensen CB, Boisen A. Adsorption kinetics and mechanical properties of thiol-modified DNA-oligos on gold investigated by micro-cantilever sensors. Ultramicroscopy 2002;91:29–36.

Masekoameng KE, Leaner J, Dabrowski J. Trends in anthropogenic mercury emissions estimated for South Africa during 2000–2006. Atmos Environ 2010;44:3007–3014.

Mason RP. Mercury emissions from natural processes and their importance in the global mercury cycle. In: Mason, R, Pirrone, N, editors. Mercury fate and transport in the global atmosphere. New York (NY): Springer; 2009. p 173–191.

McCammon CSJ, Woodfin JW. An evaluation of a passive monitor for mercury vapor. Am Ind Hyg Assoc J 1977;38:378–386.

McNamara JD, Wagner NJ. Process effects on activated carbon performance and analytical methods used for low level mercury removal in natural gas applications. Gas Sep Purif 1996;10:137–140.

McNerney JJ, Buseck PR. The detection of mercury vapor: a new use for thin gold films. Gold Bull 1973;6:106–107.

McNerney JJ, Buseck PR, Hanson RC. Mercury detection by means of thin gold films. Science 1972;178:611–612.

Metcalfe, J. 2010. United States Environmental Protection Agency (USEPA). Available at http://www.cleanairinitiative.org/portal/node/349. Accessed 2010 Dec 24.

Metzger M, Braun H. In-situ mercury speciation in flue gas by liquid and solid sorption systems. Chemosphere 1987;16:821–832.

Meyer R, Lemire C, Shaikhutdinov SK, Freund H. Surface chemistry of catalysis by gold. Gold Bull 2004;37:72–124.

Mirsky VM, Vasjari M, Novotny I, Rehacek V, Tvarozek V, Wolfbeis OS. Self-assembled monolayers as selective filters for chemical sensors. Nanotechnology 2002;13:175–178.

Mital S, MacDonald T. 2006. Environment track of the U.S.—India economic dialogue. Available at http://www.epa.gov/oia/regions/Asia/india/2006_ied.htm. Accessed 2010 Dec 24.

Mlakar TL, Horvat M, Vuk T, Stergarsek A, Kotnik J, Tratnik J, Fajon V. Mercury species, mass flows and processes in a cement plant. Fuel 2010;89:1936–1945.

Mogilevski AN, Mayorov AD, Stroganova NS, Stavrovski DB, Galkina IP, Spassov L, Mihailov D, Zaharieva R. Measurement of the concentration of mercury vapour in air through a piezoresonance method. Sens Actuators A Phys 1991;28:35–39.

Morris T, Szulczewski G. Evaluating the role of coinage metal films in the detection of mercury vapor by surface plasmon resonance spectroscopy. Langmuir 2002a;18:5823–5829.

Morris T, Szulczewski G. A spectroscopic ellipsometry, surface plasmon resonance, and x-ray photoelectron spectroscopy study of Hg adsorption on gold surfaces. Langmuir 2002b;18:2260–2264.

Morris T, Kloepper K, Wilson S, Szulczewski G. A spectroscopic study of mercury vapor adsorption on gold nanoparticle films. J Colloid Interface Sci 2002;254:49–55.

Mukherjee AB, Bhattacharya P, Sarkar A, Zevenhoven R. Mercury emissions from industrial sources in India and its effects in the environment. In: Mason, R, Pirrone, N, editors. Mercury fate and transport in the global atmosphere. New York (NY): Springer; 2009. p 81–112.

Mukherjee AB, Zevenhoven R, Bhattacharya P, Sajwan KS, Kikuchi R. Mercury flow via coal and coal utilization by-products: a global perspective. Resour Conserv Recycl 2008;52:571–591.

Narayan R. Inside mercury CEMs. Pollut Eng 2006;38: 28–31.

National pollutant inventory: Australia. Government of Australia. Available at http://www.npi.gov.au/npidata/action/load/advance-search. Accessed 2011 Jan 4.

National pollutant release inventory: Canada. Government of Canada. Available at http://www.ec.gc.ca/inrp-npri/. Accessed 2011 Jan 4.

Nelson P. 2007. Guidelines for sampling and analysis of mercury in atmospheric and source samples. Available at http://www.ccsd.biz/publications/files/TN/TN%2024%20Mercury%20Sampling%20%20Analysis_web.pdf. Accessed 2010 Nov 26.

Neville A. 2010. EPA's mercury rule: another incarnation coming. Available at http://www.powermag.com/environmental/EPAs-Mercury-Rule-Another-Incarnation-Coming_3100.html. Accessed 2011 Jan 4.

Nott BR. Intercomparison of stack gas mercury measurement methods. Water Air Soil Pollut 1995;80:1311–1314.

Nuss H, Jansen M. [Rb([18]crown-6) (NH₃)₃]Au·NH₃: gold as acceptor in N − H·Au⁻ hydrogen bonds. Angew Chem 2006;45:4369–4371.

Ohiolumex. lumex RA-915+ analyzer. Available at http://www.ohiolumex.com/product/ra915.shtml.

Pacyna EG, Pacyna JM. Global emission of mercury from anthropogenic sources in 1995. Water Air Soil Pollut 2002;137:149–165.

Pacyna JM, Pacyna EG, Steenhuisen F, Wilson S. Mapping 1995 global anthropogenic emissions of mercury. Atmos Environ 2003;37: S109–S117.

Pacyna EG, Pacyna JM, Fudala J, Strzelecka-Jastrzab E, Hlawiczka S, Panasiuk D. Mercury emissions to the atmosphere from anthropogenic sources in Europe in 2000 and their scenarios until 2020. Sci Total Environ 2006a;370:147–156.

Pacyna EG, Pacyna JM, Steenhuisen F, Wilson S. Global anthropogenic mercury emission inventory for 2000. Atmos Environ 2006b;40:4048–4063.

Paone P. Mercury controls for the cement industry. 2010 IEEE-IAS/PCA 52nd Cement Industry Technical Conference. Colorado Springs, Colorado, USA 2010. p 1–12.

Park KS, Seo YC, Lee SJ, Lee JH. Emission and speciation of mercury from various combustion sources. Powder Technol 2008;180:151–156.

Pavlish JH, Sondreal EA, Mann MD, Olson ES, Galbreath KC, Laudal DL, Benson SA. Status review of mercury control options for coal-fired power plants. Fuel Process Technol 2003;82:89–165.

Pirrone N, Cinnirella S, Feng X, Finkelman RB, Friedli HR, Leaner J, Mason R, Mukherjee AB, Stracher G, Streets DG, Telmer K. Global mercury emissions to the atmosphere from natural and anthropogenic sources. In: Mason, R, Pirrone, N, editors. Mercury fate and transport in the global atmosphere. New York (NY): Springer; 2009. p 1–47.

Pirrone N, Cinnirella S, Feng X, Finkelman RB, Friedli HR, Leaner J, Mason R, Mukherjee AB, Stracher GB, Streets DG, Telmer K. Global mercury emissions to the atmosphere from anthropogenic and natural sources. Atmos Chem Phys 2010;10:5951–5964.

Pirrone N, Keeler GJ, Nriagu JO. Regional differences in worldwide emissions of mercury to the atmosphere. Atmos Environ 1996;30:2981–2987.

Pod Technologies. Mercury monitoring. Pod Technologies. Available at http://www.podtech.com/links/hg-cems.html. Accessed 2011 Jan 7.

Powers RA. Batteries for low power electronics. Proc IEEE 1995;83:687–693.

Power & Energy. Fate-of-mercury in flue gas evaluations: the critical first step in reducing mercury emissions from coal-fired utility boilers. Available at http://www.nextgenpe.com/article/Fate-of-Mercury-in-Flue-Gas-Evaluations-the-Critical-First-Step-in-Reducing-Mercury-Emissions-from-Coal-Fired-Utility-Boilers/. Accessed 2011 Jan 11.

Prestbo EM, Bloom NS. Mercury speciation adsorption (MESA) method for combustion flue gas: methodology, artifacts, intercomparison, and atmospheric implications. Water Air Soil Pollut 1995;80:145–158.

Presto AA, Granite EJ. Survey of catalysts for oxidation of mercury in flue gas. Environ Sci Technol 2006;40:5601–5609.

Pudasainee D, Lee SJ, Lee SH, Kim JH, Jang HN, Cho SJ, Seo YC. Effect of selective catalytic reactor on oxidation and enhanced removal of mercury in coal-fired power plants. Fuel 2010;89:804–809.

Raffa V, Mazzolai B, Mattoli V, Mondini A, Dario P. Model validation of a mercury sensor, based on the resistivity variation of a thin gold film. Sens Actuators B Chem 2006;114:513–521.

Reisch M. Getting rid of mercury. Chem Eng News 2008;86:22–23.

Renzoni R, Ullrich C, Belboom S, Germain A. 2010. Mercury in the cement industry. Available at http://www.unep.org/hazardoussubstances/Portals/9/Mercury/Documents/para29submissions/CEMBUREAU-report%20Mercury%20in%20the%20cement%20the%20industry.pdf. Accessed 2011 Jan 14.

Richton RE, Farrow LA. Adsorption kinetics of ammonia on an inhomogeneous gold surface. J Phys Chem 2002;85:3577–3581.

Ritchie KA, Burke FJT, Gilmour WH, Macdonald EB, Dale IM, Hamilton RM, McGowan DA, Binnie V, Collington D, Hammersley R. Mercury vapour levels in dental practices and body mercury levels of dentists and controls. Br Dent J 2004;197:625–632.

Rocha TAP, Gomes MTSR, Duarte AC, Oliveira JABP. Quartz crystal microbalance with gold electrodes as a sensor for monitoring gas-phase adsorption/desorption of short chain alkylthiol and alkyl sulfides. Anal Commun 1998;35:415–416.

Rogers B, Bauer CA, Adams JD. Comparison of self-sensing techniques for mercury vapor detection using piezoelectric microcantilevers. J Microelectromech Syst 2003;5:663–666.

Ruys DP, Andrade JF, Guimaraes OM. Mercury detection in air using a coated piezoelectric sensor. Anal Chim Acta 2000;404:95–100.

Ryan MA, Homer ML, Shevade AV, Lara LM, Yen S-PS, Kisor AK, Manatt KS. Conductometric sensor for detection of elemental mercury vapor. ECS Meet Abstr 2008;16:431–439.

Sabri YM, Ippolito SJ, Bhargava SK. Mercury vapor sensor for alumina refinery processes. In: Bearne, G, editor. Light metals 2009. (TMS) The Minerals, Metals & Materials Society; 2009a. p 37–42.

Sabri YM, Ippolito SJ, Tardio J, Atanacio AJ, Sood DK, Bhargava SK. Mercury diffusion in gold and silver thin film electrodes on quartz crystal microbalance sensors. Sens Actuators B Chem 2009b;137:246–252.

Sabri YM, Ippolito SJ, Tardio J, Sood DK, Bhargava SK, Mullett M, Harrison I, Rosenberg S. Humidity and ammonia interference study for modified and non-modified gold based mercury vapor sensors for alumina refineries. 8th International alumina quality workshop; Darwin, Australia. 2008. p 260–266.

Sánchez Uría JE, Sanz-Medel A. Inorganic and methylmercury speciation in environmental samples. Talanta 1998;47:509–524.

Sarunac N. 2007. Evaluation and comparison of U.S. and EU reference methods for measurement of mercury, heavy metals, PMPM$_{2.5}$ and PM$_{10}$ emissions from fossil-fired power plants. U.S. Environmental Protection Agency. Available at http://www.epa.gov/ttn/emc/cem/hgpmcomp.pdf.

Sarunac N, Cipriano D, Ryan J, Schakenbach J. 2007. Field experience with mercury monitors. Available at http://www.powermag.com/instrumentation_and_controls/Field-experience-with-mercury-monitors_.html. Accessed 2011 Jan 20.

Sawant PD, Sabri YM, Ippolito SJ, Bansal V, Bhargava SK. In-depth nano-scale analysis of complex interactions of Hg with gold nanostructures using AFM-based power spectrum density method. Phys Chem Chem Phys 2009;11:2374–2378.

Scheide EP. The piezoelectric-crystal mercury dosimeter. Phys Teach 1977;15:47–51.

Scheide EP, Taylor JK. Piezoelectric sensor for mercury in air. Environ Sci Technol 1974;8:1097–1099.

Scheide EP, Taylor JK. A piezoelectric crystal dosimeter for monitoring mercury vapor in industrial atmospheres. Am Ind Hyg Assoc J 1975;36:897–901.

Scheide EP, Warnar RB. A piezoelectric crystal mercury monitor. Am Ind Hyg Assoc J 1978;39:745–749.

Schroeder WH, Hamilton MC, Stobart SR. The use of noble metals as collection media for mercury and its compounds in the atmosphere: a review. Rev Anal Chem 1985;8:179–209.

Senior C, Sarofim A, Eddings E. Behavior and measurement of mercury in cement kilns. IEEE-IAS/PCA 45th Cement industry technical conference. Dallas, Texas, USA 2003. p 233–248.

Shao R, Tan EL, Grimes CA, Ong KG. A wide-area, wireless, passive dosimeter for tracking mercury vapor exposure. Sens Lett 2007;5: 6.

Sholupov S, Pogarev S, Ryzhov V, Mashyanov N, Stroganov A. Zeeman atomic absorption spectrometer RA-915+ for direct determination of mercury in air and complex matrix samples. Fuel Process Technol 2004;85:473–485.

Sigler JM, Lee X, Munger W. Emission and long-range transport of gaseous mercury from a large-scale Canadian boreal forest fire. Environ Sci Technol 2003;37:4343–4347.

Sjöholm M, Weibring P, Edner H, Svanberg S. Atomic mercury flux monitoring using an optical parametric oscillator based lidar system. Opt Express 2004;12:551–556.

Southworth GR, Lindberg SE, Bogle MA, Zhang H, Kuiken T, Price J, Reinhart D, Sfeir H. Airborne emissions of mercury from municipal solid waste. II: potential losses of airborne mercury before landfill. J Air Waste Manag Assoc 2005;55:870–877.

Spassov L, Yankov DY, Mogilevski AN, Mayorov AD. Piezoelectric sorption sensor for mercury vapors in air using a quartz resonator. Rev Sci Instrum 1993;64:225–227.

Spiric Z, Mashyanov NR. Mercury measurements in ambient air near natural gas processing facilities. Fresenius J Anal Chem 2000;366:429–432.

Stokstad E. Environment: Uncertain science underlies new mercury standards. Science 2004;303:34–34.

Streets DG, Zhang Q, Wu Y. Projections of global mercury emissions in 2050. Environ Sci Technol 2009;43:2983–2988.

Sundseth K, Pacyna JM, Pacyna EG, Munthe J, Belhaj M, Astrom S. Economic benefits from decreased mercury emissions: projections for 2020. J Clean Prod 2010;18:386–394.

Surplice NA, Brearley W. The adsorption of carbon monoxide, ammonia, and wet air on gold. Surf Sci 1975;52:62–74.

Telmer KH, Veiga MM. World emissions of mercury from artisanal and small scale gold mining. In: Mason R, Pirrone N, editors. Mercury fate and transport in the global atmosphere. New York (NY): Springer; 2009. p 131–172.

Temmerman E, Vandecasteele C, Vermeir G, Leyman R, Dams R. Sensitive determination of gaseous mercury in air by cold vapour atomic fluorescence spectrometry after amalgamation. Anal Chim Acta 1990;236:371–376.

Thome J, Himmelhaus M, Zharnikov M, Grunze M. Increased lateral density in alkanethiolate films on gold by mercury adsorption. Langmuir 1998;14:7435–7449.

Thundat T, Wachter EA, Sharp SL, Warmack RJ. Detection of mercury vapor using resonating microcantilevers. Appl Phys Lett 1995;66:1695–1697.

Tong X, Barat RB, Poulos AT. Resonance fluorescence detection of mercury vapor in a supersonic jet. Rev Sci Instrum 2002;73:2392–2397.

The A to Z of nanotechnology 2009a: using nanotechnology to measure mercury. Available at http://www.azonano.com/Details.asp?ArticleID=2395. Accessed 2011 Jan 20.

Toth JJ, Wittman R, Schenter RE, Cooper JA. Candidate reactions for mercury detection induced by neutron and alpha particles. Nucl Instrum Methods Phys Res A 2007;572:1102–1105.

Tracy T. Cement Makers Ordered To Cut Mercury Emissions. Wall Street Journal, Tuesday, August 10, 2010.

US-EPA. 1996. Appendix A: EERC ontario-hydro and tris buffer mercury speciation methods analytical plan. Available at http://www.epa.gov/ttn/atw/combust/utiltox/mercury/aescmila.pdf. Accessed 2011 Jan 7.

US-EPA. Toxics release inventory: United States of America. Available at http://www.epa.gov/triexplorer/facility.htm. Accessed 2011 Jan 4.

US Department of State. 2009b. United States secures international consensus to develop agreement on mercury: 140 countries agree to pursue binding agreement to contain release of toxic metal. Available at http://www.state.gov/g/oes/rls/fs/2009/119961.htm. Accessed 2011 Jan 14.

UNEP. 2008a. Global atmospheric mercury assessment: sources, emissions and transport. Available at http://www.chem.unep.ch/mercury/Atmospheric_Emissions/Atmospheric_emissions_mercury.htm. Accessed 2011 Jan 14.

UNEP. 2008b. Technical background report to the global atmospheric mercury assessment. Available at http://www.chem.unep.ch/mercury/Atmospheric_Emissions/Technical_background_report.pdf. Accessed 2010 Dec 24.

UNEP. 2009. Draft decision approved by the chemicals contact group on chemicals management, including mercury. Available at http://www.unep.org/pdf/Draft_decisionapproved.pdf. 2011 Jan 14.

US-EPA. Fact sheet. Environmental technology verification program. U.S. Environmental Protection Agency. Available at http://www.epa.gov/nrmrl/std/etv/pubs/600f08012.pdf.

US-EPA. Mercury Continuous Emission Monitors (CEMs). Environmental Technology Verification Program (ETV). U.S. Environmental Protection Agency. Available at http://www.epa.gov/etv/pubs/600f07006.pdf.

US-EPA. Mercury study report to congress. Volume I, United States Environmental Protection Agency; 1997.

US-EPA. Method 29: Determination of metals emissions from stationary sources. U.S. Environmental Protection Agency. Available at http://www.epa.gov/ttn/emc/promgate/m-29.pdf.

US-EPA. Method 30B: Determination of total vapor phase mercury emissions from coal-fired combustion sources using carbon sorbent traps. U.S. Environmental Protection Agency. Available at http://www.epa.gov/ttn/emc/promgate/Meth30B.pdf.

US-EPA. Method 101: Determination of particulate and gaseous mercury emissions form chlor-alkali plants (air streams). U.S. Environmental Protection Agency. Available at http://www.epa.gov/ttn/emc/promgate/m-101.pdf.

US-EPA. Method 101A: Determination of particulate and gaseous mercury emissions form sewage sludge incinerators. U.S. Environmental Protection Agency. Available at http://www.epa.gov/ttn/emc/promgate/m-101a.pdf.

US-EPA. Performance specifications and other monitoring information. U.S. Environmental Protection Agency. Available at http://www.epa.gov/ttn/emc/monitor.html.

US-EPA. Performance Specification 12A: Specifications and test procedures for total vapor phase mercury continuous emission monitoring systems in stationary sources. U.S. Environmental Protection Agency. Available at http://www.epa.gov/ttn/emc/perfspec/ps-12A.pdf. Accessed September 2011.

US-EPA webpage. Advanced monitoring systems center verified technologies. Mercury emission monitors. U.S. Environmental Protection Agency, USA. Available at http://www.epa.gov/etv/vt-ams.html#mcem. Accessed 2010 Dec 10.

US Library of Congress. S. 1630: Clean Air Act Amendments of 1990. US Library of Congress. Available at http://thomas.loc.gov. Accessed 2011 Jan 4.

US Library of Congress. S. 2995: Clean Air Act Amendments of 2010. US Library of Congress. Available at http://thomas.loc.gov. Accessed 2011 Jan 4.

Veiga MM, Maxson PA, Hylander LD. Origin and consumption of mercury in small-scale gold mining. J Clean Prod 2006;14:436–447.

Waltisberg J. 2004. Holcim EMR list of EN standards and VDI guidelines usable for discontinuous measurements in cement plants. Available at http://www.unep.org/hazardoussubstances/Portals/9/Mercury/Documents/para29submissions/CEMBUREAU-report%20Mercury%20in%20the%20cement%20the%20industry.pdf. Accessed 2011 Jan 20.

Wang Q, Shen W, Ma Z. Estimation of mercury emission from coal combustion in China. Environ Sci Technol 2000;34:2711–2713.

Wängberg I, Edner H, Ferrara R, Lanzillotta E, Munthe J, Sommar J, Sjöholm M, Svanberg S, Weibring P. Atmospheric mercury near a chlor-alkali plant in Sweden. Sci Total Environ 2003;304:29–41.

Weibring P, Andersson M, Edner H, Svanberg S. Remote monitoring of industrial emissions by combination of lidar and plume velocity measurements. Appl Phys B 1998;66:383–388.

Weise E. EPA claps down on cement plant pollution. USA Today, Tuesday, August 10, 2010.

Weiss-Penzias P, Jaffe D, Swartzendruber P, Hafner W, Chand D, Prestbo E. Quantifying Asian and biomass burning sources of mercury using the Hg/CO ratio in pollution plumes observed at the Mount Bachelor Observatory. Atmos Environ 2007;41:4366–4379.

Weissberg BG. Determination of mercury in soils by flameless atomic absorption spectrometry. Econ Geol 1971;66:1042–1047.

Wiedinmyer C, Friedli H. Mercury emission estimates from fires: an initial inventory for the United States. Environ Sci Technol 2007;41:8092–8098.

Wilson SJ, Steenhuisen F, Pacyna JM, Pacyna EG. Mapping the spatial distribution of global anthropogenic mercury atmospheric emission inventories. Atmos Environ 2006;40:4621–4632.

Windham RL. Simple device for compensation of broad-band absorption interference in flameless atomic absorption determination of mercury. Anal Chem 1972;44:1334–1336.

Wocken CA, Holmes MJ, Laudal DL, Pflughoeft-Hassett DF, Weber GF, Ralston NVC, Miller SJ, Dunham GE, Olson ES, Raymond LJ, Pavlish JH, Sondreal EA, Benson SA. Mercury Information Clearinghouse. Final report. AAD Document Control and U.S. Department of Energy, Pittsburgh, Pennsylvania, USA 2006. Available at http://www.osti.gov. Report number: for the period October 1, 2003 through March 31, 2006.

Wu Y, Wang SX, Streets DG, Hao JM, Chan M, Jiang JK. Trends in anthropogenic mercury emissions in China from 1995 to 2003. Environ Sci Technol 2006;40:5312–5318.

Yan R, Liang DT, Tay JH. Control of mercury vapor emissions from combustion flue gas. Environ Sci Pollut Res 2003;10:399–407.

Yao S, Tan S, Nie L. Internal electrolytic determination of mercury in aqueous solution with a gold-plated piezoelectric detector. Fenxi Huaxue 1986;14:6.

Yuan CS, Lin HY, Wu CH, Liu MH. Partition and size distribution of heavy metals in the flue gas from municipal solid waste incinerators in Taiwan. Chemosphere 2005;59:135–145.

Zhang L, Wong MH. Environmental mercury contamination in China: sources and impacts. Environ Int 2007;33:108–121.

Zhao YC, Zhang JY, Chou CL, Li Y, Wang ZH, Ge YT, Zheng CG. Trace element emissions from spontaneous combustion of gob piles in coal mines, Shanxi, China. Int J Coal Geol 2008;73:52–62.

Zimmer C, McKinley D. New approaches to pollution prevention in the healthcare industry. J Clean Prod 2008;16:734–742.

PART II

SPECIATION AND TRANSFORMATION

CHAPTER 4

ATMOSPHERIC CHEMISTRY OF MERCURY

CHE-JEN LIN, PATTARAPORN SINGHASUK, and SIMO O. PEHKONEN

4.1 INTRODUCTION

The atmosphere is the most important transient reservoir of mercury released from anthropogenic emission sources and through natural processes. Once released, mercury exists primarily in three inorganic forms: (i) gaseous elemental mercury (Hg(0)); (ii) reactive gaseous mercury (RGM) that represents a mixture of gaseous mercuric (divalent) compounds; and (iii) particulate mercury (PHg) that denotes mercury species, mostly divalent, bound to airborne particles. Both RGM and PHg are operationally defined mercury forms whose chemical compositions are not clearly understood, although mercuric oxides and halides have been proposed to be the dominant species (Schroeder and Munthe, 1998; Lin et al., 2006; Lindberg et al., 2007). More than 95% of mercury in the atmosphere exists as Hg(0) because of its relatively low deposition velocity and high vapor pressure at ambient conditions (Stein et al., 1996). RGM and PHg constitute <5% combined of total mercury, although their concentrations can be significantly higher during atmospheric mercury depletion events (AMDEs) in polar springtime, in the marine boundary layer and in the upper atmosphere (Pirrone et al., 2005b; Lindberg et al., 2007). The presence of methylated mercury (MeHg) has also been reported at locations near sources such as landfill sites and in the marine boundary layer (Lindberg and Price, 1999; Lindberg et al., 2005, 2005a). The presence of Hg(I) is considered negligible as it tends to be converted into elemental or divalent forms because of its chemical instability (Lin and Pehkonen, 1999). Currently, the typical concentrations of total gaseous mercury (Hg(0) and RGM) measured at locations remote from immediate anthropogenic sources range from 1 to 4 ng/m^3, with a concentration gradient from the Northern to the Southern Hemisphere (Slemr et al., 2003).

Environmental Chemistry and Toxicology of Mercury, First Edition.
Edited by Guangliang Liu, Yong Cai, and Nelson O'Driscoll.
© 2012 John Wiley & Sons, Inc. Published 2012 by John Wiley & Sons, Inc.

Hg(0) is subject to long-range air transport because of its long atmospheric lifetime of 0.5–1.5 years (UNEP Chemicals Branch, 2008). On the other hand, RGM and PHg can be removed rapidly via dry and wet deposition because of the greater affinity to the Earth's surfaces and solubility in atmospheric droplets. These removal processes result in a much shorter atmospheric lifetime, typically ranging from minutes to weeks. Therefore, the chemical processes transforming mercury between the elemental and divalent states strongly influence the transport characteristics and deposition rate of mercury. In addition, modeling efforts that assess the global cycling of mercury (emissions, transport, and deposition) and its impacts require an in-depth knowledge of mercury chemistry in the atmosphere for appropriate model parameterization.

In this chapter, a synthesis of the current understanding of mercury chemistry in the atmosphere is presented. The up-to-date chemical reactions responsible for converting atmospheric mercury between the two primary oxidation states (0 and +2) in the gas phase, in atmospheric droplets, and on the Earth's surfaces are summarized. The uncertainties in the reported mechanisms and kinetics, as well as the current knowledge gaps in mercury chemistry, are also discussed. Future research needs to better understand mercury chemistry and its implications in the global atmospheric cycling of mercury are assessed.

4.2 THE OVERALL PICTURE

Figure 4.1 shows a simplified schematic of the redox processes of mercury, which is further detailed in the following sections. In the atmosphere, mercury partitions among gas, aqueous (e.g., cloud, fog, and rain waters), and solid (e.g., particulate matter, PM) phases. In the gas phase, the chemical processes are dominated by oxidation reactions that convert Hg(0) into RGM and PHg. Although reduction reactions have also been proposed (Schroeder et al., 1991; Seigneur et al., 1994; Pongprueksa et al., 2008), they are yet to be verified experimentally. The predominant oxidants are ozone (O_3), hydroxyl radical (OH), reactive halogen species (atomic and various molecular and radical forms of chlorine, bromine, and iodine), hydrogen peroxide (H_2O_2), and nitrate radical (NO_3). Both Hg(0) and RGM can be adsorbed onto atmospheric PM, although its quantitative information is limited because of the complex nature of atmospheric PM (e.g., the identity of the solids and the concentration variability in air).

All three mercury species can be scavenged into atmospheric droplets where redox and speciation reactions (complex formation reactions of mercuric ions with other ligands that cause changes in chemical forms without changes in oxidation state) take place. Generally, the scavenging process does not limit the reaction rates in the typical size regimes of droplets (Lin and Pehkonen, 1997). The gas–liquid equilibria are governed by Henry's law (Table 4.1). The aqueous Hg(0) level at Henry's equilibrium with gaseous Hg(0) is in the order of 10^{-14} M, which constitutes a negligible fraction of Hg concentrations in atmospheric waters. Dissolved divalent mercury species Hg(II) dominate in the aqueous phase because of their much greater Henry's constants, with a typical

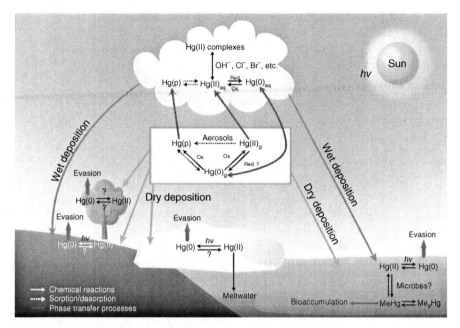

Figure 4.1 A simplified schematic illustrating the chemical processes of mercury in the atmosphere. Red., reduction; ox., oxidation.

TABLE 4.1 Gas–Liquid Equilibria of Mercury Compounds[a]

Equilibrium	H (M atm^{-1})
$Hg(0)(g) \leftrightarrow Hg(0)(aq)$	0.11
$Hg(OH)_2(g) \leftrightarrow Hg(OH)_2(aq)$	1.2×10^4
$HgCl_2(g) \leftrightarrow HgCl_2(aq)$	1.4×10^6
$HgO(g) \leftrightarrow HgO(aq)$	2.7×10^{12}
$CH_3HgCl(g) \leftrightarrow CH_3HgCl(aq)$	2.2×10^3
$CH_3HgCH_3(g) \leftrightarrow CH_3HgCH_3(aq)$	0.13

[a] $T = 25°C$. The table is adapted from Lin and Pehkonen (1999). The original references are Sanemasa (1975), Iverfeldt and Lindqvist (1982), Lindqvist and Rodhe (1985), and Schroeder and Munthe (1998).

concentration in precipitation at $10^{-9}–10^{-11}$ M (data from Mercury Deposition Network, MDN). The solid–liquid equilibria are governed by the solubility products of solid Hg compounds in water (Table 4.2). On the basis of the values in Table 4.2, Hg(II) species are not likely to be present as solids given the low aqueous concentrations of mercury in droplets. However, a significant fraction of dissolved Hg(II) may be associated with particles in the aqueous phase (e.g., soot and other insoluble particulates) through sorption processes (Seigneur et al., 1998; Lin and Pehkonen, 1999).

TABLE 4.2 Solid–Liquid Equilibria of Mercury Compounds[a]

Equilibrium	$\log(K)$
$HgO(s) + H_2O \leftrightarrow Hg^{2+} + 2OH^-$	-25.44
$HgS(s) + 2H^+ \leftrightarrow Hg^{2+} + H_2S$	-31.7
$HgCl_2(s) \leftrightarrow Hg^{2+} + 2Cl^-$	-14.57[b]
$Hg(OH)_2(s) \leftrightarrow Hg^{2+} + 2OH^-$	-24.96[b]
$Hg_2Cl_2(s) \leftrightarrow 2Hg^+ + 2Cl^-$	-17.91
$Hg_2SO_4(s) \leftrightarrow 2Hg^+ + SO_4^{2-}$	-6.13

[a] Data are from Martell et al. (1993), unless otherwise noted.
[b] Sillén and Martell (1964).

Atmospheric water droplets serve as microreactors for the redox reactions of mercury (Lin and Pehkonen, 1999). In the aqueous phase, both oxidation and reduction occur. The oxidants include dissolved O_3, OH, and molecular halogens ($HOCl/OCl^-$, $Br_2/HOBr/OBr^-$), while the reduction is mediated by hydroperoxyl radical ($HO_2^{\bullet}$), through the decomposition of mercuric (Hg^{2+}) sulfite (SO_3^{2-}) complexes (mainly through $HgSO_3$), and the photoreduction of $Hg(OH)_2$ and Hg(II)-dicarboxylic acids (C_2-C_4) complexes. Because most of the reduction pathways require the formation of specific complexes, aqueous speciation of Hg(II) has an important impact on the reduction kinetics. The speciation can be calculated by solving a series of parallel mass and charge conservation equations using the expressions of equilibrium constants and solution composition (Lin et al., 2006). Since Hg(II) has a very rapid ligand exchange rate in aqueous solutions (Brezonik, 1994), the formation of Hg(II) hydrated complexes does not limit the redox reaction rates, and can be treated separately as chemical equilibria. Table 4.3 lists the chemical equilibria and their stability constants relevant in atmospheric droplets. The total concentration of ligands and pH are the most important factors affecting Hg(II) speciation. Under typical chemical compositions in droplets, important ligands that form significant complexes are chloride (Cl^-) and sulfite (SO_3^{2-}). In both cases, the bis-complex is the most dominant species (i.e., $HgCl_2$ and $Hg(SO_3)_2^{2-}$). Owing to the short lifetime of SO_3^{2-} (several hours), Hg(II) exists primarily as $HgCl_2$ in the aqueous phase. The concentration of the reactive $HgSO_3$ peaks at about pH 4–5 with a total SO_3^{2-} concentration at about 1 µM (Lin and Pehkonen, 1998b).

As part of the air–surface exchange processes (deposition and evasion of mercury), *in situ* redox reactions at various surfaces of the Earth have also been reported. Such transformations include the oxidation/reduction at water (Mason and Sheu, 2002; Ferrara et al., 2003; Sheu and Mason, 2004; O'Driscoll et al., 2006; Whalin and Mason, 2006; Whalin et al., 2007; Selin, 2009; Qureshi et al., 2010) and vegetative surfaces (Rea et al., 2002; Graydon et al., 2006; Ariya et al., 2009); as well as reduction at soil (Carpi and Lindberg, 1997; Gustin et al., 2002) and snow (King and Simpson, 2001; Lalonde et al., 2003; Poulain et al., 2004) surfaces. These reactions are primarily derived from field observations and their mechanisms are not well defined (i.e., the oxidants and reductants have not been

TABLE 4.3 Chemical Equilibria for Calculating Aqueous Phase Hg(II) Speciation[a]

Reaction No.	Equilibrium	$\log(K_{eq})$
E1	$H_2O \cdot SO_2 \leftrightarrow H^+ + HSO_3^-$	−1.91
E2	$HSO_3^- \leftrightarrow H^+ + SO_3^{2-}$	−7.18
E3	$H_2O\ CO_3 \leftrightarrow H^+ + HCO_3$	−6.35
E4	$HCO_3^- \leftrightarrow H^+ + CO_3^{2-}$	−10.33
E5	$Hg^{2+} + OH^- \leftrightarrow Hg(OH)^+$	10.63
E6	$Hg^{2+} + 2OH^- \leftrightarrow Hg(OH)_2$	22.24
E7	$Hg^{2+} + SO_3^{2-} \leftrightarrow HgSO_3$	12.7
E8	$Hg^{2+} + 2SO_3^{2-} \leftrightarrow Hg(SO_3)_2^{2-}$	24.1
E9	$Hg^{2+} + OH^- + Cl^- \leftrightarrow HgOHCl$	18.25
E10	$Hg^{2+} + Cl^- \leftrightarrow HgCl^+$	7.30
E11	$Hg^{2+} + 2Cl^- \leftrightarrow HgCl_2$	14.0
E12	$Hg^{2+} + 3Cl^- \leftrightarrow HgCl_3^-$	15.0
E13	$Hg^{2+} + 4Cl^- \leftrightarrow HgCl_4^{2-}$	15.6
E14	$Hg^{2+} + Br^- \leftrightarrow HgBr^+$	9.07
E15	$Hg^{2+} + 2Br^- \leftrightarrow HgBr_2$	17.27
E16	$Hg^{2+} + 3Br^- \leftrightarrow HgBr_3^-$	19.7
E17	$Hg^{2+} + 4Br^- \leftrightarrow HgBr_4^{2-}$	21.2
E18	$Hg^{2+} + OH^- + Br^- \leftrightarrow HgOHBr$	19.7
E19	$Hg^{2+} + CO_3^{2-} \leftrightarrow HgCO_3$	11.0
E20	$Hg^{2+} + SO_4^{2-} \leftrightarrow HgSO_4$	1.34
E21	$Hg^{2+} + 2SO_4^{2-} \leftrightarrow Hg(SO_4)^{2-}$	2.40
E22	$Hg^{2+} + NO_3^- \leftrightarrow Hg(NO_3)^+$	0.11

[a]Data are from Smith and Martell (2004).

identified). In addition, the reported transformation rates are usually site specific and not generally applicable in the modeling assessment of environmental mercury cycling. Nevertheless, these chemical transformation pathways are important natural processes that contribute to the removal and emission from the Earth's surfaces that cover a large area and therefore are included in this synthesis.

It should be noted that our understanding of the atmospheric chemistry of mercury is still evolving. In fact, there are ongoing debates on the relative importance of various chemical transformation pathways to the transport and removal of mercury in the atmosphere. This is primarily due to the lack of knowledge in the heterogeneous chemistry of mercury (e.g., the chemical reactions induced by particulate matter and/or occurred on reactive surfaces) and the uncertainty in our current understanding of mercury chemistry. Because of the ultra-trace concentrations of mercury in the atmosphere, it is extremely difficult to verify the kinetic and mechanistic results obtained from laboratory studies, which are conducted in well-controlled but simplified chemical systems, under realistic atmospheric conditions. Data inconsistencies also exist in the literature for the same transformation pathways. In the past decade, the research community's view of mercury chemistry has changed significantly.

4.3   CHEMICAL TRANSFORMATIONS IN THE GAS PHASE

Table 4.4 lists the gas-phase oxidation reactions of Hg(0) (as well as selected reactions of dimethyl mercury) and their reported rate coefficients. Although there are other gaseous oxidants that may be responsible for Hg(0) oxidation (e.g., NO_3, HO_2, O^{1D}, O^{3P}, HOCl, HOBr; Schroeder et al. (1991); Lin and Pehkonen (1999)), the kinetic and mechanistic data are not available and therefore are not discussed here. Oxidation of Hg(0) is the first and most important step for Hg removal from the atmosphere. Understanding the oxidation processes provides important insight into the atmospheric lifetime of mercury.

4.3.1   Oxidation of Hg(0) by O_3

Ozone is a daytime oxidant produced from photochemical reactions involving volatile organic compounds (VOC), oxides of nitrogen (NO_x), and molecular oxygen. Stratospheric ozone can also enter the troposphere through vertical mixing (Shim et al., 2008).

The oxidation of Hg(0) by O_3 (G1 in Table 4.4) was first investigated by (P'yankov, 1949) using an absolute kinetic technique with very high concentrations of O_3 (5.5 mg/m^3) and Hg(0) (7.9 mg/m^3). Although the rate coefficient was not reported, P'yankov (1949) observed that a yellow-brown solid (assumed to be HgO) was produced from the reaction. P'yankov's data have been used by several groups to calculate the rate coefficient. Slemr et al. (1985) estimated a rate coefficient of 4.2×10^{-19} cm^3/molec/s at 293 K. Schroeder et al. (1991) reported a value of 4.9×10^{-18} cm^3/molec/s at 293 K (or 8.4×10^{-18} cm^3/molec/s at 303 K). Iverfeldt and Lindqvist (1986) also measured the Hg(0)–O_3 reaction kinetics using lower reactant concentrations (i.e., 0.4–1.8 μg/m^3 Hg(0) and 70–200 ppbv O_3). They reported a rate coefficient of 1.7×10^{-18} cm^3/molec/s (at 20°C and 71% relative humidity), although it is suggested that the oxidation may occur in the water film formed on the quartz reactor wall during the experiment.

To eliminate the possible contribution by reactor walls to the observed oxidation rate, Hall (1995) reexamined the kinetics of this reaction using a pseudo-first-order kinetic technique with high concentrations of O_3 (20–1500 ppm) in Teflon reactors of different surface-to-volume (S/V) ratios. By extrapolating the kinetic data to zero S/V, a rate coefficient of $(3 \pm 2) \times 10^{-20}$ cm^3/molec/s was estimated. This is the rate coefficient used by most of the global and regional models (Bullock and Brehme (2002); Travnikov (2005); Seigneur et al. (2006, 2007), Dastoor et al. (2008)). Hall also measured the oxidation rate at various temperature, humidity, and sunlight levels. Relative humidity did not have an effect on the reaction rate. This was attributed to the hydrophobicity of the Teflon reactors, which prevents the formation of a water film on reactor walls at high relative humidity. Solar irradiation increased the rate by six fold, although the cause of the increased rate is not clear. Increasing the temperature also enhanced the rate. No product identification was performed in the study. Therefore, it was unclear whether HgO was produced in the gas phase.

TABLE 4.4 Current Understanding of Mercury Reactions and Kinetic Parameters in the Gas Phase

Reaction No.	Reaction Type	Mechanism	Buffer Gas[a]	Rate Coefficient	References
G1	Ox.	$Hg(0)(g) + O_3(g) \longrightarrow$ $HgO(s) + O_2(g)$	N/A, 1 atm	4.2×10^{-19} cm³/molec/s	P'yankov (1949) and Slemr et al. (1985)
			N/A, 1 atm	4.9×10^{-18} cm³/molec/s	P'yankov (1949) and Schroeder et al. (1991)
			Air, 1 atm	1.7×10^{-18} cm³/molec/s	Iverfeldt and Lindqvist (1986)
			N_2/O_2, 1 atm	$(3 \pm 2) \times 10^{-20}$ cm³/molec/s	Hall (1995)
			N_2, 1 atm	$(7.5 \pm 0.9) \times 10^{-19}$ cm³/molec/s	Pal and Ariya (2004b)
			Air, 1 atm	$(6.4 \pm 2.3) \times 10^{-19}$ cm³/molec/s	Sumner et al. (2005)
			N_2, 1 atm	$(6.2 \pm 1.1) \times 10^{-19}$ cm³/molec/s	Snider et al. (2008)
G2	Ox.	$Hg(0)(g) + {}^{\cdot}OH(g) \longrightarrow$ $HgOH(g)$	Air, 1 atm	$(8.7 \pm 2.8) \times 10^{-14}$ cm³/molec/s	Sommar et al. (2001)
		${}^{\cdot}HgOH(g) + O_2(g) \longrightarrow$ $HgO(s) + HO$	N/A, 1 atm (343 K)	$(1.6 \pm 0.2) \times 10^{-11}$ cm³/molec/s	Miller et al. (2001)
			Air, 1 atm	$<1.2 \times 10^{-13}$ cm³/molec/s	Bauer et al. (2003)
			N/A, 1 atm (180–400 K)	$3.2 \times 10^{-13}(T/298K)^{-3.06}$ cm³/molec/s	Goodsite et al (2004)
			N/A, 1 atm (298 K)	3.2×10^{-13} cm³/molec/s	Goodsite et al. (2004)
			Air/N_2, 1 atm	$(9.0 \pm 1.3) \times 10^{-14}$ cm³/molec/s	Pal and Ariya (2004a)

(continued)

TABLE 4.4 (*Continued*)

Reaction No.	Reaction Type	Mechanism	Buffer Gas[a]	Rate Coefficient	References
G3	Ox.	$Hg(0)(g) + NO_3(g) \longrightarrow$ $HgO(g) + NO_2(g)$	N_2, $(5 - 10) \times 10^{-3}$ atm	$< 4 \times 10^{-15}$ cm^3/molec/s	Sommar et al. (1997)
			Air, 1 atm	$< 7 \times 10^{-15}$ cm^3/molec/s	Sumner et al. (2005)
G4	Ox.	$Hg(0)(g) + NO_3(g) \longrightarrow$ $HgO(g) + NO_2(g)$	N/A, 1 atm	$\leq 4.1 \times 10^{-16}$ cm^3/molec/s	Seigneur et al. (1994)
			N_2, N/A	$< 8.5 \times 10^{-19}$ cm^3/molec/s	Tokos et al. (1998)
G5	Ox.	$Hg(0)(g) + Cl(g) \longrightarrow$ $HgCl(g)$	Ar, 0.93 atm	$(3.2 \pm 1.7) \times 10^{-11}$ cm^3/molec/s	Horne et al. (1968)
			Air, NO, 1 atm	6.4×10^{-11} cm^3/molec/s	Spicer et al. (2002)
			Air, N_2, 1 atm	$(1.0 \pm 0.2) \times 10^{-11}$ cm^3/molec/s	Ariya et al. (2002)
			N/A, 1 atm	1.38×10^{-12} $\exp(208.02/T)$ cm^3/molec/s	Khalizov et al. (2003)
			N/A, 1 atm (298 K)	2.81×10^{-12} cm^3/molec/s	Khalizov et al. (2003)
			N_2 (243–298 K)	$(2.2 \pm 0.5) \times 10^{-32} \exp[(680 \pm 400)(1/T - 1/298)]$cm^6/molec^2/s^1	Donohoue et al. (2005)
			N_2, 1 atm (298 K)	5.4×10^{-13} cm^3/molec/s	Donohoue et al. (2005)
			N_2, 1 atm	1.2×10^{-10} cm^3/molec/s	Byun et al. (2010)

		Reaction	Conditions	Rate	Reference
G6	Ox.	$Hg(0)(g) + Br(g) \longrightarrow$ $HgBr(g)$	Air, N_2, 1 atm	$(3.2 \pm 0.3) \times 10^{-12}$ cm^3/molec/s	Ariya et al. (2002)
			Air, NO, 1 atm	9×10^{-13} cm^3/molec/s	Spicer et al. (2002)
			N/A, 1 atm	$1.01 \times 10^{-12} \exp(209.03/T)$cm^3/molec/s	Khalizov et al. (2003)
			N/A, 1 atm (298 K)	2.07×10^{-12} cm^3/molec/s	Khalizov et al. (2003)
			N/A, (180–400 K)	$1.1 \times 10^{-12}(T/298\mathrm{K})^{-2.37}$ cm^3/molec/s	Goodsite et al. (2004)
			N/A, 1 atm (298 K)	1.1×10^{-12} cm^3/molec/s	Goodsite et al. (2004)
			N_2, (243–298 K)	$(1.46 \pm 0.34) \times 10^{-32} \times (T/298)^{-(1.86 \pm 1.49)}$ cm^6/molec^2/s	Donohoue et al. (2006)
			N_2, 1 atm (298 K)	$(3.6 \pm 0.9) \times 10^{-13}$ cm^3/molec/s	Donohoue et al. (2006)
			Ar, 1 atm	$9.80 \times 10^{-13} \exp[401(1/T - 1/298)]$cm^3/molec/s	Shepler et al. (2007)
			Ar, 1 atm (298 K)	9.8×10^{-13} cm^3/molec/s	Shepler et al. (2007)
G7	Ox.	$HgBr(g) + Br(g) \longrightarrow$ $HgBr_2(g)$	CF_3Br, 0.26 atm	7×10^{-17} cm^3/molec/s	Greig et al. (1970)
			N/A, 1 atm (180–400 K)	$2.5 \times 10^{-10}(T/298\mathrm{K})^{-0.57}$ cm^3/molec/s	Goodsite et al. (2004)
			N/A, 1 atm (298 K)	2.5×10^{-10} cm^3/molec/s	Goodsite et al. (2004)

(continued)

TABLE 4.4 (*Continued*)

Reaction No.	Reaction Type	Mechanism	Buffer Gas[a]	Rate Coefficient	References
G8	Ox.	$Hg(0)(g) + F(g) \longrightarrow$ $HgF(g)$	N/A, 1 atm	$0.92 \times 10^{-12} \exp(206.81/T) cm^3/$ molec/s	Khalizov et al. (2003)
G9	Ox.	$Hg(0)(g) + I(g) \longrightarrow HgI(g)$	N/A, 1 atm (298 K)	$1.86 \times 10^{-12} cm^3/$ molec/s	Khalizov et al. (2003)
			N/A, 1 atm (180–400 K)	$4.0 \times 10^{-13}(T/298K)^{-2.38} cm^3/$ molec/s	Goodsite et al. (2004)
			N/A, 1 atm (298 K)	$4.0 \times 10^{-13} cm^3/molec/s$	Goodsite et al. (2004)
G10	Ox.	$Hg(0)(g) + Cl_2(g) \longrightarrow$ $HgCl_2(g)$	Air, N_2, 1 atm	$(2.6 \pm 0.2) \times 10^{-18} cm^3/molec/s$	Ariya et al. (2002)
			Air, 1 atm	$(2.5 \pm 0.9) \times 10^{-18} cm^3/molec/s$	Sumner et al. (2005)
			N_2, 1 atm	$4.3 \times 10^{-15} cm^3/molec/s$	Byun et al. (2010)
G11	Ox.	$Hg(0)(g) + Br_2(g) \longrightarrow$ $HgBr_2(g)$	Air, N_2, 1 atm	$<(0.9 \pm 0.2) \times 10^{-16} cm^3/molec/s$	Ariya et al. (2002)
G12	Ox.	$Hg(0)(g) + F_2(g) \longrightarrow$ Hg^{2+} + Products	Air, 1 atm	$(1.8 \pm 0.4) \times 10^{-15} cm^3/molec/s$	Sumner et al. (2005)
G13	Ox.	$Hg(0)(g) + ClO(g) \longrightarrow$	N_2, 1 atm	$\leq (1.27 \pm 0.58) \times$ $10^{-19} cm^3/molec/s$	Raofie et al. (2008)
G14	Ox.	$Hg(0)(g) + ClO(g) \longrightarrow$ $HgClO(g)$	N_2, 1 atm	$1.1 \times 10^{-11} cm^3/molec/s$	Byun et al. (2010)

No.		Reaction	Conditions	Rate constant	Reference
G15	Ox.	$Hg(0)(g) + BrO(g) \longrightarrow HgBrO(g)$	Air, NO, 1 atm	$(3.0\text{–}6.4) \times 10^{-14}$ cm^3/molec/s	Spicer et al. (2002)
G16		$(CH_3)_2Hg(g) + O_3(g) \longrightarrow$ Products	N_2, 1 atm	$(1\text{–}100) \times 10^{-15}$ cm^3/molec/s	Raofie and Ariya (2003)
				$<10^{-21}$ cm^3/molec/s	Niki et a. (1983b)
G17		$(CH_3)_2Hg(g) + {}^{\bullet}OH(g) \longrightarrow (CH_3)_2HgOH(g) + CH_3(g)$	Air, 0.92 atm	$(1.97 \pm 0.23) \times 10^{-11}$ cm^3/molec/s	Niki et al. (1983b)
				2.72×10^{-13} cm^3/molec/s	Meylan and Howard (1993)
G18		$(CH_3)_2Hg(g) + Cl^{\bullet}(g) \longrightarrow CH_3HgCl(g) + CH_3(g)$		$(2.75 \pm 0.30) \times 10^{-10}$ cm^3/molec/s	Niki et al. (1983a)
G19		$(CH_3)_2Hg(g) + NO_3^{\bullet}(g) \longrightarrow Hg(0)(g) + HgO(g) +$ Products		$(7.4 \pm 2.6) \times 10^{-14}$ cm^3/molec/s	Sommar et al. (1996)
G20		$(CH_3)_2Hg(g) + O(^3P)(g) \longrightarrow HgO(s) +$ Products		$(2.5 \pm 0.2) \times 10^{-11}$ cm^3/molec/s	Thomsen and Egsgaard (1986)
G21		$(CH_3)_2Hg(g) + 18F^{\bullet}(g) \longrightarrow$ Products		$(4.7 \pm 0.5) \times 10^{-10}$ cm^3/molec/s	McKeown et al. (1983)

Ox., oxidation.
[a]Room temperature, unless noted otherwise.

Later, Pal and Ariya (2004b) reinvestigated the oxidation of Hg(0) by O_3 using both absolute and relative kinetic techniques with halocarbon wax coating on reactor walls to prevent unwanted reactions on the surface. They estimated a rate coefficient of $(7.5 \pm 0.9) \times 10^{-19}$ cm^3/molec/s that accounts for a primary gas-phase reaction and possibly a secondary reaction on reactor walls with the absolute kinetic technique. With the relative kinetic approach, Hg(0) decay was observed relative to the decay of propene and 1-butene under N_2, which yielded the same rate as in the absolute approach. The rate is about 25 times greater than the value reported by Hall (1995). However, it was comparable to the value derived from a later study by Sumner et al. (2005), $(6.4 \pm 2.3) \times 10^{-19}$ cm^3/molec/s, using a pseudo-first-order kinetic technique, where a reactor with a very large volume $(17.3 \ m^3)$ was used to minimize wall reactions. In the experiments of Pal and Ariya (2004b), the oxidation produced <1% of airborne PHg with HgO on the reactor walls identified as the primary product. The gas-phase product was not confirmed. Sumner et al. (2005) suggested that 30–40% of oxidized mercury was deposited on the wall surfaces.

More recent work by Snider et al. (2008) examined the effects of S/V ratio and concentrations of $H_2O(g)$ and $CO(g)$ on the oxidation kinetics of Hg(0) by O_3 using a relative kinetic technique. The study reported a rate coefficient of $(6.2 \pm 1.1) \times 10^{-19}$ cm^3/molec/s with $\pm 20\%$ composite uncertainty on account of the experimental setup error. This is comparable to the rate reported by Pal and Ariya (2004b) and Sumner et al. (2005). Increases in the S/V ratio and CO concentrations were found to accelerate the reaction. Also, a nonlinear positive relationship was found between the rate and relative humidity. Through the use of mass spectrometry (MS) and high resolution transmission electron microscopy coupled to electron-dispersive spectrometer (HRTEM-EDS), the product was identified as HgO and the product phase was confirmed as solid on a carbon grid at 50% relative humidity, probably due to the elevated concentrations used in their experiments.

Interestingly, the agreeable kinetic data reported by the three most recent experimental studies do not seem to conform to the understanding of atmospheric lifetime of mercury. With these rate coefficients, the lifetime of Hg(0) would be about 20–30 days based on 30 ppbv of background O_3, much shorter than the accepted 0.5–1.5 years. Atmospheric modeling using the higher rate $(7.5 \times 10^{-19}$ cm^3/molec/s) also does not produce a reasonable global Hg(0) concentration distribution (Seigneur et al., 2006). These suggest that the oxidation of Hg(0) by O_3 under atmospheric conditions may be very different from what has been observed in the laboratory studies.

A number of theoretical analyses using quantum chemical computation and kinetic modeling have also been attempted to better understand this gas-phase oxidation pathway. On the basis of the results of quantum chemical kinetic analysis performed by Shepler and Peterson (2003) and Tossell (2003), Hynes et al. (2009) suggested that a homogeneous gas-phase oxidation of Hg(0) by O_3 is very unlikely to be energetically favorable. This is in agreement with another computational study (Castro et al., 2009), where the reaction was reported to be endothermic by 72.3 kJ/mol with an activation barrier of 259.4 kJ/mol, too high to be kinetically favorable.

To explain the observed "fast" kinetics in the laboratory investigations, Calvert and Lindberg (2005) hypothesized that the laboratory-observed HgO may be an artifact from the decomposition of HgO_3 intermediate on reactor walls and argued that the production of gaseous HgO is unlikely in the atmosphere because of unfavorable thermodynamics. They proposed a possible pathway of Hg(0) oxidation by O_3 via homogeneous, exothermic (about 16 kJ/mol) gas-phase reaction with an enthalpy change to produce HgO_3 as the primary product. The produced HgO_3 can survive thermal and photochemical decomposition, and then transform into $Hg(OH)_2$ or HgX_2 (X = Cl, Br) after depositing onto moist aerosols in the atmosphere or on reactor walls. However, Hynes et al. (2009) argued that the oxidation by a heterogeneous pathway is also unlikely in the atmosphere because of the ultra-trace concentrations of Hg(0). Even if the heterogeneous reaction could occur, it must be at a rate much smaller than those derived from laboratory chamber experiments in order to reproduce reasonable global Hg(0) concentration in models, because the availability of surface area in the atmosphere is limited unless in clouds and fogs (Seigneur et al., 2006).

4.3.2 Oxidation of Hg(0) by OH

The hydroxyl radical is the most important oxidant for many trace gases (both organic and inorganic) in the atmosphere. The sources of OH are from reactions of water vapor and excited atomic oxygen produced from the photolysis of O_3, nitrous acid (HONO), nitric acid (HNO_3), hydrogen peroxide (H_2O_2), and peroxynitric acid (HO_2NO_2) (Jacobson, 2005).

The gas-phase oxidation of Hg(0) by OH was first examined by Sommar et al. (2001). In their experiment, OH was produced from the photolysis of methyl nitrite, and cyclohexane (C_6H_{12}) was used as the reference molecule in a relative kinetic method. They estimated a rate coefficient of $(8.7 \pm 2.8) \times 10^{-14}$ cm^3/molec/s, and proposed the formation of $^\bullet HgOH$ as an intermediate, followed by its reaction with O_2 to produce HgO(s) and HO_2 (G2 in Table 4.4). Although there was no evaluation of possible heterogeneous reactions at reactor walls, a relatively low S/V ratio (~ 0.1 cm^{-1}) and the use of perfluorinated material were believed to minimize surface reactions. About the same time, a higher rate was reported by Miller et al. (2001), $(1.6 \pm 0.2) \times 10^{-11}$ cm^3/molec/s at 343 K without product identification in a preliminary study.

Later, Bauer et al. (2003) used a pulsed laser photolysis-pulsed laser-induced fluorescence (PLP-PLIF) approach to monitor the decay of OH using a pseudo-first-order kinetic technique with excess Hg(0) at room temperature and atmospheric pressure in both air and He buffer gases. They reported no evidence of the oxidation and estimated an upper rate limit of 1.2×10^{-13} cm^3/molec/s for the reaction. More recently, Pal and Ariya (2004a) studied the reaction using a relative kinetic technique with $^\bullet OH$ generated by the photolysis of isopropyl nitrite in the presence of air and NO in a halocarbon wax-coated reactor. Cyclohexane, n-butane and 2-methylcyclopropane were used as reference compounds. They reported a rate coefficient of $(9.0 \pm 1.3) \times 10^{-14}$ cm^3/molec/s, which is comparable to the rate estimated by Sommar et al. (2001), but more than two orders of magnitude slower compared to the rate reported by Miller et al. (2001) and also slower than a theoretically derived value by Goodsite et al. (2004), 3.2×10^{-13} cm^3/molec/s. Using mass spectroscopic detection, the oxidation products by OH were identified as 6% PHg and 10% RGM, both as HgO, the rest being various wall-sorbed species (Ariya et al., 2002; Pal and Ariya, 2004a).

However, Calvert and Lindberg (2005) reexamined the kinetic data of Pal and Ariya (2004a) and argued that the rate for the Hg(0)–OH reaction may be very much overestimated because of the presence of other reactive radicals (i.e., HO$_2$, RO, RO$_2$, NO, and NO$_2$) and O$_3$, which were also present during the generation of OH under the experimental conditions. Furthermore, since the oxidation of Hg(0) by OH may be greatly attenuated by HgOH decomposition back to Hg(0) and OH (Goodsite et al., 2004), and there are many other trace gases (with much higher concentrations than Hg(0)) competing for OH, the oxidation of Hg(0) by OH in the atmosphere is potentially unimportant (Calvert and Lindberg, 2005). Thermodynamically, Hynes et al. (2009) suggested that the reaction is not energetically favorable based on new HgO thermochemistry. More studies that can rule out the interferences caused by other reactive radicals during the experiment are clearly needed for this reaction.

4.3.3 Oxidation of Hg(0) by NO$_3^{\bullet}$

Nitrate radical (NO$_3^{\bullet}$) is a nighttime oxidant generated mainly from reaction of O$_3$ and nitrogen dioxide (NO$_2$) (Finlayson-Pitts and Pitts, 2000b). The slow photolysis of dinitrogen pentoxide (N$_2$O$_5$) can also produce NO$_3^{\bullet}$ during the day ($\lambda < 385$ nm), but it is much less important, because it can be quickly photolyzed (Jacobson, 2005).

The first investigation for NO$_3^{\bullet}$ as an oxidant for Hg(0) in the gas phase was conducted by Sommar et al. (1997) using a fast flow discharge technique in a halocarbon wax-coated reactor. The reaction of fluorine atoms discharged by microwave in excess of nitric acid was used to generate NO$_3^{\bullet}$. Without identifying the reaction products, they reported a rate coefficient of 4×10^{-15} cm^3/molec/s and found the rate to be an upper limit (G3 in Table 4.4). The rate is in agreement with the result from another recent investigation performed by Sumner et al. (2005) using a relative rate technique with dimethyl sulfide (CH$_3$)$_2$S as the reference compound (7×10^{-15} cm^3/molec/s). Sommar et al. (1997) estimated the reaction to be exothermic by 12 kJ/mol. However, on the basis of the new HgO thermochemistry, Hynes et al. (2009) estimated a significant endothermicity of 195 kJ/mol and considered this oxidation pathway not important in the atmosphere.

4.3.4 Oxidation of Hg(0) by H₂O₂

Hydrogen peroxide (H_2O_2) is produced from the photooxidation of formaldehyde and hydrocarbons in the presence of NO_x or from radical–radical reaction of HO_2. Therefore, it can exist in both polluted and clean air at 1–5 ppbv near the Earth's surface (Finlayson-Pitts and Pitts, 2000a).

The first report on the rate of Hg(0) oxidation by H_2O_2 was in a chemical modeling study by Seigneur et al. (1994) as $\leq 4.1 \times 10^{-16}$ cm³/molec/s. An experimental investigation was performed by Tokos et al. (1998) using Teflon reactors of various S/V ratios. The experiment was performed in the dark and the reaction was assumed to follow the scheme proposed by Seigneur et al. (1994) (G4 in Table 4.4). The gas-phase rate coefficient was estimated to be in the range of $3.5–8.5 \times 10^{-19}$ cm³/molec/s, about three orders of magnitude smaller than the value used by Seigneur et al. (1994). There was also no product identification in this experiment.

4.3.5 Oxidation of Hg(0) by Halogen Atoms, Molecules, and Monoxides

Gaseous reactive halogen species (i.e., Cl, Cl_2, ClO, HOCl, Br, Br_2, BrO, HOBr, I, I_2, IO, etc.) can either be produced autocatalytically from sea salt aerosols or come from the anthropogenic release of NO_x and halogenated compounds followed by atmospheric processing (Simpson et al., 2007; Mahajan et al., 2010). Given the favorable environmental conditions, their concentrations can be high enough to cause rapid oxidation of Hg(0) in the marine boundary layers (Laurier et al., 2003; Hedgecock and Pirrone, 2004; Holmes et al., 2009) or in the Polar Regions (Steffen et al., 2002; Lindberg et al., 2002a; Ariya et al., 2004; Goodsite et al., 2004; Simpson et al., 2007), and possibly in the free troposphere and stratosphere (Holmes et al., 2006; Lindberg et al., 2007). These reactions are particularly believed to play an important role during AMDEs when atmospheric Hg(0) is rapidly depleted from ~ 1.7 ng/m³ to <0.1 ng/m³ within 24–48 h after the Polar springtime sunrise (Schroeder and Munthe, 1998; Lindberg et al., 2002a; Skov et al., 2006; Steffen et al., 2008). In this section, the oxidation of Hg(0) by a number of reactive halogen species is presented.

4.3.5.1 Oxidation of Hg(0) by Cl Atoms. The Hg(0)-Cl reaction was first investigated by Horne et al. (1968) in CF_3Cl and argon gas mixture, with an estimated rate coefficient of $1.5–5.0 \times 10^{-11}$ cm³/molec/s at 383–443 K (G5 in Table 4.4). They noted an uncertainty level of three in their experiment and proposed that HgCl was formed followed by a dimerization step to form Hg_2Cl_2. Later, Spicer et al. (2002) and Ariya et al. (2002) studied the same reaction in gaseous media more relevant to the atmosphere. Spicer et al. (2002) employed a relative kinetic technique in a fairly large environmental chamber (17.3 m³) and estimated a rate coefficient of 6.4×10^{-11} cm³/molec/s. Ariya et al. (2002) studied the reaction using relative (using five reference compounds), and reported a rate coefficient of $1.0 \pm 0.2 \times 10^{-11}$ cm³/molec/s. The oxidation

products identified using MS, gas chromatography-mass spectrometry (GC-MS), and inductively coupled plasma mass spectrometry (ICP-MS) showed $HgCl_2$ as the primary product, mainly on the reactor walls, with a small fraction ($<0.5\%$) in the aerosol phase captured in a microfilter. This suggested that the reaction may be principally in the gas phase or on the surface. These three studies showed a good agreement in the kinetic estimate. However, Hynes et al. (2009) suspected that the experiment by Spicer et al. (2002) could suffer from the effects of potential side reactions of Cl and O_2, which produces ClO_2 that consumes Cl and may directly react with Hg(0). This would lead to an overestimation of the reaction rate. The results in Ariya et al. (2002) also could not rule out the effect of side reactions between the reference molecules and OH (Hynes et al., 2009).

Alternatively, Donohoue et al. (2005) used a PLP-PLIF system to measure the rate over a wide range of temperatures and pressures in a pseudo-first-order manner in excess of either Hg(0) or Cl. Concentrations of both reactants were monitored simultaneously. One challenge of the experiment was that Cl was calculated from Cl_2 photolysis, because it cannot be measured accurately so that the potential side reactions initiated by Cl and O_2 could not be ruled out. Using N_2 as a buffer gas, the rate coefficient was estimated to be $(2.2 \pm 0.5) \times 10^{-32}$ $\exp[(680 \pm 400)(1/T - 1/298)]$ $cm^6/molec^2/s$ with an uncertainty of $\pm 50\%$. This translates to 7.6×10^{-13} $cm^3/molec/s$ at 260 K, 760 Torr (Donohoue et al., 2005), two orders of magnitudes smaller than the previous studies. $HgCl_2$ was also believed to be the primary product through a two-step chlorination process.

Recently, Byun et al. (2010) revisited the Hg(0)–Cl reaction in the presence of NO. In their experiment, NO_2–$NOClO_2$ was used to produce OClO to yield OCl and NO_2 via a reaction with NO. The oxidation efficiency based on observed Hg(0) decay was found to increase with increasing NO concentration. Using kinetic simulation constrained by the experimental data, the rate coefficient of Hg(0)–Cl oxidation was estimated to be 1.2×10^{-10} $cm^3/molec/s$ with an uncertainty attributed to unknown surface reactions in addition to the gas-phase oxidation (Byun et al., 2010).

Quantum chemical computations have also been applied to estimate the rate. An excellent summary of the computational methods as well as their limitations has been summarized by Ariya et al. (2009). Khalizov et al. (2003) used Gaussian 94 and Gaussian 98 software to estimate the rate and reported a rate coefficient of 2.81×10^{-12} $cm^3/molec/s$ for a two-step chlorination process with the possibility of dissociation of HgCl. However, Hynes et al. (2009) suggested that the assumption made for Hg(0)–Cl collisions in the study overestimates the stabilization of vibrationally excited diatomic HgCl*, possibly resulting in overestimated rate constant.

4.3.5.2 Oxidation of Hg(0) by Br Atoms.

Oxidation of Hg(0) by Br follows a two-step process similar to that of Hg(0)–Cl reaction (G6 and G7 in Table 4.4). The reaction kinetics was investigated by Ariya et al. (2002) using a relative kinetic technique with the photolysis of dibromomethane as the Br source. A rate coefficient of $(3.2 \pm 0.3) \times 10^{-12}$ cm^3/molec/s was obtained. With the large amount of cyclohexane added as the OH scavenger, wall adsorption of reactants became increased and this complicated the estimate of the rate coefficient (Ariya et al., 2002). HgBr$_2$ was identified as the primary product, mainly on the reactor walls, with little in the particulate phase. It was also noted that only one reference compound was used in the relative kinetic study. Because the accuracy of such a kinetic method is dependent on the accuracy of the rate of the reference reactions, a further examination of Hg(0)–Br kinetics using additional reference compounds would be needed (Ariya et al., 2009). The reaction was also investigated by Spicer et al. (2002) using DMS and propene as the reference compounds. Both reference molecules yield somewhat slower rate coefficients compared to the value reported by Ariya et al. (2002), with the value of 9×10^{-13} cm^3/molec/s relative to propene, which was recommended because of a smaller uncertainty.

Donohoue et al. (2006) investigated the kinetics of the Hg(0)–Br combination (G7 in Table 4.4) using PLP-PLIF to monitor the decay of Br and Hg(0) in excess of Br with N$_2$ and He as third body gases. They reported a rate coefficient as a function of pressure and temperature, which translates to $(3.6 \pm 0.9) \times 10^{-13}$ cm^3/molec/s at 298 K. This is about one order of magnitude smaller than the value reported by Ariya et al. (2002). An earlier study of the HgBr–Br combination (G8 in Table 4.4) using an absolute kinetic technique estimated a rate coefficient of 7×10^{-17} cm^3/molec/s at 397 K using CF$_3$Br as the buffer gas (Greig et al., 1970).

Rate constant determination using quantum chemical computations gives rate coefficients falling between the values of experimental investigations. Khalizov et al. (2003) estimated a rate coefficient of 2.07×10^{-12} cm^3/molec/s based on the assumption of strong collisional deactivation of excited HgBr (the same assumption as for the Hg(0)–Cl reaction). Another computational study by Goodsite et al. (2004) suggested a comparable rate coefficient at 1.1×10^{-12} cm^3/molec/s at 298 K and 760 Torr based on a weaker temperature-independent deactivation. They also estimated the rate coefficient of the HgBr–Br reaction to be 2.5×10^{-10} cm^3/molec/s at 298 K, indicating that the first oxidation step is the rate-determining step. This also suggested that HgBr competes with Hg(0) for available Br during the oxidation process. Recently, Shepler et al. (2007) performed kinetic calculations based on the collision-induced dissociation (CID) of HgBr in the presence of Ar, and obtained a rate coefficient of $9.80 \times 10^{-13}\exp[401(1/T - 1/298)]$ cm^3/molec/s, equivalent to 9.8×10^{-13} cm^3/molec/s at 298 K.

4.3.5.3 Oxidation of Hg(0) by Molecular Halogens (Cl$_2$, Br$_2$, F$_2$) and Atomic Fluorine (F).

The oxidation of Hg(0) by molecular halogens was extensively studied by Ariya et al. (2002) using the absolute rate method (G10 and G11 in Table 4.4), with estimated rate coefficients of $(2.6 \pm 0.2) \times 10^{-18}$ and less than $(0.9 \pm 0.2) \times 10^{-16}$ cm^3/molec/s for the Hg(0)–Cl$_2$ and Hg(0)–Br$_2$ reaction, respectively. The identified products were HgCl$_2$ and HgBr$_2$. Sumner et al. (2005) reexamined the kinetics of Hg(0) oxidation by Cl$_2$, Br$_2$, and F$_2$ using an absolute kinetic technique in a Teflon-coated (FTP) reactor. They estimated the rate coefficient of the Hg(0)–Cl$_2$ reaction to be $(2.5 \pm 0.9) \times 10^{-18}$ cm^3/molec/s, in excellent agreement with the rate reported by Ariya et al. (2002). However, they reported no evidence of the Hg(0)–Br$_2$ reaction after 2 h of reaction time and suggested that it could be due to the large reactor and low reactant concentrations in their experiment that reduced the wall effects. More recently, Byun et al. (2010) studied the Hg(0)–Cl$_2$ reaction in the presence of NO and estimated a rate coefficient of 4.3×10^{-15} cm^3/molec/s for the Hg(0)–Cl$_2$ reaction, much faster than the values reported earlier. This was attributed to unknown surface-induced oxidation processes of the gas mixture in their experiment (Byun et al., 2010).

The rate of the Hg(0)–F$_2$ reaction (G12 in Table 4.4) was estimated to be $(1.8 \pm 0.4) \times 10^{-15}$ cm^3/molec/s using an absolute kinetic technique by Sumner et al. (2005). The reaction product was deposited on reactor walls, but not identified. The oxidation of Hg(0) by atomic fluorine (G8 in Table 4.4) was estimated computationally by Khalizov et al. (2003). The authors reported a temperature-dependent rate coefficient of $0.92 \times 10^{-12} \exp(206.81/T)$, or 1.86×10^{-12} cm^3/molec/s at 298 K.

4.3.5.4 *Oxidation of Hg(0) by Halogen Monoxides (ClO and BrO).* The oxidation of Hg(0) by BrO (G15 in Table 4.4) was investigated by Spicer et al. (2002) and Raofie and Ariya (2003), both by relative kinetic techniques. Spicer et al. (2002) generated BrO through Br$_2$ photolysis in the presence of O$_3$ with (CH$_3$)$_2$S as the reference compound, and estimated the rate coefficient to be in the range of $(3.0-6.4) \times 10^{-14}$ cm^3/molec/s. Raofie and Ariya (2003) employed visible and UV photolysis of bromine and dibromomethane in the presence of O$_3$ as the BrO source and three reference compounds (i.e., propane, butane, and DMS) for the rate determination. They estimated the rate coefficient to be in the range of (1.0×10^{-15}) and (1.0×10^{-13}) cm^3/molec/s, with HgBr, HgBrO (HgOBr), and HgO as the possible products. Both studies could not rule out the contributions from Br produced during the generation of BrO. The rate of the Hg(0)–ClO reaction (G14 in Table 4.4) was recently investigated by Byun et al. (2010) using the reaction of OClO (produced by NO$_2$ and NOClO$_2$) and NO. Using kinetic modeling constrained by the experimental data, the rate coefficient of the Hg(0)–ClO oxidation was estimated to be 1.1×10^{-11} cm^3/molec/s.

Possible mechanisms of the Hg(0)–BrO reaction were investigated using quantum chemical computations. The pathway for the production of HgBr(g) + O was unlikely to be thermodynamically favorable (Hynes et al., 2009). The production of HgO(g) + Br is also strongly endothermic (Khalizov et al., 2003; Shepler and Peterson, 2003; Peterson et al., 2007); therefore, it appeared unlikely that HgO(g) is the primary oxidation product. The production of HgBrO was proposed to be the primary first-step pathway. Although the formation of HgBrO is exothermic, being an insertion reaction, this process should be extremely slow.

4.3.5.5 *Oxidation of Hg(0) by I, I$_2$, and IO.* Raofie et al. (2008) studied the oxidation products of Hg(0) by I, I$_2$, and IO using GC-MS. The reaction products

were identified as HgI_2, HgIO (or HgOI), HgO, and HgI. The kinetic study was also performed for the Hg(0)–I_2 reaction (G13 in Table 4.4) at 740 Torr, 296 ± 2 K in the presence of N_2 and air using an absolute kinetic technique in a Teflon reactor. Again, heterogeneous reactions caused by the wall effects cannot be excluded and an upper limit of the rate coefficient was reported, $\leq$ $(1.27 \pm 0.58) \times 10^{-19}$ cm^3/molec/s.

Goodsite et al. (2004) studied the kinetics of the Hg(0)–I reaction (G9 in Table 4.4) computationally and suggested a rate coefficient of 4.0×10^{-13} cm^3/molec/s at 298 K. However, the product (HgI) was weakly bound and was likely to dissociate back to Hg(0) and I (Hynes et al., 2009). Another kinetic modeling analysis by Calvert and Lindberg (2004) demonstrated that rapid reaction of an iodine atom with ozone could indirectly enhance Hg removal by interacting with existing BrO, which results in an increase in the Br atom concentration and thus increases the rate of the Hg–Br reaction.

4.4 CHEMICAL TRANSFORMATIONS IN THE AQUEOUS PHASE

4.4.1 Oxidation Pathways

4.4.1.1 Oxidation of Hg(0) by O_3. The presence of O_3 in atmospheric water is mainly from the scavenging of gaseous O_3 (Henry's constant $= 0.013$ M atm^{-1} at 298 K). The aqueous oxidation of Hg(0) by O_3 (A1 in Table 4.5) was studied by Munthe (1992) using a relative kinetic technique with SO_3^{2-} as the reference compound at pH 5.2–6.2 and 5–35°C. He found that the reaction was independent of both pH and temperature, and reported a rate coefficient of $(4.7 \pm 2.2) \times 10^7$ M^{-1} s^{-1}. The Hg(II) produced was believed to be dissolved in the aqueous phase.

4.4.1.2 Oxidation of Hg(0) by OH. Aqueous OH can be from the scavenging of gaseous OH (Henry's constant $= 25$ M/atm at 298 K) and in-cloud production via photolysis of a number of compounds (i.e., $Fe(OH)_3$, H_2O_2, NO_3^-, HONO, etc.) (Lin and Pehkonen, 1999). The kinetics of the oxidation pathway (A2 in Table 4.5) was first investigated by Lin and Pehkonen (1997) using a steady-state kinetic technique. In this experiment, photolysis of nitrate in the presence of benzene as OH scavenger was used to maintain a steady-state concentration of OH in the aqueous phase. A rate coefficient of 2.0×10^9 M^{-1} s^{-1} was estimated for the overall reaction, which was proposed to take place in a two-step oxidation by OH, with the rate-determining step being the first step. Gårdfeldt et al. (2001) reexamined the reaction using a relative kinetic technique with CH_3Hg as the reference compound. They reported a similar rate at $(2.4 \pm 0.3) \times 10^9$ M^{-1} s^{-1}, but suggested that the reaction was mediated through the oxidation by OH followed by oxidation by dissolved O_2. The reaction is typically regarded as a single-step process in modeling analyses as shown in Table 4.5.

TABLE 4.5 Current Understanding of Mercury Reactions and Kinetic Parameters in the Aqueous Phase

Reaction NO.	Reaction Type	Mechanism	Temperature, pH	Rate Coefficient	References
A1	Ox.	$Hg(0)(aq) + O_3(aq) \xrightarrow{H^+} Hg^{2+}(aq) + OH^-(aq) + O_2(aq)$	Ambient	$(4.7 \pm 2.2) \times 10^7 M^{-1}s^{-1}$	Munthe (1992)
A2	Ox.	$Hg(0)(aq) + \cdot\ OH(aq) \longrightarrow Hg^{2+}(aq) + Products$	$298 \pm 2K$	$2.0 \times 10^9 M^{-1}s^{-1}$	Lin and Pehkonen (1997)
			$298\ K$	$(2.4 \pm 0.3) \times 10^9 M^{-1}s^{-1}$	Gårdfeldt et al. (2001)
A3	Ox.	$Hg(0)(aq) + HOCl(aq) \longrightarrow Hg^{2+}(aq) + Cl^-(aq) + OH^-(aq)$	Ambient	$(2.09 \pm 0.06) \times 10^6 M^{-1}s^{-1}$	Lin and Pehkonen (1998a)
A4	Ox.	$Hg(0)(aq) + OCl^-(aq)H^+ \xrightarrow{H^+} Hg^{2+}(aq) + Cl^-(aq) + OH^-(aq)$	Ambient	$(1.99 \pm 0.05) \times 10^6 M^{-1}s^{-1}$	Lin and Pehkonen (1998a)
A5	Ox.	$Hg(0)(aq) + HOBr(aq) \longrightarrow Hg^{2+}(aq) + Br^-(aq) + OH^-(aq)$	$295 \pm 1K$	$(0.28 \pm 0.02)M^{-1}s^{-1}$	Wang and Pehkonen (2004)
A6	Ox.	$Hg(0)(aq) + OBr^-(aq) \longrightarrow Hg^{2+}(aq) + Br^-(aq) + OH^-(aq)$	$295 \pm 1K$	$(0.27 \pm 0.04)M^{-1}s^{-1}$	Wang and Pehkonen (2004)
A7	Ox.	$Hg(0)(aq) + Br_2(aq) \longrightarrow Hg^{2+}(aq) + 2Br^-(aq)$	$295 \pm 1K$	$(0.2 \pm 0.03)M^{-1}s^{-1}$	Wang and Pehkonen (2004)
A8	Red.	$HgSO_3(aq) \longrightarrow Hg^0(aq) + S(VI)$	Ambient $279.5-307.4\ K$	$0.6s^{-1}$ $T \exp[(31.971T - 12595)/T]s^{-1}$	Munthe et al. (1991) Van Loon et al. (2000)
			$298\ K$	$(0.0106 \pm 0.0009)s^{-1}$	Van Loon et al. (2000)

A9	Red.	$Hg(SO_3)_2^{2-}(aq) \longrightarrow$ $Hg^0(aq) + S(VI)$	Ambient	$\ll 10^{-4} s^{-1}$	Munthe et al. (1991)
A10	Red.	$Hg^{2+}(aq) + HO_2(aq) \longrightarrow$ $Hg^0(aq) + Products$	275 ± 2 K	$1.7 \times 10^4 M^{-1} s^{-1}$	Pehkonen and Lin (1998)
A11	Red.	$Hg(OH)_2(aq) \overset{h\nu}{\longrightarrow} [Hg(OH)*]$ $\longleftrightarrow$ $Hg(OH)(aq) + OH(aq)$ $Hg(OH)_2(aq) \overset{h\nu}{\longrightarrow} Hg(0)(aq) +$ Products	Midday 60° N	$3 \times 10^{-7} s^{-1}$	Xiao et al. (1994)
A12	Red.	$Hg(OOC)_2 R(aq) \overset{h\nu}{\longrightarrow} Hg^+(aq) +$ $O_2 CRCO_2^-(aq)$ $^{\cdot}O_2 CRCO_2^-(aq) +$ $Hg^{2+}(aq) \overset{+H_2O}{\longrightarrow} + Hg^+(aq) +$ $CO_2(aq) + HORCO_2^-(aq) +$ $H^+(aq)$ $Hg^+(aq) + R(CO_2)_2^{2-g}(aq) \longrightarrow$ $Hg(0)(aq) + O_2 CRCO_2^-(aq)$ or $Hg^{2+}(aq) + nR(CO_2)_2^{2-} \longrightarrow$ $(Hg((OOC)_2 R)n)^{(2-2n)}$ $\overset{h\nu+H_2O}{\longrightarrow} HORCO_2 H(aq) +$ $Hg(0)(aq)$ $+CO_2(aq) + (n-1)R(CO_2)_2^{2-}$	$296 \pm 2K$, R = Oxalic acids 296 ± 2 K, R = Manolic Acids $296 \pm 2K$, R = Succinic acids	$(1.2 \pm 0.2) \times$ $10^4 M^{-1} s^{-1}$ $(4.9 \pm 0.8) \times$ $10^3 M^{-1} s^{-1}$ $(2.8 \pm 0.5) \times$ $10^3 M^{-1} s^{-1}$	Xiao et al. (1994) and Si and Ar‚ya (2008) Xiao et al. (1994) and Si and Ariya (2008) Xiao et al (1994) and Si and Ariya (2008)

Ox.. oxidation; Red.. reduction.

4.4.1.3   Oxidation of Hg(0) by Chlorine (HOCl OCl⁻). Aqueous chlorine is mainly from the scavenging of gaseous Cl_2 (Henry's constant $= 7.61 \times 10^{-2}$ M atm^{-1} at 298 K) into the aqueous phase and the oxidation of chloride by OH (Lin and Pehkonen, 1999). Once incorporated into the aqueous phase, it dissociates to form HOCl and OCl⁻ ($pK_a = 7.5$), which are the primary oxidants and also increase the solubility of total chlorine. It is a nighttime oxidant because both Cl_2 and HOCl can be readily photolyzed under solar irradiation (Impey et al., 1997).

The oxidation of Hg(0) by aqueous chlorine was first studied by Kobayashi (1987) by allowing liquid mercury to react with added chlorine. The initial rate coefficient was reported to be extremely rapid and independent of spiked chlorine concentration in the solution (Kobayashi, 1987), suggesting mass-transfer limitation from the liquid mercury droplet. The kinetic of the reaction was reevaluated by Lin and Pehkonen (1998a) using a steady-state kinetic method with chloramine as the free chlorine reservoir. They proposed two oxidation pathways (A3 and A4 in Table 4.5), with rate coefficients of $(2.09 \pm 0.06) \times 10^6$ M^{-1} s^{-1} for Hg(0)(aq)-HOCl(aq) reaction and $(1.99 \pm 0.06) \times 10^6$ M^{-1} s^{-1} Hg(0)(aq)–OCl⁻ (aq) at room temperature (23–25°C), respectively. The concentration of HOCl and OCl⁻ can be estimated from the effective Henry's constant of Cl_2 and the acid–base chemistry of dissolved chlorine as shown by Lin and Pehkonen (1999).

4.4.1.4   Oxidation of Hg(0) by Bromine (Br₂/HOBr/BrO⁻). In atmospheric water, bromine species mainly exist as HOBr, HBr, and OBr⁻ with a tendency to be converted to Br_2 and BrCl at night and photolyzed during daytime. Sources of bromine are marine aerosol, acidification of snowpack, and wave breaking on ocean surface (Wang and Pehkonen, 2004). The dissolution of Br_2 in water yields Br_2, HOBr, and OBr⁻. Their role in oxidizing aqueous Hg(0) (A5–A7 in Table 4.5) was investigated by Wang and Pehkonen (2004) at room temperature (294–296 K), with rate coefficients of (0.28 ± 0.02), (0.27 ± 0.04), and (0.2 ± 0.03) M^{-1} s^{-1} for HOBr, OBr⁻, and Br_2, respectively. The reaction rates between elemental mercury and aqueous bromine species are much slower compared to other aqueous oxidation pathways.

4.4.2   Reduction Pathways

4.4.2.1   Reduction of Hg(II) by SO_3^{2-}. Sulfite in the aqueous phase comes from the scavenging of gaseous SO_2. Dissolved SO_2 forms H_2SO_3 and undergoes acid–base chemical dissociation that yields SO_3^{2-} and HSO_3^- (E1 and E2 in Table 4.3). SO_3^{2-} is a soft ligand and forms strong complexes with dissolved Hg(II) (E7 and E8 in Table 4.3). The reduction of aqueous Hg(II) by S(IV) (A8 and A9 in Table 4.5) was first studied by Munthe et al. (1991). They found that different Hg(II)–SO_3^{2-} complexes exhibit different reactivities. Hg(SO_3)₂$^{2-}$ is very stable, while $HgSO_3$ decomposes readily to form Hg(0) and S(VI), with first-order rate constants of $<10^{-4}$ s^{-1} and 0.6 s^{-1}, respectively.

Van Loon et al. (2000) reevaluated the reduction kinetics of $HgSO_3$(aq) and reported a temperature-dependent rate coefficient of $T \times [\exp([(31.971 \times T) - 12,595]/T)]s^{-1}$, equivalent to (0.0106 ± 0.0009) s^{-1} at $25°C$. This is a much smaller rate constant than that reported by Munthe et al. (1991) and is more widely used in modeling works (Lin et al., 2006).

4.4.2.2 Reduction of Hg(II) by HO₂.

Aqueous HO_2 is a daytime oxidant from the scavenging of gaseous HO_2 into droplets, and in-cloud production (Lin and Pehkonen, 1999). HO_2 is a weak acid with a pK_a of 5.5. The reduction of aqueous Hg(II) by HO_2 was investigated by Pehkonen and Lin (1998) using photolysis of $C_2O_4^{2-}$ as the HO_2 source. They proposed a two-step reduction by HO_2/O_2^-, with an overall rate coefficient of 1.7×10^4 M^{-1} s^{-1} (A10 in Table 4.5). However, the reduction cannot rule out the possibility of direct ligand-to-metal electron transfer within HgC_2O_4 because of the near-UV absorption band of the complex (Pehkonen and Lin, 1998).

Gårdfeldt and Jonsson (2003) reexamined the reduction pathway using pulse photolysis to generate aqueous HO_2. Although no kinetic parameter was reported, they argued that the aqueous Hg(II) reduction by HO_2/O_2^- should not occur under ambient conditions because of the possible reoxidation of Hg(I) by dissolved O_2 before the second electron transfer can take place. A direct kinetic analysis of the Hg(II)–HO_2 reaction is difficult because the generation of the radical may also produce other reactive species that interfere with the reaction itself, and further studies are therefore needed.

4.4.2.3 Photoreduction of Hg(II)–Hydroxide Complex.

$Hg(OH)_2$ can be formed from the aqueous speciation of Hg(II) with hydroxide ions, particularly at pH > 7 (E5 and E6 in Table 4.3). Xiao et al. (1994) investigated the photochemical behavior of $Hg(OH)_2$ and HgS_2^{2-} in water on irradiation. They found that $Hg(OH)_2$ can be photolyzed to produce Hg(0) four times faster than HgS_2^{2-}, with a molar extinction coefficient of ~ 1 M^{-1} cm^{-1} at $\lambda > 290$ nm. Nriagu (1994) suggested that the photoreduction of $Hg(OH)_2$ undergoes an excitation of $Hg(OH)_2$ followed by an electron transfer from OH (A11 in Table 4.5). The net reaction was typically expressed as a one-step photoreduction with an overall rate coefficient of 3×10^{-7} s^{-1} at midday $60°N$ latitude (Xiao et al., 1994).

4.4.2.4 Photoreduction of Hg(II)–dicarboxylic acid complexes (C₂-C₄).

Dicarboxylic acid ligands can exist in atmospheric droplets from the scavenging of biomass burning emissions (Erel et al., 1993; Nepotchatykh and Ariya, 2002). Si and Ariya (2008) investigated the reduction kinetics and mechanisms of a number of Hg(II)–dicarboxylic acid complexes (C_2-C_4) in excess of the organic ligands at (296 ± 2) K and pH 3.0. The production of Hg(0) was monitored and product analysis was performed using matrix-assisted laser desorption ionization time of flight mass spectrometer (MALDI-TOF-MS). They observed that the reduction is of second order and reported rate coefficients of $(1.2 \pm 0.2) \times 10^4$, $(4.9 \pm 0.8) \times 10^3$, and $(2.8 \pm 0.5) \times 10^3$ M^{-1} s^{-1} for

Hg-oxalic acid, Hg–malonic acid, and Hg–succinic acid complexes, respectively (A12 in Table 4.5). The reduction was mediated through intramolecular two-electron transfer (ligand-to-metal), in agreement with a mechanism proposed by Gårdfeldt and Jonsson (2003).

4.5 REDOX CHEMISTRY AT THE INTERFACE BETWEEN THE ATMOSPHERE AND EARTH'S SURFACES

The redox chemistry of mercury at the interface of air and surfaces plays an important role in the deposition and evasion processes of mercury. These redox reactions are mostly inferred from environmental measurements and represent a special class of chemical transformations that control mercury cycling for a given eco-system. Unfortunately, these processes are very often loosely defined owing to the challenge of identifying the oxidants/reductants under specific environmental conditions because of the trace concentration of the reactants and the complexity of involved chemistry. In this section, a summary of the results from earlier studies is provided.

4.5.1 Redox at Surface Water

Input of mercury to surface waters is mainly from wet and dry deposition, and the contribution from each is comparable (Pirrone and Mahaffey, 2005). The redox processes in fresh water are dominated by phtoreduction of Hg(II) to form Hg(0) (so-called dissolved gaseous mercury, DGM) that is subject to evasion (Ferrara et al., 2003). Dissolved organic carbons and Fe(III) species have been shown to enhance the photoreduction (Zhang and Lindberg, 2001). Several field studies have been performed to determine the photoreduction rate. O'Driscoll et al. (2006) measured the rate in lake and river water under ambient conditions in the presence of UVA and UVB irradiation using incubation techniques. They reported reduction rates of 7.76×10^{-5} s^{-1} under UVA irradiation and 8.91×10^{-5} s^{-1} under UVB irradiation in lake water; and 1.78×10^{-4} s^{-1} under UVA irradiation and 1.81×10^{-4} s^{-1} under UVB irradiation in river water, probably due to the higher dissolved organic concentration in river water. Whalin and Mason (2006) evaluated the photoredox kinetics of mercury in filtered coastal and fresh water in the absence of irradiation (Whalin and Mason, 2006). The changes in concentration due to the reduction of ^{199}Hg(II) and the oxidation of ^{202}Hg(0) for both waters were measured. Oxidation rates of $(2.6–5.3) \times 10^{-4}$ s^{-1} in coastal water and $(8.0–15) \times 10^{-4}$ s^{-1} in fresh water were estimated. Reduction rates were $(4.4–11) \times 10^{-4}$ s^{-1} for coastal water and $(2.9–11) \times 10^{-4}$ s^{-1} for fresh water. They concluded that reduction and oxidation of mercury in the water system occurred simultaneously with similar rates, and the system was expected to reach equilibrium within hours. They also found that biotic processes were less important relative to sunlight in mediating the reduction of mercury in waters (Whalin et al., 2007).

In seawater, both reduction and oxidation can be important (Ariya et al., 2009). The oxidation pathway reduces the evasion of Hg(0) from oceans (Mason and Sheu, 2002; Selin, 2009; Zhang and Hsu-Kim, 2010). The oxidation is photoinduced and promoted by halogen chemistry both above and below the water/air interface (Sheu and Mason, 2004). The reduction can occur through biological and photochemical pathways (Mason and Sheu, 2002; Selin, 2009). Only a small portion of Hg(II) is converted into more toxic methylmercury and dimethylmercury (2–35% of total mercury in oceans, Selin, 2009); while demethylation is principally mediated by microbes (Whalin et al., 2007). Methyl mercury can also be readily degraded through photolytic pathways, particularly in the presence of naturally occurring organic ligands in fresh water (Zhang and Hsu-Kim, 2010).

Qureshi et al. (2010) recently evaluated the gross reduction and oxidation of mercury in oceans using a photoreactor controlled under ambient conditions and irradiation by UVA and UVB for filtered and unfiltered samples of sea water. The plot of DGM production over time suggested that the photoredox of mercury was not simple two-species reversible reactions as proposed by earlier studies (O'Driscoll et al., 2006; Whalin and Mason, 2006; Whalin et al., 2007), but the back reaction (i.e., oxidation) could produce an unidentified intermediate mercury species that lead to the formation of either Hg(0) or Hg(II), similar to the photoredox process suggested by Nriagu (1994). The pseudo-first-order reduction rate was estimated to be from 4.17×10^{-5} to 2.58×10^{-4} s^{-1}, while the oxidation rate was in the range of $(1.11–5.27) \times 10^{-4}$ s^{-1} (Qureshi et al., 2010).

4.5.2 Chemical Processes at Soil Surfaces

Mercury accumulated in soils is primarily from wet deposition (Grigal, 2003). Soils differ greatly in their adsorption capacity, organic content, and reactivity for mercury (Gabriel and Williamson, 2004). Despite the losses of mercury to runoff and leaching to groundwater (Johnson and Lindberg, 1995; Grigal, 2003), the majority of mercury accumulated in soils is potentially evaded back to the atmosphere by reduction and desorption processes (Carpi and Lindberg, 1997), the displacement of Hg(0) after watering, or the desorption of Hg(0) due to replacement of H$_2$O molecules (Gustin and Stamenkovic, 2005), and subsequent diffusion through soil pores (Zhang et al., 2001). Evasion from soils is considered as an important source of atmospheric mercury.

Several factors have an important influence on Hg(0) evasion fluxes, including the characteristics of soils (mercury, water, and organic content), air oxidant concentration (O$_3$) and meteorological parameters (solar radiation, air temperature, wind and atmospheric turbulence, etc.) (Carpi and Lindberg, 1997; Lindberg et al., 1998; Zhang et al., 2001; Gustin et al., 2002; Scholtz et al., 2003; Poissant et al., 2004; Gustin and Stamenkovic, 2005; Moore and Carpi, 2005; Wang et al., 2007). In particular, solar radiation is found to play an important role, as it is believed to accelerate the photoreduction process in soils (Carpi and Lindberg, 1997; Gustin et al., 2002). Zhang et al. 2001 hypothesized that solar radiation could decrease the energy level required for the evasion process. Soil moisture content, air temperature, and the presence of air oxidants all enhance the evasion flux (Zhang et al., 2001; Poissant et al., 2004; Gustin and Lindberg, 2005; Gustin and Stamenkovic, 2005; Moore and Carpi, 2005). These observed flux enhancements, varying significantly for different soils and environmental conditions, were attributed to hypothesized chemical processes that are still poorly understood because of the challenge of observing chemical processes at soil surfaces.

4.5.3 Chemical Processes at Vegetation Surfaces

Plants are believed to be capable of absorbing and releasing atmospheric Hg(0) through stomata pores (Lindberg et al., 1992; Hanson et al., 1995; Ericksen et al., 2003; Ericksen and Gustin, 2004; Stamenkovic and Gustin, 2009). Stomata uptake is considered to be the main pathway for the accumulation in various leaf compartments (Ericksen et al., 2003). Although all three species of atmospheric mercury contribute to the accumulation (Pirrone et al., 2005c), dry deposition of Hg(0) is considered to dominate the plant uptake via stomata pores (Rea et al., 2002; Ericksen and Gustin, 2004; Lindberg et al., 2007). Another important pathway is the deposition and adsorption of RGM and PHg on cuticle surfaces because of their higher surface reactivity (Lindberg et al., 1992, 2007; Ericksen and Gustin, 2004). The release of mercury from vegetation surfaces may proceed through two pathways. One is from the direct release of accumulated mercury in leaf (Rea et al., 2002; Ericksen et al., 2003; Frescholtz and Gustin, 2004; Graydon et al., 2006; Millhollen et al., 2006; Fay and Gustin, 2007; Gustin et al., 2008), the other is through the active uptake of Hg(II) from soils by roots and the subsequent release of Hg(0) to the atmosphere via evapotranspiration (Lindberg et al., 1998, 2002b; Gustin and Lindberg, 2005; Obrist et al., 2005). Vegetation surface was considered as a net source of mercury (Mason and Sheu, 2002). However, recent findings indicated that it could be a net sink (Millhollen et al., 2006; Gustin et al., 2008).

A number of hypothesized chemical processes have been proposed to explain the air–surface exchange of mercury over vegetation surfaces. Rea et al. (2002) suggested that after Hg(0) deposition onto leaf surface, a subsequent oxidation is required to avoid volatilization back to the atmosphere in order for surface accumulation to occur. Since the accumulated mercury is primarily in the divalent forms (Ericksen et al., 2003), it needs to go through a reduction process, possibly photochemically driven, to give volatile Hg(0) in order for the evasion to occur (Xu et al., 1999). It was also suggested that the photoreduction of Hg(II) on leaf surfaces is most effective in the UV band (Ariya et al., 2009). Although plausible in explaining the observed mercury exchange, these hypotheses require further experimental verification.

4.5.4 Chemical Processes at Snow/Ice Surfaces

In snow, mercury exists principally in Hg(II) forms consisting of HgC_2O_4, $Hg(OH)_2$, HgOHCl, HgO, and others, with a small fraction of Hg(0) ($<1\%$ of total Hg, Poulain et al. (2004)) and possibly $(CH_3)Hg$ from marine sources (Ferrari et al., 2002; Steffen et al., 2008). Oxidation of Hg(0), primarily via reactive halogens and O_3, followed by dry deposition is the primary cause of mercury accumulation in surface snow (Lu et al., 2001; Steffen et al., 2002; Lindberg et al., 2002a; Brooks et al., 2006; Sommar et al., 2007).

The primary redox processes on snow surfaces are dominated by photochemically induced reactions. For example, it was estimated that 50–80% of deposited mercury can be reemitted back to the atmosphere within a day of AMDEs (Lalonde et al., 2002; Dommergue et al., 2003; Ferrari et al., 2008). This release is driven by the photoreduction of Hg(II) to Hg(0) in the interstitial air within snowpack, mostly induced by UVB radiation (Lalonde et al., 2003). Factors influencing the reemission include sunlight and temperature (Steffen et al., 2002; Ferrari et al., 2005), although the actual processes that control the reduction have not been elucidated. On the other hand, the newly formed Hg(0) has been found to be reoxidized in snow, which was also attributed to unknown photochemical processes (Poulain et al., 2004), possibly controlled by halogen radicals in snow near coastal areas (Ariya et al., 2004). For snow surfaces in forest areas, the photochemical processes are weakened because of the attenuation of solar radiation by the canopy. This results in slower photoreduction and higher mercury concentrations in snow under canopy (Ariya et al., 2009).

The chemical processes on ice surfaces appear to be different from those on the snow surface. Douglas et al. (2008) found that ice crystals of different morphologies exhibit very different degrees of mercury scavenging. The ice crystals formed in the vapor phase tend to have higher total mercury concentrations (up to 10 times higher) than those in the snow deposit, possibly due to its greater surface area. This indicates the role of different surfaces on the heterogeneous chemistry of mercury. However, the kinetics and mechanisms of such reactions are poorly understood.

One difficulty in understanding the heterogeneous and photochemical reactions in snow and ice surfaces is the poor comprehension of light penetration and transmission in these media, because UV and visible light can be easily scattered by the surfaces (Steffen et al., 2008). However, it was estimated that 85% of the photoredox reactions take place in the top layer only (10 cm from surfaces) (King and Simpson, 2001), but the estimate could vary greatly depending on physical characteristics and the temperature of snow (Steffen et al., 2008).

4.6   ATMOSPHERIC IMPLICATIONS OF THE IDENTIFIED REDOX PATHWAYS

Oxidation followed by dry and wet deposition is the most important driving force in removing mercury from the atmosphere. Table 4.6 lists the estimated chemical lifetime of mercury resulting from each gas-phase oxidation mechanism known to date. It should be noted that the estimated lifetime in Table 4.6 is for comparing the oxidation potential of different oxidants *only* and does not represent the "actual" lifetime of Hg(0) in the atmosphere. In contrast to typical air pollutants that are irreversibly removed by oxidation processes, atmospheric mercury undergoes a redox cycle. Oxidized mercury can be reduced and therefore reemitted back into the atmosphere. The synthesis here is based on Table 4.6 and the results from a number of modeling analyses that implemented mercury chemistry in models (Pleijel and Munthe, 1995; Lin and Pehkonen, 1997, 1998b; Seigneur et al., 2001; Hedgecock and Pirrone, 2004; Seigneur et al., 2004, 2006; Travnikov, 2005; Holmes et al., 2006; Lin et al., 2006, 2007; Pan et al., 2007; Selin et al., 2007, 2008; Dastoor et al., 2008; Travnikov et al., 2010).

Among the gaseous Hg(0) oxidants, O_3, OH, and H_2O_2 are ubiquitous with well-known, consistent concentrations in the atmosphere. The reported kinetic data has a large uncertainty, though, as indicated by the wide range of rate coefficients in Table 4.4. Using the kinetic parameters implemented by atmospheric mercury models, OH and O_3 dominate Hg(0) oxidation in the continental troposphere (Seigneur et al., 2001, 2004; Lin et al., 2006). The relative importance of O_3 and OH on Hg(0) oxidation has received much attention. The two most frequently cited kinetic measurements for the O_3 pathway differ by a factor of 25 (3.0×10^{-20} cm^3/molec/s and 7.5×10^{-19} cm^3/molec/s, Table 4.6). Using the higher rate, O_3 is the most important oxidant of Hg(0). If the lower rate constant is used, OH dominates the oxidation based on the relatively consistent rate coefficient (Table 4.4). However, the occurrence of the two oxidation reactions in the atmosphere has been questioned (Calvert and Lindberg, 2005; Hynes et al., 2009), as discussed earlier. Modeling studies using the higher rate of O_3 oxidation also could not produce realistic global concentrations and distribution of mercury, and it has been suggested that the high oxidation rate should be regarded as an upper limit (Seigneur et al., 2006). In addition, the oxidation products by O_3 and OH (RGM vs PHg) in the atmosphere are uncertain because of the low saturated vapor pressure of HgO. H_2O_2 is not an important oxidant based on the slow kinetics.

Reactive halogens are important oxidants of Hg(0) in the marine boundary layer and in the Arctic, where Br is found to be most dominant oxidant. The lifetime of Hg(0) can be as short as a few hours to a few days when air is enriched with Br (Mason and Sheu, 2002; Hedgecock and Pirrone, 2004; Dastoor et al., 2008). Owing to the chemical uncertainties associated with O_3 and OH, Holmes et al. (2006) conducted a global modeling study using Br as the primary gaseous oxidant and concluded that Br is a major sink and could be the dominant oxidant of Hg(0) in the atmosphere globally. However, the global concentration distribution of Br is poorly understood and the conclusion needs to be further verified with more field data. There is limited field evidence that the oxidation product stays in the gaseous phase as RGM (Lindberg et al., 2002a) and the saturated vapor pressure of various mercuric halides also supports that such compounds should exist as RGM. NO_3 is more localized in polluted urban airsheds and is not an important oxidant on a global scale.

In the aqueous phase, the total amount of Hg(0) oxidized by various oxidants (Table 4.5) is much less significant compared to that in the gaseous phase on a

TABLE 4.6 Estimated Lifetime of Hg(0) because of Gas-Phase Reactions with Selected Atmospheric Oxidants at 298 K

Oxidant	Background/Typical Concentration (cm^{-3})	Rate Coefficient (cm^3/molec/s)	Estimated Lifetime of Hg(0) in Gas Phase	Remark
O$_3$	$7.38 \times 10^{11a,b}$	4.2×10^{-19}	37 d	Global mean background concentration
		4.9×10^{-18}	3 d	
		1.7×10^{-18}	9 d	
		3×10^{-20k}	525 d	
		7.5×10^{-19k}	21 d	
		6.4×10^{-19}	25 d	
		6.2×10^{-19}	25 d	
OH	8.0×10^{5c}	8.7×10^{-14k}	266 d	Global mean background concentration
		$<1.2 \times 10^{-13}$	>121d	
		3.2×10^{-13}	45 d	
		9.0×10^{-14}	257 d	
NO$_3$	$4.92 \times 10^{8b,d}$	$<4 \times 10^{-15}$	> 6 d	Typical urban airshed
		$<7 \times 10^{-15}$	> 3 d	
H$_2$O$_2$	$2.46 \times 10^{10b,e}$	$\leq 4.1 \times 10^{-16}$	>1 d	Typical mean concentration
		$\leq 8.5 \times 10^{-19k}$	> 553 d	
Cl	1.0×10^{4f}	3.2×10^{-11}	36 d	Remote marine boundary layer
		6.4×10^{-11}	18 d	
		1.0×10^{-11k}	116 d	
		2.81×10^{-12}	>412 d	
		5.4×10^{-13}	> 6 yr	
		1.2×10^{-10}	10 d	

(continued)

TABLE 4.6 (*Continued*)

Oxidant	Background/Typical Concentration (cm^{-3})	Rate Coefficient (cm^3/molec/s)	Estimated Lifetime of Hg(0) in Gas Phase	Remark
Br	1.0×10^{7f}	3.2×10^{-12k}	9 h	Remote marine boundary layer
		9×10^{-13}	1 d	
		2.07×10^{-12}	13 h	
		1.1×10^{-12}	1 d	
		3.6×10^{-13}	3 d	
		9.8×10^{-13}	1 d	
Cl_2	$2.46 \times 10^{8b,g}$	2.6×10^{-18k}	50 yr	Remote marine boundary layer
		2.5×10^{-18}	52 yr	
		4.3×10^{-15}	11 d	
Br_2	$<2.5 \times 10^{10f}$	$<0.9 \times 10^{-16k}$	> 5 d	Remote marine boundary layer
F_2	$2.46 \times 10^{7b,h}$	1.8×10^{-15}	261 d	Remote marine boundary layer
ClO	$8.61 \times 10^{8b,i}$	1.1×10^{-11}	2 min	Remote marine boundary layer
BrO	$3.69 \times 10^{8b,j}$	$(3.0 \sim 6.4) \times 10^{-14}$	12 h $\sim$ 1 d	Remote marine boundary layer
		$(1 \sim 100) \times 10^{-15k}$	7 h $\sim$ 31 d	

[a] 30 ppbv (Hall, 1995).
[b] 1 ppbv = 2.46×10^{10} molec/cm^3 at 298 K, 1 atm (Snider et al., 2008).
[c] Jacobson (2005).
[d] 20 pptv or 0.02 ppbv (Sumner et al., 2005).
[e] 1 ppbv (Lin and Pehkonen, 1999).
[f] Ariya et al. (2002).
[g] 10 pptv or 0.01 ppbv (Sumner et al., 2005).
[h] 1 pptv or 0.001 ppbv (Sumner et al., 2005).
[i] 35 pptv or 0.035 ppbv (Wang and Pehkonen, 2004).
[j] 15 pptv or 0.015 ppbv (Wang and Pehkonen, 2004).
[k] Values that have been widely used in atmospheric mercury models.

global scale, although those oxidation reactions can be important in a localized, two-phase environment such as in fog or cloud (Lin and Pehkonen, 1997, 1998b). The primary significance of the aqueous chemistry of mercury is its contribution to the reduction in the atmosphere. Since sulfite can be completely consumed within a few hours by a variety of oxidants (e.g., H_2O_2, $^{\bullet}OH$, and O_3) in the aqueous phase under typical atmospheric conditions, HO_2 should be the only reductant balancing all the oxidation pathways in both gaseous and aqueous phases (Lin and Pehkonen, 1999). Model results also showed that excluding the HO_2 reduction pathway cannot reproduce the global mercury concentration and distribution (Seigneur et al., 2006; Lin et al., 2007; Pan et al., 2007; Selin et al., 2007). However, the occurrence of the HO_2 reduction pathway has also been questioned as discussed earlier (Gårdfeldt and Jonsson, 2003) and including the pathway could result in an overestimate of the reduction (Hynes et al., 2009). It is evident that the aqueous reduction could be mediated photochemically from the Hg(II)–organic complexes (Si and Ariya, 2008). Field data are needed to verify this hypothesis.

4.7 FUTURE RESEARCH NEEDS

In the past two decades, much work has been devoted to understanding the atmospheric chemistry of mercury, yet many questions, particularly in the oxidation product identification, remain unanswered. Current knowledge is based on the extrapolation of limited laboratory and theoretical investigations. Because the atmosphere is a complicated dynamic system that is difficult to assimilate in laboratory studies, such extrapolations may not be appropriate and field evidence for the proposed chemical mechanisms is critically needed to enhance our understanding. Unfortunately, the present measurement techniques are not capable of identifying specific mercury compounds (both RGM and PHg are operationally defined) because of the low concentrations of mercury in the atmosphere. The development of new analytical techniques capable of deterministic mercury compound identification at ultra-trace levels in both gas and particulate phases will be very helpful to elucidate the actual chemical processes taking place in the atmosphere.

One significant knowledge gap is in the understanding of the redox transformations that occur on surfaces and in the heterogeneous phase (e.g., water, soil, snow, and vegetative surfaces as well as in aerosol). There is limited evidence that such reactions may be significant enough to alter our current view of mercury cycling in the atmosphere (Ariya et al., 2009). However, there are a few reports in the literature describing the physical and chemical interactions between mercury compounds and various surfaces in the gas phase, aqueous phases, as well as at Earth's surfaces. More studies characterizing the heterogeneous redox reactions are obviously needed. Finally, laboratory kinetic, mechanistic, and product studies that can better assimilate atmospheric conditions will yield valuable insight on the redox cycling of mercury in the atmosphere.

REFERENCES

Ariya PA, Dastoor AP, Amyot M, Schroeder WH, Barrie L, Anlauf K, Raofie F, Ryzhkov A, Davignon D, Lalonde J, Steffen A. The Arctic: a sink for mercury. Tellus B 2004;56(5):397–403.

Ariya PA, Khalizov A, Gidas A. Reactions of gaseous mercury with atomic and molecular halogens: kinetics, product studies, and atmospheric implications. J Phys Chem A 2002;106(32):7310–7320.

Ariya PA, Peterson K, Snider G, Amyot M. Mercury chemical transformations in the gas, aqueous and heterogeneous phases: state-of-the-art science and uncertainties. Mercury fate and transport in the global atmosphere. New York (NY): Springer; 2009. p 459–501.

Bauer D, D'Ottone L, Campuzano-Jost P, Hynes AJ. Gas phase elemental mercury: a comparison of LIF detection techniques and study of the kinetics of reaction with the hydroxyl radical. J Photochem Photobiol A 2003;157(2,3):247–256.

Brezonik PL. Chemical kinetics and process dynamics in aquatic systems. Boca Raton (FL): Lewis Publishers, CRC Press; 1994.

Brooks SB, Saiz-Lopez A, Skov H, Lindberg SE, Plane JMC, Goodsite ME. The mass balance of mercury in the springtime arctic environment. Geophys Res Lett 2006;33(13):4.

Bullock OR, Brehme KA. Atmospheric mercury simulation using the CMAQ model: formulation description and analysis of wet deposition results. Atmos Environ 2002;36(13):2135–2146.

Byun Y, Cho M, Namkung W, Lee K, Koh DJ, Shin DN. Insight into the unique oxidation chemistry of elemental mercury by chlorine-containing species: experiment and simulation. Environ Sci Technol 2010;44(5):1624–1629.

Calvert JG, Lindberg SE. The potential influence of iodine-containing compounds on the chemistry of the troposphere in the polar spring. II. Mercury depletion. Atmos Environ 2004;38(30):5105–5116.

Calvert JG, Lindberg SE. Mechanisms of mercury removal by O3 and OH in the atmosphere. Atmos Environ 2005;39(18):3355–3367.

Carpi A, Lindberg SE. Sunlight-mediated emission of elemental mercury from soil amended with municipal sewage sludge. Environ Sci Technol 1997;31(7):2085–2091.

Castro L, Dommergue A, Ferrari C, Maron L. A DFT study of the reactions of O-3 with Hg degrees or Br. Atmos Environ 2009;43(35):5708–5711.

Dastoor AP, Davignon D, Theys N, Van Roozendael M, Steffen A, Ariya PA. Modeling dynamic exchange of gaseous elemental mercury at polar sunrise. Environ Sci Technol 2008;42(14):5183–5188.

Donohoue DL, Bauer D, Cossairt B, Hynes AJ. Temperature and pressure dependent rate coefficients for the reaction of Hg with Br and the reaction of Br with Br: a pulsed laser photolysis-pulsed laser induced fluorescence study. J Phys Chem A 2006;110(21):6623–6632.

Donohoue DL, Bauer D, Hynes AJ. Temperature and pressure dependent rate coefficients for the reaction of Hg with Cl and the reaction of Cl with Cl: a pulsed laser photolysis-pulsed laser induced fluorescence study. J Phys Chem A 2005;109(34):7732–7741.

Dommergue A, Ferrari CP, Boutron CF. First investigation of an original device dedicated to the determination of gaseous mercury in interstitial air in snow. Anal Bioanal Chem 2003;375(1):106–111.

Douglas TA, Sturm M, Simpson WR, Blum JD, Alvarez-Aviles L, Keeler GJ, Perovich DK, Biswas A, Johnson K. Influence of snow and ice crystal formation and accumulation on mercury deposition to the Arctic. Environ Sci Technol 2008;42(5):1542–1551.

Erel Y, Pehkonen SO, Hoffmann MR. Redox chemistry of iron in fog and stratus clouds. J Geophys Res 1993;98(D10):18423–18434.

Ericksen JA, Gustin MS. Foliar exchange of mercury as a function of soil and air mercury concentrations. Sci Total Environ 2004;324(1–3):271–279.

Ericksen JA, Gustin MS, Schorran DE, Johnson DW, Lindberg SE, Coleman JS. Accumulation of atmospheric mercury in forest foliage. Atmos Environ 2003;37(12):1613–1622.

Fay L, Gustin M. Assessing the influence of different atmospheric and soil mercury concentrations on foliar mercury concentrations in a controlled environment. Water Air Soil Pollut 2007;181(1–4):373–384.

Ferrara R, Ceccarini C, Lanzillotta E, Gårdfeldt K, Sommar J, Horvat M, Logar M, Fajon V, Kotnik J. Profiles of dissolved gaseous mercury concentration in the Mediterranean seawater. Atmos Environ 2003;37(1 Suppl):85–92.

Ferrari CP, Dommergue A, Veysseyre A, Planchon F, Boutron CF. Mercury speciation in the French seasonal snow cover. Sci Total Environ 2002;287(1–2):61–69.

Ferrari CP, Gauchard PA, Aspmo K, Dommergue A, Magand O, Bahlmann E, Nagorski S, Temme C, Ebinghaus R, Steffen A, Banic C, Berg T, Planchon F, Barbante C, Cescon P, Boutron CF. Snow-to-air exchanges of mercury in an Arctic seasonal snow pack in Ny-Alesund, Svalbard. Atmos Environ 2005;39(39):7633–7645.

Ferrari CP, Padova C, Fain X, Gauchard PA, Dommergue A, Aspmo K, Berg T, Cairns W, Barbante C, Cescon P, Kaleschke L, Richter A, Wittrock F, Boutron C. Atmospheric mercury depletion event study in Ny-Alesund (Svalbard) in spring 2005. Deposition and transformation of Hg in surface snow during springtime. Sci Total Environ 2008;397(1–3):167–177.

Finlayson-Pitts BJ, Pitts JJN. Analytical methods and typical atmospheric concentrations for gases and particles. Chemistry of the upper and lower atmosphere. San Diego (CA): Academic Press; 2000a. p 547–656.

Finlayson-Pitts BJ, Pitts JJN. Rates and mechanisms of gas-phase reactions in irradiated organic-NO_x-air mixtures. Chemistry of the upper and lower atmosphere. San Diego (CA): Academic Press; 2000b. p 179–263.

Frescholtz TF, Gustin MS. Soil and foliar mercury emission as a function of soil concentration. Water Air Soil Pollut 2004;155(1–4):223–237.

Gabriel MC, Williamson DG. Principal biogeochemical factors affecting the speciation and transport of mercury through the terrestrial environment. Environ Geochem Health 2004;26(4):421–434.

Gårdfeldt K, Jonsson M. Is bimolecular reduction of Hg(II) complexes possible in aqueous systems of environmental importance. J Phys Chem C 2003;107(22):4478–4482.

Gårdfeldt K, Sommar J, Stromberg D, Feng XB. Oxidation of atomic mercury by hydroxyl radicals and photoinduced decomposition of methylmercury in the aqueous phase. Atmos Environ 2001;35(17):3039–3047.

Goodsite ME, Plane JMC, Skov H. A theoretical study of the oxidation of Hg-0 to $HgBr_2$ in the troposphere. Environ Sci Technol 2004;38(6):1772–1776.

Graydon JA, St Louis VL, Lindberg SE, Hintelmann H, Krabbenhoft DP. Investigation of mercury exchange between forest canopy vegetation and the atmosphere using a new dynamic chamber. Environ Sci Technol 2006;40(15):4680–4688.

Greig G, Gunning HE, Strausz OP. Reactions of metal atoms. II. The combination of mercury and bromine atoms and the dimerization of HgBr. J Chem Phys 1970;52:3684–3690.

Grigal DF. Mercury sequestration in forests and peatlands: a review. J Environ Qual 2003;32(2):393–405.

Gustin MS, Biester H, Kim CS. Investigation of the light-enhanced emission of mercury from naturally enriched substrates. Atmos Environ 2002;36(20):3241–3254.

Gustin MS, Lindberg S. Terrestrial Hg fluxes: is the next exchange up, down, or neither? Dynamics of mercury pollution on regional and global scales. New York (NY): Springer; 2005. p 241–259.

Gustin MS, Lindberg SE, Weisberg PJ. An update on the natural sources and sinks of atmospheric mercury. Appl Geochem 2008;23(3):482–493.

Gustin MS, Stamenkovic J. Effect of watering and soil moisture on mercury emissions from soils. Biogeochemistry 2005;76(2):215–232.

Hall B. The gas-phase oxidation of elemental mercury by ozone. Water Air Soil Pollut 1995;80(1–4):301–315.

Hanson PJ, Lindberg SE, Tabberer TA, Owens JG, Kim KH. Foliar exchange of mercury-vapor - evidence for a compensation point. Water Air Soil Pollut 1995;80:373–382.

Hedgecock IM, Pirrone N. Chasing quicksilver: modeling the atmospheric lifetime of Hg-(g)(0) in the marine boundary layer at various latitudes. Environ Sci Technol 2004;38(1):69–76.

Holmes CD, Jacob DJ, Mason RP, Jaffe DA. Sources and deposition of reactive gaseous mercury in the marine atmosphere. Atmos Environ 2009;43(14):2278–2285.

Holmes CD, Jacob DJ, Yang X. Global lifetime of elemental mercury against oxidation by atomic bromine in the free troposphere. Geophys Res Lett 2006;33(20):5.

Horne DG, Gosavi R, Strausz OP. Reactions of metal atoms: combination of mercury and chlorine atoms and the dimerization of HgCl. J Chem Phys 1968;48(10):4758–4764.

Hynes AJ, Donohoue DL, Goodsite ME, Hedgecock IM. Our current understanding of major chemical and physical processes affecting mercury dynamics in the atmosphere and at the air-water/terrestrial interfaces. Mercury fate and transport in the global atmosphere. New York (NY): Springer; 2009. p 427–457.

Impey GA, Shepson PB, Hastie DR, Barrie LA, Anlauf KG. Measurements of photolyzable chlorine and bromine during the polar sunrise experiment 1995. J Geophys Res 1997;102(D13):16005–16010.

Iverfeldt AÅ., Lindqvist O. Distribution equilibrium of methyl mercury chloride between water and air. Atmos Environ (1967) 1982;16(12):2917–2925.

Iverfeldt AÅ., Lindqvist O. Atmospheric oxidation of elemental mercury by ozone in the aqueous phase. Atmos Environ (1967) 1986;20(8):1567–1573.

Jacobson MZ. Fundamentals of atmospheric modeling. 2nd ed. Cambridge: Cambridge University Press; 2005.

Johnson DW, Lindberg SE. The biogeochemical cycling of Hg in forests: alternative methods for quantifying total deposition and soil emission. Water Air Soil Pollut 1995;80(1):1069–1077.

Khalizov AF, Viswanathan B, Larregaray P, Ariya PA. A theoretical study on the reactions of Hg with halogens: atmospheric implications. J Phys Chem A 2003;107(33):6360–6365.

King MD, Simpson WR. Extinction of UV radiation in Arctic snow at Alert, Canada (82 degrees N). J Geophys Res-Atmos 2001;106(D12):12499–12507.

Kobayashi T. Oxidation of metallic mercury in aqueous solution by hydrogen peroxide and chlorine. J Jpn Soc Air Pollut 1987;22:230–236.

Lalonde JD, Amyot M, Doyon MR, Auclair JC. Photo-induced Hg(II) reduction in snow from the remote and temperate experimental lakes area (Ontario, Canada). J Geophys Res-Atmos 2003;108(D6):8.

Lalonde JD, Poulain AJ, Amyot M. The role of mercury redox reactions in snow on snow-to-air mercury transfer. Environ Sci Technol 2002;36(2):174–178.

Laurier FJG, Mason RP, Whalin L, Kato S. Reactive gaseous mercury formation in the North Pacific Ocean's marine boundary layer: a potential role of halogen chemistry. J Geophys Res-Atmos 2003;108(D17):12.

Lin CJ, Pehkonen SO. Aqueous free radical chemistry of mercury in the presence of iron oxides and ambient aerosol. Atmos Environ 1997;31(24):4125–4137.

Lin CJ, Pehkonen SO. Oxidation of elemental mercury by aqueous chlorine (HOCl/OCl-): implications for tropospheric mercury chemistry. J Geophys Res-Atmos 1998a;103(D21):28093–28102.

Lin CJ, Pehkonen SO. Two-phase model of mercury chemistry in the atmosphere. Atmos Environ 1998b;32(14,15):2543–2558.

Lin CJ, Pehkonen SO. The chemistry of atmospheric mercury: a review. Atmos Environ 1999;33(13):2067–2079.

Lin CJ, Pongprueksa P, Lindberg SE, Pehkonen SO, Byun D, Jang C. Scientific uncertainties in atmospheric mercury models I: model science evaluation. Atmos Environ 2006;40(16):2911–2928.

Lin CJ, Pongprueksa P, Russell Bullock O, Lindberg SE, Pehkonen SO, Jang C, Braverman T, Ho TC. Scientific uncertainties in atmospheric mercury models II: sensitivity analysis in the CONUS domain. Atmos Environ 2007;41(31):6544–6560.

Lindberg SE, Brooks S, Lin CJ, Scott KJ, Landis MS, Stevens RK, Goodsite M, Richter A. Dynamic oxidation of gaseous mercury in the Arctic troposphere at polar sunrise. Environ Sci Technol 2002a;36(6):1245–1256.

Lindberg SE, Dong W, Meyers T. Transpiration of gaseous elemental mercury through vegetation in a subtropical wetland in Florida. Atmos Environ 2002b;36(33):5207–5219.

Lindberg SE, Bullock R, Ebinghaus R, Engstrom D, Feng XB, Fitzgerald W, Pirrone N, Prestbo E, Seigneur C. A synthesis of progress and uncertainties in attributing the sources of mercury in deposition. Ambio 2007;36(1):19–32.

Lindberg SE, Hanson PJ, Meyers TP, Kim KH. Air/surface exchange of mercury vapor over forests - the need for a reassessment of continental biogenic emissions. Atmos Environ 1998;32(5):895–908.

Lindberg SE, Meyers TP, Taylor GE, Turner RR, Schroeder WH Jr. Atmosphere-surface exchange of mercury in a forest: results of modeling and gradient approaches. J Geophys Res 1992;97:2519–2528.

Lindberg SE, Price JL. Airborne emissions of mercury from municipal landfill operations: a short-term measurement study in Florida. J Air Waste Manag Assoc 1999;49(5):520–532.

Lindberg SE, Southworth G, Prestbo EM, Wallschlager D, Bogle MA, Price J. Gaseous methyl- and inorganic mercury in landfill gas from landfills in Florida, Minnesota, Delaware, and California. Atmos Environ 2005;39(2):249–258.

Lindqvist O, Rodhe H. Atmospheric mercury - a review. Tellus B 1985;37B(3):136–159.

Lu JY, Schroeder WH, Barrie LA, Steffen A, Welch HE, Martin K, Lockhart L, Hunt RV, Boila G, Richter A. Magnification of atmospheric mercury deposition to polar regions in springtime: the link to tropospheric ozone depletion chemistry. Geophys Res Lett 2001;28(17):3219–3222.

Mahajan AS, Plane JMC, Oetjen H, Mendes L, Saunders RW, Saiz-Lopez A, Jones CE, Carpenter LJ, McFiggans GB. Measurement and modelling of tropospheric reactive halogen species over the tropical Atlantic Ocean. Atmos Chem Phys 2010;10(10):4611–4624.

Martell AE, Smith RM, Motekaitis RJ. NIST critical stability constants of metal complex database. Gaithersburg (MD): NIST Standard Reference Data; 1993.

Mason RP, Sheu GR. Role of the ocean in the global mercury cycle. Global Biogeochem Cycles 2002;16(4):1093.

McKeown FP, Iyer RS, Rowland FS. Methyl fluoride formation from thermal fluorine-18 reaction with dimethylmercury. J Phys Chem 1983;87(20):3972–3975.

Meylan WM, Howard PH. Computer estimation of the atmospheric gas-phase reaction rate of organic compounds with hydroxyl radicals and ozone. Chemosphere 1993;26(12):2293–2299.

Miller GC, Quashnick J, Hebert V. Reaction rate of metallic mercury with hydroxyl radical in the gas phase. Abstr Pap Am Chem Soc 2001;221:16–AGRO.

Millhollen AG, Gustin MS, Obrist D. Foliar mercury accumulation and exchange for three tree species. Environ Sci Technol 2006;40(19):6001–6006.

Moore C, Carpi A. Mechanisms of the emission of mercury from soil: role of UV radiation. J Geophys Res-Atmos 2005;110(D24):9.

Munthe J. The aqueous oxidation of elemental mercury by ozone. Atmos Environ A 1992;26(8):1461–1468.

Munthe J, Xiao Z, Lindqvist O. The aqueous reduction of divalent mercury by sulfite. Water Air Soil Pollut 1991;56(1):621–630.

Nepotchatykh OV, Ariya PA. Degradation of dicarboxylic acids (C-2-C-9) upon liquid-phase reactions with O-3 and its atmospheric implications. Environ Sci Technol 2002;36(15):3265–3269.

Niki H, Maker PS, Savage CM, Breitenbach LP. A Fourier transform infrared study of the kinetics and mechanism for the reaction $Cl + CH_3HgCH_3$. J Phys Chem 1983a;87:3722–3724.

Niki H, Maker PS, Savage CM, Breitenbach LP. A long-path Fourier transform infrared study of the kinetics and mechanism for the reaction HO-radical initiated oxidation of dimethylmercury. J Phys Chem 1983b;87:4978–4981.

Nriagu JO. Mechanistic steps in the photoreduction of mercury in natural-waters. Sci Total Environ 1994;154(1):1–8.

Obrist D, Gustin MS, Arnone JA, Johnson DW, Schorran DE, Verburg PSJ. Measurements of gaseous elemental mercury fluxes over intact tallgrass prairie monoliths during one full year. Atmos Environ 2005;39(5):957–965.

O'Driscoll NJ, Siciliano SD, Lean DRS, Amyot M. Gross photoreduction kinetics of mercury in temperate freshwater lakes and rivers: application to a general model of DGM dynamics. Environ Sci Technol 2006;40(3):837–843.

Pal B, Ariya PA. Gas-phase HO center dot-initiated reactions of elemental mercury: kinetics, product studies, and atmospheric implications. Environ Sci Technol 2004a; 38(21):5555–5566.

Pal B, Ariya PA. Studies of ozone initiated reactions of gaseous mercury: kinetics, product studies, and atmospheric implications. Phys Chem Chem Phys 2004b;6(3):572–579.

Pan L, Chai TF, Carmichael GR, Tang YH, Streets D, Woo JH, Friedli HR, Radke LF. Top-down estimate of mercury emissions in China using four-dimensional variational data assimilation. Atmos Environ 2007;41(13):2804–2819.

Pehkonen SO, Lin CJ. Aqueous photochemistry of mercury with organic acids. J Air Waste Manag Assoc 1998;48(2):144–150.

Peterson KA, Shepler BC, Singleton JM. The group 12 metal chalcogenides: an accurate multireference configuration interaction and coupled cluster study. Mol Phys 2007;105(9):1139–1155.

Pirrone N, Mahaffey KR. Where we stand on mercury pollution and its health effects on regional and global scales. Dynamics of mercury pollution on regional and global scales. New York (NY): Springer; 2005. p 1–21.

Pirrone N, Mahaffey KR, Barth H. The DG research perspective-research on Hg supported by the European Commission. Dynamics of mercury pollution on regional and global scales. New York (NY): Springer; 2005a. p 81–89.

Pirrone N, Mahaffey KR, Mason R. Air-sea exchange and marine boundary layer atmospheric transformation of Hg and their importance in the global mercury cycle. Dynamics of mercury pollution on regional and global scales. New York (NY): Springer; 2005b. p 213–239.

Pirrone N, Sprovieri F, Hedgecock IM, Trunfio GA, Cinnirella S. Dynamic processes of atmospheric Hg in the Mediterranean region. Dynamics of mercury pollution on regional and global scales. New York (NY): Springer; 2005c. p 541–579.

Pleijel K, Munthe J. Modelling the atmospheric mercury cycle-chemistry in fog droplets. Atmos Environ 1995;29(12):1441–1457.

Poissant L, Pilote M, Constant P, Beauvais C, Zhang HH, Xu X. Mercury gas exchanges over selected bare soil and flooded sites in the bay St. François wetlands (Québec, Canada). Atmos Environ 2004;38(25):4205–4214.

Pongprueksa P, Lin CJ, Lindberg SE, Jang C, Braverman T, Bullock OR, Ho TC, Chu HW. Scientific uncertainties in atmospheric mercury models III: boundary and initial conditions, model grid resolution, and Hg(II) reduction mechanism. Atmos Environ 2008;42(8):1828–1845.

Poulain AJ, Lalonde JD, Amyot M, Shead JA, Raofie F, Ariya PA. Redox transformations of mercury in an Arctic snowpack at springtime. Atmos Environ 2004;38(39):6763–6774.

P'yankov VA. O kinetike reaktsii parov rtuti s ozonom (Kinetics of the reaction of mercury vapour with ozone). Zhurmal Obscej Chem Akatemijaneuk SSSR 1949;19:224–229.

Qureshi A, O'Driscoll NJ, MacLeod M, Neuhold Y-M, Hungerbühler K. Photoreactions of mercury in surface ocean water: gross reaction kinetics and possible pathways. Environ Sci Technol 2010;44(2):644–649.

Raofie F, Ariya PA. Kinetics and products study of the reaction of BrO radicals with gaseous mercury. J Phys IV 2003;107:1119–1121.

Raofie F, Snider G, Ariya PA. Reaction of gaseous mercury with molecular iodine, atomic iodine, and iodine oxide radicals—kinetics, product studies, and atmospheric implications. Can J Chem 2008;86(8):811–820.

Rea AW, Lindberg SE, Scherbatskoy T, Keeler GJ. Mercury accumulation in foliage over time in two northern mixed-hardwood forests. Water Air Soil Pollut 2002;133(1–4):49–67.

Sanemasa I. The solubility of elemental mercury vapor in water. Bull Chem Soc Jpn 1975;48:1795–1798.

Scholtz MT, Van Heyst BJ, Schroeder W. Modelling of mercury emissions from background soils. Sci Total Environ 2003;304(1–3):185–207.

Schroeder W, Munthe J. Atmospheric mercury–An overview. Atmos Environ 1998;32(5):809–822.

Schroeder W, Yarwood G, Niki H. Transformation processes involving mercury species in the atmosphere—results from a literature survey. Water Air Soil Pollut 1991;56(1):653–666.

Seigneur C, Abeck H, Chia G, Reinhard M, Bloom NS, Prestbo E, Saxena P. Mercury adsorption to elemental carbon (soot) particles and atmospheric particulate matter. Atmos Environ 1998;32(14–15):2649–2657.

Seigneur C, Karamchandani P, Lohman K, Vijayaraghavan K, Shia RL. Multiscale modeling of the atmospheric fate and transport of mercury. J Geophys Res-Atmos 2001;106(D21):27795–27809.

Seigneur C, Vijayaraghavan K, Lohman K. Atmospheric mercury chemistry: sensitivity of global model simulations to chemical reactions. J Geophys Res 2006;111(D22):D22306.

Seigneur C, Vijayaraghavan K, Lohman K, Karamchandani P, Scott C. Global source attribution for mercury deposition in the United States. Environ Sci Technol 2004;38(2):555–569.

Seigneur C, Wrobel J, Constantinou E. A chemical kinetic mechanism for atmospheric inorganic mercury. Environ Sci Technol 1994;28(9):1589–1597.

Selin NE. Global biogeochemical cycling of mercury: a review. Annu Rev Environ Resour 2009;34(1):43–63.

Selin NE, Jacob DJ, Park RJ, Yantosca RM, Strode S, Jaeglé L, Jaffe D. Chemical cycling and deposition of atmospheric mercury: global constraints from observations. J Geophys Res 2007;112(D02308):1–14.

Selin NE, Jacob DJ, Yantosca RM, Strode S, Jaegle L, Sunderland EM. Global 3-D land-ocean-atmosphere model for mercury: present-day versus preindustrial cycles and anthropogenic enrichment factors for deposition. Global Biogeochem Cycles 2008;22(GB2011):1–13. (vol 22, artn no GB3099, 2008).

Shepler BC, Balabanov NB, Peterson KA. Hg+Br–>HgBr recombination and collision-induced dissociation dynamics. J Chem Phys 2007;127(16):164304.

Shepler BC, Peterson KA. Mercury monoxide: a systematic investigation of its ground electronic state. J Phys Chem A 2003;107(11):1783–1787.

Sheu GR, Mason RP. An examination of the oxidation of elemental mercury in the presence of halide surfaces. J Atmos Chem 2004;48(2):107–130.

Shim C, Wang Y, Yoshida Y. Evaluation of model-simulated source contributions to tropospheric ozone with aircraft observations in the factor-projected space. Atmos Chem Phys 2008;8(6):1751–1761.

Si L, Arıya PA. Reduction of oxidized mercury species by dicarboxylic acids (C-2-C-4): kinetic and product studies. Environ Sci Technol 2008;42(14):5150–5155.

Sillén LG, Martell AE. Stability constants of metal-ion complexes. 2nd ed. London: Chemical Society; 1964. Special publication, 17; Special publication (Chemical Society (Great Britain)).

Simpson WR, von Glasow R, Riedel K, Anderson P, Ariya P, Bottenheim J, Burrows J, Carpenter LJ, Friess U, Goodsite ME, Heard D, Hutterli M, Jacobi HW, Kaleschke L, Neff B, Plane J, Platt U, Richter A, Roscoe H, Sander R, Shepson P, Sodeau J, Steffen A, Wagner T, Wolff E. Halogens and their role in polar boundary-layer ozone depletion. Atmos Chem Phys 2007;7(16):4375–4418.

Skov H, Brooks SB, Goodsite ME, Lindberg SE, Meyers TP, Landis MS, Larsen MRB, Jensen B, McConville G, Christensen J. Fluxes of reactive gaseous mercury measured with a newly developed method using relaxed eddy accumulation. Atmos Environ 2006;40(28):5452–5463.

Slemr F, Brunke EG, Ebinghaus R, Temme C, Munthe J, Wangberg I, Schroeder W, Steffen A, Berg T. Worldwide trend of atmospheric mercury since 1977. Geophys Res Lett 2003;30(10):4.

Slemr F, Schuster G, Seiler W. Distribution, speciation, and budget of atmospheric mercury. J Atmos Chem 1985;3(4):407–434.

Smith RM, Martell AE. NIST critically selected stability constants of metal complexes database version 8. Gaithersburg (MD): National Institute of Standards and Technology; 2004.

Snider G, Raofie F, Ariya PA. Effects of relative humidity and CO(g) on the O-3-initiated oxidation reaction of Hg-0(g): kinetic & product studies. Phys Chem Chem Phys 2008;10(36):5616–5623.

Sommar J, Gardfeldt K, Stromberg D, Feng XB. A kinetic study of the gas-phase reaction between the hydroxyl radical and atomic mercury. Atmos Environ 2001;35(17):3049–3054.

Sommar J, Hallquist M, Ljungström E. Rate of reaction between the nitrate radical and dimethyl mercury in the gas phase. Chem Phys Lett 1996;257(5,6):434–438.

Sommar J, Hallquist M, Ljungstrom E, Lindqvist O. On the gas phase reactions between volatile biogenic mercury species and the nitrate radical. J Atmos Chem 1997;27(3):233–247.

Sommar J, Wangberg I, Berg T, Gardfelt K, Munthe J, Richter A, Urba A, Wittrock F, Schroeder WH. Circumpolar transport and air-surface exchange of atmospheric mercury at Ny-Alesund (79 degrees N), Svalbard, spring 2002. Atmos Chem Phys 2007;7:151–166.

Spicer CW, Satola J, Abbgy AA, Plastridge RA, Cowen KA. Kinetics of Gas-Phase Elemental Mercury Reaction with Halogen Species, Ozone, and Nitrate Radical Under Atmospheric Conditions. Final report to Florida Department of Environmental Protection. Columbus (OH): Battelle; 2002.

Stamenkovic J, Gustin MS. Nonstomatal versus stomatal uptake of atmospheric mercury. Environ Sci Technol 2009;43(5):1367–1372.

Steffen A, Douglas T, Amyot M, Ariya P, Aspmo K, Berg T, Bottenheim J, Brooks S, Cobbett F, Dastoor A, Dommergue A, Ebinghaus R, Ferrari C, Gardfeldt K, Goodsite ME, Lean D, Poulain AJ, Scherz C, Skov H, Sommar J, Temme C. A synthesis of atmospheric mercury depletion event chemistry in the atmosphere and snow. Atmos Chem Phys 2008;8(6):1445–1482.

Steffen A, Schroeder W, Bottenheim J, Narayan J, Fuentes JD. Atmospheric mercury concentrations: measurements and profiles near snow and ice surfaces in the Canadian Arctic during alert 2000. Atmos Environ 2002;36(15,16):2653–2661.

Stein ED, Cohen Y, Winer AM. Environmental distribution and transformation of mercury compounds. Crit Rev Environ Sci Technol 1996;26(1):1–43.

Sumner A, Spicer C, Satola J, Mangaraj R, Cowen K, Landis M, Stevens R, Atkeson T. Environmental chamber studies of mercury reactions in the atmosphere. Dynamics of mercury pollution on regional and global scales. New York (NY): Springer; 2005. p 193–212.

Thomsen EL, Egsgaard H. Rate of reaction of dimethylmercury with oxygen atoms in the gas phase. Chem Phys Lett 1986;125(4):378–382.

Tokos JJS, Hall B, Calhoun JA, Prestbo EM. Homogeneous gas-phase reaction of $Hg°$ with H2O2, O3, CH3I, and (CH3)2S: Implications for atmospheric Hg cycling. Atmos Environ 1998;32(5):823–827.

Tossell JA. Calculation of the energetics for oxidation of gas-phase elemental Hg by Br and BrO. J Phys Chem A 2003;107(39):7804–7808.

Travnikov O. Contribution of the intercontinental atmospheric transport to mercury pollution in the Northern Hemisphere. Atmos Environ 2005;39(39):7541–7548.

Travnikov O, Lin CJ, Dastoor A, Bullock OR, Hedgecock IM, Holmes C, Ilyin I, Jaeglé L, Jung G, Pan L, Pongprueksa P, Seigneur C, Skov H. Mercury - global and regional modeling. In: Pironne N, Keating T, editors. Hemispheric transport of air pollution (HTAP) 2010 assessment report. Part B: Mercury; 2010 (Vol. 18, p. 97–138).

UNEP Chemicals Branch. The global atmospheric mercury assessment: sources, emissions and transport. Geneva: UNEP-Chemicals; 2008.

Van Loon L, Mader E, Scott SL. Reduction of the aqueous mercuric ion by sulfite: UV spectrum of HgSO3 and its intramolecular redox reaction. J Phys Chem A 2000;104(8):1621–1626.

Wang S, Feng X, Qiu G, Shang L, Li P, Wei Z. Mercury concentrations and air/soil fluxes in wuchuan mercury mining district, guizhou province, China. Atmos Environ 2007;41(28):5984–5993.

Wang Z, Pehkonen SO. Oxidation of elemental mercury by aqueous bromine: atmospheric implications. Atmos Environ 2004;38(22):3675–3688.

Whalin L, Kim E-H, Mason R. Factors influencing the oxidation, reduction, methylation and demethylation of mercury species in coastal waters. Mar Chem 2007;107(3):278–294.

Whalin L, Mason RP. A new method for the investigation of mercury redox chemistry in natural waters utilizing deflatable teflon (R) bags and additions of isotopically labeled mercury. Anal Chim Acta 2006;558(1,2):211–221.

Xiao ZF, Munthe J, Stromberg D, Lindqvist O. Photochemical behavior of inorganic hg compounds in aqueous solution. In: Watras CJ, Huckabee JW, editors. Mercury as a global pollutant - integration and synthesis. Boca Taton (FL): Lewis Publishers; 1994. p 581–592.

Xu XH, Yang XS, Miller DR, Helble JJ, Carley RJ. Formulation of bi-directional atmosphere-surface exchanges of elemental mercury. Atmos Environ 1999;33(27):4345–4355.

Zhang T, Hsu-Kim H. Photolytic degradation of methylmercury enhanced by binding to natural organic ligands. Nat Geosci 2010;3(7):473–476.

Zhang H, Lindberg SE. Sunlight and iron(III)-induced photochemical production of dissolved gaseous mercury in freshwater. Environ Sci Technol 2001;35(5):928–935.

Zhang H, Lindberg SE, Marsik FJ, Keeler GJ. Mercury air/surface exchange kinetics of background soils of the tahquamenon river watershed in the Michigan Upper Peninsula. Water Air Soil Pollut 2001;126(1,2):151–169.

CHAPTER 5

MICROBIAL TRANSFORMATIONS IN THE MERCURY CYCLE

CHU-CHING LIN, NATHAN YEE, and **TAMAR BARKAY**

5.1 INTRODUCTION

Microbial chemical transformations play a key role in geochemical cycles of most elements by changing their redox states and by converting between organic and inorganic forms. As a result, the physical and chemical properties of the elements are altered, affecting their mobility and driving their partition into various reservoirs in the environment. Most importantly, microbial transformations affect the bioavailability of chemical elements. For bioessential elements (e.g., carbon, nitrogen, sulfur, phosphorous, iron, and numerous trace elements), these transformations are critical to fulfilling the biological requirements for growth. Conversely, for toxic elements, such as mercury (Hg), microbial transformations may modulate toxicity and thus the impact of these elements on public and ecosystem health. Understanding microbial transformations and their place in element cycles requires an integration of studies on the underpinning biochemical reactions, the genetic systems that specify and regulate these cellular processes, the environmental factors that modulate transformation rates, and the microbes that carry them out. The latter requires information on the taxonomic and phylogenetic affiliations of the active microbes, and the environments they live in.

As thoroughly documented in this book, Hg may be the best example of how the ecological and health effects of an element strongly depend on its chemical form (Clarkson, 1997, 1998). Although all Hg species are considered toxic, the naturally occurring organic form, methylmercury (MeHg), a potent neurotoxic substance, is the most toxic form (Robinson and Tuovinen, 1984; Boening, 2000) because of its lipophilic and protein-binding properties that enhance its bioaccumulation to high levels in aquatic food webs, making it a potential threat

Environmental Chemistry and Toxicology of Mercury, First Edition.
Edited by Guangliang Liu, Yong Cai, and Nelson O'Driscoll.
© 2012 John Wiley & Sons, Inc. Published 2012 by John Wiley & Sons, Inc.

to human health and wild life reproduction (Fitzgerald and Clarkson, 1991; Wolfe et al., 1998). Since Hg enters the environment, either from natural sources such as volcanic or geothermal activities or from anthropogenic sources, mostly in its inorganic forms, processes that directly or indirectly affect MeHg synthesis and its degradation play a key role in controlling Hg toxicity and mobility in the environment. It is from this perspective that microbial transformations are critical; microorganisms transform Hg between its organic and inorganic forms as well as partake in redox transformations of inorganic Hg and are thus an integral part of the Hg geochemical cycle (Fig. 5.1).

This chapter is focused on microbial transformations of Hg, specifically addressing developments in the last 5–10 years since the last comprehensive reviews on this topic were published (Barkay et al., 2003; Barkay and Wagner-Döbler, 2005; Silver and Phung, 2005). The major studies and findings on Hg transformations by microorganisms are described and synthesized with the purpose of (i) creating an updated picture of the role of microbial transformations in the Hg biogeochemical cycle (Fig. 5.1) and (ii) identifying research goals to improve the understanding of Hg biogeochemistry and environmental management of Hg contamination (Table 5.1).

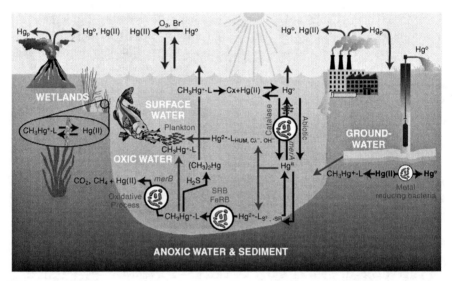

Figure 5.1 The mercury geochemical cycle. Transport (gray arrows) and transformations (black arrows) of Hg in the environments considered in this chapter are shown. Microbially mediated transformation are illustrated by microbial cells enclosed in white circles and superimposed on arrows; Hg(II) represent all ionic Hg complexes and when the ligands are known, the annotation used is $Hg^{2+}-L_X$; names of organisms and gene/enzymes that are responsible for each transformation appear alongside arrows.

TABLE 5.1 The Current State of Knowledge on Microbial Mercury Transformations (See Text for Details)

Transformation	Important Findings in the Last Decade	Important Pending Research Questions
Methylation	• Methylation by iron-reducing bacteria (FeRB) (Fleming et al., 2006; Kerin et al., 2006) • Passive transport of $HgS(0)_{(aq)}$ is still the paradigm for Hg transport through cell membranes, but facilitated transport (Golding et al., 2003) and active transport of Hg–cysteine complexes (Schaefer and Morel, 2009) are also possible • There are at least two pathways for methylation among SRB; complete oxidizers use the B_{12}-containing methyltransferases and incomplete oxidizers do not use the acetyl-coA pathway for methylation (Ekstrom et al., 2003; Ekstrom and Morel, 2008) • Interactions between DOC, Hg, and sulfide modulate methylation rates in anoxic sediment (Miller et al., 2007)	• What are the phylogenetic and taxonomic affiliations of methylating strains? • Do active and facilitated transport of Hg(II) occur in methylating strains? • What are the pathways that lead to the formation of MeHg in SRB and FeRB? • What is the role of syntrophy in methylation? • How interactions among the Hg, sulfur, and iron cycles affect MeHg production?
Demethylation	• Detailed understanding of the molecular mechanism by which MeHg is degraded reductively by the organomercury lyase	• What is the mechanism of oxidative MeHg degradation?
Hg(II) reduction	• Mechanistic and molecular details of the *mer* system have been described (Gue et al., 2010; Miller, 2007; Parks et al., 2009) • Anaerobic reduction of Hg(II) by DMRB (Wiatrowski et al., 2006) and a biotic/abiotic reduction pathway initiated by the reduction of iron oxyhydroxide to ferrous iron by FeRB (Widdel and Bak, 1992)	• What is the contribution of *mer*-mediated Hg(II) reduction to volatilization of Hg in the environment? • What is the contribution of Hg(II) reduction by DMRB to Hg geochemistry in anoxic environments?
Hg(0) oxidation	• Microbial oxidation of Hg(0) suggested by correlating oxidase activities with concentrations of DGM in freshwater lakes (Siciliano et al., 2002)	• What are the mechanisms of microbial Hg(0) oxidation? • Does oxidation of Hg(0) occur under anoxic conditions, and if so, what is its effects on Hg mobility in subsurface environments?

5.2   MERCURY METHYLATION

Research on Hg methylation was initiated in late 1960s after the Hg-toxicosis incident in Minamata Bay, Japan, when local people were poisoned by the consumption of MeHg-contaminated fish (Abelson, 1970; Bakir et al., 1973). Transformation of inorganic Hg to MeHg by microorganisms was first demonstrated by Jensen and Jernelov (1969), who showed that bottom sediments from freshwater aquaria methylated $HgCl_2$, whereas the sterilized sediment did not. A large body of work has since explored various aspects of microbial Hg methylation. These studies are summarized below. One should also be aware of the abiotic methylation associated with humic substances (Weber, 1993; Siciliano et al., 2005), though their importance relative to microbial methylation is arguable.

5.2.1   Who Methylates Hg in the Environment?

Early studies on microbial methylation of Hg focused on methanogens as a model and were based on the assumptions that (i) methylcorrinoid derivatives would be the only methylating agents because in biological systems they are the only ones known to transfer a negatively charged methyl group, the carbanion (i.e., CH_3^-), to the positively charged mercuric ion (Hg^{2+}) and (ii) anaerobic bacteria must perform the alkylation of Hg (Wood et al., 1968b; Wood, 1974). Cell-free extracts of a methanogenic bacterium were first shown to methylate Hg (Wood et al., 1968a); however, since vitamin B_{12} was known to spontaneously react with inorganic Hg to form MeHg (Wood, 1984), it was unclear whether methylation was an enzymatic transformation rather than the spontaneous transfer of biochemically formed carbanion to Hg^{2+}.

The notion that methanogenic microbes were responsible for environmental Hg methylation lasted until the mid-1980s. It was then that the question "who methylates Hg in anoxic sediments?" was asked by Richard Bartha and his students. Salt marsh sediments, where the formation of MeHg was predominantly microbial (Berman and Bartha, 1986), were incubated with specific metabolic inhibitors and stimulators to reveal that dissimilatory sulfate-reducing bacteria (SRB), rather than methanogens, were the principle Hg methylators (Compeau and Bartha, 1985). In this early study, Hg methylation dramatically decreased when the sediments were incubated with molybdate, a specific inhibitor of sulfate reduction. In contrast, when bromoethane sulfonate (BES), a specific inhibitor of methanogens, was added, MeHg production increased, presumably by shifting the flow of energy and growth substrates from methanogens to SRB. The point that is clearly made by these seminal experiments is that in order to connect activities to specific group of microbes, it is not enough to show that representatives of this group can carry out the function in the test tube but one also has to demonstrate the activity of this group in environmental samples and under environmentally relevant conditions. Thus, many microbes were shown to methylate Hg *in vitro* (Robinson and Tuovinen, 1984), including anaerobes (e.g., *Clostridium cochlearium*), facultative anaerobes and aerobes (e.g., *Pseudomonas* spp,

Bacillus megaterium, Escherichia coli, and *Enterobacter aerogenes*), and even fungi (*Neurospora crassa, Aspergillus niger*, and *Scopularis brevicaulis*) methylated Hg (Landner, 1971; Robinson and Tuovinen, 1984). These early studies were conducted with high Hg concentrations not comparable to those in the environment (Fitzgerald and Lamborg, 2005) and many of the test microbes could not even live in anoxic sediments where methylation was known to take place. Indeed, a recent survey of various metabolically different anaerobes showed that *Clostridium* spp and *Pseudomonas* spp could not produce MeHg when tested at low Hg(II) concentrations as encountered by microbes in the environment (Ranchou-Peyruse et al., 2009).

Since the 1980s, a number of field and laboratory studies have confirmed the importance of SRB as the key Hg methylators in a wide range of aquatic systems using molybdate inhibition (Gilmour et al., 1992; Chen et al., 1997; King et al., 1999), sulfate stimulation (Steffan et al., 1988; Gilmour and Henry, 1991; Gilmour et al., 1992; Choi and Bartha, 1994; Branfireun et al., 1999), microbial community analysis (Devereux et al., 1992, 1996; King et al., 2000, 2001; Macalady et al., 2000), as well as positive correlations between sulfate reduction and Hg-methylation rates in sediment incubations (Gilmour et al., 1998; Cleckner et al., 1999; King et al., 1999, 2000, 2001). In addition, pure cultures of Hg-methylating SRB have been isolated for mechanistic studies of Hg methylation (Compeau and Bartha, 1985; Rooney-Varga et al., 1998; Pak and Bartha, 1998; King et al., 2000; Jay et al., 2002; Ekstrom et al., 2003; Lin and Jay, 2007). It is noted that all known Hg-methylating SRB, including those that completely oxidize acetate (e.g., the family Desulfobacteriacea) and those that incompletely oxidize carbon substrates to acetate (e.g., the family Desulfovibrionaceae), fall in the subclass Deltaproteobacteria (Widdel and Bak, 1992). However, the ability to methylate Hg is not ubiquitous among SRB (Choi and Bartha, 1993; Ullrich et al., 2001; Benoit et al., 2003). Moreover, when SRB strains representing two genera, *Desulfovibrio* and *Desulfomicrobium*, were recently tested for their ability to methylate Hg that was provided at 10 µg/L, the results revealed that Hg-methylation potentials were neither genus nor species dependent (Ranchou-Peyruse et al., 2009), consistent with a previous study showing that Hg methylation was randomly scattered through the SRB phylogenetic tree (Devereux et al., 1992). One conclusion from this observation is that using microbial community analysis of environmental samples to explain or predict MeHg formation in natural ecosystems by the presence of SRB or of genes encoding for sulfate reduction should always be conducted together with actual measurements of the impact of metabolic stimulators and inhibitors of anaerobic respiratory pathways (King et al., 2001; Yu et al., 2010).

Recent research has suggested that dissimilatory iron-reducing bacteria (FeRB) also play a significant role in Hg methylation in the environment (Fleming et al., 2006; Kerin et al., 2006). The first evidence that Hg methylation may be attributed to FeRB came from an observation that riverine sediments where iron reduction was the dominant terminal electron-accepting (TEA) process had Hg-methylation potentials comparable to those in sulfate-reducing sediments (Warner et al., 2003).

Similarly, Fleming et al. (2006) observed that in sediments from Clear Lake, CA, where microbial iron reduction rates were significant, addition of molybdate to levels that fully inhibited sulfate reduction did not result in complete inhibition of Hg methylation. The authors isolated a bacterial strain, *Geobacter* sp CLFeRB, from Clear Lake sediments, which methylated Hg at rates similar to those of Hg-methylating SRB (Fleming et al., 2006). To further assess the role of FeRB in Hg methylation, Kerin et al. (2006) tested pure cultures of several FeRB strains belonging to the genera *Geobacter, Desulfuromonas*, and *Shewanella* for their methylation activities. Representative of the first two, both belonging to the Deltaproteobacteria, produced MeHg at levels exceeding those of abiotic controls when grown with Fe(III) as the TEA process, while *Shewanella* spp, belonging to the Gammaproteobacteria, did not methylate under either Fe(III) or nitrate-reducing conditions. Moreover, *Geobacter metallireducens* and *Geobacter sulfurreducens* methylated while respiring either fumarate or nitrate (Kerin et al., 2006), suggesting that iron reduction is not essential for Hg methylation. Together with the findings of Fleming et al. (2006), these results point out that (i) Hg-methylation capacity may be common in the family Geobacteraceae; (ii) the ability to methylate Hg is not ubiquitous among FeRB, as evidenced by the lack of methylating capacity among *Shewanella* strains; and (iii) MeHg can be produced by FeRB under various TEA conditions in addition to dissolved or solid Fe(III) phases. Notably, most tested pure cultures of Hg-methylating SRB and FeRB belong to the Deltaproteobacteria. Therefore, further research is warranted to ascertain whether Hg-methylating activity is randomly distributed among the Proteobacteria or is correlated with phylogenetic affiliation. Such information may provide insight into the biochemical pathways of Hg methylation, as well as the relationships between microbial community structure and methylation potentials in the environment (Kerin et al., 2006).

How important is methylation by FeRB in the environment? In the absence of specific inhibitors of iron reduction, similar to those of sulfate reduction and methanogenesis (see above), the answer to this question is not forthcoming. Correlations between potential methylation and iron reduction rates and high potential methylation observed in environments where iron reduction is the dominant TEA process support the involvement of FeRB in methylation (Fleming et al., 2006; Kerin et al., 2006; Mitchell and Gilmour, 2008). Similarly, a role for FeRB may also be suggested by increased methylation rates upon the addition of ferric iron to environmental incubations (Gilmour et al., 2007) (Yu and Barkay, in preparation). In summary, while some FeRB that belong to the Gammaproteobacteria methylate Hg in culture, their role in Hg methylation and the relative importance of SRB versus FeRB in environmental MeHg production remains to be determined.

5.2.2   Mechanisms of Microbial Mercury Methylation

It is generally accepted that the methylation of Hg is an intracellular process in bacteria (Benoit et al., 2003), which implies that the passage of inorganic Hg across the bacterial cell wall before methylation is a pivotal step in this process. For this reason, we start our consideration of the mechanism of methylation with a discussion on Hg transport and follow with a description of what is known about the biochemical mechanisms of microbial Hg methylation.

5.2.2.1 Transport of Inorganic Hg through the Cell Membranes of Methylating Microbes.

Mercury has no known biological function in living organisms. To date, the most well-characterized interaction between Hg and microbes is conferred by the Hg-resistance (*mer*) operon (see below) and this system has not been found in SRB and FeRB that methylate Hg (Benoit et al., 2003; Barkay et al., 2010). Considering that (i) MeHg is at least as toxic as inorganic Hg to microbes and their communities (Robinson and Tuovinen, 1984; Boening, 2000) and (ii) MeHg is not likely to readily diffuse away from the cells owing to its strong affinity for intracellular sulfur-containing compounds (Stumm and Morgan, 1996), methylation of inorganic Hg as a detoxification mechanism among SRB and FeRB seems questionable. Indeed, experiments with SRB have suggested that Hg methylation was not linked to resistance (Henry, 1992), making it unlikely that an active transport pathway for inorganic Hg has evolved as a part of the methylation mechanism. Rather, passive diffusion of inorganic Hg across cell membranes has been proposed (Benoit et al., 1999a,b, 2001a,b) implying that the extracellular chemical speciation of Hg is an important determinant of Hg bioavailability for methylation. In fact, passive diffusion was shown to govern the transport of inorganic Hg species with high lipid solubility through artificial membranes and in phytoplankton cells under aerobic conditions (Gutknekt, 1981; Mason et al., 1995b, 1996; Barkay et al., 1997).

As Hg is a classical chalcophilic element, its geochemical cycle is intimately linked to the sulfur cycle (Morel and Hering, 1993; Stumm and Morgan, 1996). In anoxic environments, a variety of dissolved Hg–sulfide complexes exist in pore waters, including both neutral species, that is, $HgS(0)_{(aq)}$ and $Hg(SH)_2$, and charged species, that is, $Hg(SH)^+$, HgS_2^{2-}, and $HgHS_2^-$ (Dyrssen and Wedborg, 1991; Benoit et al., 1999b; Jay et al., 2000). It is possible that soluble uncharged Hg complexes, such as $HgS(0)_{(aq)}$ and $Hg(SH)_2$, passively diffuse through the membranes of methylating bacteria, while charge can hinder partitioning into (and thus diffusion through) a lipid-bilayered cell membrane (Madigan et al., 2002). According to chemical speciation models, when the total Hg in the system is limiting and sulfide level is relatively low, uncharged species, such as $HgS(0)_{(aq)}$, are the dominant chemical form, whereas Hg speciation tends to shift toward charged complexes, such as $HgHS_2^-$, when sulfide levels increase (Morel et al., 1998; Benoit et al., 1999b; Jay et al., 2000). Although higher levels of sulfate can enhance the activity of Hg-methylating SRB in sediments, the excess sulfide released during sulfate respiration may limit inorganic Hg availability by increasing the fraction of extracellular charged Hg–sulfide complexes.

Observations from many field studies have supported the hypothesis of the passive diffusion of neutral Hg species in Hg-methylating bacteria. In freshwater sediments, it has been shown that methylation was optimal when sulfate concentrations ranged from 10 to about 300 μM, or when sulfide concentration was as low as 10 μM; above these levels, Hg-methylation rate and/or the MeHg concentration was inversely related to the dissolved sulfide concentration or the sulfate reduction rate (Gilmour et al., 1992, 1998; Benoit et al., 1998).

Building on these field observations, as well as the coordination chemistry between Hg and sulfide, Benoit et al. (1999a) developed a model that allowed for the accurate prediction of the magnitude and trend in total dissolved Hg concentration at the Florida Everglades and Patuxent River field sites. This model also showed a strong correlation between dissolved $HgS(0)_{(aq)}$ and ambient MeHg concentrations. It is noted, however, that a thorough analysis of bioavailability of neutral species needs to consider a species concentration by its membrane permeability, which depends on both the octanol–water partition coefficient (K_{ow}) and the species molar volume (Stein and Lieb, 1986). By determining the overall octanol–water partitioning coefficients (D_{ow}) for neutral dissolved inorganic Hg across a sulfide gradient, Benoit et al. (1999b) later experimentally demonstrated the existence of neutrally charged Hg in sulfidic solutions, and the data suggested that $HgS(0)_{(aq)}$ rather than $Hg(SH)_2$ was the dominant dissolved Hg complex determining the lipid solubility in sulfidic solutions at near neutral pH (Benoit et al., 1999b). Subsequently, when the model was applied in pure culture experiments of *Desulfobulbus propionicus* with Hg supplied in the form of mineral ores, a strong correlation between the estimated $HgS(0)_{(aq)}$ and measured MeHg production was shown (Benoit et al., 2001a,b). Together, both modeling and experimental results identified $HgS(0)_{(aq)}$ as a major species to permeate lipid-bilayered membranes. For the past 10 years, passive diffusion of uncharged, small-sized Hg complexes has been widely considered as the mechanism that controls cellular transport of Hg in methylating microbes (Benoit et al., 2003). Notably, Hg–polysulfide experiments showed that while their presence increased the solubility of cinnabar and changed Hg speciation by shifting the dominant dissolved Hg from Hg–disulfide to Hg–polysulfide complexes (Jay et al., 2000), Hg methylation by *Desulfovibrio desulfuricans* ND132 was unaffected, consistent with the passive diffusion model (Jay et al., 2002).

The paradigm of the passive diffusion of neutrally charged Hg–sulfide complexes has been challenged in recent years. First, a facilitated uptake of charged Hg species by microbes has been proposed on the basis of experiments with a *Vibrio anguillarum* bioreporter containing a *mer–lux* plasmid that showed a strong pH dependence of mercury uptake between pH 6.3 and 7.3, which could not be explained by differences in the concentration of neutral species (Kelly et al., 2003). Golding et al. (2008) showed that the neutral or positively charged complexes between Hg and small organic ligands were equally available for mercury uptake. However, the bioavailability of negatively charged complexes of Hg to *mer–lux* bioreporter strains was reduced relative to the uncharged forms (Barkay et al., 1997; Crespo-Medina et al., 2009). These studies indicate that both the concentration of the available species (which can include both charged and uncharged species) and the particular facilitated uptake system are important for Hg transport into bacterial cells (Kelly et al., 2003). However, it should be noted that the uptake of charged Hg complexes has never been demonstrated in a known Hg-methylating bacterium so far.

Second, a recent study with *G. sulfurreducens* showed that Hg methylation was greatly enhanced in the presence of low concentrations of cysteine, suggesting that Hg-methylating microbes may take up inorganic Hg through the transport of strong Hg complexes with specific thiol-containing compounds and/or sulfide, instead of merely by diffusion of neutral species through cellular membranes (Schaefer and Morel, 2009). This study pointed out that the transport of Hg may be controlled more tightly by biological mechanisms than previously thought, thus more study on Hg transport by Hg-methylating bacteria is warranted.

5.2.2.2 Biochemical Pathways of MeHg Formation in Methylating Microbes.

Methylation of Hg by anaerobic microorganisms was discovered more than 40 years ago (Jensen and Jernelöv. 1969) and yet the biochemical pathways that lead to methylation are still unknown. This lack of knowledge is not due to lack of trying (Wood et al., 1968a; Wood, 1974; Berman et al., 1990; Choi and Bartha, 1993; Choi et al., 1994a,b; Ekstrom and Morel, 2008). Rather, the absence of an identified genetic system for methylation and of a clear relationship between methylation and the taxonomic affiliation of methylating strains (see above) are the major contributors to this gap in our knowledge. However, many studies have revealed physiological details associated with, and mechanistic aspects of, methylation, advancing our knowledge even though a clear paradigm for this process has not yet emerged.

To methylate Hg, microbes need an intracellular methylating agent, for example, an enzyme that mediates methyl transfer reactions, in addition to methyl-group donors. As stated above, only methylcorrinoids, that is, vitamin B_{12}, may transfer a carbanion (CH_3^-) to mercuric (Hg^{2+}) salts (Wood, 1974; Ridley et al., 1977). Thus, Bartha and coworkers conducted a series of experiments with one model sulfate reducer, *D. desulfuricans* LS, to address the role of methylcorrinoids in Hg methylation (Berman et al., 1990; Choi and Bartha, 1993; Choi et al., 1994a,b). Their results suggested that methyl groups that had originated either from C-3 serine or from formate was donated to tetrahydrofolate (Berman et al., 1990); methylation later proceeded through the acetyl-coenzyme A (acetyl-CoA) pathway, involving a methyl-group transfer from tetrahydrofolate to a corrinoid protein and enzymatic transmethylation to Hg^{2+} (Choi and Bartha, 1993; Choi et al., 1994a,b).

The finding that Hg methylation in *D. desulfuricans* LS involved the acetyl-CoA pathway was surprising because this sulfate-reducing strain does not completely oxidize acetate and thus does not use acetyl-CoA in its major carbon metabolism (Widdel and Bak, 1992; Muyzer and Stams, 2008). Indeed, Choi et al. (1994b) who had shown low levels of activities of acetyl-CoA pathway enzymes in crude extracts of strain LS, relative to those activities in acetogens, suggested that the acetyl-CoA pathway was involved in minor reactions that required methyl-group transfer in strain LS. The involvement of the acetyl-CoA pathway in MeHg synthesis by SRB was further pursued by Ekstrom et al.

who conducted enzyme-inhibition (Ekstrom et al., 2003) and cobalt-limitation (Ekstrom and Morel, 2008) assays. The majority of the tested incomplete oxidizers of carbon methylated Hg via a pathway that was independent of the acetyl-CoA pathway (Ekstrom et al., 2003). Furthermore, growth under cobalt-limited conditions did not affect MeHg production by the incomplete oxidizer strain *Desulfovibrio africanus*, while it declined threefold with the complete oxidizer strain *Desulfococcus multivorans* (Ekstrom and Morel, 2008). Thus, there are at least two methylation pathways in SRB and only one of them is associated with the acetyl-CoA pathway. Other proposed pathways for methylation include methionine biosynthesis in the fungus *N. crassa* (Landner, 1971) and possibly the degradation of dimethylsulfoniopropionate (DMSP) to dimethylsulfide and methanthiol (Larose et al., 2010).

Since not all SRB/FeRB are capable of Hg methylation, processes that are unique to methylating strains must partake in MeHg synthesis. Because (i) not all Hg(II) that enters the bacterial cell is methylated and (ii) estimated transport rates are greatly in excess of methylation rates as revealed by pure culture studies (Benoit et al., 2003), it seems that in the cytoplasm, Hg may be bound to ligands and placed in the correct orientation to accept the carbanion group, or that steric hindrance prevents that transfer in some organisms but not in others (Benoit et al., 2003). When tested in crude cell extracts of *G. sulfurreducens*, Hg–cysteine complexes were methylated, while complexes with other Hg–thiol compounds such as penicillamine, glutathione, and dithioerythritol (DTE) were not (Schaefer and Morel, 2009), suggesting that the physical and chemical properties of the substrate may have a critical effect on Hg methylation *in vivo*. Thus, the large differences in methylation rates among various strains of SRB/FeRB may result from differences in Hg partitioning within cells, which would depend on a number of factors including differences in physiology, size, and membrane composition (Benoit et al., 2003).

Clearly, further studies on the physiology and the molecular characterization of the biochemical pathways that methylate Hg is a high priority, as elucidating these processes can provide novel mechanistic insights into the factors that control environmental MeHg formation.

5.2.3 Environmental Factors That Influence Microbial Hg Methylation

The overall efficiency of microbial Hg methylation depends on a number of factors that can influence the bioavailability of Hg, the activity of methylating bacteria, and the structure of the microbial community. These environmental parameters include temperature, pH, redox potentials, availability of nutrients and electron acceptors, as well as the presence of ligands and adsorbing surfaces. However, these parameters cannot be viewed independently, as they often interact with one another, thereby resulting in a complex system of synergistic and antagonistic effects (see Ullrich et al. (2001) for a review). Here, we briefly discuss recent advances in the understanding of the effects of dissolved organic carbon (DOC), iron chemistry, and microbial physiology on MeHg formation.

5.2.3.1 Dissolved Organic Carbon. The impact of DOC on microbial Hg methylation appears to be complex. While organic nutrients generally stimulate microbial activity and thus enhance the amount of MeHg produced (St Louis et al., 1994), the degradation of organic matter in aquatic environments may lead to the formation of low-molecular-weight, thiol-containing molecules that can complex with Hg and hence influence Hg bioavailability. For example, using a microbial bioreporter, Barkay et al. (1997) demonstrated that DOC reduced Hg bioavailability and that this effect was more pronounced under neutral than under acidic conditions. However, in a recent study with *G. sulfurreducens*, a Hg–cysteine complex promoted both the efficiency of Hg uptake by intact cells and the methylation rates by crude cell extracts (Schaefer and Morel, 2009). Interestingly, enhanced formation of MeHg by whole cells in the presence of other dissolved thiols including DTE, L/D-penicillamine, and glutathione were not observed. Thus, the composition and structure of DOC should be taken into account when evaluating the methylation potential.

It is noted that according to the conventional thermodynamic models, the complexation of Hg by DOC has been predicted to dominate the speciation of Hg under oxygenated conditions, but under sulfidic conditions, the interaction between DOC and Hg is outcompeted by inorganic sulfide as a result of stronger affinity of Hg for sulfide relative to its affinity for DOC (Morel et al., 1998). Indeed, studies using isolated DOC have verified that Hg–DOC binding is unlikely to be important in Hg complexation in sediment porewaters under typical concentrations of DOC and sulfide (Benoit et al., 2001a). Consistent with this hypothesis, a marked reduction in methylation rates were observed in the presence of cysteine when 10 µM of sulfide was added to the assays with *G. sulfurreducens* (Schaefer and Morel, 2009). However, using octanol–water partitioning extractions and centrifuge ultrafiltration techniques to separate complexes by charge and size, respectively, Miller et al. (2007) showed that Hg–sulfide complexes did not dominate in natural samples where concentrations of neutrally charged Hg–sulfide complexes were lower than predicted. The authors suggested the existence of a previously unknown ternary complex, DOC-S-Hg-S-DOC, which is not included in the current thermodynamic models (Miller et al., 2007).

Taken together, the role of DOC in environmental microbial Hg methylation needs to be reconsidered, and additional research on the interactions between Hg, sulfide, and DOC, as well as on the relationship between Hg methylation and the physical/chemical properties of DOC is necessary.

5.2.3.2 Iron. To date, the biogeochemistry of iron has been poorly linked to Hg methylation. However, the finding that FeRB methylate Hg (Fleming et al., 2006; Kerin et al., 2006) highlighted its critical role in Hg biogeochemistry. Similar to DOC and sulfides, iron, on one hand, impacts Hg methylation through chemical controls on Hg redox state/solubility/bioavailability, leading to decreases in MeHg production; on the other hand, it may enhance Hg methylation by stimulating the activities of methylating FeRB. As a result, levels of iron in soils and sediments should be examined and incorporated into environmental methylation models.

Iron minerals with strong reducing power have been used for remediation of environmental contaminants (Larese-Casanova and Scherer, 2008). In fact, both ferrous-containing minerals, such as green rust (O'Loughlin et al., 2003) and magnetite (Wiatrowski et al., 2009), and sorbed ferrous species (Charlet et al., 2002) converted Hg(II) to Hg(0) in laboratory studies. Given that the substrate for Hg methylation is Hg(II), not Hg(0), reduction of Hg(II) directly decreases the methylation potential. In addition, iron minerals may sorb and complex Hg. For instance, in efforts to find a simple approach that can mitigate MeHg production in restored and constructed wetlands, Mehrotra et al. (2003) and Mehrotra and Sedlak (2005) tested the hypothesis that adding ferrous iron to sulfidic wetland sediments would decrease net methylation by affecting the formation of neutrally charged complexes of Hg with sulfides (see above). Indeed, methylation rates by both pure cultures of *D. propionicus* 1pr3 (Mehrotra et al., 2003) and wetland sediment slurries from San Francisco Bay, CA (Mehrotra and Sedlak, 2005) declined along with the addition of ferrous iron. This effect was attributed to a decrease in sulfide activity and a concomitant decrease in the concentration of dissolved Hg. Thus, interactions between iron and sulfur cycles affect methylation where sulfate reduction is the dominating TEA process.

In contrast, ferric iron is a substrate for FeRB and may potentially enhance Hg methylation. Indeed, enhanced methylation was observed in zones of microbial iron reduction in a Chesapeake Bay salt marsh (Mitchell and Gilmour, 2008). However, amending soil mesocosms with iron oxyhydroxide had concentration-dependent effect; at the highest dose, it inhibited methylation while at the lowest dose, it stimulated methylation (Gilmour et al., 2007). The authors hypothesized that iron may have affected Hg availability for methylation as suggested by reduction in filterable Hg concentrations, possibly by sorption of ionic Hg to iron mineral phases. Similarly, rates of methylation were lower in wetland sediments where iron reduction was the dominant TEA process as compared to those in sulfate-reducing or methanogenic sediments (Warner et al., 2003, 2005).

5.2.3.3 Microbial Physiology.

While Hg methylation is closely linked to sulfate reduction, some pure cultures of SRB can methylate Hg under fermentative conditions and while growing in syntrophy with methanogens (Compeau and Bartha, 1985; Choi and Bartha, 1993; Pak and Bartha, 1998; Benoit et al., 2001a). The discovery of Hg methylation by SRB while growing fermentatively has led to the hypothesis that in sulfate-limited environments, SRB may stay active and methylate Hg, particularly when grown syntrophically with methanogens. This hypothesis was tested in experiments with cocultures of sulfidogens (*D. desulfuricans* strains LS and ND132) and a methanogen (*Methanococcus maripaludis* ATCC 43000) in a sulfate-free lactate medium (Pak and Bartha, 1998). Neither bacterium could grow or methylate Hg individually, whereas the cocultures showed vigorous growth and Hg methylation. Thus, the removal of the sulfidogen fermentation products, H_2 and acetate or CO_2, by the methanogen enabled the consumption of lactate even though lactate fermentation is not a thermodynamically favorable reaction (Madigan et al., 2002). Such interspecies hydrogen transfer between organisms in anoxic environments has been used to explain Hg methylation under methanogenic conditions (Warner et al., 2003), and may shed light on MeHg formation in certain environments, for example, groundwater (Stoor et al., 2006) and northern wetlands (Yu et al., 2010). Studies that specifically evaluate the contribution of syntrophic relationship to methylation in intact environmental samples are clearly needed.

As stated above, not all sulfate reducers and iron reducers methylate Hg, and phylogenetically similar organisms methylate at different rates. King et al. (2000) showed that methylation rates normalized to sulfate reduction rates by pure cultures were in the following order: *Desulfobacterium* > *Desulfobacter* ~ *Desulfococcus* > *Desulfovibrio* ~ *Desulfobulbus*. Thus, cultures of complete oxidizers had higher methylation rates compared to incomplete oxidizers. Consistent with these pure culture experiments, acetate-amended estuarine sediments, which were dominated by members of the *Desulfobacterium* and *Desulfobacter* groups, as shown by oligonucleotide 16S rRNA gene probing, produced more MeHg than lactate-amended and control slurries (King et al., 2000). Similarly, *Desulfobacter*-like organisms were found by lipid fatty acid analysis to be important methylators in sediments of a Hg-contaminated freshwater system, Clear Lake, CA (Macalady et al., 2000). Together with the results of Ekstrom et al. (2003), these studies identify SRB that completely oxidize acetate as efficient methylators of Hg. Thus, studies on the mechanisms of methylation should focus on this group of microbes where methylation is associated with the acetyl-CoA pathway (Ekstrom et al., 2003; Ekstrom and Morel, 2008).

Because microorganisms in natural aquatic environments potentially live in attached communities where they retain and recycle elements, biofilms may play a critical role in MeHg production in the environment. Studies conducted in tropical ecosystems in Brazil (Mauro et al., 1999, 2001, 2002; Guimar aes et al., 2000; Achá et al., 2005) and in the Florida Everglades (Cleckner et al., 1999) have reported that biofilms associated with submerged or floating macrophytes had a high potential for Hg methylation. In the Everglades, it was posited that the cooperation between phototrophic sulfide oxidizers that grow proximal to sulfate reducers in biofilms lead to the cycling of sulfur and localized regions of Hg methylation (Cleckner et al., 1999). This may partially explain the high rates of methylation commonly observed in wetlands, and may implicate aquatic macrophytes in lakes as important sites of methylation (Fig. 5.1). Consistent with this hypothesis, when grown as a biofilm, pure cultures of *D. desulfuricans* strains methylated Hg at rates that were approximately an order of magnitude higher than the rates of the same cultures grown as planktonic cells (Lin and Jay, 2007). Physiological differences between biofilm and planktonic cultures may explain the enhancement of methylation in biofilms (Lin and Jay, 2007). In contrast, a recent study with natural communities showed higher methylation efficiencies for planktonic microbes relative to biofilms from the same water reservoir; furthermore, the addition of biofilm components inhibited methylation by planktonic microbes (Huguet et al., 2010). Interpretation of these results is complicated because of the likely different populations in planktonic and biofilm microbial consortia.

Nevertheless, the role of biofilms in Hg methylation in different ecosystems and characterization of methylating biofilm communities should be a high priority considering the magnitude of periphyton associated MeHg production.

5.3 METHYLMERCURY DEGRADATION

The degradation of MeHg is the other half, next to methylation, of the balance that determines the production of this neurotoxic substance. The contribution of demethylation to net MeHg production is arguable because of the positive correlations that are usually observed between total Hg and MeHg concentrations in environmental samples (Schaefer et al., 2004; Heim et al., 2007). Furthermore, Drott et al (2008) who observed a positive correlation of potential methylation rate constants and the percentage of the total Hg present as MeHg in surficial lake sediments suggested that methylation rather than demethylation was driving net MeHg production. In contrast, a clear role for demethylation was proposed by a relationship between the potential demethylation rates and the percentage of the total Hg present as MeHg in oxic water column incubations (Schaefer et al., 2004), and higher potential demethylation than methylation rates were reported for many environmental incubations (Hines et al., 2000; Marvin-DiPasquale et al., 2003; Gray and Hines, 2009).

Three processes, photodegradation (Sellers et al., 1996) and two microbially mediated ones (Schaefer et al., 2004; Barkay and Wagner-Döbler, 2005), are known for the degradation of MeHg. Photodegradation, a process mediated by ultraviolet radiation (Lehnherr and St Louis, 2009) and enhanced by the presence of organic ligands (Zhang and Hsu-Kim, 2010), is the dominant demethylation mechanism in riverine (Bonzongo et al., 2002), estuarine (Hines et al., 2006), and freshwater (Hammerschmidt et al., 2006) surface water.

Microbial pathways for the degradation of MeHg are distinguished by the gaseous carbon products of the degradation process; in oxidative demethylation, carbon dioxide and methane are produced and in the reductive process, the only product is methane. We (Schaefer et al., 2004) and others (Marvin-Dipasquale et al., 2000; Gray et al., 2004) have shown that the choice between these processes is to a large extent controlled by environmental factors. Reductive demethylation, an activity that is mediated by the organomercury lyase enzyme, a part of the Hg-resistance (*mer*) system in bacteria (see below), is favored at concentrations of Hg that select for Hg-resistant bacteria and induce *mer* operon expression (see below) (Schaefer et al., 2004). Oxidative demethylation is favored at low redox and under a broad range of Hg concentrations. The importance of both methanogens and SRB in oxidative demethylation was demonstrated with pure cultures (Oremland et al., 1991) and in environmental incubations (Marvin-Dipasquale and Oremland, 1998; Hines et al., 2000). Marvin-Dipasquale and Oremland (1998) proposed that methanogens oxidatively degrade MeHg by cometabolic pathways related to the consumption of monomethylamines:

$$4CH_3Hg^+ + 2H_2O + 4H^+ \rightarrow 3CH_4 + CO_2 + 4Hg^{2+} + 4H_2$$

and that SRB do so by pathways related to acetate oxidation:

$$SO_4^{2-} + CH_3Hg^+ + 3H^+ \rightarrow H_2S + CO_2 + Hg^{2+} + 2H_2O$$

Oxidative demethylation by these proposed pathways would, therefore, result in a mixture of methane and carbon dioxide in proportion to the relative contribution of methanogens and SRB to this process. Thus, methane production upon MeHg degradation does not necessarily mean degradation by *mer*-carrying microbes. Unfortunately, the results of the experiments testing the role of these reactions in demethylation have not been reported, although they were proposed over a decade ago (Marvin-Dipasquale and Oremland, 1998). Moreover, as most demethylation experiments now employ MeHg with stable Hg isotopes as a tracer, rather than ^{14}C-MeHg, the two pathways are no longer distinguished. Because oxidative demethylation, leading to the formation of Hg^{2+} and possibly to subsequent methylation, is the dominant pathway in many environments, studies on the physiology and biochemistry of this process is a high priority for future research.

5.4   REDOX CYCLING OF INORGANIC Hg

The cycling of inorganic Hg between its two stable states, Hg(0) and Hg(II), affects MeHg production by controlling the amount of substrate that is available for methylation. Thus, processes that stimulate conversion of Hg(II) to Hg(0) may limit (Vandal et al., 1991; Schaefer et al., 2004), while oxidation of Hg(0) to Hg(II) may enhance (Dominique et al., 2007) MeHg production.

5.4.1   Reduction of Hg(II)

Photoreduction is the dominant pathway for the reduction of Hg(II) to Hg(0) in sunlit environments (Nriagu, 1994), a process that may be indirectly affected by biological activities owing to its dependence on DOC (O'Driscoll et al., 2004; Ravichandran, 2004), which is often biogenically formed, for example, by photosynthesis (Bade et al., 2007). The reduction of Hg(II) in the dark has been known for a long time (Mason et al., 1995a; Amyot et al., 1997) and has been attributed to the activities of heterotrophic and chemotrophic microorganisms (Mason et al., 1995a; Monperrus et al., 2007). With the exception of the *mer*-mediated mechanism (see below), little is known about the dark Hg(II) reduction and while the *mer* pathway contributes to Hg cycling in some environments (Siciliano et al., 2002; Schaefer et al., 2004; Poulain et al., 2007b), understanding of other reduction mechanisms is clearly needed for the successful management of Hg-contaminated environments.

5.4.1.1   *Reduction by Hg-Resistant Microorganisms.*   The microbial *mer* operon (Fig. 5.2) specifies an elaborate Hg-resistance system whereby Hg(II) and some organomercury compounds are actively transported into the cell's cytoplasm

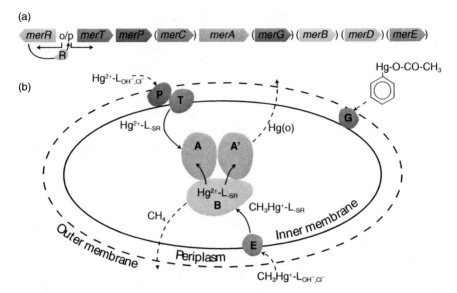

Figure 5.2 The microbial Hg detoxification system. (a) A generic *mer* operon structure; genes enclosed by parentheses are not present in all operons. (b) The resistance mechanism to Hg and organic Hg compounds. The outer cell wall is depicted by a broken line circle illustrating that not all microbes have an outer membrane in their cell wall; broken line arrows indicate diffusion; solid line arrows indicate transformations; annotations of Hg speciation follows the rationale that is described in the legend to Fig. 5.1. Gray tones of various Mer proteins correspond with the gray tones of the gene that encodes for these proteins in (a).

where they are converted by enzymes to volatile Hg(0) that diffuses out of the cell because of its low aqueous solubility (6 µg/100 mL; water at 25°C) and high vapor pressure (Henry's coefficient of 0.3), allowing for the commencement of growth (Barkay et al., 2003). Most functions of the *mer* system depend on the interactions of Hg with thiol groups, for example, cysteines, in Mer proteins, and thus, the *mer* pathway has been likened to a "thiol bucket brigade" (Silver and Hobman, 2007).

Mer Functions and Activities. The Mer detoxification system is the main Hg-resistance mechanism among the Bacteria and Archaea. The following is a general description of the various *mer* operon functions (for a detailed description, which is beyond the scope of this chapter, see Barkay et al. (2003) and Silver and Hobman (2007)). The first Mer protein to interact with Hg(II) as it enters the periplasmic space is MerP, a protein that is structurally related to other metal chaperons, such as copper (Atx1, CopA), and cadmium (CadA) transport proteins and includes a conserved GlyMetCysXXCys metal-binding motif (Steele and Opella, 1997). MerP then transfers Hg(II) to MerT, a membrane-spanning protein with three α-helical hydrophobic membrane-embedded domains, the first of which contains a cysteine pair that accepts Hg from MerP and transfers it to a second cysteine pair at the carboxy terminal on the cytoplasmic side of the membrane (Barkay et al., 2003; Silver and Hobman, 2007). Additional Hg transporters are known, all having a similar structure to MerT, albeit with varying number of predicted membrane-spanning domains; MerC (Sahlman et al., 1997) and the recently described MerH (Schuè et al., 2009) with four, and MerF (Wilson et al., 2000) and MerE (Kiyono et al., 2009) with two. Recent work has began to elucidate the substrate specificity of various transporters. Thus, Kiyono et al. (2009) and Sone et al. (2010) clearly showed that MerE of Tn*21* is a MeHg and Hg(II) transporter, while MerT of the soil bacterium *Pseudomonas* sp. K62, previously shown to transport both Hg(II) and the arylmercury compound phenylmercury acetate (PMA), could not transport MeHg (Uno et al., 1997). An additional transport function that specifically targets PMA is MerG in strain K62. When deleted, *merG* mutants are more sensitive to, yet accumulate less, PMA, suggesting that MerG is a periplasmic protein that limits the entry of PMA into the cytoplasm and thus reduces its toxicity (Kiyono and Pan-Hou, 1999).

The Mer transporters are broadly distributed among *mer* operons from diverse environments and microbial taxa (see Table S1 in Barkay et al. (2010) for distribution patterns). The mechanism of Hg transport across the membrane is not clear, but is likely based on simple binding (Sahlman et al., 1997) and possibly facilitated diffusion (Barkay et al., 2003). Similarly, how Hg transport is energized remains to be resolved, even though the inhibition of Hg transport by respiratory chain uncouplers, such as NaCN and mCCCP, has been known for a long time (Nakahara et al., 1979).

Once Hg(II) is transported into the cytoplasm, it is reduced by the mercuric reductase, MerA, an FAD-containing disulfide oxidoreductase and the homodimeric product of *merA*. This process involves the sequential transfer of Hg(II) through the cytoplasm, or possibly from the periplasmic domain of MerT (Schuè et al., 2008), to the N-terminal domain of MerA, NmerA, a 70 amino acid extension related to other metal chaperones such as CopZ. Next, Hg(II) is transferred via a vicinal Cys pair at the carboxy terminal of the opposite MerA monomer to the redox active Cys pair at the active site where electrons derived from NAD(P)H via the FAD cofactor reduce the thiol bound Hg to Hg(0) (Engst and Miller, 1999; Barkay et al., 2003).

Bacteria that are resistant to and reduce Hg from organomercury compounds possess the enzyme organomercury lyase, MerB, the gene product of *merB* (Fig. 5.2). The enzymatic mechanism is based on the coordination of R-Hg(II) by three nucleophilic groups, one of which donates the proton that cleaves the C–Hg bond to produce a reduced organic moiety and Hg(II) (Engst and Miller, 1999) that is then reduced to Hg(0) by MerA. Recent studies have shown that the two conserved cysteine residues in positions 96 and 159 (numbering according to MerB on the plasmid R831b) and a conserved aspartic acid at position 99 are the three residues that partake in this interaction (Melnick and Parkin, 2007; Miller, 2007; Lafrance-Vanasse et al., 2009; Parks et al., 2009), consistent with *in vivo* evidence showing loss of activity when these residues are replaced by site-specific mutagenesis (Pitts and Summers, 2002; Parks et al., 2009). Using hybrid density functional theory calculations, Parks et al. (2009) recently suggested a two-step proton transfer from Cys96 or Cys159 to Asp99, the formation of Cys96–Hg(II)–Cys159, and the protonation of the leaving carbanion group by Asp99. Interestingly, Benison et al. (2004) who employed NMR and X-ray absorption fine structure spectroscopy to study the properties of a MerB/Hg/DTT (dithiothreitol) complex suggested a model whereby the carboxy terminal vicinal Cys pair of MerA is involved in the direct transfer of Hg(II) between the active sites of MerB and MerA.

The expression of *mer* operons is controlled by the MerR regulator, both a repressor and an activator, depending on the absence or presence of Hg^{2+}, respectively. In the absence of Hg^{2+}, a homodimer of MerR forms a ternary closed complex with the operator/promoter region and RNA polymerase to prevent the initiation of transcription. Hg^{2+}, when present, binds to the metal-binding domains of both MerR monomers to alter the confirmation of the DNA allowing for the commencement of transcription and expression of *mer* functions (Barkay et al., 2003; Song et al., 2004, 2007; Silver and Hobman, 2007; Guo et al., 2010). An additional regulatory function encoded by *merD* is found in *mer* operons of the *Beta*- and *Gammaproteobacteria* (Barkay et al., 2010) with the documented role of displacing the Hg^{2+}/MerR/RNA polymerase complex from the operator/promoter region allowing for occupancy by apo-MerR and repression of *mer* expression once Hg has been removed from the cell (Champier et al., 2004).

The Taxonomic and Environmental Diversity of Hg-Resistant Microorganisms. Mercury-resistant bacteria are ubiquitous; they and homologs of *mer* genes have often been isolated from contaminated environments, those impacted by industrial activities as well as from deep sea and terrestrial hot springs where Hg is enriched due to geothermal activities (Barkay et al., 2003; Schelert et al., 2004; Simbahan et al., 2004, 2005; Vetriani et al., 2005; Ní Chadhain et al., 2006; Poulain et al., 2007b; Wang et al., 2009). The distribution of the *mer* system, however, was recently shown to be limited to specific microbial phyla and guilds (Barkay et al., 2010). A survey of 213 MerA sequences obtained from complete microbial genomes and other sequences deposited in databases showed most to belong to aerobic heterotrophic microbes, while MerA was conspicuous in its absence among anaerobic microbes and those that obtain energy phototrophicaly. The authors suggested that this distribution pattern could be explained by the impact of redox and pH on Hg(II) speciation and the existence of alternative Hg-resistance mechanisms among phototrophic microbes, respectively. The stability zones of inorganic Hg species in Eh–pH diagrams that simulate the aqueous speciation of Hg(II) at high and low sulfide concentrations showed that below Eh of +450 to +250 mV, Hg(0) dominated at low sulfide, while soluble and insoluble complexes with sulfur dominated at high sulfide (Barkay et al., 2010). The reduced toxicity of these inorganic Hg forms relative to the toxicity of $HgCl_2$ or $Hg(OH)_2$ (Rooney, 2007) suggested that microbes that possess *mer* systems are only selected in environments that are characterized by high Eh (Barkay et al., 2010).

The Significance of mer *Functions to Hg Geochemical Cycling.* The depen-dence of *mer* operon gene expression on induction by Hg(II) (see above), in the laboratory requiring nanomolar to micromolar concentrations of the inducer, has led to a consensus that *mer* has a limited role in Hg geochemistry (Morel et al., 1998). However, this consensus is challenged by observing MerA activi-ties in protein extracts of lake biomass (Siciliano et al., 2002), the presence of *merA* gene transcripts in microbial biomass collected in the High Arctic from environments with picomolar Hg concentrations (Poulain et al., 2007b), and by correlations of *mer* transcript abundance with reductive demethylation and a reduced MeHg accumulation in a contaminated wetland ecosystem (Schaefer et al., 2004). Moreover, chemical modeling of Hg cycling in the High Arctic suggested that MerA-mediated reduction could account for 90% of Hg(0) pro-duction at depth where photoreduction could not take place owing to reduced light penetration (Poulain et al., 2007b). Thus, *mer* operons may be induced at very low concentrations of Hg(II) (Kelly et al., 2003) to affect the methylation rates by substrate competition in diverse environments.

The Significance of mer *Functions to Environmental Management and Remediation.* The detailed knowledge of the *mer* operon, its functions, and regulation has been exploited in various strategies toward management and reme-diation of Hg contamination. These strategies are described here briefly; cited references contain more information to be used by the interested reader.

First, bioreactors inoculated with Hg-resistant heterotrophic bacteria (Wagner-Döbler et al., 2000), or by genetically engineered pseudomonads that express *mer* functions constitutively (Horn et al., 1994), remove Hg(II) from waste streams to levels that allow disposal of bioreactor effluents to local sewage systems (von Canstein et al., 1999, 2001a; Wagner-Döbler et al., 2000, 2003). Concentrations of Hg were reduced from as high as 10 mg/L in raw wastewater to < 50 µg/L (Wagner-Döbler et al., 2000) and such bioreactors removed >75% of the influent Hg over a 16-month operation with chlor-alkali plant wastes producing effluents with as low as 140 µg/L Hg (von Canstein et al., 2001b). Either fluidized (Deck-wer et al., 2004) or fixed (Wagner-Döbler, 2003) bed bioreactors were engineered allowing for the recovery of Hg(0) in the vapor phase or as globules within the fixed bed material, respectively. This approach therefore results in reducing the Hg content of the waste effluents and the concentration of Hg into a small volume that can be safely disposed or recycled.

Second, plants, including *Arabidopsis thaliana* (Bizily et al., 1999, 2000), tobacco, poplar trees (Rugh et al., 1998), and *Spartina alterniflora* (Czako et al., 2006), have been engineered for Hg phytoremediation by cloning of *mer* systems into their genomes (Meagher, 2000). Intact *mer* operons modified to optimize expression in plants and cloned into the nuclear genome (Rugh et al., 1996; Bizily et al., 2003), or unmodified ones cloned into the chloroplast genome (Ruiz et al., 2003), have increased Hg tolerance of transgenic plants by 10–100 fold relative to the wild-type plants. For example, transgenic tobacco grew in soils containing 400-µM PMA, while the growth of wild-type plant was stunted at 50 µM (Ruiz et al., 2003). Furthermore, transgenic plants accumulated up to 2 mg/g Hg in their roots and shoots and formed Hg(0) at fast rates (Hussein et al., 2007). While the development of the *mer* transgenic plants is impressive, results of mass balance calculations, that is, how much of the soil Hg is removed by sorption to plant material or volatilization, have not been reported and, furthermore, no cases of a successful reclamation of contaminated soils are known.

Third, biosorbing cells and macromolecules were developed using various *mer* functions. MerR, the regulator of the *mer* operon, with its high affinity (10^{-8} M; (Ralston and O'Halloran, 1990) and specificity to the binding of Hg^{2+}, was used to construct engineered microbial sorbents where MerR was exposed on the surface of the cells. Such cells sorbed sixfold more Hg(II) from solution than the unengineered *E. coli* strain (Bae et al., 2003). In a different approach, Kostal et al. (2003) engineered biopolymers consisting of MerR and repeat units of elastine-like polypeptides that removed almost all of the Hg from a solution containing 218-nM $HgCl_2$. Polymer-bound Hg(II) and the MerR-elastine-like polymer were recovered by heating, which led to the precipitation of the polymer with its bound Hg, extraction of the Hg with mercaptoethanol, and dissolution of the Hg-free polymer in the cold. At least five subsequent rounds of sorption, precipitation, extraction, and dissolutions were carried out without much reduction in the efficiency of Hg removal (Kostal et al., 2003).

In a different approach, biosorbing cells were developed by genetically engineering bacteria with *mer* transport functions, that is, MerP and MerT, together with macromolecules with a high capacity for intracellular sequestration of Hg(II). *E. coli* containing plasmids encoding for *merR, merT, merP*, and sometimes *merB* together with a gene encoding for polyphosphate kinase (pkk) accumulated 6 times more Hg and MeHg from solution than the unengineered strain presumably owing to the binding of Hg(II) by polyphosphates (Pan-Hou et al., 2001). Alginate-immobilized cells reduced the concentration of Hg(II) in wastewater fivefold in interactions that were relatively insensitive to variation in the composition of wastewater (Kiyono et al., 2003). Similar removal efficiencies were reported for *E. coli* cells engineered to produce MerT and MerP together with metallothioneins (Chen and Wilson, 1997) and these cells when immobilized in hollow fiber bioreactors reduced the concentration of Hg in wastewater from 2 mg/L to 5 µg/L (Chen et al., 1998). Similar to the *mer* transgenic plants (see above), there are no reports documenting the use of these "smart" constructs in the reclamation of Hg-laden wastes.

Finally, the regulatory circuit of the *mer* operon is integrated into the biore-porter bacterial strains for the detection of Hg that is bioavailable to microorganisms (Barkay et al., 1998). These bioreporters contain gene fusions between a sensing element, consisting of MerR, and the operator/promoter region of the *mer* operon (Fig. 5.2) cloned upstream of a reporting element, a gene that specify a readily detected protein (Barkay et al., 1998). The gene fusions are delivered into the bacterial cells, the bioreporter hosts, by genetic methods, and the genetically transformed cells produce the reporting protein when Hg(II) enters the cytoplasm and interacts with MerR to initiate transcription of the reporting gene. Since MerR responds to Hg^{2+} quantitatively (Ralston and O'Halloran, 1990), the more Hg^{2+} is present inside the cell, the higher is the reporting signal (Condee and Summers, 1992; Rasmussen et al., 1997). Using calibration curves, it is therefore possible to measure how much Hg(II) enters the cells (but see below).

Available bioreporters for Hg(II) (Selifonova et al., 1993; Hansen and Sørensen, 2000; Virta et al., 1995) and organomercury (Ivask et al., 2001) vary in the nature of their reporting element. The luminescence (*lux*) system from marine vibrios is the most commonly used reporter as it allows for nondisruptive "real-time on-line" monitoring (Selifonova et al., 1993; Hansen and Sørensen, 2000). Other reporting elements are the green fluorescence protein (Hansen and Sørensen, 2000), firefly luciferase (*luc*) (Virta et al., 1995; Ivask et al., 2001), and the bacterial enzyme β-galactosidase (Hansen and Sørensen, 2000) and each of these has advantages and disadvantages. The Hg bioreporters were developed for the purpose of measuring bioavailable Hg in environmental samples (Selifonova et al., 1993; Virta et al., 1995; Kelly et al., 2003); indeed, the sensitivity of some of them reaches subpicomolar concentrations (Virta et al., 1995; Kelly et al., 2003) as required for measuring Hg(II) in environments where methylation takes place (Fitzgerald et al., 2007). Because Hg that is freshly added to environmental samples is more bioavailable than Hg(II) that has equilibrated with environmental matrices over time (Hintelmann et al., 2002) and observations suggesting that the rate of Hg(II) transport through the cell wall is higher than the rate of methylation (see above and Benoit et al. (2003)), this goal has not been achieved. However, the Hg bioreporters have been useful in determining how environmental factors affect Hg(II) bioavailability (Barkay et al., 1997; Kelly et al., 2003), how Hg(II) speciation affects Hg(II) transport into cells (Selifonova and Barkay, 1994; Golding et al., 2002, 2008; Crespo-Medina et al., 2009), and in documenting that Hg(II) in soils (Rasmussen et al., 2000; Ivask et al., 2002), Arctic snow (Scott, 2001), and rain water (Selifonova et al., 1993) was bioavailable to microorganisms.

5.4.1.2   *Mercury Reduction by Hg-Sensitive Metal-Reducing Bacteria.*

A newly discovered mechanism for the reduction of Hg(II) to Hg(0) was recently described among Hg-sensitive dissimilatory metal-reducing bacteria (DMRB), which use iron and/or manganese as TEA in respiration (Wiatrowski et al., 2006). When the DMRB, *Shewanella oneidensis* MR-1 and *G. sulfurreducens* PCA and *G. metallireducens* GS-15, were incubated with fumarate or ferric oxyhydroxide, as much as 36% of Hg(II), added at an initial 825 nM, was reduced and volatilized in 3 h (Fig. 5.3a) and this activity depended on the availability of both electron donors and acceptors. However, other strains of metal reducers did not reduce Hg(II) when incubated under similar conditions showing that this activity was not common to all DMRB. Mercury reduction by strain MR-1 was constitutively expressed, that is, induction was not needed for the initiation of activity, and when its rate was compared with that of the *mer*-mediated pathway, it was significantly faster under noninducing conditions (2.53 ± 0.17 as compared to 1.60 ± 0.32 nmol/min/mg protein) but lower when cells were preexposed to

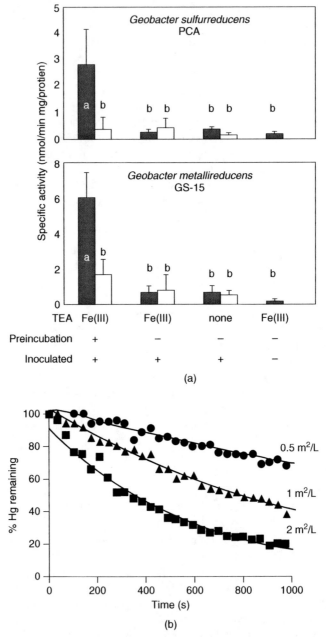

Figure 5.3 The reduction of Hg(II) by DMRB and by magnetite. (a) The effect of preincubation on reduction of Hg(II) by two *Geobacter* spp during growth on iron ferrihydroxide. Treatments are indicated below the X axis; black bars indicate live cultures; white bars indicate autoclaved controls. *Source*: Reproduced with permission from Wiatrowski et al. (2006). (b) The effect of magnetite surface area on Hg(II) loss from aqueous incubations. *Source*: Reproduced with permission from Wiatrowski et al. (2009).

Hg(II) (2.0 ± 0.6 as compared to 16.3 ± 1.3 nmol/min/mg protein) (Wiatrowski et al., 2006). These results suggested that Hg(II) reduction by DMRB may be a significant process in anoxic environments where Hg concentrations are too low for *mer* operon induction (Morel et al., 1998) and where ferric iron phases are abundant, such as in saturated sediments of groundwater aquifers (Fig. 5.1).

When Hg(II) reduction by DMRB was carried out with iron oxyhydroxide as a TEA, activity required an overnight preincubation period before the addition of Hg(II) (Fig. 5.3a) and it was 5 times higher than when tested with fumarate as a TEA (specific Hg[II] reduction rates by strain MR-1 where 13.3 ± 3.9 and 2.6 ± 0.2 nmol/min/mg protein when grown with iron oxyhydroxide and fumarate, respectively). This observation suggested that a process that takes place during growth on solid iron oxyhydroxide enhanced Hg(II) reduction. The hypothesis that ferrous iron formed during iron respiration reduced Hg(II)—both readily adsorb to iron oxide surfaces (Mac Naughton and James, 1974; Appelo et al., 2002) and as previously described for the reduction of metals including Hg by green rust (O'Loughlin et al., 2003)—was then tested by following the production of Hg(0) during incubations of magnetite with $HgCl_2$ in aqueous solution (Wiatrowski et al., 2009). Close to 80% of 100-nM $HgCl_2$ were lost during a 2-h incubation with magnetite in distilled water and the lost Hg(II) was fully recovered as Hg(0) in trapping solutions. The rate of Hg(II) loss from solution was increased with the magnetite surface area that was added to reactions (Fig. 5.3b) as well as with increasing pH from 4.77 to 6.73 and with decreasing chloride concentration. Further characterization by X-ray photoelectron spectroscopy showed that Hg(II) was adsorbed to the magnetite mineral surface and [57]Fe-specific Mössbauer spectroscopy indicated that ferrous iron was oxidized during incubations suggesting that Hg(II) was reduced by electrons that had been derived from ferrous iron (Wiatrowski et al., 2009). Together, the results suggest a biotic/abiotic process whereby ferrous iron formed during ferric iron respiration by DMRB remains attached to the surface of the iron oxide minerals and spontaneously reduces Hg(II). This reaction is favored because of the half cell potentials of the Fe(III)/Fe(II) pair, -0.34 to -0.65 V, relative to that of the Hg(II)/Hg(0) pair, +0.85 V. This mechanism may significantly affect inorganic Hg speciation in subsurface environments limiting the substrate availability for methylation and enhancing the production of Hg(0), a public health concern as it leads to high levels of Hg(0) in water distribution systems (Barringer et al., 2006).

5.4.2 Oxidation of Hg(0)

The oxidation of Hg(0) is one of the least explored steps in the Hg biogeochemical cycle. Oxidation is an important process that decreases dissolved gaseous mercury (DGM) levels in aquatic settings and increases the concentration of Hg(II), the substrate for methylation. In surface waters, Hg(0) oxidation is known to be facilitated by sunlight. Laboratory investigations of natural and artificial waters have shown that the oxidation of Hg(0) by solar ultraviolet radiation is linked to photochemically produced reactive compounds such as hydroxyl radicals (Lalonde et al., 2001, 2004). This indirect photochemical process appears to require the presence of a complexing agent such as chloride. Lalonde et al. (2001) hypothesized that chloride ions affected Hg(0) photooxidation by stabilizing Hg(I) and decreasing the Hg(I)/Hg(0) redox potential. In this model, the photoproduced hydroxyl radicals act as an electron acceptor in the oxidation of Hg(0) to Hg(I), and the subsequent Hg(I)–chloride complex is then oxidized by oxygen.

Dark oxidation of Hg(0) can also occur in lakes and coastal waters. In the absence of light, Hg(0) is subject to chemical oxidization in the presence of oxygen, chloride, and thiol compounds (de Magalhaes and Tubino, 1995; Yamamoto, 1995, 1996; Amyot et al., 2005). Amyot et al. (2005) showed that liquid drops of Hg(0) oxidized significantly faster than dissolved Hg(0), with oxidation rates increasing with increasing chloride and oxygen concentrations. As such, the chemical oxidation of Hg(0) in anoxic freshwaters is expected to be slow, with faster reaction rates in oxygenated seawater.

The biological oxidation of Hg(0) to Hg(II) is also known to occur. In animals and plants, catalase, an enzyme that degrades harmful hydrogen peroxide, oxidizes Hg(0) vapor (Magos et al., 1978; Kim et al., 1997). Smith et al. (1998) showed that the catalase activity of the intestinal bacterium *E. coli* oxidized dissolved Hg(0) in water. The oxidation activity in *E. coli* was associated with the catalase/hydroperoxidases KatG and KatE. However, a double mutant, lacking both the *katG* and *katE* genes, retained some of the ability to oxidize Hg(0) suggesting the existence of other bacterial oxidation pathways that are currently uncharacterized. The aerobic soil bacteria *Bacillus* and *Streptomyces* also exhibited high levels of Hg(0) oxidizing activity (Smith et al., 1998) thus illustrating the potential for microbial oxidation in the cycling of Hg in soils. In lake water, a field study by Siciliano et al. (2002) showed that a strong correlation exists between microbial Hg(0) oxidase activity and a decrease in DGM. Recently, experiments by Poulain et al. (2007a) demonstrated that biogenic organic material produced by marine algae can oxidize Hg(0). Together, these studies suggest that microorganisms play an important role in catalyzing the oxidation of Hg(0) to Hg(II) in a range of different environmental settings.

Although previous work has begun to elucidate the biological oxidation of Hg(0) in oxic environments, the subsurface microbial processes that catalyze Hg(0) oxidation remain poorly understood. In the vadose zone, the loss of gaseous Hg(0) into the atmosphere decreases the amount of Hg remaining in the watershed (Selvendiran et al., 2008). In saturated sediments where gas exchange is restricted, Hg(0) can remain dissolved in water and mobilized by groundwater advection. A field study in New Jersey reported groundwater aquifers supersaturated with Hg(0) that were found to discharge into the drinking water wells (Murphy et al., 1994). In submarine discharge, mobile Hg(0) in groundwater has been found to be a significant source of Hg to surface waters (Bone et al., 2007). Although the chemical oxidation of Hg(0) in anoxic waters is kinetically slow (Amyot et al., 2005), anaerobic microbial action may greatly enhance the rates of Hg(0) oxidation in these environments. Unfortunately, there is currently a dearth of knowledge of the potential microbial processes that may impact the fate of

Hg(0) in groundwater. Addressing this knowledge gap is particularly important as anaerobic bacteria isolated from groundwater aquifers (Coates et al., 2001) have been shown to methylate Hg (Kerin et al., 2006). Therefore, the biological processes that mediate the oxidation of Hg(0) to Hg(II) in anoxic freshwater may have significant implications for the production of MeHg in terrestrial groundwater environments.

5.5   CONCLUSIONS

The production of MeHg in the environment is determined by its synthesis and degradation, processes that are directly or indirectly impacted by microbial transformations. While paradigm-changing studies have been reported for some transformations in recent years, research on others has been lagging (Table 5.1). Thus, our concept on microbial Hg methylation has been expanded with the discovery that FeRB methylate Hg at rates similar to those of SRB and with the demonstration that there are at least two pathways for Hg methylation among SRB and only one of them is related to acetyl-CoA biosynthesis. Studies on the transport of Hg(II) across cell membranes have questioned the exclusivity of passive diffusion by neutrally charged aqueous complexes of mercuric sulfide. In contrast, the mechanism of oxidative demethylation remains unknown even though research has consistently pointed out to this process as a major pathway for the degradation of MeHg in environmental samples. Our understanding of Hg transformations that are mediated by Hg-resistant bacteria have progressed significantly, shading light on the reductive degradation of MeHg and on the reduction of Hg(II), while the microbial oxidation of Hg(0) to Hg(II) and its impact on Hg geochemistry is a topic few have considered.

Together, the present status of knowledge suggests that when a Hg transformation is a cometabolic process, for example, methylation and likely oxidative demethylation, characterizing specific pathways are a challenging task. Very low concentrations of MeHg in the environment become a serious public health problem when MeHg is bioaccumulated and biomagnified in food chains. Therefore, the targets of our investigations are reactions that are kinetically slow, are performed by a few microbes in large and complex microbial communities, and are a part of these microbes' central metabolism. These challenges highlight the importance of the progress that has been achieved in recent years and of the unanswered questions regarding how Hg is methylated in the environment and how this process is affected by microbial activities and interactions.

ACKNOWLEDGMENTS

Britta Munter is acknowledged for creating some of the illustrations that accompany this chapter. Research in the authors' laboratories is supported by the Office of Science (BER), US Department of Energy Grant No. DE-FG02-08ER64544 and by a European Union Marie Curie Actions—International Incoming Fellowship (to TB).

REFERENCES

Abelson PH. Methyl mercury. Science 1970;169:237.

Achá D, Iniguez V, Roulet M, Guimarãaes JRD, Luna R, Alanoca L, Sanchez S. Sulfate-reducing bacteria in floating macrophyte rhizospheres from an Amazonian floodplain lake in Bolivia and their association with Hg methylation. Appl Environ Microbiol 2005;71:7531–7535.

Amyot M, Gill GA, Morel FMM. Production and loss of dissolved gaseous mercury in coastal seawater. Environ Sci Technol 1997;31:3606–3611.

Amyot M, Morel FM, Ariya PA. Dark oxidation of dissolved and liquid elemental mercury in aquatic environments. Environ Sci Technol 2005;39:110–114.

Appelo CA, Van Der Weiden MJ, Tournassat C, Charlet L. Surface complexation of ferrous iron and carbonate on ferrihydrite and the mobilization of arsenic. Environ Sci Technol 2002;36:3096–3103.

Bade DL, Carpenter SR, Cole JJ, Pace ML, Kritzberg K, Van de Bogert MC, Cory RM, McKnight DM. Sources and fates of dissolved organic carbon in lakes as determined by whole-lake carbon isotope additions. Biogeochemistry 2007;84:115–129.

Bae W, Wu CH, Kostal J, Mulchandani A, Chen W. Enhanced mercury biosorption by bacterial cells with surface-displayed MerR. Appl Environ Microbiol 2003;69:3176–3180.

Bakir F, Damluji SF, Amin-Zaki L, Murtadha M, Khalidi A, Al-Rawi NY, Tikriti S, Dhahir HI, Clarkson TW, Smith JC, Doherty RA. Methylmercury poisoning in Iraq. Science 1973;181:230–241.

Barkay T, Gillman M, Turner RR. Effects of dissolved organic carbon and salinity on bioavailability of mercury. Appl Environ Microbiol 1997;63:4267–4271.

Barkay T, Kritee K, Boyd E, Geesey G. A thermophilic bacterial origin and subsequent constraints by redox, light and salinity on the evolution of the microbial mercuric reductase. Environ Microbiol 2010;12:2904–2917.

Barkay T, Miller SM, Summers AO. Bacterial mercury resistance from atoms to ecosystems. FEMS Microbiol Rev 2003;27:355–384.

Barkay T, Turner RR, Rasmussen LD, Kelly CA, Rudd JW. Luminescence facilitated detection of bioavailable mercury in natural waters. Methods Mol Biol 1998;102:231–246.

Barkay T, Wagner-Döbler I. Microbial transformations of mercury: potentials, challenges, and achievements in controlling mercury toxicity in the environment. Adv Appl Microbiol 2005;57:1–53.

Barringer JL, Szabo Z, Schneider D, Atkinson WD, Gallagher RA. Mercury in ground water, septage, leach-field effluent, and soils in residential areas, New Jersey coastal plain. Sci Total Environ 2006;361:144–162.

Benison GC, Di Lello P, Shokes JE, Cosper NJ, Scott RA, Legault P, Omichinski JG. A stable mercury-containing complex of the organomercurial lyase MerB: catalysis, product release, and direct transfer to MerA. Biochemistry 2004;43:8333–8345.

Benoit JM, Gilmour CC, Heyes A, Mason RP, Miller CL. Geochemical and biological controls over methylmercury production and degradation in aquatic ecosystems. In: Chai Y, Braids OC, editors. Biogeochemistry of environmentally important trace elements. Washington (DC): American Chemical Society; 2003. p 262–297.

Benoit JM, Gilmour CC, Mason RP, Riedel GS, Riedel GF. Behavior of mercury in the Patuxent River estuary. Biogeochemistry 1998;40:249–265.

Benoit JM, Gilmour CC, Mason RP, Heyes A. Sulfide controls on mercury speciation and bioavailability to methylating bacteria in sediment pore waters. Environ Sci Technol 1999a;33:951–957.

Benoit JM, Mason RP, Gilmour CC. Estimation of mercury-sulfide speciation in sediment pore waters using octanol-water partitioning and implications for availability to methylating bacteria. Environ Toxicol Chem 1999b;18:2138–2141.

Benoit JM, Gilmour CC, Mason RP. Aspects of bioavailability of mercury for methylation in pure cultures of *Desulfobulbus propionicus* (1pr3). Appl Environ Microbiol 2001a;67:51–58.

Benoit JM, Gilmour CC, Mason RP. The influence of sulfide on solid phase mercury bioavailability for methylation by pure cultures of *Desulfobulbus propionicus* (1pr3). Environ Sci Technol 2001b;35:127–132.

Berman M, Bartha R. Levels of chemical versus biological methylation of mercury in sediments. Bull Environ Contam Toxicol 1986;36:401–404.

Berman M, Chase T, Bartha R. Carbon flow in mercury biomethylation by *Desulfovibrio desulfuricans*. Appl Environ Microbiol 1990;56:298–300.

Bizily SP, Kim T, Kandasamy MK, Meagher RB. Subcellular targeting of methylmercury lyase enhances its specific activity for organic mercury detoxification in plants. Plant Physiol 2003;131:463–471.

Bizily SP, Rugh CL, Meagher RB. Phytodetoxification of hazardous organomercurials by genetically engineered plants. Nat Biotechnol 2000;18:213–217.

Bizily SP, Rugh CL, Summers AO, Meagher RB. Phytoremediation of methylmercury pollution: *merB* expression in *Arabidopsis thaliana* confers resistance to organomercurials. Proc Natl Acad Sci USA 1999;96:6808–6813.

Boening DW. Ecological effects, transport, and fate of mercury: a general review. Chemosphere 2000;40:1335–1351.

Bone SE, Charette MA, Lamborg CH, Gonneea ME. Has submarine groundwater discharge been overlooked as a source of mercury to coastal waters? Environ Sci Technol 2007;41:3090–3095.

Bonzongo JC, Lyons WB, Hines ME, Warwick JJ, Faganeli J, Horvat M, Lechler PJ, Miller JR. Mercury in surface waters of three mine-dominated river systems: Idrija River, Slovenia; Carson River, Nevada; and Madeira River, Brazilian Amazon. Geochem Explor Environ Anal 2002;2:111–119.

Branfireun BA, Roulet NT, Kelly CA, Rudd JWM. *In situ* sulphate stimulation of mercury methylation in boreal peatland: toward a link between acid rain and methylmercury contamination in remote environments. Global Biogeochem Cycles 1999;13:743–750.

von Canstein H, Li Y, Timmis KN, Deckwer WD, Wagner-Döbler I. Removal of mercury from chloralkali electrolysis wastewater by a mercury-resistant *Pseudomonas putida* strain. Appl Environ Microbiol 1999;65:5279–5284.

von Canstein HF, Li Y, Felske A, Wagner-Döbler I. Long-term stability of mercury-reducing microbial biofilm communities analyzed by 16S-23S rDNA interspacer region polymorphism. Microb Ecol 2001a;42:624–634.

von Canstein H, Li Y, Wagner-Döbler I. Long-term performance of bioreactors cleaning mercury-contaminated wastewater and their response to temperature and mercury stress and mechanical perturbation. Biotechnol Bioeng 2001b;74:212–219.

Champier L, Duarte V, Michaud-Soret I, Coves J. Characterization of the MerD protein from *Ralstonia metallidurans* CH34: a possible role in bacterial mercury resistance by switching off the induction of the *mer* operon. Mol Microbiol 2004;52:1475–1485.

Charlet L, Bosbach D, Peretyashko T. Natural attenuation of TCE, As, Hg linked to the heterogeneous oxidation of Fe(II): an AFM study. Chemical Geology 2002;190:303–319.

Chen Y, Bonzongo J-CJ, Lyons WB, Miller GC. Inhibition of mercury methylation in anoxic freshwater sediment by group VI anions. Environ Toxicol Chem 1997;16:1568–1574.

Chen S, Kim E, Shuler ML, Wilson DB. Hg^{2+} removal by genetically engineered *Escherichia coli* in a hollow fiber bioreactor. Biotechnol Prog 1998;14:667–671.

Chen S, Wilson DB. Construction and characterization of *Escherichia coli* genetically engineered for bioremediation of Hg^{2+}-contaminated environments. Appl Environ Microbiol 1997;63:2442–2445.

Choi SC, Bartha R. Cobalamin-mediated mercury methylation by *Desulfovibrio desulfuricans* LS. Appl Environ Microbiol 1993;59:290–295.

Choi SC, Bartha R. Environmental factors affecting mercury methylation in estuarine sediments. Bull Environ Contam Toxicol 1994;53:805–812.

Choi SC, Chase T, Bartha R. Enzymatic catalysis of mercury methylation by *Desulfovibrio desulfuricans* LS. Appl Environ Microbiol 1994a;60:1342–1346.

Choi SC, Chase T, Bartha R. Metabolic pathways leading to mercury methylation in *Desulfovibrio desulfuricans* LS. Appl Environ Microbiol 1994b;60:4072–4077.

Clarkson TW. The toxicology of mercury. Crit Rev Clin Lab Sci 1997;34:369–403.

Clarkson TW. Human toxicology of mercury. J Trace Elem Exp Med 1998;11:303–317.

Cleckner L, Gilmour CC, Hurley L, Krabbenhoft D. Mercury methylation in periphyton of the Florida Everglades. Limnol Oceanogr 1999;44:1815–1825.

Coates JD, Bhupathiraju VK, Achenbach LA, McLnerney MJ, Lovley DR. *Geobacter hydrogenophilus, Geobacter chapellei* and *Geobacter grbiciae*, three new, strictly anaerobic, dissimilatory Fe(III)-reducers. Int J Syst Evol Microbiol 2001;51:581–588.

Compeau GC, Bartha R. Sulfate-reducing bacteria: principal methylators of mercury in anoxic estuarine sediment. Appl Environ Microbiol 1985;50:448–502.

Condee CW, Summers AO. A *mer-lux* transcriptional fusion for real-time examination of *in vivo* gene expression kinetics and promoter response to altered superhelicity. J Bacteriol 1992;174:8094–8101.

Crespo-Medina M, Chatziefthimiou AD, Bloom NS, Luther GW 3rd, Reinfelder JR, Vetriani C, Barkay T. Adaptation of chemosynthetic microorganisms to elevated mercury concentrations in deep-sea hydrothermal vents. Limnol Oceanogr 2009;54:41–49.

Czako M, Feng X, He Y, Liang D, Marton L. Transgenic *Spartina alterniflora* for phytoremediation. Environ Geochem Health 2006;28:103–110.

De Magalhaes ME, Tubino M. A possible path for mercury in biological systems: the oxidation of metallic mercury by molecular oxygen in aqueous solutions. Sci Total Environ 1995;170:229–239.

Deckwer WD, Becker FU, Ledakowicz S, Wagner-Döbler I. Microbial removal of ionic mercury in a three-phase fluidized bed reactor. Enviorn Sci Technol 2004,38.1858–1865.

Devereux R, Kane MD, Winfrey MR, Stahl DA. Genus- and group-specific hybridization probes for determinative and environmental studies of sulfate-reducing bacteria. Syst Appl Microbiol 1992;15:601–609.

Devereux R, Winfrey MR, Winfrey J, Stahl D. Depth profile of sulfate-reducing bacterial ribosomal RNA and mercury methylation in an estuarine sediment. FEMS Microbiol Ecol 1996;20:23–31.

Dominique Y, Muresan B, Duran R, Richard S, Boudou A. Simulation of the chemical fate and bioavailability of liquid elemental mercury drops from gold mining in Amazonian freshwater systems. Environ Sci Technol 2007;41:7322–7329.

Drott A, Lambertsson L, Bjorn E, Skyllberg U. Do potential methylation rates reflect accumulated methyl mercury in contaminated sediments? Environ Sci Technol 2008;42:153–158.

Dyrssen D, Wedborg M. The sulfur-mercury(II) system in natural-waters. Water Air Soil Pollut 1991;56:507–519.

Ekstrom EB, Morel FMM. Cobalt limitation of growth and mercury methylation in sulfate-reducing bacteria. Environ Sci Technol 2008;42:93–99.

Ekstrom EB, Morel FMM, Benoit JM. Mercury methylation independent of the acetyl-coenzyme a pathway in sulfate-reducing bacteria. Appl Environ Microbiol 2003;69:5414–5422.

Engst S, Miller SM. Alternative routes for entry of HgX_2 into the active site of mercuric ion reductase depend on the nature of the X ligands. Biochemistry 1999;38:3519–3529.

Fitzgerald WF, Clarkson TW. Mercury and monomethylmercury: present and future concerns. Environ Health Perspect 1991;96:159–166.

Fitzgerald WF, Lamborg CH. Geochemistry of mercury in the environment. In: Lollar BS, editor. Environmental geochemistry. Oxford: Elsevier; 2005. p 107–148.

Fitzgerald WF, Lamborg CH, Hammerschmidt CR. Marine biogeochemical cycling of mercury. Chem Rev 2007;107:641–662.

Fleming EJ, Mack EE, Green PG, Nelson DC. Mercury methylation from unexpected sources: molybdate-inhibited freshwater sediments and an iron-reducing bacterium. Appl Environ Microbiol 2006;72:457–464.

Gilmour CC, Henry EA. Mercury methylation in aquatic systems affected by acid deposition. Environ Pollut 1991;71:131–169.

Gilmour CC, Henry EA, Mitchell R. Sulfate stimulation of mercury methylation in freshwater sediments. Environ Sci Technol 1992;26:2281–2287.

Gilmour C, Krabbenhoft D, Orem W, Aiken G, Roden E. Appendix 3B-2: status report on ACME studies on the control of mercury methylation and bioaccumulation in the Everglades. Volume I, The South Florida environment. South Florida Water Management District and Florida Department of Environmental Protection, West Palm Beach, FL; 2007.

Gilmour CC, Riedel GS, Ederington MC, Bell JT, Benoit JM, Gill GA, Stordal MC. Methylmercury concentrations and production rates across a trophic gradient in the northern Everglades. Biogeochemistry 1998;40:327–345.

Golding GR, Kelly CA, Sparling R, Loewen PC, Rudd JWM, Barkay T. Evidence for facilitated uptake of Hg(II) by *Vibrio anguillarum* and *Escherichia coli* under anaerobic and aerobic conditions. Limonol Oceanogr 2002;47:967–975.

Golding GR, Sparling R, Kelly CA. Effect of pH on intracellular accumulation of trace concentrations of Hg(II) in *Escherichia coli* under anaerobic conditions, as measured using a *mer-lux* bioreporter. Appl Environ Microbiol 2008;74:667–675.

Gray JE, Hines ME. Biogeochemical mercury methylation influenced by reservoir eutrophication, Salmon Falls Creek Reservoir, Idaho, USA. Chem Geol 2009;258:157–167.

Gray JE, Hines ME, Higueras PL, Adatto I, Lasorsa BK. Mercury speciation and microbial transformations in mine wastes, stream sediments, and surface waters at the Almaden Mining District, Spain. Environ Sci Technol 2004;38:4285–4292.

Guimar aes JRD, Meili M, Hylander LD, Silva EDE, Roulet M, Mauro JBN, de Lemos RA. Mercury net methylation in five tropical flood plain regions of Brazil: high in the root zone of floating macrophyte mats but low in surface sediments and flooded soils. Sci Total Environ 2000;261:99–107.

Guo HB, Johs A, Parks JM, Olliff L, Miller SM, Summers AO, Liang L, Smith JC. Structure and conformational dynamics of the metalloregulator MerR upon binding of Hg(II). J Mol Biol 2010;398:555–568.

Gutknekt J. Inorganic mercury (Hg^{2+}) transport through lipid bilayer membranes. J Membr Biol 1981;61:61–66.

Hammerschmidt CR, Fitzgerald WF, Lamborg CH, Balcom PH, Tseng CM. Biogeochemical cycling of methylmercury in lakes and tundra watersheds of Arctic Alaska. Environ Sci Technol 2006;40:1204–1211.

Hansen LH, Sørensen SJ. Versatile biosensor vectors for detection and quantification of mercury. FEMS Microbiol Ecol 2000;193:123–127.

Heim WA, Coale KH, Stephenson M, Choe KY, Gill GA, Foe C. Spatial and habitat-based variations in total and methyl mercury concentrations in surficial sediments in the San Francisco Bay-Delta. Environ Sci Technol 2007;41:3501–3507.

Henry EA. The role of sulfate-reducing bacteria in environmental mercury methylation. Cambridge (MA): Engineering Sciences, Harvard University; 1992.

Hines ME, Faganeli J, Adatto I, Horvat M. Microbial mercury transformations in marine, estuarine and freshwater sediment downstream of the Idrija Mercury Mine, Slovenia. Appl Geochem 2006;21:1924–1939.

Hines ME, Horvat M, Faganeli J, Bonzongo JCJ, Barkay T, Major EB, Scott KJ, Bailey EA, Warwick JJ, Lyons WB. Mercury biogeochemistry in the Idrija River, Slovenia, from above the mine into the Gulf of Trieste. Environ Res 2000;83:129–139.

Hintelmann H, Harris R, Heyes A, Hurley JP, Kelly CA, Krabbenhoft DP, Lindberg S, Rudd JW, Scott KJ, St Louis VL. Reactivity and mobility of new and old mercury deposition in a boreal forest ecosystem during the first year of the METAALICUS study. Enviorn Sci Technol 2002;36:5034–5040.

Horn JM, Brunke M, Deckwer WD, Timmis KN. *Pseudomonas putida* strains which constitutively overexpress mercury resistance for biodetoxification of organomercurial pollutants. Appl Environ Microbiol 1994;60:357–362.

Huguet L, Castelle S, Schafer J, Blanc G, Maury-Brachet R, Reynouard C, Jorand F. Mercury methylation rates of biofilm and planktonic microorganisms from a hydroelectric reservoir in French Guiana. Sci Total Environ 2010;408:1338–1348.

Hussein HS, Ruiz ON, Terry N, Daniell H. Phytoremediation of mercury and organomercurials in chloroplast transgenic plants: enhanced root uptake, translocation to shoots, and volatilization. Enviorn Sci Technol 2007;41:8439–8446.

Ivask A, Hakkila K, Virta M. Detection of organomercurials with sensor bacteria. Anal Chem 2001;73:5168–5171.

Ivask A, Virta M, Kahru A. Construction and use of specific luminescent recombinant bacterial sensors for the assessment of bioavailable fraction of cadmium, zinc, mercury and chromium in the soil. Soil Biol Biochem 2002;34:1439–1447.

Jay JA, Morel FMM, Hemond HF. Mercury speciation in the presence of polysulfides. Environ Sci Technol 2000;34:2196–2200.

Jay JA, Murray KJ, Roberts AL, Mason RP, Gilmour CC, Morel FMM, Hemond HF. Mercury methylation by *Desulfovibrio desulfuricans* ND 132 in the presence of polysulfides. Appl Environ Microbiol 2002;68:5741–5745.

Jensen S, Jernelöv A. Biological methylation of mercury in aquatic organisms. Nature 1969;223:753–754.

Kelly CA, Rudd JW, Holoka MH. Effect of pH on mercury uptake by an aquatic bacterium: implications for Hg cycling. Enviorn Sci Technol 2003;37:2941–2946.

Kerin EJ, Gilmour CC, Roden E, Suzuki MT, Coates JD, Mason RP. Mercury methylation by dissimilatory iron-reducing bacteria. Appl Environ Microbiol 2006;72:7919–7921.

Kim K-H, Hanson PJ, Barnett MO, Lindberg SE. Biogeochemistry of mercury in the air-soil-plant system. In: Sigel A, Sigel H, editors. Mercury and its effects on environment and biology. New York (NY): Marcel Dekker; 1997. p 185–212.

King JK, Kostka JE, Frischer ME, Saunders FM. Sulfate-reducing bacteria methylate mercury at variable rates in pure culture and in marine sediments. Appl Environ Microbiol 2000;66:2430–2437.

King JK, Kostka JE, Frischer ME, Saunders FM, Jahnke RA. A quantitative relationship that demonstrates mercury methylation rates in marine sediments are based on the community composition and activity of sulfate-reducing bacteria. Environ Sci Technol 2001;35:2491–2496.

King JK, Saunders FM, Lee RF, Jahnke RA. Coupling mercury methylation rates to sulfate reduction rates in marine sediments. Environ Toxicol Chem 1999;18:1362–1369.

Kiyono M, Omura H, Omura T, Murata S, Pan-Hou H. Removal of inorganic and organic mercurials by immobilized bacteria having *mer-ppk* fusion plasmids. Appl Microbiol Biotechnol 2003;62:274–278.

Kiyono M, Pan-Hou H. The merG gene product is involved in phenylmercury resistance in *Pseudomonas* strain K-62. J Bacteriol 1999;181:726–730.

Kiyono M, Sone Y, Nakamura R, Pan-Hou H, Sakabe K. The MerE protein encoded by transposon Tn*21* is a broad mercury transporter in *Escherichia coli*. FEBS Lett 2009;583:1127–1131.

Kostal J, Mulchandani A, Gropp KE, Chen W. A temperature responsive biopolymer for mercury remediation. Environ Sci Technol 2003;37:4457–4462.

Lafrance-Vanasse J, Lefebvre M, Di Lello P, Sygusch J, Omichinski JG. Crystal structures of the organomercurial lyase MerB in its free and mercury-bound forms: insights into the mechanism of methylmercury degradation. J Biol Chem 2009;284:938–944.

Lalonde JD, Amyot M, Kraepiel AM, Morel FM. Photooxidation of Hg(0) in artificial and natural waters. Environ Sci Technol 2001;35:1367–1372.

Lalonde JD, Amyot M, Orvoine J, Morel FM, Auclair JC, Ariya PA. Photoinduced oxidation of Hg0$_{aq}$ in the waters from the St. Lawrence estuary. Environ Sci Technol 2004;38:508–514.

Landner L. Biochemical model for the biological methylation of mercury suggested from methylation studies *in vivo* with *Neurospora crassa*. Nature 1971;230:452–454.

Larese-Casanova P, Scherer MM. Abiotic reduction of hexahydro-1,3,5-trinitro-1,3,5-triazine by green rusts. Environ Sci Technol 2008;42:3975–3981.

Larose C, Dommergue A, De Angelis M, Cossa D, Averty B, Marusczak N, Soumis N, Schneider D, Ferrari CP. Springtime changes in snow chemistry lead to new insights into mercury methylation in the Arctic. Geochim Cosmochim Acta 2010;74:6263–6275.

Lehnherr I, St Louis VL. Importance of ultraviolet radiation in the photodemethylation of methylmercury in freshwater ecosystems. Environ Sci Technol 2009;43:5692–5698.

Lin C-C, Jay JA. Mercury methylation by planktonic and biofilm cultures of *Desulfovibrio desulfuricans*. Environ Sci Technol 2007;41:6691–6697.

St Louis VL, Rudd JWM, Kelly CA, Beaty KG, Bloom NS, Flett RJ. Importance of wetlands as sources of methyl mercury to boreal forest ecosystems. Can J Fish Aquat Sci 1994;51:1065–1076.

Mac Naughton MG, James RO. Adsorption of aqueous mercury (II) complexes on the oxide/water interface. J Colloid Interface Sci 1974;46:151–166.

Macalady JL, Mack EE, Nelson DC, Scow KM. Sediment microbial community structure and mercury methylation in mercury-polluted Clear Lake, California. Appl Environ Microbiol 2000;66:1479–1488.

Madigan MT, Martinko JM, Parker J. Brock biology of microorganisms. 10th ed. Upper Saddle River (NJ): Prentice Hall; 2002.

Magos L, Halbach S, Clarkson TW. Role of catalase in the oxidation of mercury vapor. Biochem Pharmacol 1978;27:1373–1377.

Marvin-DiPasquale MC, Agee JL, Bouse RM, Jaffe BE. Microbial cycling of mercury in contaminated pelagic and wetland sediments of San Pablo Bay, California. Environ Geol 2003;43:260–267.

Marvin-Dipasquale MC, Agee J, McGowan C, Oremland RS, Thomas M, Krabbenhoft D, Gilmour CC. Methyl-mercury degradation pathways: a comparison among three mercury-impacted ecosystems. Environ Sci Technol 2000;34:4908–4917.

Marvin-Dipasquale MC, Oremland RS. Bacterial methylmercury degradation in Florida Everglades peat sediment. Environ Sci Technol 1998;32:2556–2563.

Mason RP, Morel FMM, Hemond HF. The role of microorganisms in elemental mercury formation in natural waters. Water Air Soil Pollut 1995a;80:775–787.

Mason RP, Reinfelder JR, Morel FMM. Bioaccumulation of mercury and methylmercury. Water Air Soil Pollut 1995b;80:915–921.

Mason RP, Reinfelder JR, Morel FMM. Uptake, toxicity, and trophic transfer of mercury in a coastal diatom. Environ Sci Technol 1996;30:1835–1845.

Mauro JBN, Guimar aes JRD, Melamed R. Mercury methylation in a tropical macrophyte: influence of abiotic parameters. Appl Organomet Chem 1999;13:631–636.

Mauro JBN, Guimar aes JRD, Hintelmann H, Watras CJ, Haack EA, Coelho-Souza SA. Mercury methylation in macrophytes, periphyton, and water- comparative studies with stable and radio-mercury additions. Anal Bioanal Chem 2002;374:983–989.

Mauro JBN, Guimar aes JRD, Melamed R. Mercury methylation in macrophyte roots of a tropical lake. Water Air Soil Pollut 2001;127:271–280.

Meagher RB. Phytoremediation of toxic elemental and organic pollutants. Curr Opin Plant Biol 2000;3:153–162.

Mehrotra AS, Horne AJ, Sedlak DL. Reduction of net mercury methylation by iron in *Desulfobulbus propionicus* (1pr3) cultures: implications for engineered wetlands. Environ Sci Technol 2003;37:3018–3023.

Mehrotra AS, Sedlak DL. Decrease in net mercury methylation rates following iron amendment to anoxic wetland sediment slurries. Environ Sci Technol 2005;39:2564–2570.

Melnick JG, Parkin G. Cleaving mercury-alkyl bonds: a functional model for mercury detoxification by MerB. Science 2007;317:225–227.

Miller SM. Cleaving C-Hg bonds: two thiolates are better than one. Nat Chem Biol 2007;3:537–538.

Miller CL, Mason RP, Gilmour CC, Heyes A. Influence of dissolved organic matter on the complexation of mercury under sulfidic conditions. Environ Toxicol Chem 2007;26:624–633.

Mitchell CPJ, Gilmour CC. Methylmercury production in a Chesapeake Bay salt marsh. J Geophys Res 2008;113:G00C04.

Monperrus M, Tessier A, Amouroux D, Leynaert A, Huonnic P, Donard OFX. Mercury methylation, demethylation and reduction rates in coastal and marine surface waters of the Mediterranean Sea. Mar Chem 2007;107:46–63.

Morel FMM, Hering JG. Principles and applications of aquatic chemistry. New York: John Wiley & Sons, Inc.; 1993.

Morel FMM, Kraepiel AML, Amyot M. The chemical cycle and bioaccumulation of mercury. Annu Rev Ecol Syst 1998;29:543–566.

Murphy EA, Dooley J, Windom HL, Smith RG Jr. Mercury species in potable groundwater in southern New Jersey. Water Air Soil Pollut 1994;78:61–72.

Muyzer G, Stams AJM. The ecology and biotechnology of sulphate-reducing bacteria. Nat Rev Microbiol 2008;6:441–454.

Nakahara H, Silver S, Miki T, Rownd RH. Hypersensitivity to Hg^{2+} and hyperbinding activity associated with cloned fragments of the mercurial resistance operon of plasmid NR1. J Bacteriol 1979;140:161–166.

Ní Chadhain SM, Schaefer JK, Crane S, Zylstra GJ, Barkay T. Analysis of mercuric reductase (*merA*) gene diversity in an anaerobic mercury-contaminated sediment enrichment. Environ Microbiol 2006;8:1746–1752.

Nriagu JO. Mechanistic steps in the photoreduction of mercury in natural waters. Sci Total Environ 1994;154:1–8.

O'Driscoll NJ, Lean DRS, Loseto LL, Carignan R, Siciliano SD. Effect of dissolved organic carbon on the photoproduction of dissolved gaseous mercury in lakes: potential impacts of forestry. Environ Sci Technol 2004;38:2664–2672.

O'Loughlin EJ, Kelly SD, Kemner KM, Csencsits R, Cook RE. Reduction of Ag(I), Au(III), Cu(II), and Hg(II) by Fe(II)/Fe(III) hydroxysulfate green rust. Chemosphere 2003;53:437–446.

Oremland RS, Culbertson CW, Winfrey MR. Methylmercury decomposition in sediments and bacterial cultures: involvement of methanogens and sulfate reducers in oxidative demethylation. Appl Environ Microbiol 1991;57:130–137.

Pak K-R, Bartha R. Mercury methylation by interspecies hydrogen and acetate transfer between sulfidogens and methanogens. Appl Environ Microbiol 1998;64:1987–1990.

Pan-Hou H, Kiyono M, Kawase T, Omura T, Endo G. Evaluation of *ppk*-specified polyphosphate as a mercury remedial tool. Biol Pharm Bull 2001;24:1423–1426.

Parks JM, Guo H, Momany C, Liang L, Miller SM, Summers AO, Smith JC. Mechanism of Hg-C protonolysis in the organomercurial lyase MerB. J Am Chem Soc 2009;131:13278–13285.

Pitts KE, Summers AO. The roles of thiols in the bacterial organomercurial lyase (MerB). Biochemistry 2002;41:10287–10296.

Poulain AJ, Garcia E, Amyot M, Campbell PG, Raofie F, Ariya PA. Biological and chemical redox transformations of mercury in fresh and salt waters of the high arctic during spring and summer. Environ Sci Technol 2007a;41:1883–1888.

Poulain AJ, Ní Chadhain SM, Ariya PA, Amyot M, Garcia E, Campbell PGC, Zylstra GJ, Barkay T. A potential for mercury reduction by microbes in the High Arctic. Appl Environ Microbiol 2007b;73:2230–2238.

Ralston DM, O'Halloran TV. Ultrasensitivity and heavy-metal selectivity of the allosterically modulated MerR transcription complex. Proc Natl Acad Sci USA 1990;87:3846–3850.

Ranchou-Peyruse M, Monperrus M, Bridou R, Duran R, Amouroux D, Salvado JC, Guyoneaud R. Overview of mercury methylation capacities among anaerobic bacteria including representatives of the sulphate-reducers: implications for environmental studies. Geomicrobiol J 2009;26:1–8.

Rasmussen LD, Sørensen SJ, Turner RR, Barkay T. Application of a *mer-lux* biosensor for estimating bioavailable mercury in soil. Soil Biol Biochem 2000;32:639–646.

Rasmussen LD, Turner RR, Barkay T. Cell-density-dependent sensitivity of a *mer-lux* bioassay. Appl Environ Microbiol 1997;63:3291–3293.

Ravichandran M. Interactions between mercury and dissolved organic matter–a review. Chemosphere 2004;55:319–331.

Ridley WP, Dizikes LJ, Wood JM. Biomethylation of toxic elements in the environment. Science 1977;197:329–332.

Robinson JB, Tuovinen OH. Mechanisms of microbial resistance and detoxification of mercury and organomercury compounds: physiological, biochemical, and genetic analyses. Microbiol Rev 1984;48:95–124.

Rooney JP. The role of thiols, dithiols, nutritional factors and interacting ligands in the toxicology of mercury. Toxicology 2007;234:145–156.

Rooney-Varga JN, Genthner BRS, Devereux R, Willis SG, Friedman SD, Hines ME. Phylogenetic and physiological diversity of sulfate-reducing bacteria isolated from a salt marsh sediment. Syst Appl Microbiol 1998;21:557–568.

Rugh CL, Senecoff JF, Meagher RB, Merkle SA. development of transgenic yellow-poplar for mercury phytoremediation. Nat Biotechnol 1998;33:616–621.

Rugh CL, Wilde HD, Stack NM, Thompson DM, Summers AO, Meagher RB. Mercuric ion reduction and resistance in transgenic *Arabidopsis thaliana* plants expressing a modified bacterial *merA* gene. Proc Natl Acad Sci USA 1996;93:3182–3187.

Ruiz ON, Hussein HS, Terry N, Daniell H. Phytoremediation of organomercurial compounds via chloroplast genetic engineering. Plant Physiol 2003;132:1344–1352.

Sahlman L, Wong W, Powlowski J. A mercuric ion uptake role for the integral inner membrane protein, MerC, involved in bacterial mercuric ion resistance. J Biol Chem 1997;272:29518–29526.

Schaefer JK, Morel FMM. High methylation rates of mercury bound to cysteine by *Geobacter sulfurreducens*. Nat Geosci 2009;2:123–126.

Schaefer JK, Yagi J, Reinfelder JR, Cardona T, Ellickson KM, Tel-Or S, Barkay T. Role of the bacterial organomercury lyase (MerB) in controlling methylmercury accumulation in mercury-contaminated natural waters. Environ Sci Technol 2004;38:4304–4311.

Schelert J, Dixit V, Hoang V, Simbahan J, Drozda M, Blum P. Occurrence and characterization of mercury resistance in the hyperthermophilic archaeon *Sulfolobus solfataricus* by use of gene disruption. J Bacteriol 2004;186:427–437.

Schuè M, Dover LG, Besra GS, Parkhill J, Brown NL. Sequence and analysis of a plasmid-encoded mercury resistance operon from *Mycobacterium marinum* identifies MerH, a new mercuric ion transporter. J Bacteriol 2009;191:439–444.

Schuè M, Glendinning KJ, Hobman JL, Brown NL. Evidence for direct interactions between the mercuric ion transporter (MerT) and mercuric reductase (MerA) from the Tn *501 mer* operon. Biometals 2008;21:107–116.

Scott KJ. Bioavailable mercury in Arctic snow determined by a light-emitting *mer-lux* bioreporter. Arctic 2001;54:92–95.

Selifonova OV, Barkay T. Role of Na$^+$ in transport of Hg^{2+} and induction of the Tn*21* mer operon. Appl Environ Microbiol 1994;60:3503–3507.

Selifonova O, Burlage R, Barkay T. Bioluminescent sensors for detection of bioavailable Hg(II) in the environment. Appl Environ Microbiol 1993;59:3083–3090.

Sellers P, Kelly CA, Rudd JWM, MacHutchon AR. Photodegradation of methylmercury in lakes. Nature 1996;380:694–697.

Selvendiran P, Driscoll CT, Montesdeoca MR, Bushey JT. Inputs, storage, and transport of total and methyl mercury in two temperate forest wetlands. J Geophys Res Biogeosci 2008;113:G00C01.

Siciliano SD, O'Driscoll NJ, Lean DRS. Microbial reduction and oxidation of mercury in freshwater lakes. Environ Sci Technol 2002;36:3064–3068.

Siciliano SD, O'Driscoll NJ, Tordon R, Hill J, Beauchamp S, Lean DR. Abiotic production of methylmercury by solar radiation. Environ Sci Technol 2005;39:1071–1077.

Silver S, Hobman JL. Mercury microbiology: resistance systems. environmental aspects, methylation, and human health. In: Nies DH, Silver S, editors. Molecular microbiology of heavy metals. Berlin, Heidelberg: Springer-Verlag; 2007. p 357–370.

Silver S, Phung LT. A bacterial view of the periodic table: genes and proteins for toxic inorganic ions. J Ind Microbiol Biotechnol 2005;32:587–605.

Simbahan J, Drijber R, Blum P. *Alicyclobacillus vulcanalis* sp. nov., a thermophilic, acidophilic bacterium isolated from Coso Hot Springs, California, USA. Int J Syst Evol Microbiol 2004;54:1703–1707.

Simbahan J, Kurth E, Schelert J, Dillman A, Moriyama E, Jovanovich S, Blum P. Community analysis of a mercury hot spring supports occurrence of domain-specific forms of mercuric reductase. Appl Environ Microbiol 2005;71:8836–8845.

Smith T, Pitts K, McGarvey JA, Summers AO. Bacterial oxidation of mercury metal vapor, Hg(0). Appl Environ Microbiol 1998;64:1328–1332.

Sone Y, Pan-Hou H, Nakamura R, Sakabe K, Kiyono M. Roels played by MerE and MerT in the transport of inorganic and organic mercury compounds in Gram-negative bacteria. J Health Sci 2010;56:123–127.

Song L, Caguiat J, Li Z, Shokes J, Scott RA, Olliff L, Summers AO. Engineered single-chain, antiparallel, coiled coil mimics the MerR metal binding site. J Bacteriol 2004;186:1861–1868.

Song L, Teng Q, Phillips RS, Brewer JM, Summers AO. 19F-NMR reveals metal and operator-induced allostery in MerR. J Mol Biol 2007;371:79–92.

Steele RA, Opella SJ. Structures of the reduced and mercury-bound forms of MerP, the periplasmic protein from the bacterial mercury detoxification system. Biochemistry 1997;36:6885–6895.

Steffan RJ, Korthals ET, Winfrey MR. Effects of acidification on mercury methylation, demethylation, and volatilization in sediments from an acid-susceptible lake. Appl Environ Microbiol 1988;54:2003–2009.

Stein W, Lieb W. Transport and diffusion across cell membranes. New York (NY): Academic Press; 1986.

Stoor RW, Hurley JP, Babiarz CL, Armstrong DE. Subsurface sources of methyl mercury to Lake Superior from a wetland-forested watershed. Sci Total Environ 2006;368:99–110.

Stumm W, Morgan JJ. Aquatic chemistry - Chemical equilibria and rates in natural waters. 3rd ed. New York: John Wiley & Sons, Inc.; 1996.

Ullrich SM, Tanton TW, Abdrashitova SA. Mercury in the environment: a review of the factors affecting methylation. Crit Rev Environ Sci Technol 2001;31:241–293.

Uno Y, Kiyono M, Tezuka T, Pan-Hou H. Phenylmercury transport mediated by *merT-merP* genes of *Pseudomonas* K-62 plasmid pMR26. Biol Pharm Bull 1997;20:107–109.

Vandal GM, Mason RP, Fitzgerald WF. Cycling of volatile mercury in temperate lakes. Water Air Soil Pollut 1991;56:791–803.

Vetriani C, Chew YS, Miller SM, Yagi J, Coombs J, Lutz RA, Barkay T. Mercury adaptation among bacteria from a deep-sea hydrothermal vent. Appl Environ Microbiol 2005;71:220–226.

Virta M, Lampinen J, Karp M. A luminescence-based mercury biosensor. Anal Chem 1995;67:667–669.

Wagner-Döbler I. Pilot plant for bioremediation of mercury-containing industrial wastewater. Appl Microbiol Biotechnol 2003;62:124–133.

Wagner-Döbler I, von Canstein HF, Li Y, Timmis KN, Deckwer WD. Removal of mercury from chemical wastewater by microorganisms in technical scale. Environ Sci Technol 2000;34:4628–4634.

Wang Y, Freedman Z, Lu-Irving P, Kaletzky R, Barkay T. The initial characterization of mercury resistance (*mer*) in the thermophilic bacterium *Thermus thermophilus* HB27. FEMS Microbiol Ecol 2009;67:118–129.

Warner KA, Bonzongo J-CJ, Roden EE, Ward GM, Green AC, Chaubey I, Lyons WB, Arrington DA. Effect of watershed parameters on mercury distribution in different environmental compartments in the Mobile Alabama River Basin, USA. Sci Total Environ 2005;347:187–207.

Warner KA, Roden EE, Bonzongo J-C. Microbial mercury transformation in anoxic freshwater sediments under iron-reducing and other electron-accepting conditions. Environ Sci Technol 2003;37:2159–2165.

Weber JH. Review of possible paths for abiotic methylation of mercury(II) in the aquatic environment. Chemosphere 1993;26:2063–2077.

Wiatrowski HA, Das S, Kukkadapu R, Ilton E, Barkay T, Yee N. Reduction of Hg(II) to Hg(0) by Magnetite. Environ Sci Technol 2009;42:5307–5313.

Wiatrowski HW, Ward PM, Barkay T. Novel reduction of mercury(II) by mercury-sensitive dissimilatory metal reducing bacteria. Environ Sci Technol 2006;40:6690–6696.

Widdel F, Bak F. Gram-negative mesophilic sulfate-reducing bacteria. In: Balows A, Truper HG, Dowrkin M, Harder W, Schleifer KH, editors. The prokaryotes: a handbook on the biology of bacteria: ecophysiology, isolation, identification, applications. 2nd ed. New York (NY): Springer-Verlag; 1992. p 3352–3378.

Wilson JR, Leang C, Morby AP, Hobman JL, Brown NL. MerF is a mercury transport protein: different structures but a common mechanism for mercuric ion transporters? FEBS Lett 2000;472:78–82.

Wolfe MF, Schwarzbach S, Sulaiman RA. Effects of mercury on wildlife: a comprehensive review. Environ Toxicol Chem 1998;17:146–160.

Wood JM. Biological cycles for toxic elements in the environment. Science 1974;183:1049–1052.

Wood JM. Alkylation of metals and the activity of metal-alkyls. Toxicol Environm Chem 1984;7:229–240.

Wood JM, Kennedy FS, Rosen CG. Synthesis of methyl-mercury compounds by extracts of a methanogenic bacterium. Nature 1968a;220:173–174.

Wood JM, Kennedy FS, Wolfe RS. The reaction of multihalogenated hydrocarbons with free and bound reduced vitamin B12. Biochemistry 1968b;7:1707–1713.

Yamamoto M. Possible mechanism of elemental mercury oxidation in the presence of SH compounds in aqueous solution. Chemosphere 1995;31:2791–2798.

Yamamoto M. Stimulation of elemental mercury oxidation in the presence of chloride ion in aquatic environments. Chemosphere 1996;32:1217–1224.

Yu R-Q, Adatto I, Montesdeoca MR, Driscoll CT, Hines ME, Barkay T. Mercury methylation in Sphagnum moss mats and its association with sulfate-reducing bacteria in an acidic Adirondack forest lake wetland. FEMS Microbiol Ecol 2010;74:655–668.

Zhang T, Hsu-Kim H. Photolytic degradation of methylmercury enhanced by binding to natural organic ligands. Nat Geosci 2010;3:473–476.

CHAPTER 6

PHOTOREACTIONS OF MERCURY IN AQUATIC SYSTEMS

EMMA E. VOST, MARC AMYOT, and **NELSON J. O'DRISCOLL**

6.1 SIGNIFICANCE OF MERCURY PHOTOREACTIONS

Mercury photoreactions are a significant part of the mercury cycle controlling several important processes that affect mercury fate. Two of these critical processes are (i) mercury volatilization, transport, and atmospheric deposition in remote ecosystems and (ii) the production and destruction of bioavailable methylmercury.

Mercury is present in several different species in ecosystems, and this speciation largely controls its movements and fate both regionally and globally (O'Driscoll et al., 2005a). Elemental mercury (Hg(0)) is a global contaminant that has an approximate atmospheric residence time of six months to 1 year when derived from anthropogenic sources (Selin et al., 2008); thus through long-range atmospheric transport, it can be found in the atmosphere of remote ecosystems that have no proximal point sources (O'Driscoll et al., 2005b). Through many photochemical atmospheric mechanisms, elemental mercury is oxidized to a more soluble inorganic form (e.g., monovalent (Hg(I)) and divalent mercury (Hg(II)), which are readily removed from the atmosphere and deposited in ecosystems. Monovalent mercury quickly dissociates to divalent mercury under normal atmospheric conditions (Baltisberger et al., 1979); thus divalent mercury is generally the most abundant form of mercury in aquatic ecosystems. In addition, it is highly soluble and readily binds to particles and other abundant ligands such as chloride or dissolved organic matter (DOM) (Allard and Arsenie, 1991; Xiao et al., 1995; Ravichandran, 2004).

Photochemical reactions also contribute to mercury losses from ecosystems. Photoreduction results in the production of aqueous Hg(0) (operationally defined as dissolved gaseous mercury (DGM)) from inorganic forms of mercury. This

Environmental Chemistry and Toxicology of Mercury, First Edition.
Edited by Guangliang Liu, Yong Cai, and Nelson O'Driscoll.
© 2012 John Wiley & Sons, Inc. Published 2012 by John Wiley & Sons, Inc.

aqueous Hg(0) can then volatilize to the atmosphere (a process known as *water-to-air flux*) facilitated by wind and surface layer disturbances (O'Driscoll et al., 2003a,b), thus removing mercury that would otherwise be available for methylation and bioaccumulation (Orihel et al., 2007).

Several studies have highlighted the importance of this loss process. Rolfhus and Fitzgerald (2001), using a gas exchange model, estimated that 35% of the total annual mercury inputs to Long Island Sound in New York was volatilized to the atmosphere. Mason et al. (1994) and Amyot et al. (1994) have observed that mercury volatilization can equal the rate of wet deposition, while O'Driscoll et al. (2005a,b), using quantitative data in a mass balance, observed that the mass of mercury volatilized is more than double that deposited direct to a freshwater lake. Mason et al. (1994, 2002) found that volatilization from the world's oceans may account for ~40% of the total global mercury emissions to the atmosphere. Ultraviolet radiation (UVR) has been shown to be a key factor in this reversible reaction (Amyot et al., 1994, 1997c; O'Driscoll et al., 2007), in combination with lakewater characteristics (particularly, dissolved organic carbon (DOC) concentration and structure) (Allard and Arsenie, 1991; O'Driscoll et al., 2005a,b). The relationships between UVR attenuation, the effect of DOC, and the presence of photoreactive ions or biological organisms in the water column are difficult processes to control in field experiments and may explain the conflicting findings in much of the literature.

Divalent mercury in aquatic systems may also accumulate in lake sediment where it can be methylated by bacteria and ultimately bioaccumulate in the aquatic food chain (Fig. 6.1). Methylmercury is an acute neurotoxin (Chang and Hartmann, 1972) and endocrine disrupting chemical (Zhu et al., 2000; Crump and Trudeau, 2009) that biomagnifies in food webs to such a degree that higher level trophic organisms suffer sever neurological and reproductive effects (Kim and Burggraaf, 1999; Hammerschmidt et al., 2002; Klaper et al., 2006). Several studies have indicated that photoreactions have a significant role in the demethylation of methylmercury and may also affect the abiotic methylation of mercury (Sellers et al., 1996; Siciliano et al., 2005), thereby partially regulating the biomagnification of mercury in aquatic ecosystems.

There have been many recent advances in our knowledge of mercury photochemistry in aquatic systems. A recent work by Zhang (2006) provided a review of all photochemical reactions of mercury. This chapter will specifically review the current state of the science for mercury photoreactions in aquatic systems. More quantitative measurements of these processes will lead to a better understanding of a lake's sensitivity to mercury inputs and may improve the management of mercury-sensitive ecosystems.

6.2 CONCEPTS IN MERCURY PHOTOREACTIONS

6.2.1 Photoreduction of Divalent Inorganic Mercury (Hg^{2+})

Photoreduction of divalent mercury is a significant process in aquatic ecosystems as it provides a mechanism for the production of aqueous Hg(0), which can

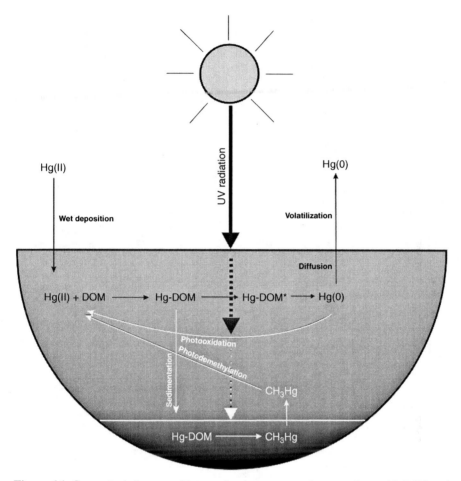

Figure 6.1 Conceptual diagram of intramolecular mercury photoreactions with DOC and fluxes in the mercury cycle of a freshwater system.

be removed from lakes through volatilization (Vandal et al., 1991; Schroeder et al., 1992). Analysis of mercury photoreduction rates has shown them to be consistent with pseudo-first-order reaction kinetics (Xiao et al., 1995; O'Driscoll et al., 2006a,b), suggesting that other reactants are in excess of the photoreducible mercury availability. There is a wide range of variability in the measured rate constants for mercury reduction in freshwater and saltwater sites as shown in Table 6.1. Since the reactions are primarily assumed to be pseudo-first-order in nature, this wide variability observed in rate constants is presumably due to the differences in the availability of reducible mercury at each site (O'Driscoll et al., 2004a,b); however, Xiao et al. (1995) found more consistent kinetic relationships when separate ligands were assumed. While the exact nature of reducible mercury is unknown, published research suggests

TABLE 6.1 Rate of Mercury Volatilization Reported in Published Literature for Freshwater and Saltwater Sites

Site Description	Mean Mercury Reduction or Oxidation Rate Constant (Standard Deviation)	Units	N	Irradiation Source	Measurement System	References
Lake N70; Central Quebec, Canada	1.01	h^{-1}	20	Natural sunlight, diurnal pattern	Batch analysis, irradiation in closed Teflon containers	O'Driscoll et al. (2004)
Spring Lake with Hg(II) spike	0.39–0.76	h^{-1}	—	Mercury arc lamp irradiation	Continuous irradiation, Tekran 2500	Hines and Brezonik (2004)
Milli-Q water with OH + Hg(II)	0.52					
Milli-Q water with Hg(II)	0.30–0.51					
Synthetic solutions with Hg(0), Photooxidation	0.6	h^{-1}	—	UV-B lamp	Continuous irradiation, Tekran 2500 AFS	Lalonde et al. (2001)
St. Lawrence river with Hg(0)	0.58					
Gouffre River	0.26					
Freshwater	0.25 (0.02)					
Sea water	0.67 (0.10)					
Pondwater spiked with Fe(III)	0.1	h^{-1}	4	Natural solar radiation, diurnal pattern	Tekran 2537A CV-AFS Continuous analysis	Zhang and Lindberg (2001)
Lakewater with Fe(III)	0.2					

Sample	Rate	Units	n	Irradiation system	Analysis	Reference
River water, UV-B only, UV-A only	1.81×10^{-4} (0.57×10^{-4}), 1.78 (1.03)	s^{-1} $\times 10^{-4}$ s^{-1}	3	LuzChem UV-B and UV-A irradiation system	Continuous irradiation and analysis CV-AFS; gross reduction only	O'Driscoll et al. (2006b)
Lakewater, UV-B only, UV-A only	8.91 (3.31), 7.76 (18.8)	$\times 10^{-5}$ s^{-1} $\times 10^{-5}$ s^{-1}				
DI Milli-Q water enhanced with algae	$0.0871 + 0.00129C_0$; $C_0 = [Hg]_{initial}$	h^{-1}	3	Metal halide lamps	CV-AAS: $[Hg]_{total}$ at 1-h intervals	Deng et al. (2008)
Chesapeake Bay, coastal seawater, Paxtuent river water, estuarine water, filtered	6.5 (1.5), 7.0 (2.0), 6.5 (2.6), respectively	$\times 10^{-4}$ s^{-1}	4	Natural sunlight, addition of $^{199}Hg(II)$ spike	Degassing, gold trap amalgamation, CV-AFS	Whalin et al. (2007)
Artificial mercury solutions			24 23	Artificial solar radiation	AAS on-line mercury monitor with zeem-effect (Semtech)	Xiao et al. (1995)
A humic substances, B humic substances	1.63 (0.29), $\times 10^{-2}$ s^{-1} 2.38 (0.40) $\times 10^{-4}$ s^{-1}					
River water: UV and visible light, Visible light only	2.2 (0.2), 1.0 (0.1), 0.183	h^{-1} s^{-1}	14 2	UV and visible radiation; visible radiation only 254-nm lamp UV irradiation	PS Analytical Merlin Mercury Monitor Total Hg (EPA 245.1) using $SnCl_2$ and AAS	Amyot et al. (2000) Byrne et al. (2009)
Mercury nitrate in deionized water						
Atlantic ocean water (3-m depth), UV-B, UV-A	0.38–0.93 h^{-1}, 0.15–0.24		—	UV-B or UV-A irradiation with lamps	Tekran 2537 continuous analysis	Qureshi et al. (2010)

AFS-atomic fluorescence spectroscopy; CVAFS-cold vapour atomic fluorescence spectroscopy; CVAAS-cold vapour atomic absorption spectroscopy; EPA-Environmental Protection Agency; AAS-atomic absorption spectroscopy.

that its availability is affected by three key variables: (i) irradiation intensity and spectrum; (ii) the quantity and structure of DOM; and (iii) the presence of dissolved ions.

6.2.1.1 Effects of Solar Radiation Intensity and Quality.

Solar radiation intensity and quality have both been shown to be important variables in the process of mercury photoreduction (Amyot et al., 1994; Zhang and Lindberg, 2001; Garcia et al., 2005a). Solar radiation spans a range of wavelengths that interact with dissolved molecules in aquatic systems; the most important wavelengths for these interactions include visible radiation (400–700 nm) and UVR (spanning 100–400 nm). UVR is subdivided into UV-C (100–280 nm), UV-B (280–320 nm), and UV-A (320–400 nm) radiation. However, the ozone layer surrounding the earth effectively absorbs all radiation below 290 nm (Kirk, 1994); thus, the incoming UVR is between 290 and 400 nm. UV-B radiation is shorter in wavelength and higher in energy than UV-A radiation, although the availability of UV-A is much greater, with 95% of the UVR reaching the earth's surface comprised of UV-A radiation, and only 5% UV-B (Blumthaler and Ambach, 1990). Photochemical reactions can be either primary or secondary in nature. Primary photochemical reactions result from the absorption of radiation by the reactant, which may result in dissociation into reactive subunits, direct reactions, ionization, or isomerization (Zhang, 2006). Secondary photochemical reactions include processes such as the absorption of radiation energy by an intermediate molecule (such as DOC) followed by secondary reactions with a reactant molecule and either the excited intermediate or subsequently produced excited subunits or free radicals (Zhang, 2006). UVR is important in aquatic chemistry because of its ability to efficiently induce primary and secondary photochemical reactions in natural waters, particularly to provide energy to bonds in complex molecules such as DOM (Häder et al., 2007). Although the mechanism for mercury photoreduction is still unclear, most recent studies suggest DOM as a required photomediator with direct photolysis being explored to a lesser extent. Nriagu (1994) suggested a general mechanism for the direct photolysis of mercury species; however, recent research has shown that direct photolysis is too slow to be a significant pathway in aquatic systems (Zhang, 2006).

Initial work in the field of mercury photochemistry was performed with broad-spectrum irradiation sources such as natural solar radiation or xenon lamps; however, recent research has focused on the effects of radiation wavelength on mercury reduction. Several studies have indicated the importance of the UV portion of the spectrum. Garcia et al. (2005a), working in freshwaters with a wide range of DOM, demonstrated that UVR can account for 61% to 73% of DGM production, while visible light can account for a maximum of 27% of DGM production in lakewater. Amyot et al. (2001) showed evidence of a relationship between solar radiation and mercury reduction in the field; solar radiation increased the ambient DGM by 2.6 times in St. Lawrence River water, with rapid increases observed at sunrise. Amyot et al. (2001) also observed a diel pattern that varied with seasonal intensity changes, whereby increased hours of sunlight in the summer result in more irradiation time. Removal of UV-B radiation using a Mylar screen did not significantly change the DGM production rates (t-test, $p > 0.05$, $N = 3$) (Amyot et al., 1994), which suggests that UV-A radiation is primarily responsible for mercury reactions. Vette (1998) found that the rate of formation of DGM is significantly reduced in the absence of UV-A (320–400 nm) radiation. Finally, the strong correlation between DGM production and photobleaching (primarily caused by UV-A radiation) found by Garcia et al. (2005a) suggests the importance of UV-A radiation in DGM photoreduction.

In recent years, research has suggested that UV-B radiation is a key portion of the electromagnetic spectrum responsible for mercury reduction in freshwaters. O'Driscoll et al. (2006a,b) performed controlled irradiation experiments in freshwaters for both UV-B and UV-A radiation and found that the rate constants were higher for UV-B irradiations (ranging from 6.00×10^{-5} s^{-1} to 4.40×10^{-4} s^{-1}) than for UV-A irradiations (ranging from 5.26×10^{-5} s^{-1} to 3.04×10^{-4} s^{-1}). O'Driscoll et al. (2006a,b) also noted a close to 50% decrease in dissolved organic carbon fluorescence (DOCF) for UV-A irradiation with no change in DOC concentration, while UV-B irradiation showed little ($<10\%$) change in DOCF or DOC, suggesting that UV-A was the primary driver for DOC structural changes resulting in fluorescence loss. Qureshi et al. (2010) observed similar mercury photoreduction results in irradiated surface water from the central North Atlantic Ocean with rate constants being higher for UV-B (ranging from 0.38 to 0.93 h^{-1}) than for UV-A (ranging from 0.15 to 0.24 h^{-1}).

The rates of photoreactions are most likely affected by a combination of the quality and intensity of radiation, the concentration and structure of chromophores in the natural water, and the rate of attenuation of specific radiation wavebands. Amyot et al. (1997b) found that the effects of irradiation on DGM formation were dependent on the DOC composition of the high Arctic lakes they examined. In medium to high DOC lakes, for example, visible radiation induced DGM formation, while UVR was mainly responsible for DGM formation in clearer lakes. They hypothesized that higher levels of DOC interfered with the availability of UVR for photochemical processes. Garcia et al. (2005a) also suggested that the type of irradiation that is most influential on DGM production depends on the DOM content. They found that clearer lakes (lower concentration of DOM chromophores) had a higher rate of DGM production under UV-B irradiation, while more humic lakes (higher concentration of DOM chromophores) had a higher rate of DGM production under UV-A irradiation.

Radiation attenuation is highly correlated with both DOM concentration and structure in freshwaters (Lean, 1998a) and has been shown to be important in the development of whole lake models for mercury photoreduction (O'Driscoll et al., 2007). The vertical attenuation coefficient (K_d) is a measure of the attenuation of light with depth in the water column (Scully and Lean, 1994), and its calculation using Equation 6.1 was outlined by Scully and Lean (1994) using the Beer–Lambert law:

$$I_d = I_0 \, e^{-K_d \times D} \tag{6.1}$$

where I_d is the intensity of radiation at any depth, I_o is the intensity of radiation at the surface of the water body, K_d is the diffuse vertical attenuation coefficient, and D is the depth.

Humic substances in DOM contain aromatic rings that readily absorb shorter wavelengths of radiation; thus UV-B has a higher attenuation coefficient than UV-A radiation in typical freshwaters (Kirk, 1994; Morris et al., 1995; Lean, 1998a). Freshwaters typically have higher concentrations of DOM than marine waters; thus UV attenuation is greater and the photoactive layer is confined to shallower depths. For instance, typically 90% of UV-B radiation is attenuated in the first 20 cm for lakes with DOM >10 mg L^{-1}, while photochemical activity can take place in the top 15 m for Pacific or Antarctic Ocean water (Lean, 1998a). Radiation intensity will therefore be distributed to deeper areas of freshwaters with lower DOM concentrations and may affect the translocation of volatile mercury to surface waters as observed in the St. Lawrence River by O'Driscoll et al. (2007).

Whalin et al. (2007) noted that a coastal shelf site with higher total suspended solids (TSSs) and a higher DOC concentration than other offshore sites had a lower reduction rate constant. They attributed this to decreased penetration of solar radiation due to the elevated levels of particles in the water. Lean (1998a,b) ascertains that particulates are more likely to have an effect on attenuation in marine waters, where light can penetrate to deeper depths because of lower concentrations of DOM.

Of recent interest is the effect of radiation on mercury reactions in frozen aquatic systems. O'Driscoll et al. (2008) observed that the St. Lawrence River has substantial contributions of volatile elemental mercury from snow and ice. Dommergue et al. (2003) examined the cycling of mercury in a snowpack and the availability of radiation; they observed that while infrared radiation is absorbed by snow, visible and UVR are scattered, leading to better penetration of these wavelengths. The absorption of UV irradiation and the depth of the photochemically active snowpack are dependent on the characteristics of the snow—crystal shape, size, structure, and composition. Mercury research in polar environments has been very active since the discovery of atmospheric mercury depletion events (MDEs) in the Arctic (Schroeder et al., 1998). With respect to photochemistry, studies have focused mostly on atmospheric and snow redox chemistry, and less on aquatic photochemistry. The interested reader is referred to the recent review by Steffen et al. (2008).

6.2.1.2 Role of Dissolved Organic Matter and Particulates.

Several researchers have examined the effects of DOM (measured as DOC concentration) on mercury reduction; however, the results are conflicting. Some researchers report that DOM has no effect on DGM concentration. Wollenberg and Peters (2009), for instance, reported no significant effect of DOM on DGM production; however, only a small range of DOC concentrations were examined (3.3–4.7 mg L^{-1}), which is on the low end of most freshwater DOC concentrations. Other scientists have reported that DGM production was not influenced by the amount of DOC present (Amyot et al., 1997c; Matthiessen, 1998; Ahn et al., 2010). In a few studies, DGM production was higher in lower DOC lakes than in higher DOC lakes (Watras et al., 1995; Amyot et al., 1997c; Garcia et al., 2005a); this could suggest a negative relationship between DOC concentrations and DGM production. One explanation for these discrepancies could be that DGM production is positively related to DOC; however, it reaches a threshold and is inhibited at higher DOC concentrations. Whatever is the exact mechanism, it is likely that the relationship between DOC concentration and DGM production is more complex than a linear relationship.

O'Driscoll et al. (2006b) suggested that the contradictions in published literature may be because of the unaccounted for variances in DOM structure in field experiments. Ideally, future research exploring this relationship should normalize reduction rates to key DOM structures involved in the mercury photoreaction. However, the DOM structures involved and the DOM-mediated mechanisms controlling mercury photoreactions under field conditions are currently unknown. A study by O'Driscoll et al. (2004a,b) controlled DOM structure and dissolved ions using tangential ultrafiltration to alter DOM concentration within a lake and found a positive relationship between DOC concentration and the rate of mercury photoreduction.

While the exact mechanism of DOM-facilitated mercury reduction is unknown, some research has suggested that DOM structure has an indirect effect on the rate of mercury photoreactions through changes in the availability of photoreducible mercury species (O'Driscoll et al., 2006b) and secondary photoreactants (Nriagu, 1994). A few researchers have tried to separate the effects of DOM structure on mercury reduction. Amyot et al. (1997b) hypothesized that mercury complexes to DOM; thus in higher DOM lakes, there is less total mercury available for photoreduction. Rolfhus et al. (2003) found that higher DOC river water more rapidly scavenged reactive mercury (mercury available for photoreactions and binding to other compounds) than estuarine water with lower DOC. However, O'Driscoll et al. (2006a,b) suggest that mercury bound to specific DOM functional groups may represent the photoreducible fraction of mercury, in which case, DOM is critical to facilitating the reduction process (Fig. 6.1).

Several researchers have pointed out that carboxylic functional groups are important structures in DOM, which affect mercury photoreactions (O'Driscoll et al., 2005a,b; Si and Ariya, 2008). As previously mentioned, it is unknown whether carboxylic acids facilitate an intramolecular (Fig. 6.1) or intermolecular (Fig. 6.2) photoreduction process; however, it is clear that both DOC concentration and structure are important in determining mercury photoreduction rates in aquatic systems (O'Driscoll et al., 2004a,b, 2006a,b).

Si and Ariya (2008) found that small (C2–C4) dicarboxylic acids play an important role in mediating the reduction of Hg(II) through complexes that are formed between these two species and that competition for complexation by chloride reduced the reduction rate, thus suggesting an intramolecular reduction process within the carboxylic acid–mercury structure. The importance of carboxylic functional groups was also observed by O'Driscoll et al. (2006b)

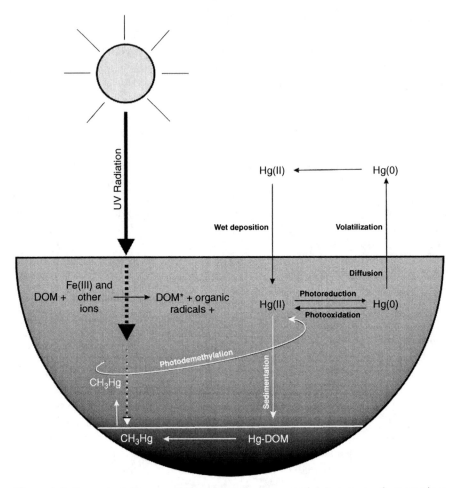

Figure 6.2 Conceptual diagram of intermolecular (or secondary) mercury photoreactions with DOC and fluxes in the mercury cycle of a freshwater system.

who found that significant differences in carboxylic acid functional groups were observable between lakes with a range of clear-cutting levels in their catchments. Although the sample size was small ($n = 4$), it was found that clear-cut lakes had lower rates of DGM photoproduction (20 fg L^{-1} $(kJ/m^2)^{-1}$) and increased levels of carboxylic functional groups on the DOM, thus supporting the concept of an intramolecular photoreduction reaction. Variations in dissolved ions between lakes and the low sample size, however, may have had an impact on this result.

Allard and Arsenie (1991) found that Hg(II) was reduced to Hg(0) by soluble humic substances, likely because of the intermediates such as semiquinones found in humic acids. Xiao et al. (1994) noted that for deionized water spiked with 20 ng L^{-1} $Hg(OH)_2$, the addition of humic and fulvic acids resulted in rate constants for photoreduction that were slightly higher ($1.3 \pm 0.3 \times 10^{-2}$ s^{-1} to 2.3×10^{-2} s^{-1})

than for natural water ($1.8 \pm 0.1 \times 10^{-2}$ s^{-1} to 4.1×10^{-3} s^{-1}). Costa and Liss (1999) observed that seawater spiked with 5 mg L^{-1} of humic acid had higher average photoreduction rates (2% per h) with natural solar irradiation over an 8-h incubation than those samples spiked with less DOC (2.5 mg L^{-1} resulting in 1.9% per h and 1 mg L^{-1} resulting in 1.16% per h) or with natural amounts of DOC (<1 mg L^{-1} resulting in 0.52% per h). Lin and Pehkonen (1997) found that mercury reactions with organic acids containing oxalates resulted in an increased mercury photoreduction rate (loss of mercury from 1.0×10^{-5} M to 1.7×10^{-6} M in ~360 min). The mechanism was hypothesized to be a result of photoproduced HO$_2$ radicals and may be further enhanced in the presence of iron oxides (loss of mercury from 1.0×10^{-5} M to below detection limits in ~100 min).

The effects of DOM on mercury reduction have been observed to vary with acidity of the water. Matthiessen (1998) related the reducing properties of humic acid to pH, with mercury reduction increasing with increasing pH. This was attributed by the author to the increases in dissociation of phenolic functional groups in the humic acid, which corresponds to a decrease in redox potential. However, it could also indicate increased mercury binding and an intramolecular reduction process. A more recent study agrees with this notion; Ahn et al. (2010) found that DGM concentrations generally increase as pH levels increase in freshwater lakes. This was attributed to the fact that nearly all the Hg(II) was bound to ligands such as DOM, and in low pH waters, the functional groups are more likely to be protonated, thus reducing the availability of complexation sites; this suggests an intramolecular process with DOM.

Organic particulates (including microbial surfaces (Daughney et al., 2002) also likely affect mercury photoreactions; however, there have been few studies to separate these effects from dissolved reactions. Effects on photoreactions from organic particles may be due to either (i) binding of photoreactants to the particle surface or (ii) to changes in quality and intensity of solar radiation because of absorption or scattering by particles. Several studies have suggested a surface binding effect. Beucher et al. (2002) determined that filtration did not have a significant effect on the production of DGM in tropical waters; they hypothesized that mercury reactions thus involve soluble species (based on the similarities between filtration and the previously studied Fe^{3+} reactions). In addition, it was suggested by Lean (1998a,b) that particles have minimal effects on UVR absorption in lakes owing to the fact that freshwater DOC concentrations are 2–40 times higher than particulate organic carbon concentrations. However, Garcia et al. (2005a) noted that the DGM production plateau was 30% higher for filtered lakewater samples. This is supported by many other researchers such as Tseng et al. (2002) who found that lakes with greater suspended particulate matter and DOC had lower rates of DGM formation. Amyot et al. (1997c) observed that filtration lowered DGM production by 26%, concluding that DGM production was associated with the dissolved and colloidal phases; however, a later study by Amyot et al. (2000) found that filtration did not decrease photoreduction. Other studies have supported the idea that particulates may have an indirect effect on mercury photoreactions through the blocking or absorption of radiation. Castelle et al. (2009) related lower DGM levels in a French estuary to higher attenuation of light due to elevated suspended particulate matter concentrations. O'Driscoll et al. (2007) explored the influence of UV attenuation on DGM production and found that 50% of volatilized DGM was produced at a depth below 0.3 m. They also related the lower UV attenuation in St. Lawrence River to low concentrations of both DOC and TSS.

The relationship between DOM and mercury reduction is thus very complex, as organic compounds can influence mercury reduction at different points in the reaction. It is clear that some DOM is needed to bind the mercury in aqueous solution and to provide photoproduced radicals; yet too much DOM can either block incoming radiation or complex mercury, making it less available for reduction. Further studies on carbon structure and how organic acids react with metals are required to better determine their effects on mercury reduction rates.

6.2.1.3 Effects of Dissolved Ions.

Several researchers have indicated that inorganic ions affect mercury photoreduction in aquatic systems. Again, the mechanisms of this may involve direct interaction with radiation or displacement of mercury from photoactive sites on DOM (Fig. 6.2). Fe oxides, Al oxides, Mn oxides, and ZnO are semiconducting phases of these metals. When dissolved in water, radiation can excite the electrons in these compounds, which are then likely available for the reduction of Hg compounds (Nriagu, 1994).

One dissolved ion that may play an important role in creating secondary photoreactants involved in mercury reduction is Fe(III). Zhang and Lindberg (2001) found that freshwater spiked with Fe(III) and then exposed to sunlight had dramatically higher increases in DGM (380% in 1 h, 420% in 2h, and 470% in 4h) than samples exposed to sunlight without the Fe(III) spike. Zhang and Lindberg (2001) suggest that highly reducing organic free radicals are created through photolysis of Fe(III)–organic acid coordination compounds (OACCs) in the mechanism outlined in Equations 6.2–6.4.

$$\text{Fe(III)} + \text{natural organic acids(OA)} \rightarrow \text{Fe(III)}-\text{(OACC)} \qquad (6.2)$$

$$\text{Fe(III)}-\text{(OACC)} + hv \rightarrow \text{Fe(II)} + \text{organic free radicals(OFR)} \qquad (6.3)$$

$$\text{OFR} + \text{Hg(II)} \rightarrow \text{Hg(0)} + \text{products} + CO_2 \qquad (6.4)$$

Zhang and Lindberg (2001) also postulated that elemental mercury oxidation may be mediated by iron in the mechanism outlined in Equations 6.5–6.8.

$$\text{Organic free radicals} + O_2 \rightarrow O_2^- + \text{products} + CO_2 \qquad (6.5)$$

$$O_2^- + O_2^- + 2H^+ \rightarrow H_2O_2 + O_2 \qquad (6.6)$$

$$H_2O_2 + \text{Fe(II)} \rightarrow OH + OH^- + \text{Fe(III)} \qquad (6.7)$$

$$OH + \text{Hg(0)} \rightarrow \text{Hg(II)} \qquad (6.8)$$

Deng *et al*. (2009) found that the photoreduction rate of divalent mercury was increased with an increasing concentration of Fe(III) and humic substances, supporting the hypothesis of Zhang and Lindberg (2001). However, the role of iron still requires some clarification as a later study by Wollenberg and Peters (2009) found no significant *in situ* correlation between total iron and Fe(III) with dissolved mercury concentrations or mercury emissions in surface water. This discrepancy may be due to a wide variety of ecosystem variables such as changes in the DOM composition of the natural water between studies or variations in the dissolved absorbance of a water body. Maloney et al. (2005) found that Fe(III) may increase UV absorbance of humic lakewater for extended time periods through binding with DOM. Lin and Pehkonen (1997) also observed that the addition of iron oxides or aerosols in aqueous solution increased the photoreduction of Hg(II) under Xenon lamp radiation. The authors identified oxalate (but not formate or acetate) as being a key facilitator of the reduction reactions through its photolysis and formation of the HO_2 radical.

The role of chloride in mercury reduction has been observed in a number of studies, which suggest that it hinders photoreduction through binding of Hg(II) in solution. Si and Ariya (2008) observed that chloride significantly reduced the reduction of mercury by small dicarboxylic acids by competing for complexation sites with the carboxylic acids. Allard and Arsenie (1991) also determined that competing ions such as chloride inhibit the reduction of mercury. However, both Matthiessen (1998) and Whalin et al. (2007) found that chloride ions did not affect the amount of Hg(II) reduced. The effect of chloride on mercury reduction may be more notable in saltwaters, where DOC concentrations are lower and chloride ions are abundant; Rolfhus et al. (2003) noted that estuarine waters were more likely to contain reactive Hg(II), which in turn enhanced the production of Hg(0), than river water. An alternate explanation for the apparent inhibitory effect of chloride on photoreduction is its role in promoting the reverse reaction, that is, Hg(0) photooxidation (Lalonde, 2001).

6.2.1.4 *Biological Influences.*

6.2.1.4 Biological Influences. The photoreduction of divalent mercury may be influenced by biological processes. Organisms may affect the concentration and structure of DOM available, thereby changing the chemical conditions of the photoreaction, or the photoreaction may be directly mediated by biological processes. When no relationship between radiation and DGM production in an artificial reservoir in Korea was observed, Ahn et al. (2010) hypothesized that the increase in DGM was attributed to the presence of microbes. A number of authors have reported a relationship between the production of DGM and phytoplanktonic pigments (Vandal et al., 1991; Baeyens and Leermakers, 1998; Poulain et al., 2004), algal physiology (Ben-Bassat and Mayer, 1978), or algal cell densities (Deng et al., 2008; Morelli et al., 2009) suggesting that plankton species may play a role in the production of Hg(0). Laboratory experiments indicate that photobiological reduction by algae is mainly controlled by the excretion of small organic molecules and free electrons. Indeed, Lanzillotta et al. (2004) have reported that at environmentally relevant Hg(II) levels (picomolar range), DGM was produced at similar rates in the presence of a marine diatom or of its isolated exudates. Deng et al. (2008) found similar results while working at high Hg(II) levels (nanomolar range), in which case, the nature of the exudates may have been altered by mercury exposure (Morelli et al., 2009). Siciliano et al. (2002) detailed a photobiological process for the reduction and oxidation of mercury, whereby microbes reduce mercury and are stimulated to oxidize mercury by the presence of photoproduced hydrogen peroxide. This mechanism was shown to be capable of resulting in the diel dynamics of DGM observed in the surface waters of lakes. However, in all these studies, the relative amount of photobiological and abiotic mercury reduction has yet to be quantified.

6.2.2 Photooxidation of Elemental Mercury

Photooxidation of elemental mercury is a process that has only recently been quantified in both freshwaters and coastal waters (Lalonde et al., 2001, 2004; Whalin et al., 2007). As such, there is much less information available on this process. There are several inherent difficulties with making these analyses: (i) the concentrations are generally at ultratrace levels ($<1 \, ng \, L^{-1}$) and subject to reproducibility errors and contamination; (ii) photooxidation tends to occur in tandem with photoreduction, making it difficult to separate out the individual rates of this reversible reaction; (iii) while the product of reduction (Hg(0)) can be easily identified and removed from solution, the oxidation of Hg(0) results in many possible complexes of inorganic mercury that join the natural pool of inorganic mercury. Finally, photooxidation measurements are also complicated by the fact that oxidation of Hg(0) has also been found to occur in the dark (Amyot et al., 1997a), and is affected by Cl^- concentrations, particles, and colloids.

6.2.2.1 Effect of Dissolved Ions on Photooxidation. Halogen elements have been implicated as key dissolved ions and atmospheric radicals controlling photoredox reactions of mercury. Bromine and chlorine atoms have been shown to be integral to the reoxidation of mercury in the atmosphere. Mason and Sheu (2004) have suggested that this process causes 40% of atmospheric Hg(0) to be reoxidized in the area where the atmosphere meets the ocean's surface (the marine boundary layer or MBL). Holmes et al. (2009) determined that bromine atoms are a significant atmospheric oxidant, as they account for 35–60% of the reactive gaseous mercury in a marine environment, while oxidation by chlorine atoms accounts for only 3–7%. Although the photoredox reaction mechanisms of halogens in the atmosphere and in aqueous solution are not entirely understood, the predominant role seems to be to enhance oxidation such that marine environments are likely to support faster oxidation than freshwater environments (Poulain *et al*., 2007; Ariya et al., 2009; Qureshi et al., 2010).

In the aqueous environment, halogen ions are also seen to play an important role in mercury photochemistry. The role of these ions as either a ligand for mercury or a direct photoreactant is still unclear. Lalonde et al. (2001) suggested that chloride ions are not an oxidant of Hg(0), but their presence is necessary to stabilize the mercury ions in solution and thus allow the transfer of an electron to an electron acceptor (such as a semiquinone). The effect of chloride ion on mercury oxidation is somewhat disputed in the literature and is an area that could use clarification. Amyot et al. (2005) found that dissolved Hg(0) under dark conditions did not rapidly oxidize in the presence of chloride ion or O_2, thus agreeing with Lalonde et al. (2004) who observed no significant loss of Hg(0) over time when brackish waters were kept in the dark. Amyot et al. (2005) did find that liquid droplets of Hg(0) were rapidly oxidized in the presence of chloride ions and that these reaction rates increased with more oxygen. This suggests that the presence of pure Hg(0) liquid surface is more important in the dark oxidation of Hg(0) than the presence of chloride ion or O_2. Lalonde et al. (2001) noted the presence of dark oxidation of coastal seawaters observed by Amyot et al. (1997a), but ascertained that photooxidation must also exist in order to explain the plateau that is observed in Hg(0) photoproduction experiments. Lalonde et al. (2001) found that oxidation of Hg(0) requires the presence of chloride ions, a photoreactive compound (such as a benzoquinone), and radiation. A photochemically produced intermediate promotes the oxidation of Hg(0) in the presence of chloride ions; therefore, the oxidation of mercury is indirectly photochemically mediated. Lalonde et al. (2001) observed that the photooxidation of Hg(0) was significant in aquatic systems with no added chloride ions, suggesting that there was either enough chloride, or another photochemically active complexing agent was present.

Hines and Brezonik (2004) determined the average first-order mercury photooxidation rate to be 0.58 h^{-1} in a small Northern Minnesota lake, and found that photooxidation rates increased with higher concentrations of chloride ions. However, it is possible that the mercury photoredox reactions in this study were affected more by the high levels of hydroxyl radicals observed than the relatively low concentrations of chloride.

Whalin et al. (2007) determined that the oxidation rate constants of freshwaters ($4.1 \pm 0.89 \times 10^{-4}$ s^{-1}) and ocean waters ($12 \pm 4.1 \times 10^{-4}$ s^{-1}) spiked with mercury were on the same order of magnitude as the reduction rate constants ($6.5 \pm 1.5 \times 10^{-4}$ s^{-1}, $7.0 \pm 2.1 \times 10^{-4}$ s^{-1}, respectively). Using Hg isotopes (^{202}Hg(0) for examining oxidation and ^{199}Hg(II) for examining reduction), they also found that oxidation rates were highest during sampling periods with exposure to sunlight ($4.7 \pm 1.2 \times 10^{-4}$ s^{-1} at midday compared to $2.1 \pm 0.4 \times 10^{-4}$ s^{-1} in morning). Since oxidation was previously thought to be a negligible process, this study was important in demonstrating that oxidation and reduction occur simultaneously and with potentially equal influence on the fate of mercury. Garcia et al. (2005b) observed that mercury photooxidation rates in a freshwater lake on the Canadian Shield ranged from 0.02 to 0.07 h^{-1} with a peak occurring near midday. In contrast to Whalin et al. (2007), Garcia *et al*. (2005b) noted that reduction was the predominant process during the day even during peak photooxidation periods. When examining the role of dicarboxylic acids in the dark reduction of divalent mercury, Si and Ariya (2008) observed that the presence of chloride ions and dissolved oxygen promoted the reoxidation of reduced Hg species to Hg(II).

6.2.2.2 Effect of Hydrogen Peroxide. Hydrogen peroxide (H_2O_2) can be a source of photochemically produced hydroxide radicals, which are thought to be the dominant oxidants of Hg(0) in natural water (Gardfeldt et al., 2001; Hines and Brezonik, 2004). However, in two field experiments examining the effects of solar radiation, Amyot et al. (1994, 1997b) added H_2O_2 to lakewater during incubation and did not observe significant changes in mercury photoreduction. Schroeder et al. (1992) suggest that the H_2O_2 may oxidize (at higher pH; Eq. 6.9) or reduce (at lower pH; Eq. 6.10) depending on the concentration of complex-forming species (such as DOM).

$$H_2O_2 + 2H^- + Hg(0) \rightarrow 2H_2O + Hg^{2+} \tag{6.9}$$

$$H_2O_2 + 2OH^- + Hg^{2+} \rightarrow O_2 + 2H_2O + Hg(0) \tag{6.10}$$

It has also been suggested that the effect of H_2O_2 on mercury photoreactions may be indirect through biological mechanisms. Siciliano et al. (2002) determined that microbial enzymes inducing oxidation were stimulated in the presence of hydrogen peroxide. H_2O_2 follows a strong diel pattern in lakewater because of its photochemical production through reactions with DOM as outlined by Scully et al. (1996). As such, Siciliano et al. (2002) suggest that the photoproduction of H_2O_2 may partially regulate the oxidation of elemental mercury in freshwaters through microbial mechanisms.

6.2.3 Photoreactions of Methylmercury

Much research has been done examining microbial methylation of mercury. Sulfate-reducing bacteria have been identified as principal methylators (Gilmour et al., 1992) with other bacterial populations (e.g., iron-reducing bacteria) recently being explored as significant methylators in some ecosystems (Fleming et al., 2006; Kerin et al., 2006). While there is very little evidence of mercury pho-tomethylation, Siciliano et al. (2005) observed that methylmercury concentrations peaked at solar noon in two contracting lakes in Kejimkujik Park, Nova Scotia, showing a diurnal pattern over a 48-h measurement period. Siciliano et al. (2005) also found that the photoproduction of methylmercury was dependent on the DOM structure present in the freshwater.

The photodegradation of methylmercury is a process significantly affecting the budget of methylmercury in aquatic systems and can account for as much as 80% of MeHg flux out of lakes (Sellers et al., 2001). Sellers et al. (1996) were the first to detail the degradation of methylmercury by solar radiation in freshwater lakes and to highlight the importance of this process. A few recent studies have confirmed these results. Notably, Hammerschmidt and Fitzgerald (2006) calculated that this process was very significant in Arctic lakes, accounting for about 80% of the methylmercury mobilized annually from *in situ* sedimentary production. They further showed that sterilization or filtration of the lake samples before exposure to solar radiation did not affect degradation rates, therefore suggesting that photodemethylation was mainly abiotic. Recent work by Hammerschmidt and Fitzgerald (2010) showed that the photodegradation of MeHg in Arctic lakes is not a result of direct photolysis or reactions with DOM, instead secondary oxidants such as the hydroxyl radical produced by photo-Fenton reactions are key reactants, with photon flux being the primary control. For northern temperate lakes, Hg photodemethylation is largely driven by UVR, with demethylation rates an order of magnitude greater in their presence (Lehnherr and St.Louis, 2009), when compared to exposure to visible radiation only. Indeed, UVR can account for 58% and 79% of methylmercury photodemethylation in clear and colored lakes, respectively.

The potential mechanisms involved in photodemethylation have been recently reviewed by Chen et al. (2003) and Zhang et al. (2006). Although methylmercury can be directly degraded by UVR, this photolysis occurs at wavelengths not encountered at the earth's surface (Inoko, 1981); therefore, photodemethylation is mainly driven by indirect processes. Suda et al. (1993) reported that methyl and ethyl mercury can be dealkylated by reactive oxygen species, such as hydroxyl radicals and singlet oxygen. Chen et al. (2003) demonstrated through laboratory studies that methylmercury photodemethylation by hydroxyl radicals, produced via photo-Fenton reactions or photolysis of nitrate, followed pseudo-first-order kinetics, and the rates were increased in the presence of chloride. The authors proposed that both hydroxyl and chlorine radicals could attack the C–Hg bond, resulting in demethylation and this is supported by the recent work of Hammerschmidt and Fitzgerald (2010). Most studies report inorganic Hg(II) as the main product of the reaction (Gardfeldt et al., 2001). Assuming that this is correct in a natural ecosystem, this Hg(II) would then be available for photoreduction processes (Figs 6.1 and 6.2).

Although photodemethylation rates in laboratory studies are often enhanced by the presence of chloride ions, Zhang and Hsu-Kim (2010) recently noted that photodemethylation measured in the field was often slower in seawater than in lakewater. They argued that the steady-state concentrations of hydroxyl radicals needed to sustain photodegradation in aquatic systems could only be achieved under very specific conditions, such as in agriculturally impacted waters (with nitrate available for hydroxyl formation) or in acidic waters, and that other photoreaction intermediates, such as singlet oxygen, are probably more important than previously acknowledged. A key discovery of their study is that the speciation of methylmercury with DOM has a direct impact on its photochemical degradation. Specifically, when methylmercury is complexed to small nonprotein sulfur-containing ligands such as glutathione or mercaptoacetate, degradation rates are faster than when methylmercury is present as chloride complexes. This argues for more research on Hg and MeHg–thiol complexation and the photochemistry in aquatic systems (Moingt et al., 2010).

6.3   CURRENT METHODS IN MERCURY PHOTOCHEMISTRY

In most remote environments, elemental mercury exists in water at trace-level concentrations that can fluctuate substantially in short periods of time (O'Driscoll et al., 2003b). It is therefore important to develop accurate and precise analytical methods that are capable of high temporal resolution. Several important factors in method development include the type of materials used, the means of sample collection and storage, and the temporal resolution of the analysis.

Teflon or glass analysis vessels are most commonly used for elemental mercury analysis owing to low binding affinity for trace ions. FEP Teflon®, however, may increase error through Hg(0) absorption (Whalin and Mason, 2006), unless it is prerinsed with acid. Discrete or individual sample methods involving Teflon containers and transport to an on-site lab were commonly used in many studies of DGM production (Amyot et al., 1994; O'Driscoll et al., 2004a,b). These methods suffer from transportation issues and poor temporal resolution. Transportation of samples typically involves dark cold storage in either dark plastic Teflon containers or aluminum foil coverings inside a cooler (Amyot et al., 1994; Whalin and Mason, 2006). The necessity of storage and transport protocol has recently been removed by the development of *in situ* methods (Amyot et al., 2001). For instance, O'Driscoll et al. (2003a,b, 2007) monitored the *in situ* creation of DGM production under the influence of natural solar radiation using a glass sparger connected to a peristaltic pump to sample surface water and a continuous gaseous mercury monitoring system (Tekran 2537) to achieve a 5-min analysis resolution.

In situ methods for analyzing mercury photoreactions have several advantages: (i) there is less possibility for sample contamination or degradation during transport and (ii) it allows for real-time analysis often with high temporal resolution. This is particularly important when analyzing for subparts-per-trillion concentrations of mercury. These methods provide environmentally realistic data; however, they suffer the disadvantage of having little control of environmental variables. As such, a detailed analysis of mechanisms is often not possible.

O'Driscoll et al. (2004b,2007) noted that many methods of DGM analysis involve the measurement of mercury that has been previously formed in the sample. The DGM concentrations thus represent the net production of elemental mercury, as mercury photooxidation partially balances the reduction process. Continuous physical removal of DGM as it is formed thereby pushes this reversible photoreaction predominantly toward reduction that has been labeled gross reduction by O'Driscoll et al. (2004b). Using controlled irradiation and continuous DGM analysis (Fig. 6.3) and plotting the gross cumulative elemental mercury production, O'Driscoll et al. (2004b) observed that the reaction follows pseudo-first-order kinetics. As such, the reaction rate constant can be quantified through curve fitting the integrated first-order reaction equation. Table 6.1 summarizes the rate constants obtained from a variety of net reduction and gross reduction studies. It can be seen that the values typically span a wide range (from 0.2 to 2.2 h^{-1}) likely because of the variations in DOM, dissolved ions, and irradiation characteristics as previously discussed.

Through the measurement of both net photoreduction kinetics and gross photoreduction kinetics, the gross photooxidation kinetics can be calculated and accurately quantified (Qureshi et al., 2010). Another method was developed by

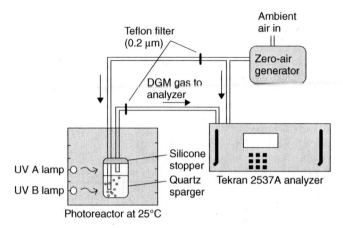

Figure 6.3 Schematic of the gross reduction analysis system using Tekran 2537A analyzer, quartz sparger, and photoincubator.

Whalin and Mason (2006) to concurrently measure mercury reduction and oxidation by adding isotopically labeled ^{199}Hg(II) and ^{202}Hg(0) and measuring the final ratios of ^{199}Hg and ^{202}Hg species relative to ^{201}Hg using inductively coupled plasma-mass spectrometry (ICP-MS) such that simultaneous processes can be examined. These methodology advancements will allow for the identification of specific factors that control both the reduction and oxidation half reactions; such relationships may have not been observable using net reduction measurements.

In addition to using Hg isotopes as conservative tracers, a number of recent studies have established that Hg fractionation can occur in the environment. For instance, the discovery that photochemical reduction of aqueous mercury leads to both mass-dependent fractionation of Hg isotopes and mass-independent fractionation (MIF) of the odd-mass isotopes provides a new set of tools for tracing Hg biogeochemical pathways (Bergquist and Blum, 2007). Early results from this emerging field suggest that MIF signals in fish can be used as a record of the amount of mercury lost from a lake or the ocean as a result of photoreduction and water–air exchange (Bergquist and Blum, 2007). This type of technique can also provide insights related to photochemical mechanisms. For instance, results from Zheng and Hintelmann (2010) suggest that opposite magnetic isotope effects are produced by S-containing ligands (e.g., cysteine, glutathione) as opposed to other ligands (serine, oxalic acid). These isotopic effects specifically can be used to distinguish the role of different organic functional groups during Hg phototransformations.

6.4 SUMMARY

Photoreactions are an integral component of the mercury cycle, controlling processes such as deposition, volatilization, and availability of methylmercury. However, many of these processes have been poorly studied and many research gaps remain. One of the key research gaps concerns the interaction between DOM and mercury species, specifically the form of mercury available for photoreactions. The most recent research suggests that DOM structure may be a key factor influencing the rates of mercury photoreduction (and possibly photooxidation). Much of the previous theory on this subject has treated mercury reduction as an intermolecular (Fig. 6.2) reaction involving DOM as a charged species and resulting in the creation of secondary photoreducing agents that facilitate the electron transfer to mercury. In this review, we suggest that it is equally likely that mercury reduction may be an intramolecular process (Fig. 6.1), with mercury bound to specific DOM functional groups receiving the electron transfer from photoactive DOM groups. However, the exact relationship between DOM structure and these processes has to be quantified yet. Currently, the term *photoreducible mercury* is used in models to represent the mercury available for reduction; however, it is not yet clear if this represents mercury bound to DOM or other mercury species in freshwater. This will be a key area for future research.

Another gap includes the mechanisms of mercury photooxidation, where many similar processes require clarification. A large number of publications on Hg(II) oxidation have focused on atmospheric chemistry and, as a result, most proposed photochemical intermediates are important atmospheric oxidants such as hydroxyl radicals. The role of longer-lived oxidants associated with DOM needs to be better ascertained. Examples of these include phenolic radicals, excited triplet states of DOM, and other DOM-derived radicals (Zhang, 2006).

Much work is also required in the area of modeling. Mechanistic models may lead to new insights into these processes. For example, recent work by Qureshi et al. (2010) demonstrated that mercury photoreduction reactions in ocean water are seemingly more complex than freshwaters, resulting in the production of an unknown mercury species that is not readily available for photoreduction.

The role of irradiation quality still requires more effort, in particular, the development of more realistic models that incorporate the effects of solar attenuation of specific wavebands in aquatic systems. This has been performed to a limited extent at specific sites (O'Driscoll et al., 2007); however, no whole lake depth-integrated models have been developed over a range of sites.

REFERENCES

Ahn M-C, Holsen TB, Yi S-M, Han Y-J. Factors influencing concentrations of dissolved gaseous mercury (DGM) and total mercury (TM) in an artificial reservoir. Environ Pollut 2010;158:347–355.

Allard B, Arsenie I. Abiotic reduction of mercury by humic substances in aquatic system-an important process for the mercury cycle. Water Air Soil Pollut 1991;56:457–464.

Amyot M, Auclair JC, Poissant L. In situ high temporal resolution analysis of elemental mercury in natural waters. Anal Chim Acta 2001;447:153–159.

Amyot M, Mierle G, Lean DRS, McQueen DJ. Sunlight-induced formation of dissolved gaseous mercury in lake waters. Environ Sci Technol 1994;28:2366–2371.

Amyot M, Gill GA, Morel FMM. Production and loss of dissolved gaseous mercury in coastal seawater. Environ Sci Technol 1997a;31(12):3603–3611.

Amyot M, Lean DRS, Mierle G. Photochemical formation of volatile mercury in high Arctic lakes. Environ Toxicol Chem 1997b;16(10):2054–2063.

Amyot M, Mierle G, Lean DRS, McQueen DJ. Effect of solar radiation on the formation of dissolved gaseous mercury in temperate lakes. Geochim Cosmochim Acta 1997c;61:975–987.

Amyot M, Lean DRS, Poissant L, Doyon M-R. Distribution and transformation of elemental mercury in the St. Lawrence River and Lake Ontario. Can J Fish Aquat Sci 2000;57:155–163.

Amyot M, Morel FMM, Ariya PA. Dark oxidation of dissolved liquid elemental mercury in aquatic environments. Environ Sci Technol 2005;39: 110–114.

Ariya PA, Peterson K, Snider G, Amyot M. Mercury chemical transformations in the gas, aqueous and heterogeneous phases: state-of-the-art science and uncertainties. In: Mason R, Pirrone N, editors. Mercury fate and transport in the global atmosphere. New York (NY): Springer; 2009. p 459–501.

Baeyens W, Leermakers M. Elemental mercury concentrations and formation rates in the Scheldt Estuary and the North Sea. Mar Chem 1998;60:257–266.

Baltisberger RJ, Hildebrand DA, Grieble D, Ballintine TA. A study of the disproportionation of mercury (I) induced by gas sparging in acidic aqueous solutions for cold-vapor atomic absorption spectrometry. Anal Chim Acta 1979;111:111–122.

Ben-Bassat D, Mayer AM. Light induced volatilization and O2 evolution in *chlorella* and the effect of DCMU and methylamine. Physiol Plant 1978;42: 33–38.

Bergquist BA, Blum JD. Mass-dependent and-independent fractionation of Hg isotope by photo-reduction in aquatic systems. Science 2007;318(5849):417–420.

Beucher C, Wong-Wah-Chung P, Richard C, Mailhot G, Bolte M, Cossa D. Dissolved gaseous mercury formation under UV irradiation of unamended tropical waters from French Guyana. Sci Total Environ 2002;290: 131–138.

Blumthaler M, Ambach W. Indication of increasing solar ultraviolet-B radiation flux in Alpine regions. Science 1990;248: 206–208.

Castelle S, Schäfer J, Blanc G, Dabrin A, Lanceleur L, Masson M. Gaseous mercury at the air-water interface of a highly turbid estuary (Gironde Estuary, France). Mar Chem 2009;117: 42–51.

Chang LW, Hartmann HA. Ultrastructural studies of the nervous system after mercury intoxication. Acta Neuropathol 1972;20: 122–138.

Chen J, Pehkonen SO, Lin C-J. Degradation of monomethylmercury chloride by hydroxyl radicals in simulated natural waters. Water Res 2003;37(10):2496–2504.

Costa M, Liss PS. Photo-reduction of mercury in sea water and its possible implications for Hg^0 air-sea fluxes. Mar Chem 1999;68:87–95.

Crump KL, Trudeau VL. Mercury-induced reproductive impairment in fish. Environ Toxicol Chem 2009;28(5):895–907.

Daughney CJ, Siciliano SD, Rencz AN, Lean D, Fortin D. Hg(II) adsorption by bacteria: a surface complexation model and its application to shallow acidic lakes and wetlands in Kejimkujik National Park, Nova Scotia, Canada. Environ Sci Technol 2002;36(7):1546–1553.

Deng L, Fu D, Deng N. Photo-induced transformation of mercury (II) species in the presence of algae, *Chlorella vulgaris*. J Hazard Mater 2009;164:798–805.

Deng L, Wu F, Deng N, Zuo Y. Photo-reduction of mercury (II) in the presence of algae, *Anabaena cylindrical*. J Photochem Photobiol B 2008;91:117–124.

Dommergue A, Ferrari CP, Poissant L, Gauchard P-A, Boutron CF. Diurnal cycles of gaseous mercury at Kuujjuarapik/Whapmagoostui, Québec, Canada. Environ Sci Technol 2003;37(15):3289–3297.

Fleming EJ, Mack EE, Green PG, Nelson DC. Mercury methylation from unexpected sources: molybdate-inhibited freshwater sediments and an iron-reducing bacterium. Appl Environ Microbiol 2006;72(1):457–464.

Garcia E, Amyot M, Ariya P. Relationship between DOC photochemistry and mercury redox transformation in temperate lakes and wetlands. Geochim Cosmochim Acta 2005a;69(8):1917–1924.

Garcia E, Poulain AJ, Amyot M, Ariya PA. Diel variations in photoinduced oxidation of Hg^0 in freshwater. Chemosphere 2005b;59:977–981.

Gardfeldt K, Sommar J, Stromberg D, Feng X. Oxidation of atomic mercury by hydroxyl radicals and photoinduced decomposition of methylmercury in the aqueous phase. Atmos Environ 2001;35:3039–3047.

Gilmour CC, Henry EA, Mitchell R. Sulfate stimulation of mercury methylation in freshwater sediments. Environ Sci Technol 1992;26(11):2281–2287.

Häder D-P, Kumar HD, Smith RC, Worrest RC. Effects of solar UV radiation on aquatic ecosystems and interactions with climate change. Photochem Photobiol Sci 2007;6:267–285.

Hammerschmidt CR, Fitzgerald WF. Photodecomposition of methylmercury in an arctic Alaskan lake. Environ Sci Technol 2006;40(4):1212–1216.

Hammerschmidt CR, Fitzgerald WF. Iron-mediated photochemical decomposition of methylmercury in an Arctic Alaskan lake. Environ Sci Technol 2010;44:6138–6143.

Hammerschmidt CR, Sanderheinrich MB, Wiener JG, Rada RG. Effects of dietary methylmercury on reproduction of fathead minnows. Environ Sci Technol 2002;36:877–883.

Hines NA, Brezonik PL. Mercury dynamics in a small Northern Minnesota lake: water to air exchange and photoreactions of mercury. Mar Chem 2004;90:137–149.

Holmes CD, Jacob DJ, Mason RP, Jaffe DA. Sources and deposition of reactive gaseous mercury in the marine atmosphere. Atmos Environ 2009;43:2278–2285.

Inoko M. Studies on the photochemical decomposition of organomercurials-methylmercury (II) chloride. Environ Pollut B 1981;2(1):3–10.

Kerin EJ, Gilmour CC, Roden E, Suzuki MT, Coates JD, Mason RP. Mercury methylation by dissimilatory iron-reducing bacteria. Appl Environ Microbiol 2006;72(12):7919–7921.

Kim JP, Burggraaf S. Mercury bioaccumulation in rainbow trout (*Oncorhynchus mykiss*) and the trout food web in Lakes Okareka, Okarom Tarawera, Rotomahana, and Rotorua, New Zealand. Water Air Soil Pollut 1999;115:535–546.

Kirk JTO. Optics of UV-B radiation in natural waters. Arch Hydrobiol Beih Ergeb Limnol 1994;43:1–16.

Klaper R, Rees CB, Drevnick P, Weber D, Sandheinrich M, Carvan MJ. Gene expression changes related to endocrine function and decline in reproduction in fathead minnow (*Pimpephales promelas*) after dietary methylmercury exposure. Environ Health Perspect 2006;114(9):1337–1343.

Lalonde JD, Amyot M, Kraepiel AM, Morel FMM. Photo-oxidation of Hg(0) in artificial and natural waters. Environ Sci Technol 2001;35:1367–1372.

Lalonde JD, Amyot M, Orvoine J, Morel FMM, Ariya PA. Photoinduced oxidation of Hg(0)(aq) in the waters from the St. Lawrence estuary. Environ Sci Technol 2004;38:508–514.

Lanzillotta E, Ceccarini C, Ferrara R, Dini F, Frontini FP, Banchetti R. Importance of the biogenic organic matter in photo-formation of dissolved gaseous mercury in a culture of the marine diatom Chaetoceros sp. Sci Total Environ 2004;318(1–3):211–221.

Lean DRS. Attenuation of solar radiation in humic waters. In: Hessen DO, Tranvik LJ, editors. Aquatic humic substances. New York (NY): Springer-Verlag; 1998a;109–124.

Lean DRS. Influence of UVB radiation on aquatic ecosystems. In: Little EE, DeLonay AJ, Greenberg BM, editors. Environmental toxicology and risk assessment. Volume 7, American Society for Testing and Materials. Philadelphia (PA); 1998b. ASTM STP 1333.

Lehnherr I, St.Louis VL. Importance of ultraviolet radiation in the photodemethylation of methylmercury in freshwater ecosystems. Environ Sci Technol 2009;43(15):5692–5698.

Lin CJ, Pehkonen SO. Aqueous free radical chemistry of mercury in the presence of iron oxides and ambient aerosol. Atmos Environ 1997;31(24):4125–4237.

Maloney KO, Morris DP, Moses CO, Osburn CL. The role of iron and dissolved organic carbon in the absorption of ultraviolet radiation in humic lake water. Biogeochemistry 2005;75(3):393–407.

Mason RP, Fitzgerald WF, Morel FMM. The biogeochemical cycling of elemental mercury, anthropogenic influences. Geochim Cosmochim 1994;58(15):3191–3198.

Mason RP, Sheu G-R. Role of the ocean in the global mercury cycle. Biogeochem Cycles 2002;16(4):1093–2010.

Mason RP, Sheu GR. An examination of the oxidation of elemental mercury in the presence of halide surfaces. J Atmos Chem 2004;48:107–130.

Matthiessen A. Reduction of divalent mercury by humic substances—kinetic and quantitative aspects. Sci Total Environ 1998;213:177–183.

Moingt M, Bressac M, Bélanger D, Amyot M. Role of ultra-violet radiation, mercury and copper on the stability of dissolved glutathione in natural and artificial freshwater and saltwater. Chemosphere 2010;80(11):1314–1320.

Morelli E, Ferrara R, Bellini B, Dini F, Giuseppe G, Fantozzi L. Changes in the non-protein thiol pool and production of dissolved gaseous mercury in the marine diatom Thalassiosira weissflogii under mercury exposure. Sci Total Environ 2009;408(2):286–293.

Morris DP, Zagarese H, Williamson CE, Balseiro EG, Hargreaves BR, Modenutti B. The attenuation of solar UV radiation in lakes and the role of dissolved organic carbon. Limnol Oceanogr 1995;40(8):1381–1391.

Nriagu JO. Mechanistic steps in the photo-reduction of mercury in natural waters. Sci Total Environ 1994;154:1–8.

O'Driscoll NJ, Beauchamp S, Rencz AN, Lean DRS. Continuous analysis of dissolved gaseous mercury (DGM) and mercury flux in two freshwater lakes in Kejimkujik National Park, Nova Scotia, evaluating mercury flux models with quantitative data. Environ Sci Technol 2003a;37:2226–2235.

O'Driscoll NJ, Siciliano SD, Lean DRS. Continuous analysis of dissolved gaseous mercury in freshwater lakes. Sci Total Environ 2003b;304:285–294.

O'Driscoll NJ, Lean DRS, Loseto LL, Carignan R, Siciliano SD. Effect of dissolved organic carbon on the photoproduction of dissolved gaseous mercury in lakes: potential impacts of forestry. Environ Sci Technol 2004a;38: 2664–2672.

O'Driscoll NJ, Siciliano SD, Lean DRS, Amyot M. Gross photo-reduction kinetics of mercury in temperate freshwater lakes and rivers: application to a general model of DGM dynamics. Environ Sci Technol 2004b;40:837–843.

O'Driscoll, NJ, Rencz, AN, Lean, DRS. The biogeochemistry and fate of mercury in natural environments. In: Sigel A, Sigel H, Sigel RKO, editors. Metal ions in biological systems. Volume 43, New York (NY): Marcel Dekker, Inc; 2005a.

O'Driscoll NJ, Rencz AN, Lean DRS, editors. Mercury Cycling in a Wetland Dominated Ecosystem, A Multidisciplinary Study. Pensacola (FL): SETAC Publishers; 2005b.

O'Driscoll NJ, Siciliano SD, Lean DRS, Amyot M. Gross photo-reduction kinetics of mercury in temperate freshwater lakes and rivers: application to a general model of DGM dynamics. Environ Sci Technol 2006a;40:837–843.

O'Driscoll NJ, Siciliano SD, Peak D, Carignan R, Lean DRS. The influence of forestry activity on the structure of dissolved organic matter in lakes: implications for mercury photoreactions. Sci Total Environ 2006b;366:880–893.

O'Driscoll NJ, Poissant L, Canário J, Ridal J, Lean DRS. Continuous analysis of dissolved gaseous mercury and mercury volatilization in the upper St. Lawrence River: exploring temporal relationships and UV attenuation. Environ Sci Technol 2007;41:5342–5348.

O'Driscoll NJ, Poissant L, Cañario J, Lean DRS. Dissolved gaseous mercury concentrations and mercury volatilization in a frozen freshwater fluvial lake. Environ Sci Technol 2008;42(14):5125–5130.

Orihel DM, Paterson MJ, Blanchfield PJ, Bodaly RA, Hintelmann H. Experimental evidence of a linear relationship between inorganic mercury loading and methylmercury accumulation by aquatic biota. Environ Sci Technol 2007;47:4952–4958.

Poulain AJ, Amyot M, Findlay D, Telor S, Barkay T, Hintelmann H. Biological and photochemical production of dissolved gaseous mercury in a boreal lake. Limnol Oceanogr 2004;49(6):2265–2275.

Poulain AJ, Garcia E, Amyot M, Campbell PGC, Raofie F, Ariya PA. Biological and chemical redox transformations of mercury in fresh and salt waters of the high arctic during spring and summer. Environ Sci Technol 2007;41(6):1883–1888.

Qureshi A, O'Driscoll NJ, MacLoed M, Neuhold Y-M, Hungerbuhler K. Photoreactions of mercury in surface ocean water, gross reaction kinetics and possible pathways. Environ Sci Technol 2010;44(2):644–649.

Ravichandran M. Interactions between mercury and dissolved organic matter—a review. Chemosphere 2004;55:319–331.

Rolfhus KR, Fitzgerald WF. The evasion and spatial/temporal distribution of mercury species in Long Island Sound, CT-NY. Geochim Cosmochim Acta 2001;65(3):407–418.

Rolfhus KR, Lamborg CH, Fitzgerald WF, Balcom PH. Evidence for enhanced mercury reactivity in response to estuarine mixing. J Geophys Res 2003;108:3353–3364.

Schroeder WH, Anlauf KG, Barrie LA, Lu JY, Steffen A, Schneeberger DR, Berg T. Arctic springtime depletion of mercury. Nature 1998;394:331–332.

Schroeder WH, Lindqvist O, Munthe J, Xiao Z. Volatilisation of mercury from lake surfaces. Sci Total Environ 1992;125:47–66.

Scully NM, Lean DRS. The attenuation of ultraviolet radiation in temperate lakes. Arch Hydrobiol 1994;43:135–144.

Scully NM, McQueen DJ, Lean DRS, Cooper WJ. Hydrogen peroxide formation: the interaction of ultraviolet radiation and dissolved organic carbon in lake waters along a 43–75°N gradient. Limnol Oceanogr 1996;41(3):540–548.

Selin, NE, Jacob, DJ, Yiantosca, RW, Strode, S, Jaeglé, L, Sunderland, EM. Global 3-D land-ocean-atmosphere model for mercury: present-day versus preindustrial cycles and anthropogenic enrichment factors for deposition. Global Biogeochem Cycles 2008;22, GB2011, 13 pp.

Sellers P, Kelly CA. Fluxes of methylmercury to the water column of a drainage lake: the relative importance of internal and external sources. Limnol Oceanogr 2001;46(3):623–631.

Sellers P, Kelly CA, Rudd JWM, MacHutchon AR. Photodegradation of methylmercury in lakes. Nature 1996;380:694–697.

Si L, Ariya P. Reduction of oxidized mercury species by dicarboxylic acids (C2–C4): kinetic and product studies. Environ Sci Technol 2008;42:5150–5155.

Siciliano SD, O'Driscoll NJ, Lean DRS. Microbial reduction and oxidation of mercury in freshwater lakes. Environ Sci Technol 2002;36:3064–3068.

Siciliano SD, O'Driscoll NJ, Tordon R, Hill J, Beauchamp S, Lean DRS. Abiotic production of methylmercury by solar radiation. Environ Sci Technol 2005;39:1071–1077.

Steffen A, Douglas T, Amyot M, Ariya P, Aspmo K, Berg T, Bottenheim J, Brooks S, Cobbett F, Dastoor A, Dommergue A, Ebinghaus R, Ferrari C, Gardfeldt K, Goodsite ME, Lean D, Poulain AJ, Scherz H, Sommar J, Temme C. A synthesis of atmospheric mercury depletion event chemistry in the atmosphere and snow. Atmos Chem Phys 2008;8(6):1445–1482.

Suda I, Suda M, Hirayama K. Degradation of methyl and ethyl mercury by singlet oxygen generated from sea water exposed to sunlight or ultraviolet radiation. Arch Toxicol 1993;67:365–368.

Tseng CM, Lamborg C, Fitzgerald WF, Engstrom DR. Cycling of dissolved elemental mercury in Arctic Alaskan lakes. Geochim Cosmochim Acta 2002;68:1173–1184.

Vandal GM, Mason RP, Fitzgerald WF. Cycling of volatile mercury in temperate lakes. Water Air Soil Pollut 1991;56:791–803.

Vette AF. Photochemical influences on the air-water exchange of mercury [thesis]. Michigan: University of Michigan; 1998. UMI Dissertation Services, Bell and Howell.

Watras CJ, Morrison KA, Host JS. Concentrations of mercury species in relationship to other site-specific factors in the surface waters of Northern Wisconsin lakes. Limnol Oceanogr 1995;40:556–565.

Whalin L, Kim E-H, Mason R. Factors influencing the oxidation, reduction, methylation and demethylation of mercury species in coastal waters. Mar Chem 2007;107(3):278–294.

Whalin LM, Mason RP. A new methos for the investigation of mercury redox chemistry in natural waters utilizing deflatable Teflon(R) bags and additions of isotopically labelled mercury. Anal Chim Acta 2006;558:211–221.

Wollenberg JL, Peters SC. Mercury emission from a temperate lake during autumn turnover. Sci Total Environ 2009;407(8):2909–2918.

Xiao ZF, Munthe J, Stromberg D, Lindqvist O. Photochemical behaviour of inorganic mercury compounds in aqueous solution. In: Watras CJ, Huckabee JW, editors. Mercury pollution: integration and synthesis. Florida: Lewis Publishers, CRC Press; 1994. p 581–592.

Xiao ZF, Stromberg D, Lindqvist O. Influence of humic substances on photolysis of divalent mercury in aqueous solution. Water Air Soil Pollut 1995;80:789–798.

Zhang H. Photochemical redox reactions of mercury. Struct Bond 2006;120:37–79.

Zhang T, Hsu-Kim H. Photolytic degradation of methylmercury enhanced by binding to natural organic ligands. Nat Geosci 2010;3(7):473–476.

Zhang H, Lindberg S. Sunlight and iron(III)-induced photochemical production of dissolved gaseous mercury in freshwater. Environ Sci Technol 2001;35:928–935.

Zheng W, Hintelmann H. Isotope fractionation of mercury during its photochemical reduction by low-molecular-weight organic compounds. J Phys Chem A 2010;114(12):4246–4253.

Zhu X, Kusaka Y, Sato K, Zhang Q. The endocrine disruptive effects of mercury. Environ Health Prev Med 2000;4:174–183.

CHAPTER 7

CHEMICAL SPECIATION OF MERCURY IN SOIL AND SEDIMENT

ULF SKYLLBERG

7.1 INTRODUCTION

Reactions of mercury and its chemical speciation in soils and sediments have been covered in several reviews over the years (Andersson, 1979; Benes and Havlik, 1979; Schuster, 1991). The latest comprehensive review of the chemical speciation, linked to the bioaccumulation of mercury, in aquatic and terrestrial environments was published in 1998 (Morel et al., 1998). Since then, experimental and field-oriented studies have contributed significant new findings. Especially, the role of natural organic matter (NOM) has been updated. Spectroscopic and binding affinity studies conducted at environmentally relevant conditions have provided new information on the stability and structure of inorganic mercury (Hg) and methyl mercury (MeHg) complexes with thiol groups in NOM. Studies have pointed out the stabilizing effect of NOM on nanoparticulate HgS(s). This has not only led to an improved understanding of the mobility of mercury but has also questioned methods used to separate aqueous and solid phases, as well as stability constants relying on those methods. Studies on chemical reactions between Hg and iron sulfides have provided quantitative data that could be incorporated in chemical equilibrium models. Despite these significant advances there is still a long way to go before the chemical speciation and solubility of mercury is fully understood. It is noteworthy that there is still not a single study in which the absolute concentration of Hg in the pore water of a soil or sediment has been satisfactorily explained by thermodynamic models, covering molecular species pertaining to aqueous and solid phases. A remaining important challenge is to determine the aqueous phase chemical speciation of Hg in equilibrium with solid phases of HgS(s) at total concentrations of sulfides less than 10 μM. Also the issues of polysulfide formation and the interaction between Hg and MeHg

Environmental Chemistry and Toxicology of Mercury, First Edition.
Edited by Guangliang Liu, Yong Cai, and Nelson O'Driscoll.
© 2012 John Wiley & Sons, Inc. Published 2012 by John Wiley & Sons, Inc.

and various types of metal sulfides need to be resolved before thermodynamic models are good enough to be used for explanatory and predictive purposes in soils and sediments.

7.2 PHYSICOCHEMICAL PROPERTIES, OXIDATION STATES, CHEMICAL FORMS, STRUCTURES, AND CONCENTRATIONS OF MERCURY IN THE ENVIRONMENT

The Greek name "hydrarguros" means liquid silver, thereof the name "quicksilver." The unique physicochemical properties, as reflected by its low melting ($-38.87°C$) and boiling ($356.57°C$) points, have facilitated the extraction and use of mercury by man since ancient times. Its electronic configuration, with filled f and d orbitals ($[Xe]4f^{14}5d^{10}6s^2$), makes elemental Hg somewhat similar in stability to noble gas elements. Because of weak interatomic attraction, mercury is the only liquid metal at room temperature, and its vapor is monoatomic. Elemental mercury Hg^0 occurs in liquid, gaseous, and aqueous phases (Table 7.1). It is quite soluble in water (60 µg/L at $25°C$) and is oxidized to the metastable dimer Hg_2^{2+}, Hg(I), and to more stable Hg(II) forms. In natural environments, the mercurous ion Hg_2^{2+} may be an intermediate in the oxidation of Hg^0 to the mercuric ion Hg^{2+}, but it is not long-lived enough to be detected by conventional methods. Release of $Hg^0(g)$ into the atmosphere by combustion of fossil fuels and natural sources such as evasion from the sea (Mason and Sheu, 2002) and volcanic eruptions, are the major sources of mercury in the environment. In the atmosphere, 95% of the total mercury is in the form of $Hg^0(g)$, and it is eventually oxidized and deposited as Hg(II) on land and in water as particles or dissolved in rain water. Mercury(II) may also be present in organic forms (often referred to as "organic mercury" or "alkylated mercury") such as monomethyl and dimethyl mercury molecules. Monomethyl mercury (commonly referred to as methyl mercury, CH_3Hg^+, MMHg, or MeHg) is by far the most abundant organic form of mercury in the environment. During the methylation process, inorganic Hg(II) is transformed to the MeHg molecule by the action of mainly iron (III) reducing bacteria (FeRB) and sulfate reducing bacteria (SRB) (see Chapter 5). Dimethyl mercury (DMHg) is encountered in deep sea water, beneath the thermocline, but

TABLE 7.1 Oxidation States and Chemical Forms of Mercury Occurring in the Environment

Chemical Form	Oxidation State	Environment
Hg(g, l, aq)	0	Aquatic–terrestrial
Hg_2^{2+}	+I	Metastable
Hg^{2+}	+II	Aquatic–terrestrial
CH_3Hg^+	+II	Aquatic–terrestrial
$(CH_3)_2Hg(aq)$	+II	Marine

it has not been detected in the mixed layer where gas exchange with the atmosphere takes place (Fitzgerald et al., 2007). Phenylmercury acetate has been used extensively as a pesticide in agriculture and pulp and paper industry but is not stable in the environment and degrades to inorganic Hg(II).

The biogeochemistry of mercury in soils and sediments is dominated by inorganic and organic mercury(II) complexes. Redox processes involving Hg(II) and Hg^0 and the partitioning of Hg^0 between liquid, aqueous, and gaseous phases are also of great importance. These processes are covered in Chapter 6. Because of its large size and stable electronic configuration ($[Xe]4f^{14}5d^{10}$), Hg(II) is easily polarized by interacting atoms. The strong covalent character of the C–Hg bond is the reason for the high stability of the MeHg molecule. Similarly, the Hg^{2+} ion forms very strong covalent bonds with soft Lewis bases (ligands) such as halides and sulfur compounds, but relatively weak bonds with hard Lewis bases such as fluorine (Fig. 7.1). These exceptional properties make Hg the "softest" of all metals (a so-called "Type B metal"). Typical for Hg(II) complexes is a low coordination number (2, 3, or 4). The linear two-coordination of Hg(II) is caused by relativistic effects (Tossell and Vaughan, 1981) and is a very unusual structure for a metal.

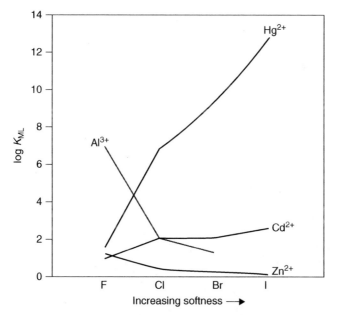

Figure 7.1 Formation constants for metal–ligand complexes illustrate the "hard–soft–acid–base" (HSAB) principle. Mercury(II) is the softest of all metal ions (Lewis acids = electron acceptor), cadmium(II) is slightly less soft, zinc is on the borderline between soft and hard acids, and aluminum is one of the hardest Lewis acids. Fluorine is a hard Lewis base (electron donor), and chlorine, bromine, and iodine are increasingly soft Lewis bases. *Source*: Figure modified from Sposito (1994).

The total concentration of Hg(II) in the aqueous phase of soils and sediments is normally in the range 5–100 pM, and solid phase concentrations are often in the range 50–500 ng/g (250–2500 pmol/g). In contaminated sediments, concentrations may be 50 times higher in the aqueous phase and up to 1000 times higher in the solid phase. Concentrations of MeHg contribute in general to 0.1–10% of the total Hg (sum of Hg and MeHg) in solid phases and 5–80% of total Hg in aqueous phases of soil and sediment.

7.3 AQUEOUS PHASE: MAJOR LIGANDS AND THEIR AFFINITIES FOR MERCURY(II)

Below I will briefly cover the Hg and MeHg aqueous species recognized as quantitatively important and that can be considered relevant for thermodynamic modeling in soil and sediment. In Appendix I, stability constants are listed for species for which the reliability of the value of the constant is considered fair. As will be explained, some stability constants are under debate, and for those I have taken a conservative standpoint and excluded them from Appendix I.

7.3.1 Oxygen-Containing Inorganic Ligands and Halides

The hydrated $Hg(H_2O)_6^{2+}$ (octahedral six-coordination) ion is an exception to the rule of low coordinated Hg(II) complexes. This complex will undergo hydrolysis with $Hg(OH)_2^0$ as the dominant protolyte at neutral pH. As expected for soft "Type B metals", the stability of Hg(II)–halide complexes increases with the atomic number of the halide (Fig. 7.1). Because of the abundance of chloride ions ($[Cl^-]$ ranging between 10^{-5} M in some freshwaters and 0.6 M in marine environments), Hg–chloride complexes are always in great excess over bromine and iodine complexes. For MeHg, the strong C–Hg bond strongly favors the formation of linear two-coordinated structures, and therefore, only the neutral forms $MeHgOH^0$ and $MeHgCl^0$ are quantitatively important.

7.3.2 Reduced Sulfur Ligands

7.3.2.1 Organic Thiols and Organic Sulfides. Recent studies show that low molecular mass (LMM) thiols (e.g., mercaptoacetic and mercaptopropionic acids, cysteine, and glutathione) are produced and build up under suboxic and anoxic conditions in hypolimnetic bottom waters. Total concentrations on the order of 10–100 nM (and sometimes even in the micromolar range) can be expected to be normal (Zhang et al., 2004; Hu et al., 2006). Thiol groups (RSH) associated with dissolved organic matter (DOM) are normally in the micromolar range and are generally more resistant to oxidation than LMM thiols. Both Hg and MeHg form very stable complexes with organic thiols. Spectroscopic studies and thermodynamic modeling conclusively show that the two-coordinated

$Hg(SR)_2$ complex is highly dominant over the one-coordinated $HgSR^+$ complex. At neutral and alkaline pH, with great excess of thiols in relation to Hg(II) and in absence of steric hindrance, three- and four-coordinated complexes can form (Koszegi-Szalai and Paal, 1999; Jalilehvand et al., 2006; Leung et al., 2007). The stability constant for these complexes are, however, not well established. The steric hindrance likely makes three- and four-coordinated Hg less abundant when complexed with thiol molecules associated with DOM or particulate NOM, as indicated by spectroscopic studies (Skyllberg et al., 2006). Studies on the complexation of Hg and MeHg with organic thiols were recently summarized (Skyllberg, 2008). In Appendix I, stability constants for the formation of the $Hg(SR)_2$ and MeHgSR molecules are listed. These constants should be seen as representative for complexes with both LMM and DOM-associated thiols. It should be noted that methodological difficulties have resulted in a number of incorrectly determined stability constants for LMM Hg–thiol complexes reported in the literature, as described in Casas and Jones (1980). Stability constants for the complexation of Hg and MeHg with organic mono- and bisulfides such as methionine (RSR) and cystine (RSSR) are much smaller (Latha et al., 2007), and these complexes are not quantitatively important in soils and sediments.

In Fig. 7.2a–d, the outcome of thermodynamic modeling of Hg and MeHg speciation under oxic conditions is illustrated. For comparative reasons, no organic ligands are present in Fig. 7.2a, which is the traditional way to illustrate the aqueous phase speciation of Hg. In the presence of LMM thiols, $Hg(SR)_2$ complexes will dominate even at quite modest concentrations of thiols (10 nM in Fig. 7.2b). In the presence of DOM, complexes with thiols [$Hg(SR-DOM)_2$ and MeHgSR-DOM] will dominate the speciation of Hg and MeHg (Fig. 7.2c and 7.2d). Even at concentrations of dissolved organic carbon (DOC) as low as 1 mg/L (corresponding to 46 nM of thiol groups if DOC is assumed to contain on average 0.15% thiol groups on a mass basis, Skyllberg (2008) $Hg(SR-DOM)_2$ complexes dominate in marine environments with chloride concentrations of 0.6 M.

7.3.2.2 Inorganic Sulfides, Bisulfides, and Mixture of Hydroxides and Sulfides.
The current theory for the formation of aqueous phase Hg–sulfide species follows the classical study of Schwarzenbach and Widmer (1963). They measured the solubility of Hg^{2+} in equilibrium with "black HgS" (metacinnabar), taking advantage of the reaction $Hg^{2+} + Hg^0(l) = Hg_2^{2+}$ ($\log K = 2.0$) occurring at the surface of an elemental mercury electrode. The total solubility of Hg was determined as the radioactivity of ^{203}Hg (after a three-day procedure during which the aqueous phase was slowly forced by N_2 gas through an 8-μm filter). Contamination by HgS particles passing the filter was recognized by the authors as a major problem in the experiment, and precautions were taken to get reproducible results. The solubility of HgS(s) in the presence of dissolved HS^- and H_2S at pH 0–10.7 (in 1.0 M KCl) was explained by the formation of the mononuclear complex $Hg(SH)_2^0$ and its two protolytes HgS_2H^- and HgS_2^{2-}.

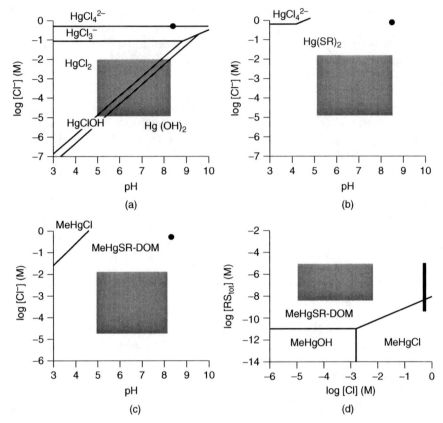

Figure 7.2 Dominance diagram for aqueous phase species of Hg under oxic conditions in the absence (a) and in the presence (b) of 10 nM of LMM thiols (RS_{tot}), and for MeHg under oxidized conditions in the presence of DOC 50 mg/L (having 2.3 μM of thiol functional groups, DOM-RS_{tot}) (c) and a pH of 7.0 (d). Marine conditions are indicated by black areas, and freshwater conditions by gray areas. Stability constants used in the calculations were taken from Appendix I, without correction for ionic strength and temperature effects.

Barnes et al. (1967) argued that in the acidic region HgS(s) should react primarily with H_2S(aq) (the dominant form of the $H_2S-HS^--S^{2-}$ system at pH below ~7), suggesting that $HgS(H_2S)_2^0$(aq) rather than $Hg(SH)_2^0$(aq) (the difference being one H_2S molecule) was the likely form of the major dissolved Hg-sulfide molecule. After deprotonation, $Hg(HS)_3^-$ and $HgS(HS)_2^{2-}$ molecules were suggested to be the dominating molecules at neutral pH and HgS_2^{2-} at alkaline pH. Recent extended x-ray absorption fine structure (EXAFS) spectroscopic studies (Lennie et al., 2003; Bell et al., 2007) have shown that Hg is two-coordinated at pH 9–11.5, which is in agreement with both studies. So far, no spectroscopic studies have been conducted at lower pH.

Stability constants for mixed chloride-bisulfide ($HgClSH^0(aq)$) and hydroxide-bisulfide ($HgOHSH^0(aq)$) listed in Appendix I are taken from Dyrssén and Wedborg (1991). It should be noted that these constants are not experimentally determined but estimated by linear free energy relationshipsLinear Free Energy Relationships (LFERs). The reported log K for the reaction $HgS(s) \mid H_2O -$ $HgOHSH^0(aq)$ is -22.3. A complication is that Dyrssén and Wedborg (1991), in an ambition to evaluate their theoretically determined constants by experimental data, also reported a log K of -10.0 for the above reaction. The difference of 12.3 log units between the two constants is due to a correction made from literature data from solubility experiments on $CdS(s)$ and $ZnS(s)$. Dyrssén and Wedborg made this correction, despite noting that the solubility data of CdS and ZnS were biased by colloidal contamination of the aqueous phase, which later was verified (Daskalakis and Helz, 1993). The reported log K of -10.0 for the reaction $HgS(s) + H_2O = HgOHSH^0(aq)$ was later used to explain the partitioning of Hg(II) in equilibrium with $HgS(s)$ between octanol and water (Benoit et al., 1999b; Jay et al., 2000). The concentration of Hg in the octanol phase was calculated by difference after determination of Hg in the aqueous phase. Particulates of $HgS(s)$ were separated from dissolved forms of Hg by 0.2- (Benoit et al., 1999b) and 0.02-μm filters (Jay et al., 2000). Because colloidal HgS has been shown to readily pass 0.1-μm filters (see below), it cannot be ruled out that K_{OW} distribution constants derived for $HgOHSH^0(aq)$ were biased by colloidal contamination. This was shown to be the case in a similar experiment in which 96% of $HgS(s)$ in nanoparticulate form was partitioned into the octanol phase when mixed with water at pH 7.0 (Deonarine and Hsu-Kim, 2009). Because of the uncertainties associated with experimental data, a conservative approach is taken in this chapter, and the theoretically derived log K of -22.3 for the reaction $HgS(s) + H_2O = HgOHSH^0(aq)$ is used in the thermodynamic modeling (corresponding to a log K of 30.3 for the reaction $HS^- + OH^- + Hg^{2+} = HgOHHS^0(aq)$, Appendix I).

7.3.2.3 Polysulfides.

7.3.2.3 Polysulfides. Polysulfides are neutral or, when deprotonated, negatively charged ions that form chains consisting of 2–8 sulfur atoms. Often the formation of polysulfides is expressed as a reaction between elemental S (rhombic S_8^0) and bisulfide: $(n - 1)/8 S_8^0 + HS^- = S_n^{2-} + H^+$, Kamyshny et al. (2004) but polysulfides exist also in the absence of S_8^0 (albeit at a much lower concentration), and the formation can then be expressed as a reaction between bisulfide and sulfate: $SO_4^{2-} + 7HS^- + H^+ = 4S_2^{2-} + 4H_2O$ (Rickard and Luther, 2007). Polysulfides are considered to be metastable in the environment, as they are commonly formed during redox fluctuations when oxidized and reduced forms of sulfur get into contact. If the more stable forms of mono- and disulfides are disregarded, polysulfides with $n > 4$ sulfur atoms dominate in the pH–Eh space where rhombic S_8^0 is the stable form (Fig. 7.3a and 7.3b). In fact, as illustrated in Fig. 7.3c, polysulfides with 3–8 S atoms show concentrations roughly similar to or higher than HS^- in the presence of rhombic S_8^0 at pH values above 8. In the absence of S_8^0, polysulfide concentrations are much lower (Fig. 7.3d).

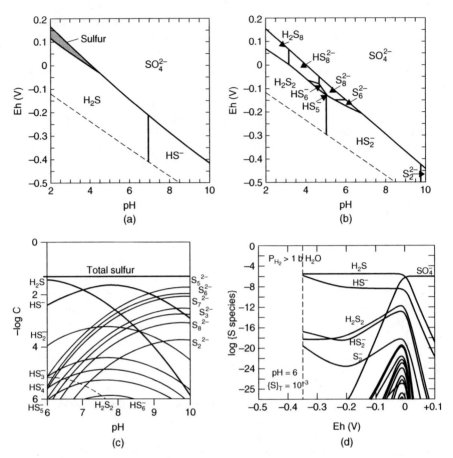

Figure 7.3 (a) Stable sulfur species in aqueous solution at 1 mM total concentration ((25)°C). (b) Stable phases removed, emphasizing the regions of dominance if only the metastable polysulfide species are considered. (c) Mono-, di-, and polysulfide distribution in the presence of excess S_8^0. (d) Mono-, di-, and polysulfide distribution in the absence of S_8^0. Thermodynamic data for polysulfide formation are taken from Kamyshny et al. (2004). *Source*: Reprinted from Rickard and Luther (2007) with permission from American Chemical Society.

Even if Schwarzenbach recognized the importance of polysulfide formation (Schwarzenbach and Fischer, 1960) before his classic work on HgS(s) solubility, it was not until the work of Paquette and Helz (1997) that the significant contribution from Hg–polysulfides was recognized. Building on the study by Schwarzenbach and Widmer (1963), Paquette and Helz explained the higher solubility of HgS(s) in the presence of S_8^0 by the formation of a polysulfide with the general form HgS_nSH^-. This species can be considered an analog to the first protolyte of the disulfide species (HgS_2H^-) and consequently dominates the speciation in the mid pH range (5.5–9.5). The number of S atoms in the HgS_nSH^- species could not be specified, but according to Kamyshny et al. (2004), $n = 4-8$ is a possible range. By ^{199}Hg NMR spectroscopy, synthesis of HgS_4S^{2-}, $HgS_4S_5^{2-}$, and $Hg(S_5)_2^{2-}$ has been verified in laboratory experiments (Bailey et al., 1991). Theoretical calculations performed by Tossell (1999) suggest that the dissolution of cinnabar through the formation of a polysulfide with $n = 4$ (HgS_4SH^-) is an energetically favorable process. So far no spectroscopic evidence exists for aqueous phase Hg–polysulfides in equilibrium with HgS(s), despite studies at the high pH range of 9–11.5, where polysulfides should dominate (Lennie et al., 2003; Bell et al., 2007).

Jay et al. (2000) extended the experimental work to lower sulfide concentrations, and at high pH two additional polysulfide species, $Hg(S_n)_2^{2-}$ and HgS_nOH^-, were suggested to explain their and Paquette and Helz's solubility data (Fig. 7.4a and 7.4b). The first species is an analog to the second protolyte of the disulfide species (HgS_2^{2-}), whereas the second species may be seen as a polysulfidic analog to $HgSHOH^0$. Jay and coworkers showed that the stability constant for the formation of $Hg(S_n)_2^{2-}$ improved the model substantially at pH values up to 8.5. The stability constant suggested for the HgS_nOH^- species ($HgS(s) + HS^- + (n - 1)S_8^0 + H_2O = HgS_nOH^- + H^+$; $\log K = -15.7(I = 0.3M)$ was less well-constrained, and the data support was restricted to pH values above 9.0 and sulfide <100 μM. Similar to the uncertainty regarding the stability assigned to $HgSHOH^0$, it could be questioned whether a mixed polysulfide/hydroxide complex would have the high stability suggested by Jay and coworkers. Even if a 0.02-μm filter was used to separate the aqueous and solid phases in the study by Jay et al. (2000), the large increase in the formation of colloidal HgS observed above pH 8 (Ravichandran et al., 1999) may call into question HgS(s) solubility data obtained above pH 9 owing to a possible colloidal contamination of filtrates by HgS(s) (see Section 7.4.2.1).

The importance of polysulfide formation for HgS(s) solubility at pH values above 4.0 is illustrated at two levels of aqueous phase sulfide concentrations in Fig. 7.4c. In this figure, the species $HgOHSH^0$ and HgS_nOH^- are not included. The great influence on the HgS(s) solubility by inclusion of a $\log K$ of 20.8 for the reaction $HS^- + (n - 1)S_8^0 + H_2O + Hg^{2+} = HgS_nOH^- + 2H^+$ and a $\log K$ of -10.0 for the reaction $HgS(s) + H_2O = HgOHSH^0(aq)$ is illustrated in Fig. 7.4d. At 1 μM S(-II), the $HOHgSH^0$ molecule dominates the solubility below pH 8 and HgS_nOH^- dominates at alkaline conditions. As can be noted in Fig. 7.4a and 7.4b, data collected at S(-II) <30 μM ($\sim10^{-4.5}$ M), which could give support for a significant contribution from $HgOHSH^0(aq)$ and HgS_nOH^-, are currently lacking. Solubility experiments conducted at sulfide concentrations lower than 30 μM under the prevention of colloidal contamination and independent spectroscopic studies are needed before stability constants for these two species can be fully established. I have therefore taken a conservative approach and excluded the HgS_nOH^- molecule and its proposed stability constant in Appendix I.

If all relevant components are considered under anoxic conditions, there will be a competition among organic thiols, inorganic sulfides, and polysulfides for Hg and MeHg in the aqueous phase, as illustrated for a soil/sediment having 50-mg

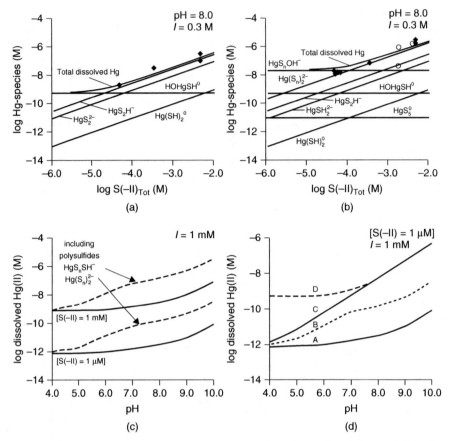

Figure 7.4 Solubility of HgS(s) in the absence (a) and presence (b) of elemental S (activity set to unity) as a function of total dissolved sulfide concentrations [S(-II)] at pH 8.0. The open circles and solid diamonds represent data points from Paquette and Helz (1997) and Jay et al. (2000), respectively, and solid lines illustrate constants reported in ref Jay et al. (2000). The solubility as a function of pH is illustrated with (broken lines) and without (solid lines) consideration of the polysulfides HgS_nSH^- and $Hg(S_n)_2^{2-}$ in (c). In (d), the sum of concentrations of $Hg(SH)_2^0 + HgS_2H^- + HgS_2^{2-}$ is represented by line A, with successive addition the polysulfides $Hg(S_n)SH^-$ and $Hg(S_n)_2^{2-}$ (line B), the polysulfide HgS_nOH^- (line C), and the species $HgOHSH^0$ (line D). Stability constants used in the calculations were taken from Jay et al. (2000), after correction for ionic strength effects.

DOC per liter in the pore water (Fig. 7.5). At 2.3 μM of RS_{tot}, concentrations of $Hg(SR-DOM)_2$ and Hg–sulfides will be roughly equal at 0.5 μM of $S(-II) = [H_2S] + [HS^-]$, and if polysulfides form, less than 0.1 μM of S(-II) is required to outcompete $Hg(SR-DOM)_2$ at pH values above 6.5. At pH less than 5, the $Hg(SH)_2^0$ molecule will be the dominant inorganic complex even if polysulfides are present. The relative competitiveness between inorganic and organic sulfur

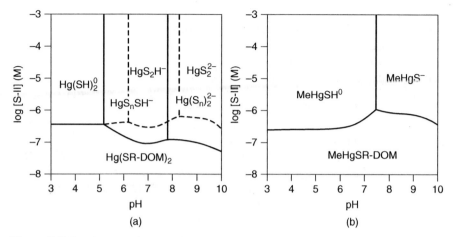

Figure 7.5 Dominance diagrams for aqueous phase species of Hg (a) and MeHg (b) as a function of pH and concentrations of $S(-II)(= [H_2S] + [HS^-])$ in the presence of DOC 50 mg/L (having 2.3 µM of thiol functional groups; DOM-RS$_{tot}$). In (a), dotted lines illustrate a situation without polysulfides, and solid lines with polysulfides (and the activity of elemental S set to unity). Stability constants used in the calculations were taken from Appendix I, without correction for ionic strength and temperature effects.

ligands for MeHg (Fig. 7.5b) is quite similar to their competitiveness for Hg, with a maximum contribution from thiol complexation when pH equals the pK_a of MeHgSH^0 (7.5).

7.4 LIQUID AND SOLID PHASES OF MERCURY IN SOILS AND SEDIMENTS

In geological deposits and in mine tailings after processing of ore, mercury is known to occur in many different mineral forms, in association with oxygen, sulfur, and chloride. The principal minerals are cinnabar (α-HgS) and metacinnabar (β-HgS), but minerals such as montroydite (HgO), mercuric chloride (HgCl$_2$), terlinguite (Hg$_2$OCl), eglestonite (Hg$_3$Cl$_3$O$_2$H), corderoite (Hg$_3$S$_2$Cl$_2$), and schuetteite (Hg$_3$O$_2$SO$_4$) are also quite abundant in mine wastes (Kim et al., 2000). At sites without direct deposition of mercury from industrial or mining processes, and in presence of NOM, sulfides are the only stable solid phases of mercury(II).

7.4.1 Elemental Mercury

Elemental mercury in gaseous and aqueous forms are well known to be ubiquitous in the environment, and the reduction of Hg(II) to Hg^0 and subsequent evasion into the atmosphere is an important source to the global mercury cycle (Mason and Sheu, 2002). The liquid form, Hg^0(l), however, is practically unknown except in soils and sediments heavily contaminated by local industry such as chlor-alkali plants from which $Hg^0(l)$ has been released into the environment. By thermodesorption analysis it has been shown that only traces of $Hg^0(l)$ persist in these highly contaminated soils and sediments (Biester et al., 2002). In marine and brackish water environments, the major degradation of $Hg^0(l)$ is rapid oxidation by chlorine ions (Yamamoto, 1996). Interestingly enough, the oxidation of $Hg^0(l)$ stops immediately when the liquid phase [droplets of $Hg^0(l)$] is removed, even if the concentration of $Hg^0(aq)$ is close to saturation with the solid phase (Amyot et al., 2005). Obviously the oxidation takes place at the interface between $Hg^0(l)$ droplets and water. The $Hg^0(aq)$ form is resistant to oxidation by chlorine but is rapidly transformed to Hg(II) by photolytic reactions (Lalonde et al., 2004). For a detailed discussion on photochemical reactions of mercury, I refer to Chapter 6.

7.4.2 Mercury(II) Sulfides

Mercury(II) sulfides exist as two polymorphs; cubic metacinnabar (β-HgS), which is considered metastable under low temperature conditions, and the more stable hexagonal cinnabar (α-HgS). Likely because of natural redox fluctuations, β-HgS(s) seems to be the predominant form in anoxic soils and sediments (Barnett et al., 1997). It has been shown by X-ray diffraction (XRD) and X-ray absorption spectroscopy (XAS) that Hg^{2+} in the initial reaction with HS^- forms an unstable low coordinated complex, with Hg–S bond distances similar to that in cinnabar. This structure is explained by a gradual clustering of the predominant two-coordinated complexes $Hg(SH)_2^0$, $HgHS_2^-$, and HgS_2^{2-} in solution. Already after 5 s a cluster is formed with a local four-coordinated structure similar to β-HgS. After hours of further aging, it is graded into a more crystalline β-HgS structure, which was not changed after 12 months of aging at $\sim20°C$ (Charnock et al., 2003). The structure of β-HgS is also consistent with an indicated fourfold coordination of Hg with polysulfides (Bailey et al., 1991) at suboxic conditions.

7.4.2.1 Colloidal Contamination of Filtrates in Studies on Mercury(II) Sulfide Solubility.
Studies on HgS(s) solubility encounter the difficulty of separating truly dissolved Hg species from colloidal forms of HgS clusters and HgS nanoparticles. Ravichandran et al. (1999) showed that the fraction of colloidal HgS passing a 0.1-μm filter increased from less than 1% to 90% when pH was increased from 8.0 to 10.0. In this experiment, HgS(s) was precipitated by mixing solutions of Na_2S and $HgCl_2$. The same problem was recognized when starting with a solid black metacinnabar phase and dissolving it in sulfidic solution (Schwarzenbach and Widmer, 1963). This means that the solubility of HgS(s) will be overestimated, especially at pH values above 8. Whether the fine 0.02-μm filters used in recent studies on HgS(s) solubility (Paquette and Helz, 1997; Jay et al., 2000) are fine enough to completely separate the finest colloids produced at alkaline conditions from the true aqueous phase we simply do not know.

7.4.2.2 *Solubility Product of Hg(II) Sulfide.* The solubility product of mercury(II) sulfides has been determined in a few studies. Schwarzenbach and Widmer (1963) determined the log solubility product of a black HgS (the structure was not determined, but it is generally assumed to be equivalent to metacinnabar) to be -36.8 ($HgS(s) + H^+ = HS^- + Hg^{2+}$) in a 1.0 M KCl ionic medium. For red HgS(s), cinnabar, a solubility product of -36.5 was determined at 0.7 M ionic strength (Paquette and Helz, 1997), Thus, despite the different structures of α- and β-polymorphs, their solubilities do not seem to differ significantly. LFERs suggests that the solubility product of metacinnabar would be 0.4 log units lower (more soluble) than cinnabar (Potter and Barnes, 1978).

As can be seen in Fig. 7.4a and b, solubility data collected for HgS(s) have been restricted by the detection limit of methods used to determine total Hg in the aqueous phase and no data points exist at total S(-II) concentrations lower than approximately 30 μM. This means that the solubility at lower sulfide concentrations is extrapolated from the chemical speciation determined at higher sulfide concentrations. Considering the uncertainty in analytical methods used for determination of Hg in aqueous phase, the problems of separating truly dissolved species from clusters and colloidal HgS, as well as the variation in crystallinity and structure of HgS(s) formed in natural soils and sediments in presence of NOM, a log K value in the range -36 to -38 seems justified for the reaction $HgS(s) + H^+ = HS^- + Hg^{2+}$ at this point.

7.5 REACTIONS OF MERCURY(II) WITH SOIL AND SEDIMENT PARTICLE SURFACES

As a consequence of the strong affinity for reduced sulfur groups, Hg^{2+} and $MeHg^+$ ions will be adsorbed to functional groups associated with NOM and to metal sulfides. Because sulfur groups almost always are in great excess of total concentrations of Hg and MeHg, oxygen functional groups at Fe and Al oxyhydroxides and at the edges of phyllosilicates only play a role as indirect adsorbents of Hg and MeHg complexes. There are a number of experimental studies on the direct adsorption of Hg to oxidized surfaces, which are useful and relevant for certain highly contaminated conditions (Kim et al., 2004; Skyllberg, 2010), but they will not be discussed further in this chapter.

7.5.1 Complex Formation with Natural Organic Matter

The role of NOM as an important complexing agent for Hg has been known for many decades, as reflected by numerous reports on the significant, positive correlation between total concentrations of Hg and DOC in stream water (Mierle and Ingram, 1991). The relationship is so strong that it was recently suggested that DOC (or even better the UV absorption of DOC) can be used as a proxy for total Hg concentrations in streams (Dittman et al., 2009). The last decade Hg, L_{III}-edge EXAFS studies (Xia et al., 1999; Hesterberg et al., 2001; Qian et al., 2002;

Yoon et al., 2005; Skyllberg et al., 2006) and binding affinity studies (Lovgren and Sjoberg, 1989; Hintelmann et al., 1997; Skyllberg et al., 2000; Karlsson and Skyllberg, 2003; Black et al., 2007; Gasper et al., 2007) have revealed that the bonding of Hg and MeHg to NOM pertaining to solid and aqueous phases is due to the complexation with thiol groups.

7.5.1.1 *Inorganic Mercury.* The current view is that Hg forms a two-coordinated linear complex with two thiol groups, $Hg(SR)_2$, having a Hg–S distance of approximately 2.33 Å (Skyllberg et al., 2006). A third sulfur group, which may be a mono- or disulfide group (–S–S–), is involved in a weaker bond (at ~3.0 Å), Fig. 7.6a. This structure has been established by increasing the Hg concentration to 100 µg/g, which is 300–1000 times higher than that in most soils and sediments. Still, at this Hg concentration only about 1% of the thiol groups, as determined by a combination of Hg EXAFS and S K-edge XANES, were saturated by Hg.

The spectroscopic results have been complemented by binding affinity studies conducted at much lower concentrations of Hg and MeHg in isolates of NOM from soil and natural water samples. Because of the very low aqueous concentrations of Hg in equilibrium with the $Hg(SR)_2$ complexes at natural conditions, the binding affinity can be determined only after addition of a competing ligand. This method is known as *competing ligand exchange* (CLE) or *competitive complexation*. To separate Hg complexes formed with NOM and with the competing ligand, liquid–liquid, solid phase, or dialysis separation methods are used. Because of dissimilarities in methods, samples, conditions, and conventions used to calculate conditional constants it is quite difficult to compare and evaluate the relevance of reported results. For such an evaluation I refer to compilations made by Black et al. (2007), Gasper et al. (2007), and Skyllberg (2008). Overall, most CLE studies conducted at reasonably low Hg to NOM molar ratios have resulted in a log K on the order of ~20–32 ($Hg^{2+} + L' = HgL'$, where L' represents a deprotonated ligand with a concentration calculated by a fitting procedure or set

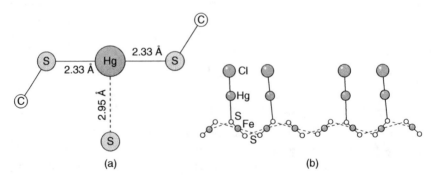

(a) (b)

Figure 7.6 Proposed structure for complex formation between Hg and thiol in NOM (Skyllberg et al., 2006) (a) and Hg with pyrite surface groups in presence of 0.2 M of chloride ions (b). *Source*: Figure (b) reprinted from Bower et al. (2008) with permission from Elsevier.

equal to NOM). Small values are generally obtained at high additions of Hg in relation to RSH groups, and values of log K on the order of ~ 10 are obtained if Hg is more than saturating the thiol groups and complexation by carboxyl groups is dominant (Lovgren and Sjoberg, 1989).

As shown by Skyllberg (2008), a log $K \sim 27$, for the reaction $Hg^{2+} + NOM = Hg-NOM$, or a log $K \sim 30$, for the reaction $Hg^{2+} + L' = HgL'$ at a total ligand concentration of 1 μM, is indicative of Hg–thiol complexation. The LMM thiols L-cysteine, DL-penicillamine, and mercaptoacetic acid have a log β_2 for the reaction $Hg^{2+} + 2RS^- = Hg(SR)_2$ in the range 37.8–44.5 (Skyllberg, 2008). If the pK_a values assigned to RSH and RNH$_2$ groups for the former two molecules (7.9, 8.5 and 10.4, 10.5, respectively) are considered macroscopic in nature, an average of 42 ± 2 can be considered the current best available estimate of log β_2 for thiol groups associated with short carbon chains and having carboxyl and amino groups in the near vicinity.

From combined measurements using S K-edge XANES and Hg L$_{III}$-edge EXAFS, the concentration of thiol groups in NOM from a soil and stream with a high affinity for Hg and MeHg has been calculated to be on the order of 0.15% of organic C on a mass basis, or 45 nmol/mg (C) (Skyllberg et al., 2005). Using this estimate in combination with data from Skyllberg et al. (2000), log β_2 values for the reaction $Hg^{2+} + 2RS^- = Hg(SR)_2$ were calculated to be in the range 43.3–47.7 for organic soils along an upland peat gradient (Skyllberg, 2008), as well as for extracted and purified humic substances from soils taken along the same gradient (Khwaja et al., 2006). The molar RS$_{tot}$ to Hg ratio was between $\sim 10^{-4}$ and 10^{-5} in the former and between $\sim 10^{-3}$ and 10^{-1} in the latter study. Thus, both the size of the stability constants and spectroscopic observations strongly point at the formation of Hg(SR)$_2$ complexes associated with NOM in the aqueous and solid phases of soils. There is a current lack of spectroscopic studies on the interaction between Hg and NOM in aquatic ecosystems; however, binding affinity studies suggest an interaction with thiols, presumably in a similar linear RS–Hg–SR configuration as established for terrestrial environments.

7.5.1.2 *Methyl Mercury.*

Similar to Hg–NOM complexes, MeHg forms a linear two-coordinated complex with one Hg–C bond of 2.05 Å (the bonding between the methyl group and mercury within the methyl mercury molecule) and one Hg–S bond of 2.35 Å with the thiol group (Qian et al., 2002; Yoon et al., 2005). The number of CLE studies on MeHg–NOM interactions is smaller than for Hg (Hintelmann et al., 1997; Amirbahman et al., 2002; Karlsson and Skyllberg, 2003; Khwaja et al., 2010), but since the affinity of MeHg is lower, the methodological problems are less expressed and results are quite consistent. Even if many studies report results pointing at a complex formation with thiols in DOM and particulate NOM from soils, few have actually measured these groups. Karlsson and Skyllberg (2003) and Khwaja et al. (2010) made independent determinations of RSH groups using S XANES and calculated stability constants at MeHg to RSH molar ratios less than 2×10^{-6} and 8×10^{-3}, respectively. Using a model with $pK_a = 9.96$ (similar to mercaptoacetic acid), a log K in the range

15.6 (pH 5.1)–17.1 (pH 2.0) at 0.25 M ionic strength (Karlsson and Skyllberg, 2003), and 15.5–16.0 at pH 3 and $I = 0$ (Khwaja et al., 2010), was reported for the reaction $MeHg^+ + RS^- = MeHgSR$ in an organic soil and Suwanee River fulvic acid, respectively. Considering experimental errors, these constants are well in agreement with stability constants in the range 15.7–17.5 as reported for the formation of MeHgSR complexes with LMM thiols, having pK_a values in the range 8.5–9.96. However, in order to fully account for the pH dependency of the data collected in the above two studies, a thiol group with a pK_a value of 4.0 is needed (Khwaja et al., 2010). Thiols with such a high acidity have been determined for clustered cysteine groups (Freisinger, 2008) and thiophenols (Summa et al., 2007). Thus, there are indications that Hg and MeHg may be bound to different types of thiol groups in NOM, something that needs to be further investigated.

7.5.2 Reactions with Iron(II) Sulfides

Pyrite (FeS_2) is generally considered the most abundant iron sulfide in soils, sediments, and waters (Rickard and Luther, 2007). It is a crystalline mineral, which is quite resistant to short-term oxidation events in sediments and soils. Mackinawite (FeS_m) is a short-range ordered, nanocrystalline iron sulfide, which readily forms in sediments and soils as a reaction between Fe^{2+} and HS^- ions. In terrestrial and freshwater environments it is considered just as abundant as pyrite (Rickard and Morse, 2005). Experimental studies show that the tetragonal crystalline structure of FeS_m forms within milliseconds. Black iron(II) monosulfides (mackinawite) is commonly referred to as amorphous, even though truly amorphous FeS(s) has not been identified (Rickard and Luther, 2007). Because of fluctuating redox conditions and kinetic constraints, pyrite and mackinawite exist side by side in sediments. Although several different reaction paths have been suggested for the formation of $FeS_2(s)$, a two-step oxidation of mackinawite to FeS_2 via greigite (Fe_3S_4), through reactions with sulfur species with intermediate oxidation states (e.g., elemental S, polysulfides, or thiosulfate) or with Fe(III), has been frequently argued as being of major importance in sediments (Wilkin and Barnes, 1996). In laboratory experiments, FeS_m and $FeS_2(s)$ have been shown to actively remove Hg from solution (Bower et al., 2008; Liu et al., 2008), and in order to model the chemical speciation of Hg, the mechanisms and thermodynamics of these reactions need to be resolved. At this point, no studies have covered interactions between MeHg and iron sulfides.

7.5.2.1 Reactions with Pyrite. The reaction between Hg and $FeS_2(s)$ has been studied by use of adsorption–desorption and spectroscopic studies. Despite HgS(s) being thermodynamically more stable than $FeS_2(s)$, significant dissolution of $FeS_2(s)$ under the formation of HgS(s) has not been observed during the timeframe of any experimental study (Hyland et al., 1990; Ehrhardt et al., 2000; Behra et al., 2001; Bower et al., 2008). This may be explained by the high kinetic stability of pyrite. Adsorption–desorption experiments have shown that

surface bonds formed between Hg and $\equiv$Fe$-$S$-$S surface groups are relatively weak (e.g., in comparison to Hg$-$S bonds in NOM) and 40% of surface-bound Hg was desorbed by the addition of 0.1 M of chloride (Behra et al., 2001). X-ray photoelectron spectroscopy (XPS) Suggested the formation of a linear $\equiv$Fe$-$S$-$S$-$Hg$-$OH surface complex in the absence (Behra et al., 2001) and a lincar $\equiv$Fe$-$S$-$S$-$Hg$-$Cl in the presence of 0.1 M NaCl (Behra et al., 2001; Bower et al., 2008) (Fig. 7.6b). In contrast to several other metals (Huerta-Diaz and Morse, 1992), there are no indications that Hg is pyritized, that is, incorporated into the FeS$_2$ structure.

7.5.2.2   Reactions with Mackinawite.

In contrast to reactions with pyrite, Hg has been shown to react with and dissolve FeS$_m$ during the formation of β-HgS(s) (Jeong et al., 2007, 2010; Skyllberg and Drott, 2010). In another study, a four-coordinated HgS compound (in agreement with β-HgS(s) formation) was formed under partly oxidized conditions, whereas at strictly reducing conditions a distorted surface complex was suggested to form Wolfenden et al. (2005). As shown with pyrite, the ability of iron sulfide to withstand dissolution by Hg likely is related to its kinetic stability and crystallinity. Therefore, the time of FeS$_m$ ageing could be important for whether reactions with Hg will lead to surface complex formation, dissolution$-$precipitation reactions, or a mixture of these processes. In the study by Skyllberg and Drott (2010), FeS$_m$ was allowed to age for 8 h, and no significant surface complexation was observed by Hg L$_{III}$-edge EXAFS at Hg to FeS$_m$ molar ratios of 0.002$-$0.012. In contrast, surface complexation of Hg onto FeS$_m$ aged for three days was observed at a Hg to FeS$_m$ molar ratio less than 0.05 in an adsorption experiment (Jeong et al., 2007). At higher molar ratios, FeS$_m$ was dissolved and β-HgS formed (as determined by XRD). Substitution of Hg^{2+} for Fe^{2+} ions in the FeS$_m$ structure has not been observed in any spectroscopic study. In order to resolve at which conditions surface adsorption, dissolution, and β-HgS(s) formation occurs, more strictly designed time-dependent experiments are needed in which adsorption is followed by spectroscopic methods. Furthermore, the influence of NOM on the reaction between Hg and FeS(s) need to be considered in order for results to be relevant under natural conditions in soils and sediments.

7.5.2.3   Reactions with Mackinawite in the Presence of Natural Organic Matter.

In soils and sediments NOM and FeS$_m$ may coexist, acting as very important components in the control of pH and pe. The binding of Hg to thiol groups in NOM is well studied, but what will happen in the presence of FeS$_m$? In the only existing study, it was shown that FeS$_m$ aged for five days was dissolved by Hg in the presence of NOM under the formation of Hg(SR)$_2$ complexes and β-HgS(s) (Skyllberg and Drott, 2010) at pH 5.7$-$6.1. Hg(SR)$_2$ complexes and β-HgS(s) (as determined by Hg EXAFS) coexisted after 30 h of equilibration. An increase in FeS$_m$ from 2 to 20 mass% (and decrease in NOM from 98 to 80 mass%) resulted in a change of Hg speciation from 43 to 100% β-HgS(s) (consequently, Hg(SR)$_2$ decreased from 47% to 0%). A simple thermodynamic calculation based on the composition of the two components was shown to be in reasonable agreement with a log solubility product of β-HgS(s) of -37 and a log β_2 for the formation of Hg(SR)$_2$ of 42 or greater. Results from this experiment suggest that in the presence of NOM, Hg complex formation at the surface of FeS$_m$ is of minor importance as compared to secondary precipitation of β-HgS(s).

7.5.3   Reactions with Other Metal Sulfides

By using XPS and Auger electron spectroscopy it was observed that Hg readily dissolved galena (PbS) under the formation of HgS(s) (Hyland et al., 1990). This is explained by the higher solubility of the lead(II) sulfide. Some Hg also formed weak complexes that passivated the galena surface from continued formation of HgS(s). Studies on the adsorption of mercury to metal sulfides such as CuS, Cu$_2$S, and ZnS have so far not been conducted.

7.5.4   Indirect Adsorption to Oxygen Groups at Mineral Surfaces

Abundant and reactive oxygen functional groups associated with the surfaces of clay minerals, Mn, Al, and Fe oxyhydroxides, are known to be of major importance for the complexation of transition metals, such as Mn, Co, Ni, Cu, and Pb, in soils. These metals form inner- and outersphere bonds with hydrated $\equiv$XOH surface groups (where X = Mn, Fe, Al, Si). Because of ubiquitous NOM and the strong affinity for thiol groups, Hg and MeHg will not bind directly to oxygen functional groups, except at exceptionally contaminated conditions in very low organic matter environments. However, reactive $\equiv$XOH surface groups may form ternary complexes with low- and high-molecular-mass Hg(SR-DOM)$_2$ and MeHgSR-DOM molecules. The most likely interaction is a "Type B" ternary surface complex formation where the $\equiv$XOH surface group interacts with an oxygen (carboxyl) and/or nitrogen functional group of the organic molecule. Using Hg-cysteine ($^-$OOCHN$_3$$^+CH_2$S)$_2$Hg as a model, depending on pH and the point of zero charge of the mineral surface, the negatively charged carboxyl group, the positively charged amino group, or both groups may interact with the $\equiv$XOH surface group. There are numerous studies on the interaction between Hg and oxidized mineral surfaces such as illite (Hamilton et al., 1995), kaolinite (Sarkar et al., 2000), and goethite (Barrow and Cox, 1992), but only a few on the interaction with MeHg (Gunneriusson et al., 1995; Desauziers et al., 1997). In the few studies in which NOM- (Yin et al., 1996) or thiol- (Senevirathna et al., 2011) containing molecules have been included, the conclusion has been that Hg(II) does not adsorb directly to $\equiv$XOH surface groups. There is so far only one study in which Hg, thiols, and mineral surfaces have been considered in a mixed system, highlighting the importance of ternary surface complexes for the regulation of adsorption and desorption of Hg-thiols onto surfaces of kaolinite (Senevirathna et al., 2011). Desorption of Hg(SR-DOM)$_2$ and MeHgSR$-$DOM complexes is likely responsible for the observed concurrent release of Hg and MeHg together with Fe and Mn from lake sediments into the bottom water (Regnell et al., 2001). Reduction of Fe(III) and Mn(III, IV) oxyhydroxides during summer or winter stratification results in a degradation of the surfaces of these minerals and a subsequent release of Hg and MeHg complexed by organic substances. Under anoxic conditions, iron(II) sulfide surfaces may be important adsorbents for $Hg(SR-DOM)_2$ as well as Hg complexes with inorganic sulfides and polysulfides. These processes still remain to be studied in controlled experiments.

7.6 STABILIZATION OF NANOPARTICULATE MERCURY(II) SULFIDES BY NATURAL ORGANIC MATTER

From a thermodynamic point of view, NOM associated thiols will compete with inorganic sulfides for Hg under anoxic conditions. Thus, in the presence of DOM the dissolution of HgS(s) will be enhanced as a consequence of $Hg(SR-DOM)_2$ complex formation. In addition to this process, nanoparticulate HgS(s) physicochemically stabilized by DOM has been shown to contribute to an apparent dissolution of HgS(s) (Ravichandran et al., 1999; Deonarine and Hsu-Kim, 2009). Thus, in experiments where HgS(s) has been allowed to precipitate out from solution, DOM has been demonstrated to have a dual role of decreasing the growth rate and aggregation of HgS polymers and at the same time stabilizing HgS colloids (Deonarine and Hsu-Kim, 2009; Slowey, 2010). Results from solubility experiments with cinnabar and DOM may suggest that hydrophobic fractions of DOM enhance the apparent solubility more than hydrophilic fractions of DOM (Ravichandran et al., 1998; Waples et al., 2005), independent of the concentration of thiol groups in these fractions. In apparent contrast, LMM amino acids with thiol groups have been shown to be much more efficient than molecules with amino and carboxyl groups alone to inhibit aggregation and to stabilize HgS nanoparticulates in experiments where metacinnabar has been allowed to precipitate after reaction between HS^- and Hg^{2+} (Deonarine and Hsu-Kim, 2009). In the latter type of experiment, it has been shown that reactions between DOM, Hg^{2+}, and HS^- and the formation of metacinnabar are dynamic over time and do not seem to reach equilibrium even after weeks (Slowey, 2010).

7.7 SOLUBILITY AND CHEMICAL SPECIATION OF MERCURY(II) IN SOILS AND SEDIMENTS

7.7.1 Linkage to the Biogeochemistry of Natural Organic Matter, Sulfur, and Iron

Natural dynamics in the formation and degradation of inorganic and organic sulfur species and their reactions with NOM and iron, to a large extent, determine the speciation of Hg and MeHg in soils, sediments, and waters. During oxic conditions, Hg and MeHg exist exclusively as organic complexes with low- and high-molecular-mass thiols, but when redox conditions are lowered to the regimes of Fe(III) and sulfate reduction, the situation gets more complex. A typical situation in sediments of estuaries and lakes is the formation of an oxic–anoxic interface in surface sediments where terrestrial sources of Fe(III), transported by streams and rivers, react with H_2S–HS^-, produced by SRB in anoxic sediments, under the formation of sulfur species with intermediate oxidation states (elemental S, polysulfides, thiosulfate) (Fig. 7.7). Under such circumstances, formation of organic thiols will take place because of diagenetic incorporation of H_2S into organic substances (Anderson and Pratt, 1995). In the presence of zero-valent sulfur, Hg-polysulfides will form and increase the solubility of Hg (Fig. 7.4). Indications of an increased solubility caused by the formation of Hg-polysulfides have been observed in controlled sulfurization experiments in the presence of iron oxyhydroxides (Slowey and Brown, 2007). Yet, these reactions remain to be demonstrated in natural soils and sediments.

During periods with high flow conditions, as well as during spring and autumn circulation in dimictic lakes, the oxic–anoxic interface in lake sediments moves downward, and during low flow conditions, such as summer and winter water stratification, the oxic–anoxic interface moves upward. These fluctuations cause

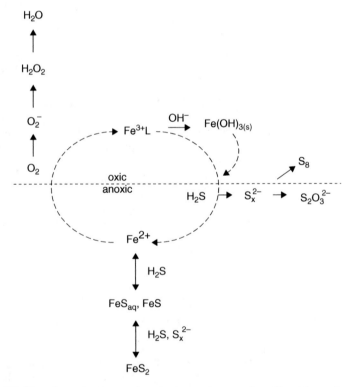

Figure 7.7 The dynamic interaction between iron and sulfur biogeochemistry at oxic–anoxic sediment or soil interfaces. *Source*: Reprinted from Rickard and Luther (2007) with permission from American Chemical Society.

dynamic changes in the speciation of Hg and MeHg, as well as in the transportation processes between the sediment pore water and bottom water. Also
methylation and demethylation reactions, which are tightly associated with the
activity of FeRB and SRB, will greatly affect the quantity of MeHg. The dynamics of Hg and MeHg solubility and mass transfer within sediments and in the
interface between pore and bottom waters have been frequently studied (Hurley
et al., 1994; Regnell et al., 2001; Goulet et al., 2007; Merritt and Amirbahman,
2007). However, because of an incomplete understanding of reactions with not
only NOM and polysulfides but also with sulfides such as FeS_m and pyrite, there
have been few attempts to determine the chemical speciation of Hg and MeHg in
these dynamic environments. Dissolved and particulate concentrations and partitioning coefficients (log K_d) have been reported for total Hg and MeHg in
numerous studies, but there are so far very few in which the partitioning of Hg
or MeHg between aqueous and solid phases of soils or sediments has been used
to evaluate chemical speciation models.

7.7.2   Dominance Diagram for Solid and Surface Phases

On the basis of the stability constants reported in Appendix I, the dominating Hg
species in the solid phase of soils and sediments can be calculated as a function
of pe and pH (Fig. 7.8a). This diagram differs from traditionally published
diagrams by including Hg complexed by thiol groups associated with NOM.
The $Hg(SR-NOM)_2$ complex dominates over the whole pH scale, and the border
to $HgS(s)$ formation coincides with the $H_2S/HS^- - SO_4^{2-}$ redox transition. It is
known since at least 35 years (Andrén and Harriss, 1975) that the complexation
of Hg to NOM, under all except extreme conditions of contamination,
outcompetes solid phases such as HgO and $HgCl_2$, as well as their aqueous
phase analogs $Hg(OH)_2^0(aq)$ and $HgCl_2^0(aq)$. Despite this insight, a lack of
proper methods has until recently restricted the possibility to determine stability
constants for Hg-NOM complexes. Furthermore, the convention to express
Hg–NOM complexes as conditional HgL' or Hg–NOM complexes, rather than
having a defined molecular structure, has precluded the use of stability constants
for Hg–NOM complexes together with well-defined inorganic molecules in
thermodynamic modeling. Therefore, recent spectroscopic information on
Hg–NOM complexes (using Hg L_{III}-edge EXAFS), and a quantification of thiol
groups in NOM by use of S K-edge XANES, has not only provided chemical
structures but also facilitated the formulation of stoichiometric reactions and
thermodynamic modeling of Hg and MeHg in soils, sediments, and waters.

It can be noted in Fig. 7.8a that Hg^0, which in traditional pH-pe diagrams
has been illustrated as the dominant form both at pe values above and below the
stability field of $HgS(s)$ (Andersson (1979), is outcompeted by $Hg(SR-NOM)_2$
complexes. Thus, the stability of $Hg^0(l)$ is restricted to highly anoxic conditions
where the boundary between $HgS(s)$ and $Hg^0(l)$ depends on the solubility product
chosen for the former. In Fig. 7.8a, a log K_{sp} of $-37.6(I = 0)$ for metacinnabar
is used. If instead a solubility product of -39.1 (Martell et al., 2003) is used,

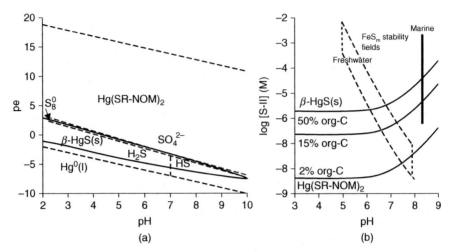

Figure 7.8 Dominance diagrams for soils and sediments with 100 ng Hg/g dry mass and 90 mass% pore water content. (a) The solid phase contains 15% organic C (NOM having a concentration of thiol functional groups corresponding to 0.8 mM on a pore water basis): the concentration of inorganic sulfur is 0.1 mM. Solid lines show the stability of mercury species, black broken lines show the stability of water and grey broken lines show the stability of sulfur species. (b) Limiting concentrations of $S(-II)(= [H_2S] + [HS^-])$ for the precipitation of metacinnabar in sediments with different concentrations of organic C. Regulation of $S(-II)$ by the solubility of FeS_m is indicated at freshwater (area bordered by dotted line) and marine conditions (black field). The stability of FeS_m is in equilibrium with Fe^{2+} concentrations of 10^{-3} to 5×10^{-5} M in freshwater and 10^{-6} to 5×10^{-8} in marine environments. Stability constants used in the calculations were taken from Appendix I, without correction for ionic strength and temperature effects. The stability constant $(\log K)$ for $FeS_m + H^+ = Fe^{2+} + HS^-$ is -3.5 (Rickard, 2006).

the boundary between $HgS(s)$ and $Hg^0(l)$ will coincide with the lower boundary for the stability of water. The suggested stability of $Hg^0(l)$ in sediments is in agreement with thermodesorption analyses showing that traces of elemental Hg released by chlor-alkali industry may still persist under highly anoxic conditions (Biester et al., 2002).

The stability constants for β-HgS(s) and $Hg(SR\text{-}NOM)_2$ can be used to calculate environmental conditions at which β-HgS(s) starts to precipitate. As illustrated in Fig. 7.8b, the limiting concentration of $S(-II) = [H_2S] + [HS^-]$ needed to precipitate β-HgS(s) is 0.004, 0.25, and 2.5 µM at pH 6 and less in soils/sediments with 2%, 15%, and 50% of organic C, respectively. At pH values below 6.2, $Hg(SH)_2{}^0(aq)$ is the dominant dissolved Hg–sulfide complex, and the solubility of β-HgS(s) is practically independent of pH (Fig. 7.4c). When the pH is raised above 6.2, the solubility of Hg increases because of an increasing dominance of HgS_2H^- and HgS_2^{2-} in solution. Because of this, the limiting $S(-II)$ concentration for precipitation of β-HgS(s) increases above pH 6.2. At pH 7 in a pure organic peat soil (having 50% organic C), 4 µM of $S(-II)$ will be needed to precipitate β-HgS(s); in a marine sediment (pH 8.3) with 2% organic

C, only 0.1 μM of S(-II) is required, whereas in a salt marsh (pH 8.3) with 15% organic C, 5.0 μM of S(-II) would be required. It should be noted that these values are highly dependent on the stability constants chosen. The K_{sp} reported for β-HgS(s) varies by roughly three orders of magnitude, and the uncertainty in the log K for the formation of $Hg(SR-NOM)_2$ may be even greater.

The formation of β-HgS(s) in sediments and soils is due to an interplay among organic matter, sulfides, and iron. If HS^- is regulated by FeS_m, β-HgS(s) likely will be found as a precipitate in most acid wetland soils as noted from Fig. 7.8b. However, in neutral soils and freshwater sediments containing FeS_m (having intermediate or high concentrations of Fe^{2+}), whether β-HgS will form or not depends on the organic matter content. Under marine conditions (having low concentrations of Fe^{2+}), the presence of FeS_m under almost all circumstances would indicate the formation of β-HgS(s). In salt marsh soils, high organic matter contents and relatively high concentrations of Fe^{2+} will counteract the formation of β-HgS.

7.7.3 Modeling of Mercury(II) Speciation in the Aqueous Phase of Soils and Sediments

Two different types of thermodynamic modeling procedures may be recognized:

1. Calculation of dissolved Hg and MeHg species from total concentrations in the aqueous phase without taking reactions with solid phases into consideration.
2. Calculation of the Hg and MeHg solubility reactions, validated by actual data from soils and sediments.

The first type of model is frequently used to calculate concentrations of Hg and MeHg aqueous species involved in diffusion and biouptake by methylating bacteria and higher organisms in soils and sediments. Pure bacterial culture experiments have shown that Hg complexed by DOM decreases the uptake of Hg (Kelly et al., 2003), obviously by lowering the concentration of small Hg molecules available for uptake. The current view is that Hg uptake may be both passive, by a diffusion of neutral forms of Hg through cell membranes of methylating bacteria (Barkay et al., 1997; Morel et al., 1998), as well as active, by the uptake of Hg complexed by LMM organic thiols (Schaefer and Morel, 2009). For passive uptake, first-order uptake rates will be directly related to the concentration of neutral forms of Hg (Benoit et al., 2003). This means that only chemical forms with reasonably high concentrations will be of quantitative importance for a passive uptake.

A thermodynamic calculation, using the constants in Appendix I, at anoxic conditions (under which HS^- is regulated by the solubility of FeS_m) in freshwater, brackish water, and marine conditions shows that the highly dominant neutral form is $Hg(SH)_2^0$. Possibly, $HgClSH^0$ and $HgOHSH^0$ can be included as candidates for passive uptake under certain conditions (Table 7.2). Under oxic conditions, $HgCl_2^0$, $Hg(OH)_2^0$ and $HgOHCl^0$ are the only known neutral forms, and neither of them reaches concentrations at a reasonable level for passive uptake. This result is partly in contradiction to previous perceptions (Morel et al., 1998), when much smaller stability constants were used for Hg bound to organic thiols in NOM. Under oxic (and suboxic) conditions, the lack of neutral forms showing a reasonable concentration ($>10^{-20}$ M) leaves active uptake of LMM organic complexes with thiols as the only realistic uptake mechanism by methylating bacteria. Mercury in these complexes may be two-coordinated, and mixed complexes with chloride and hydroxyl ions reach concentrations that may be of quantitative importance for biouptake (Table 7.2). It is noteworthy that the LMM HgClSR(aq) complex may reach higher concentrations than $Hg(SR)_2$(aq) under marine conditions. This may suggest that mixed thiol–chloride Hg complexes could contribute to bacterial uptake under high-salinity conditions.

7.7.4 Chemical Speciation Models Validated by Solubility Data in Soils and Sediments

Very few Hg speciation models have been validated by actual data from soils, sediments, or waters. An attempt was made with the mercury cycling model (MCM); (Hudson et al., 1994), a thermodynamic model for Hg and MeHg partitioning between seston (particulate NOM and plankton) and DOM in the water column of lakes linked to a kinetic model for biouptake. Owing to the lack of stability constants for Hg and MeHg interactions with particulate and dissolved organic matter (OM), log K for the reactions $Hg^{2+} + L^- = HgL^+$ and $MeHg^+ + L^- = MeHgL$ and the concentration of organic ligands (HL) were optimized. The fitted log K values of 17.5 and 12.5 for Hg and MeHg binding to DOM were compared to log K values of 22.1 and 15.7, respectively, reported for $HgSR^+$ and MeHgSR complexes (Dyrssén and Wedborg, 1991). Because the optimization included facilitated Hg^{2+} and $MeHg^+$ uptake by plankton, it was not a true validation of the thermodynamic part of the model. It should be noted that a log β_2 of 42 for the formation of $Hg(SR\text{-}NOM)_2$ corresponds to a log K of $\sim$33 if written as $Hg^{2+} + L^- = HgL^+$ (Skyllberg, 2008). Thus, even if the outcome of the modeling was interpreted as an involvement of thiols in the binding of Hg and MeHg, data were not consistent with the formation of two-coordinated Hg-thiol complexes.

In order to explain octanol–water partitioning of Hg in equilibrium with HgS(s) (Benoit et al., 1999b) and observations of an inverse relationship between MeHg concentrations in sediments and dissolved inorganic sulfides (Benoit et al., 2003) along a nutrient gradient in the Florida Everglades (Gilmour et al., 1998) and the Patuxent River (Benoit et al., 1998), Benoit et al. (1999a) developed a semiempirical thermodynamic model for Hg. The theory behind the model builds on the hypothesis that the net formation of MeHg is related to an uptake of neutral forms of Hg-sulfides by methylating

TABLE 7.2 Aqueous Phase Concentrations (Moles per Liter) of Major Chemical Species of Hg (Excluding Polysulfide Complexes) and Possible Candidates for Diffusion, Evasion, and Biouptake in the Sediment–Bottom Water Interface Under Oxic and Anoxic Conditions

	Freshwater/ Wetland Soil		Brackish Water		Marine Conditions	
pH	7.0		7.5		8.3	
Cl$^-$	10^{-4}		0.1		0.6	
DOC	4.2×10^{-3} (50 mg/L)		8.3×10^{-4} (10 mg/L)		4.2×10^{-4} (5 mg/L)	
	Oxic	Anoxic	Oxic	Anoxic	Oxic	Anoxic
DOM thiols	3.8×10^{-6}	3.8×10^{-6}	1.2×10^{-6}	1.2×10^{-6}	6.3×10^{-7}	6.3×10^{-7}
LMM thiols	10^{-9}	10^{-7}	10^{-9}	10^{-7}	10^{-9}	10^{-7}
HS$^-$	0	3.2×10^{-8}	0	2.0×10^{-6}	0	3.2×10^{-5}
S(-II)tot	0	3.3×10^{-7}	0	2.6×10^{-6}	0	3.4×10^{-5}
HgCl$_2{}^0$	3.8×10^{-29}	1.4×10^{-29}	1.9×10^{-24}	1.3×10^{-27}	1.1×10^{-23}	2.2×10^{-29}
Hg(OH)$_2{}^0$	2.4×10^{-29}	8.7×10^{-30}	1.2×10^{-27}	8.2×10^{-31}	7.6×10^{-27}	1.5×10^{-32}
HgOHCl^0	4.8×10^{-29}	1.7×10^{-29}	7.6×10^{-26}	5.9×10^{-29}	4.6×10^{-25}	9.2×10^{-31}
HgOHSH^0	0	8.2×10^{-21}	0	1.6×10^{-21}	0	7.8×10^{-23}
HgClSH^0	0	2.4×10^{-21}	0	1.5×10^{-20}	0	6.9×10^{-22}
Hg(SH)$_2{}^0$	0	3.9×10^{-12}	0	4.1×10^{-13}	0	4.0×10^{-14}
Hg(SR-LMM)$_2$	1.5×10^{-18}	5.5×10^{-15}	3.8×10^{-17}	2.6×10^{-16}	1.5×10^{-16}	3.1×10^{-18}
HgClSR-LMM	1.2×10^{-19}	4.3×10^{-18}	6.0×10^{-18}	4.1×10^{-19}	5.7×10^{-16}	1.2×10^{-21}
HgOHSR-LMM	6.0×10^{-20}	2.2×10^{-18}	9.5×10^{-18}	6.5×10^{-23}	9.6×10^{-20}	1.9×10^{-23}
Hg(SR-DOM)$_2$	1.0×10^{-11}	3.6×10^{-12}	1.0×10^{-11}	5.5×10^{-15}	1.0×10^{-11}	2.0×10^{-17}
HgS$_2$SH$^-$	0	2.5×10^{-12}	0	8.3×10^{-12}	0	5.0×10^{-12}
HgS$_2{}^{2-}$	0	1.2×10^{-14}	0	1.3×10^{-12}	0	5.0×10^{-12}

^{a}The total concentration of Hg is 10^{-11} M. The concentration of organic thiol groups associated with DOM is calculated as 0.15 mass% of DOC (Skyllberg, 2008). The concentration of LMM thiols is set to 1 nM under oxic conditions and 100 nM under anoxic conditions. The pK_a of thiols is set to 10.0. Under anoxic conditions, the concentration of HS$^-$ is regulated by the solubility of FeS$_m$ + H$^+$ = Fe^{2+} + HS$^-$; log $K_{2,SP}$ = −3.5(I = 0; Rickard, 2006) with [Fe^{2+}] = 1×10^{-3}, 5×10^{-6}, and 5×10^{-8} M in freshwater, brackish water, and marine conditions, respectively. Stability constants in Appendix I, corrected for the ionic strength effect by Davies equation, are used in the calculation. Temperature effects are not considered.

bacteria. It was also observed that while the solubility of Hg, as would be expected (c.f. Fig. 7.4a and b), increased with increasing concentrations of dissolved sulfides along the Patuxent River gradient, this was not the case in Florida Everglades. By including a reaction for diagenetic incorporation of HS$^-$ into an organic matter solid phase (ROH + HS$^-$ = RSH + OH$^-$), and a complexation reaction between Hg^{2+} and organic thiols [HgSR$^+$ and Hg(SR)$_2$], a model was created in which the Hg solubility was roughly independent of the dissolved sulfide concentration. Furthermore, by using a log K of 40.5 for the reaction HS$^-$ + OH$^-$ + Hg^{2+} = HgOHSH^0(aq), which corresponds to a log K of -10.0 for the reaction $HgS(s) + H_2O = HgOHSH^0(aq)$, the $HgOHSH^0$ molecule became quantitatively dominant and was significantly positively correlated to the sediment concentration of MeHg at both sites.

The model proposed by Benoit and coworkers can be said to be one of the few that has been validated by Hg solubility data (even if a strict validation with calculation of merit of fit was not conducted) from natural sediments. It is also the first that considered a solid phase of organic thiols associated with NOM as important components regulating the solubility of Hg, even if the concentration of thiols were not determined. There are, however, several uncertainties in the model. The diagenetic incorporation of HS^- in NOM is a complicated reaction that has not been verified by experimental data, neither in terms of kinetics nor thermodynamics. The log K for this reaction can therefore be regarded as a fitting parameter in the model. It may be plausible that (if other factors are being constant) the diagenetic formation of organic thiols increases with the concentration of dissolved sulfide, but this remains to be shown. Furthermore, as discussed in Section 7.3.2.2, the log K of 40.5 set for the formation of $HgOHSH^0$, is likely substantially overestimated.

Drott and coworkers, using a model including DOM-associated thiols, reported a positive relationship between the sum of the calculated concentrations of $Hg(HS)_2^0(aq)$ and $HgOHSH^0(aq)$ and the methylation rate constant (k_m), as well as total concentrations of MeHg, in contaminated sediments (Drott et al., 2007). Similar to that of Benoit et al. (1999a), this model was biased by an unsubstantiated, large log K for the formation of $HgOHSH^0(aq)$, even if the uncertainty in this constant was recognized and its size varied in order to account for this. Reactions with $HgS(s)$ were considered in the regulation of the concentration of $HgOHSH^0(aq)$, but reactions with solid phases were not allowed to limit the overall solubility of Hg. Thus, the model was not validated by solubility data.

7.7.5 Thermodynamic Modeling of Partitioning Coefficients ((K_d) for Hg and MeHg in Soil and Sediment

The partitioning of Hg and MeHg between solid (particulate) and aqueous phases is commonly reported for soils, sediments, and waters. The distribution coefficient K_d (L/kg) is defined as the concentration in the solid (or particulate) phase (mol/kg or g/kg) divided by the concentration in the aqueous phase (mol/L or g/L). In an oxic environment, the partitioning of Hg and MeHg will be determined by the binding to thiol groups and in turn their partitioning between solid and aqueous phases of NOM. If we assume that the binding affinity of Hg to thiols is independent of whether RS belongs to the solid (designated RS (ads)) or aqueous (designated DOM-RS (aq)) phase, the stability constant log K for Equation 7.1 is 1.0 (all concentrations are expressed as moles per liter solution).

$$Hg(SR - DOM)_2(aq) + 2RS^-(ads) =$$

$$2DOM\text{-}RS^-(aq) + Hg(SR)_2(ads); \quad K = 1 \tag{7.1}$$

$$K_d = [Hg(SR)_2(ads)]/[Hg(SR - DOM)_2(aq)]$$

$$= [RS^-(ads)]^2/[DOM - RS^-(aq)]^2 \tag{7.2}$$

If the concentration of thiols in relation to organic C is assumed to be equal in solid and aqueous phases, concentrations of solid and dissolved organic carbon (SOC and DOC) can be used as proxies for thiols in solid $[RS^-$ (ads)] and aqueous phases [DOM-RS^- (aq)], respectively. The range of SOC concentrations in most soils and sediments is roughly 10–500 g/kg, and the range of DOC concentrations in pore waters is roughly 10–300 mg/L, with concentrations of SOC and DOC more or less positively correlated. This means that a log K_d for Hg calculated by Equation 7.2 should roughly cover a range of 6.0–6.4 L/kg $[(10 \times 10^{-3})^2/(10 \times 10^{-6})^2 = 10^6$ with SOC 10 g/kg and DOC 10 mg/L and $(500 \times 10^{-3})^2/(300 \times 10^{-6})^2 = 10^{6.4}$ with SOC 500 g/kg and DOC 300 mg/L]. This means that K_d for Hg under oxic conditions can be approximated as K_d for organic carbon raised to 2. For MeHg, which forms monodentate complexes with thiols, the partitioning of MeHg simply follows the partitioning of organic C. Thus, K_d for MeHg is equal to K_d for organic C, which results in a range of log K_d between 3.0 and 3.2 if the above data on SOC and DOC are applied to Equations 7.3 and 7.4.

$$MeHgSR - DOM(aq) + RS^-(ads) =$$

$$DOM - RS^-(aq) + MeHgSR(ads); \quad K = 1 \tag{7.3}$$

$$K_d = [MeHgSR(ads)]/[MeHgSR - DOM(aq)]$$

$$= [RS^-(ads)]/[DOM - RS^-(aq)] \tag{7.4}$$

In agreement with the above calculation, log K_d for Hg is generally observed to be in the range 5.0–6.5, whereas the log K_d for MeHg often is reported to be in the range 2.5–3.5 in soils and sediments. The roughly three orders of magnitude greater K_d for Hg is thus attributed to the exponent of 2 in Equation 7.2, caused by the requirement of two independent thiol groups for the formation of the $Hg(SR)_2$ molecule. If the complexation of Hg with RS^- instead would have been expressed as a bidentate complex (i.e., the thiol groups belonging to the same molecule; HgS_2R), which has been proposed (Khwaja et al., 2006), the log K_d for Hg would have been 3.0–3.2, similar to MeHg. Even if the activity of surface complexes is not a trivial issue, the fair correspondence between measured and theoretical log K_d may therefore be taken as support for an involvement of two independent thiol groups in the complexation of Hg.

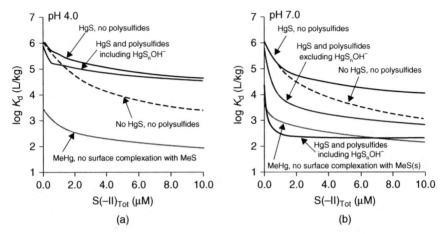

Figure 7.9 Theoretical modeling of the partitioning of Hg and MeHg between solid and aqueous phases in a hypothetical wetland soil or sediment having 15% organic C, DOC 50 mg/L, and an ionic strength of 0.5 mM. The concentration of thiols (RS) was set to 0.15 mass% of organic C in both aqueous and solid phases. The water content was 90% of wet soil mass. Total concentrations of Hg and MeHg were 100 and 0.1 ng/g, respectively. The figures were modified from Skyllberg (2008). Stability constants used in the calculations were taken from Appendix I, without correction for ionic strength and temperature effects. The stability constant for the formation of HgS_nOH^- is taken from Jay et al. (2000). In presence of polysulfides, the activity of elemental S is set to 1.0.

As illustrated in Fig. 7.9, the maximum log K_d is obtained under oxic conditions, in the absence of inorganic sulfides. When sulfides are formed and build up in solution, log K_d will decrease because of the formation of soluble Hg-sulfides and polysulfides. Thus, even at the point when HgS(s) is formed, which occurs at ~0.6 μM S(-II) in the hypothetical soil/sediment shown in Fig. 7.9a and at 1.2 μM S(-II) in Fig. 7.9b, log K_d will continue to decrease with increasing concentrations of S(-II) in solution. It can be noted by comparing Fig. 7.9a and 7.9b that a greater solubility of Hg increases at higher pH, which is in opposition to the general notion that the solubility of metals increase with decreasing pH. Even if the free Hg^{2+} ion increases at lower pH, the shift in speciation of sulfides from HS^- to H_2S results in decreased concentrations of dissolved Hg-sulfides. Another effect is the formation of polysulfides, which contributes to an increased solubility at higher pH. In Fig. 7.9b, the dramatic effect on the solubility caused by the stability constant suggested for the HgS_nOH^- molecule (Jay et al., 2000) is illustrated, increasing the solubility of Hg similar to levels of MeHg. In summary, under strong acidic conditions, the log K_d for Hg is predicted to be in the range of 4.5–6.0, whereas in neutral and alkaline soils and sediments, log K_d would vary roughly between 3 and 6, depending on whether polysulfides are formed or not.

In a review of studies from marine and estuarine sediments, log K_d for Hg was reported to vary between 5 and 6 (Fitzgerald et al., 2007); a similar range was reported in freshwater sediments (Turner et al., 2001). Most of these studies cover true anoxic conditions (sulfide concentrations exceeding 10–20 μM), and polysulfides may not be anticipated to form. There are, however, several studies in which a log K_d on the order of 3.5–4.5 has been reported, under conditions in which polysulfide formation can be suspected. Goulet et al. (2007) reported an average log K_d of 4.2 in the sediment of a riverine wetland in which elemental S was measured (concentrations up to 8 μM in pore water). Similarly, an abrupt decrease in log K_d from 4.5–5.7 in the oxidized water column (where Hg would be complexed by particulate and dissolved organic thiols alone) to a log K_d of 3.4–4.1 in the top 30 cm of the underlying sediment of Little Rock lake (Hurley et al., 1994) may be explained by polysulfide formation in the sediment (elemental S was not measured). The observation that log K_d dropped markedly from 4–5 to 3–4 when the concentration of acid volatile sulfur (AVS) decreased from above 20 to 0–10 μmol/kg (Hammerschmidt and Fitzgerald, 2004) in a near-shore marine sediment may be taken as an indication that polysulfide formation under suboxic conditions contributed to the solubility.

The log K_d for MeHg varies roughly between 1.5 and 5.4 in marine sediments (Hammerschmidt and Fitzgerald, 2004; Fitzgerald et al., 2007). Values in the low end may be consistent with the model used in Fig. 7.9b, whereas values above 4.0 are not. An obvious weakness of the proposed model is the lack of thermodynamic data on surface complexation of MeHg to iron sulfides and other metal sulfides. The formation of such complexes could counteract the decrease in log K_d with an increase in dissolved sulfide concentrations, but it remains to be shown that they are strong enough to explain log K_d values on the order of five or above, as reported in some studies. Another explanation for some unexpectedly high log K_d for MeHg may be related to the hydrophobicity of MeHg, recently proposed to increase the affinity for certain types of thiols (Khwaja, et al., 2010). These thiols may show different concentrations in relation to organic C of solid and aqueous phases. Furthermore, the fact that the highest log K_d for MeHg (up to 6.0) has been reported as a partitioning between the aqueous phase and suspended particles (including living organisms) in freshwaters (Watras et al., 1998; Babiarz et al., 2001) suggests that the partitioning of MeHg may include Hg methylation and buildup of MeHg in bacteria and phytoplankton.

Even if there are numerous studies in which log K_d has been reported, few includes measurements of all parameters needed for modeling Hg and MeHg solubility. As illustrated in Fig. 7.9, in addition to concentrations of sulfide, elemental S is the most important parameter behind Hg solubility, which often is missing. It would also be useful to determine the concentration of LMM and macromolecular organic thiols (using, e.g. S K-edge XANES). Also, total concentrations of Hg and MeHg in the sediment will influence the log K_d. If HgS(s) is present, log

K_d will increase with one order of magnitude if the total concentration increase 10 times. As discussed above, salinity (chloride concentrations) may not be a factor affecting log K_d of either Hg or MeHg through chloride complexation. But salting out of Hg-DOM and MeHg-DOM complexes is an important indirect effect that may contribute to a higher log K_d in saline environments (Babiarz et al., 2001; Turner et al., 2001).

7.8 METHODS FOR STUDYING THE CHEMISTRY OF MERCURY(II) IN SOILS AND SEDIMENTS

A complete chemical characterization of Hg and MeHg in soils and sediments requires methods for the determination of total concentrations, as well as concentrations of chemical species pertaining to aqueous, solid, surface, and gaseous phases. Total concentrations of mercury (Hg + MeHg + traces of other Hg forms) can be determined after complete digestion of the soil or sediment sample, or in aqueous phase, after reduction of mercury to Hg^0 followed by cold vapor atomic fluorescence spectroscopy (CVAFS). In contrast, a separate determination of MeHg and Hg requires combinations of extraction, liquid–liquid separation, clean-up, derivatization, separation, and detection steps, preferably using stable MeHg and Hg isotopes as internal standard for quality control (Björn et al., 2007).

Individual chemical species of Hg and MeHg are much more difficult to quantify. Selective wet chemical extraction has been used to get approximate information about Hg species pertaining to solid phases and surfaces (Bloom et al., 2003). With this method, organically bound Hg (extracted by strong acid or base) may be semiquantitatively separated from HgS(s)-dominated phases (dissolved by aqua regia) in soils and sediments. In highly contaminated mine wastes also $HgCl_2$, HgO(s), and Hg^0(l) phases may be identified and semiquantitatively determined (by dissolution in deionized water, acetate, and strong acid, respectively). A comparison with Hg L_{III}-edge EXAFS spectroscopy revealed that HgS(s) was most accurately determined by extraction, whereas the quantification of the more soluble Hg-phases such as $HgCl_2$ and HgO(s) were dependent on the overall matrix, particle size, and crystallinity of the mine waste samples (Kim et al., 2003). In less contaminated samples, such as most soils and sediments, concentrations are too low to be quantified by Hg L_{III}-edge EXAFS spectroscopy. However, if the concentration of reduced S groups is in great excess, additions of Hg (or MeHg) may give an idea of the chemical speciation also at ambient concentrations. A parallel determination of the binding ligands by, for example, S K-edge XANES is in many cases very useful. Mercury L_{III}-edge EXAFS is the only available method for the direct determination of the local binding environment (molecular structure) of Hg and MeHg in environmental samples. A recent summary of XAS study conducted on mercury in soils and sediments is given in Skyllberg (2010). The more or less distinct release of gaseous Hg as a consequence of increased temperature has been used to semiquantitatively separate $Hg^0(l)$, organically bound Hg, and HgS(s) by the thermodesorption method (Biester and Scholz, 1997). This is currently the best available method for the determination of $Hg^0(l)$ in contaminated sediments.

Because of the very low concentrations and methodological difficulties, there are currently no methods for a direct determination of dissolved Hg and MeHg species in soils and sediment pore water. Thus, the concentration of these species needs to be indirectly calculated from stability constants. Ligand-exchange methods have been successfully used to determine conditional constants for the interaction between Hg, MeHg, and organic or inorganic sulfur-containing ligands in aqueous and solid phases of soils and sediments (Gasper et al., 2007; Skyllberg, 2008).

7.9 FUTURE RESEARCH NEEDS

In order to understand the critical processes in mercury biogeochemistry, such as methylation, demethylation, gaseous evasion, diffusion, solubilization, mobilization, bioaccumulation, and biomagnification, a correct determination of the chemical speciation of Hg and MeHg in aqueous and solid phases of soils, sediments, and waters is required. Major knowledge gaps include molecular interactions of Hg and MeHg with not only the most abundant metal sulfides such as $FeS_2(s)$, FeS(s) but also the less abundant ZnS(s), CuS(s), and $Cu_2S(s)$. The interaction between MeHg and HgS(s) and FeS(s) is currently unknown. It is likely that the observed $\log K_d$ for MeHg on the order of four to six in some environments is partly due to these types of interactions. The aging of FeS_m, which is affected by the dynamics of reduction and oxidation and presence of NOM, seems to play a major role. When it comes to aqueous species, the solubility of β-HgS(s) needs to be studied at S(-II) concentrations below 30 μM. In these studies, the problem of separating truly dissolved species from nanoparticulate HgS(s) needs to be addressed. A combination of solubility modeling and independent spectroscopic studies is required to resolve the stability constants for the formation of various Hg-polysulfides and the $HgOHSH^0$ complex. To improve the understanding of critical processes such as methylation and demethylation, we need multidisciplinary approaches in which the chemical speciation of Hg and MeHg is linked to the biogeochemistry of organic C, S, and Fe and the biological activity of FeRB and SRB.

APPENDIX

Acidity and Thermodynamic Constants Used in the Thermodynamic Modeling of Soils and Sediments Reported in Table 7.2 and Figs 7.2, 7.5, 7.8, and 7.9.

Chemical Reaction	Log K	References
Proton dissociation of ligands		
$H_2O(l) = OH^- + H^+$	13.7	
$H_2S(aq) - HS^- + H^+$	7.0	
$RSH(aq) = RS^- + H^+$	9.96	Skyllberg (2008)
Formation of inorganic Hg(II) complexes		
$OH^- + Hg^{2+} - = HgOH^+$	10.3 ($I = 0$ M)	Powell et al. (2004)
$2OH^- + Hg^{2+} = Hg(OH)_2^0(aq)$	21.4 ($I = 0$ M)	Powell et al. (2004)
$3OH^- + Hg^{2+} = Hg(OH)_3^-$	20.3 ($I = 0$ M)	Powell et al. (2004)
$Cl^- + Hg^{2+} = HgCl^+$	7.3 ($I = 0$ M)	Powell et al. (2004)
$2Cl^- + Hg^{2+} = Hg(Cl)_2^0(aq)$	14.0 ($I = 0$ M)	Powell et al. (2004)
$3Cl^- + Hg^{2+} = Hg(Cl)_3^-$	14.9 ($I = 0$ M)	Powell et al. (2004)
$4Cl^- + Hg^{2+} = Hg(Cl)_4^{2-}$	15.5 ($I = 0$ M)	Powell et al. (2004)
$Cl^- + OH^- + Hg^{2+} = HgClOH^0(aq)$	18.0 ($I = 0$ M)	Powell et al. (2004)
$HS^- + Hg^{2+} = HgSH^+$	20.6 (LFER)	Dyrssén and Wedborg (1991)
$2HS^- + Hg^{2+} = Hg(SH)_2^0(aq)$	37.7 ($I = 1.0$ M)	Schwarzenbach and Widmer (1963)
$2HS^- + Hg^{2+} = HgS_2H^- + H^+$	31.5 ($I = 1.0$ M)	Schwarzenbach and Widmer (1963)
$2HS^- + Hg^{2+} = HgS_2^{2-} + 2H^+$	23.2 ($I = 1.0$ M)	Schwarzenbach and Widmer (1963)
$HS^- + OH^- + Hg^{2+} = HgOHSH^0(aq)$	30.3 (LFER)	Dyrssén and Wedborg (1991)
$HS^- + Cl^- + Hg^{2+} = HgClSH^0(aq)$	25.8 (LFER)	Dyrssén and Wedborg (1991)

Chemical Reaction	Log K	References
$2HS^- + (n\text{-}1)S^0 + Hg^{2+} = HgS_nSH^- + H^+$	32.6 ($I = 0.3$ M)	Jay et al. (2000)
$2HS^- + 2(n - 1)S^0 + Hg^{2+} = Hg(S_n)_2{}^{2-} + 2H^+$ S^0	24.8 ($I = 0.3$ M)	Jay et al. (2000)
$RS^- + Hg^{2+} = HgSR^+$	22.7 (LFER)	Dyrssén and Wedborg (1991)
$2RS^- + Hg^{2+} = Hg(SR)_2$	42.0	Skyllberg (2008)
$HgOHSR + Cl^- = HgClSR + OH^-$	-3.7	Hilton et al. (1975)
$RS^- + OH^- + Hg^{2+} = HgOHSR$	32.2 (LFER)	Dyrssén and Wedborg (1991)
Formation of MeHg(II) complexes		
$OH^- + CH_3Hg^+ = CH_3HgOH^0$	9.5	Loux (2007)
$Cl^- + CH_3Hg^+ = CH_3HgCl^0$	5.4	Loux (2007)
$SH^- + CH_3Hg^+ = CH_3HgSH^0$	14.5 (LFER)	Dyrssén and Wedborg (1991), Loux (2007)
$SH^- + CH_3Hg^+ = CH_3HgS^- + H^+$	7.0 ($I = 0.1$ M)	Schwarzenbach and Schellenberg (1965)
$RS^- + CH_3Hg^+ = CH_3HgSR$	16.5 ($I = 0$ M)	Loux (2007), Karlsson and Skyllberg (2003)
Solubility of solid phases		
Black $HgS(s) + H^+ = HS^- + Hg^{2+}$	-36.8 ($I = 1.0$ M)	Schwarzenbach and Widmer (1963)
Red $HgS(s) + H^+ = HS^- + Hg^{2+}$	-36.5 ($I = 0.7$ M)	Paquette and Helz (1997)

(continued)

Chemical Reaction	Log K	References
Formation, dissolution, volatilization, and dismutation of Hg^0		
$Hg^{2+} + 2e^- = Hg^0(l)$	28.7	Sillén and Martell (1971)
$Hg^0(l) = Hg^0(aq)$	-6.48 (I = 0 M)	Clever et al. (1985)
$Hg^0(g) = Hg^0(aq)$	-2.59 (I = 0 M)	Sanemasa (1975)
$Hg^{2+} + Hg^0(aq) = Hg_2^{2+}$	8.46 (I = 0 M)	Hietanen and Sillén (1956)

The ionic strength is reported for experimentally determined constants. LFER = constant determined by linear free energy relationships. Some constants were recalculated using the acidity constants for H_2S and H_2O and for solubilities of HgS(s) as reported in the original work or in this table.

REFERENCES

Amirbahman A, Reid AL, Haines TA, Kahl JS, Arnold C. Association of methylmercury with dissolved humic acids. Environ Sci Technol 2002;36:690–695.

Amyot M, Morel FMM, Ariya PA. Dark oxidation of dissolved and liquid elemental mercury in aquatic environments. Environ Sci Technol 2005;39:110–114.

Anderson TF, Pratt LM. Isotopic evidence for the origin of organic sulfur and elemental sulfur in marine sediments. In: Vairavamurthy MA, Schoonen MAA, editors. Geochemical transformations of sedimentary sulfur. American Chemical Society Symposium Series 612, Washington; 1995. p 378–396.

Andersson A. Mercury in soils. In: Nriagu J, editor. The biogeochemistry of mercury in the environment. New York: Elsevier/North Holland Biomedical Press; 1979. p 79–112.

Andrén AW, Harriss RC. Observations on the association between mercury and organic matter dissolved in natural waters. Geochim Cosmochim Acta 1975;39:1253–1258.

Babiarz CL, Hurley JP, Hoffmann SR, Andren AW, Shafer MM, Armstrong DE. Partitioning of total mercury and methylmercury to the colloidal phase in freshwaters. Environ Sci Technol 2001;35:4773–4782.

Bailey TD, Banda RMH, Craig DC, Dance IG, Ma INL, Scudder ML. Mercury polysulfide complexes, $[Hg(S_x)(S_y)]^{2-}$: Syntheses, [199]Hg NMR studies in solution, and crystal structure of $(Ph_4P)_4[Hg(S_4)_2]Br_2$. Inorg Chem 1991;30:187–191.

Barkay T, Gillman M, Turner RR. Effects of dissolved organic carbon and salinity on bioavailability of mercury. Appl Environ Microbiol 1997;63:4267–4271.

Barnes HL, Romberger SB, Stemprok M. Ore solution chemistry; [Part] 2, Solubility of HgS in sulfide solutions. Econ Geol Bull Soc Econ Geol 1967;62:957–982.

Barnett MO, Harris LA, Turner RR, Stevenson RJ, Henson TJ, Melton RC, Hoffman DP. Formation of mercuric sulfide in soil. Environ Sci Technol 1997;31:3037–3043.

Barrow NJ, Cox VC. The effects of pH and chloride concentration on mercury sorption. I. By goethite. J Soil Sci 1992;43:295–304.

Behra P, Bonnissel-Gissinger P, Alnot M, Revel R, Ehrhardt JJ. XPS and XAS study of the sorption of Hg(II) onto pyrite. Langmuir 2001;17:3970–3979.

Bell AMT, Charnock JM, Helz GR, Lennie AR, Livens FR, Mosselmans JFW, Pattrick RAD, Vaughan DJ. Evidence for dissolved polymeric mercury(II)-sulfur complexes. Chem Geol 2007;243:122–127.

Benes P, Havlik B. Speciation of mercury in natural waters. In: Nriagu J, editor. The biogeochemistry of mercury in the environment. New York: Elsevier/North Holland Biomedical Press; 1979. p 79–112.

Benoit JM, Gilmour CC, Mason RP, Riedel GS, Riedel GF. Behavior of mercury in the patuxent river estuary. Biogeochemistry 1998;40:249–265.

Benoit JM, Gilmour CC, Mason RP, Heyes A. Sulfide controls on mercury speciation and bioavailability to methylating bacteria in sediment pore waters. Environ Sci Technol 1999a;33:1780–1780.

Benoit JM, Mason RP, Gilmour CC. Estimation of mercury-sulfide speciation in sediment pore waters using octanol–water partitioning and implications for availability to methylating bacteria. Environ Toxicol Chem 1999b;18:2138–2141.

Benoit JM, Gilmour CC, Heyes A, Mason RP, Miller CL. Geochemical and biological controls over methylmercury production and degradation in aquatic ecosystems. ACS Symp Ser 2003;835:262–297.

Biester H, Muller G, Scholer HF. Binding and mobility of mercury in soils contaminated by emissions from chlor-alkali plants. Sci Total Environ 2002;284:191–203.

Biester H, Scholz C. Determination of mercury binding forms in contaminated soils: mercury pyrolysis versus sequential extractions. Environ Sci Technol 1997;31:233–239.

Björn E, Larsson T, Lambertsson L, Skyllberg U, Frech W. Recent advances in mercury speciation analysis with focus on spectrometric methods and enriched stable isotope applications. Ambio 2007;36:443–451.

Black FJ, Bruland KW, Flegal AR. Competing ligand exchange-solid phase extraction method for the determination of the complexation of dissolved inorganic mercury (II) in natural waters. Anal Chim Acta 2007;598:318–333.

Bloom NS, Preus E, Katon J, Hiltner M. Selective extractions to assess the biogeochemically relevant fractionation of inorganic mercury in sediments and soils. Anal Chim Acta 2003;479:233–248.

Bower J, Savage KS, Weinman B, Barnett MO, Hamilton WP, Harper WF. Immobilization of mercury by pyrite (FeS_2). Environ Pollut 2008;156:504–514.

Casas JS, Jones MM. Mercury(II) complexes with sulfhydryl containing chelating agents: stability constant inconsistencies and their resolution. J Inorg Nucl Chem 1980;42:99–102.

Charnock JM, Moyes LN, Pattrick RAD, Mosselmans JFW, Vaughan DJ, Livens FR. The structural evolution of mercury sulfide precipitate: an XAS and XRD study. Am Mineral 2003;88:1197–1203.

Clever HL, Johnson SA, Derrick ME. The solubility of mercury and some sparingly soluble mercury salts in water and aqueous electrolyte solutions. J Phys Chem Ref Data 1985;14:631–680.

Daskalakis KD, Helz GR. The solubility of sphalerite (ZnS) in sulfidic solutions at 25°C and 1atm pressure. Geochim Cosmochim Acta 1993;57:4923–4931.

Deonarine A, Hsu-Kim H. Precipitation of mercuric sulfide nanoparticles in NOM-containing water: implications for the natural environment. Environ Sci Technol 2009;43:2368–2373.

Desauziers V, Castre N, Cloirec PL. Sorption of methylmercury by clays and mineral oxides. Environ Technol 1997;18:1009–1018.

Dittman JA, Shanley JB, Driscoll CT, Aiken GR, Chalmers AT, Towse JE. Ultraviolet absorbance as a proxy for total dissolved mercury in streams. Environ Pollut 2009;157:1953–1956.

Drott A, Lambertsson L, Bjorn E, Skyllberg U. Importance of dissolved neutral mercury sulfides for methyl mercury production in contaminated sediments. Environ Sci Technol 2007;41:2270–2276.

Dyrssén D, Wedborg M. The sulphur-mercury(II) system in natural waters. Water Air Soil Pollut 1991;56:507–519.

Ehrhardt J-J, Behra P, Bonnissel-Gissinger P, Alnot M. XPS study of the sorption of Hg(II) onto pyrite FeS_2. Surf Interface Anal 2000;30:269–272.

Fitzgerald WF, Lamborg CH, Hammerschmidt CR. Marine biogeochemical cycling of mercury. Chem Rev 2007;107:641–662.

Freisinger E. Plant MTs-long neglected members of the metallothionein superfamily. Dalton Trans 2008;47: 6663–6675.

Gasper JD, Aiken GR, Ryan JN. A critical review of three methods used for the measurement of mercury (Hg^{2+})-dissolved organic matter stability constants. Appl Geochem 2007;22:1583–1597.

Gilmour CC, Riedel GS, Edrington MC, Bell JT, Benoit JM, Gill GA, Stordal MC. Methylmercury concentrations and production rates across a trophic gradient in the northern Everglades. Biogeochemistry 1998;40:327–345.

Goulet RR, Holmes J, Page B, Poissant L, Siciliano SD, Lean DRS, Wang F, Amyot M, Tessier A. Mercury transformations and fluxes in sediments of a riverine wetland. Geochim Cosmochim Acta 2007;71:3393–3406.

Gunneriusson L, Baxter D, Emteborg H. Complexation at low concentrations of methyl and inorganic mercury(II) to a hydrous goethite (α-FeOOH) surface. J Colloid Interface Sci 1995;169:262–266.

Hamilton WP, Turner RR, Ghosh MM. Effect of pH and iodide on the adsorption of mercury(II) by illite. Water Air Soil Pollut 1995;80:483–486.

Hammerschmidt CR, Fitzgerald WF. Geochemical controls on the production and distribution of methylmercury in near-shore marine sediments. Environ Sci Technol 2004;38:1487–1495.

Hesterberg D, Chou JW, Hutchison KJ, Sayers DE. Bonding of Hg(II) to reduced organic sulfur in humic acid as affected by S/Hg ratio. Environ Sci Technol 2001;35:2741–2745.

Hietanen S, Sillén LG. On the standard potentials of mercury, and the equilibrium $Hg^{2+}+Hg^0(l)=Hg_2^{2+}$ in nitrate and perchlorate solutions. Ark Kemi 1956;10:103–125.

Hilton BD, Man M, Hsi E, Bryant RG. NMR studies of mercurial-halogen equilibria. J Inorg Nucl Chem 1975;37:1073–1077.

Hintelmann H, Welbourn PM, Evans RD. Measurement of complexation of methylmercury(II) compounds by freshwater humic substances using equilibrium dialysis. Environ Sci Technol 1997;31:489–495.

Hu H, Mylon SE, Benoit G. Distribution of the thiols glutathione and 3-mercaptopropionic acid in connecticut lakes. Limnol Oceanogr 2006;51:2763–2774.

Hudson RJM, Gherini SA, Watras CJ, Porcella DB. Modeling the biogeochemical cycle of mercury in lakes: the mercury cycling model (MCM) and its application to the MTL study lakes. In: Watras CJ, editor. Mercury pollution integration and synthesis. Florida: Lewis Publishers, CRC Press; 1994. p 473–523.

Huerta-Diaz MA, Morse JW. Pyritization of trace metals in anoxic marine sediments. Geochim Cosmochim Acta 1992;56:2681–2702.

Hurley JP, Krabbenhoft DP, Babiarz CL, Andrén AW. Cycling of mercury across the sediment-water interface in seepage lakes. In: Baker LA, editor. Environmental chemistry of lakes and reservoirs. Washington (DC): ACS Publishers; 1994. p 425–449.

Hyland MM, Jean GE, Bancroft GM. XPS and AES studies of Hg(II) sorption and desorption reactions on sulphide minerals. Geochim Cosmochim Acta 1990;54:1957–1967.

Jalilehvand F, Leung BO, Izadifard M, Damian E. Mercury(II) cysteine complexes in alkaline aqueous solution. Inorg Chem 2006;45:66–73.

Jay JA, Morel FMM, Hemond HF. Mercury speciation in the presence of polysulfides. Environ Sci Technol 2000;34:2196–2200.

Jeong HY, Klaue B, Blum JD, Hayes KF. Sorption of mercuric ion by synthetic nanocrystalline mackinawite (FeS). Environ Sci Technol 2007;41:7699–7705.

Jeong HY, Sun K, Hayes KF. Microscopic and spectroscopic characterization of Hg(II) immobilization by mackinawite (FeS). Environ Sci Technol 2010;44:7476–7483.

Kamyshny A, Goifman A, Gun J, Rizkov D, Lev O. Equilibrium distribution of polysulfide ions in aqueous solutions at 25°C: a new approach for the study of polysulfides' equilibria. Environ Sci Technol 2004;38:6633–6644.

Karlsson T, Skyllberg U. Bonding of ppb levels of methyl mercury to reduced sulfur groups in soil organic matter. Environ Sci Technol 2003;37:4912–4918.

Kelly CA, Rudd JWM, Holoka MH. Effect of pH on mercury uptake by an aquatic bacterium: implications for Hg cycling. Environ Sci Technol 2003;37:2941–2946.

Khwaja AR, Bloom PR, Brezonik PL. Binding constants of divalent mercury (Hg^{2+}) in soil humic acids and soil organic matter. Environ Sci Technol 2006;40:844–849.

Khwaja AR, Bloom PR, Brezonik PL. Binding strength of methylmercury to aquatic NOM. Environ Sci Technol 2010;44:6151–6156.

Kim CS, Bloom NS, Rytuba JJ, Brown GE Jr. Mercury speciation by x-ray absorption fine structure spectroscopy and sequential chemical extractions: a comparison of speciation methods. Environ Sci Technol 2003;37:5102–5108.

Kim CS, Brown GE Jr, Rytuba JJ. Characterization and speciation of mercury-bearing mine wastes using X-ray absorption spectroscopy. Sci Total Environ 2000;261:157–168.

Kim CS, Rytuba JJ, Brown GE Jr. EXAFS study of mercury(II) sorption to Fe- and Al-(hydr)oxides: I. Effects of pH. J Colloid Interface Sci 2004;271:1–15.

Koszegi-Szalai H, Paal TL. Equilibrium studies of mercury(II) complexes with penicillamine. Talanta 1999;48:393–402.

Lalonde JD, Amyot M, Orvoine J, Morel FMM, Auclair JC, Ariya PA. Photoinduced oxidation of Hg^0 (aq) in the waters from the St Lawrence Estuary. Environ Sci Technol 2004;38:508–514.

Latha MP, Rao VM, Rao TS, Rao GN. Chemical speciation of Pb(II), Cd(II), Hg(II), Co(II), Ni(II), Cu(II) and Zn(II) binary complexes of L-methionine in 1,2-propanediol-water mixtures. Bull Chem Soc Ethiop 2007;21:363–372.

Lennie AR, Charnock JM, Pattrick RAD. Structure of mercury(II)-sulfur complexes by EXAFS spectroscopic measurements. Chem Geol 2003;199:199–207.

Leung BO, Jalilehvand F, Mah V. Mercury(II) penicillamine complex formation in alkaline aqueous solution. Dalton Trans 2007;41:4666–4674.

Liu J, Valsaraj KT, Devai I, DeLaune RD. Immobilization of aqueous Hg(II) by mackinawite (FeS). J Hazard Mater 2008;157:432–440.

Loux NT. An assessment of thermodynamic reaction constants for simulating aqueous environmental monomethylmercury speciation. Chem Speciat Bioavailab 2007;19:193–206.

Lovgren L, Sjoberg S. Equilibrium approaches to natural water systems–7. Complexation reactions of copper(II), cadmium(II) and mercury(II) with dissolved organic matter in a concentrated bog-water. Water Res 1989;23:327–332.

Martell AE, Smith RM, Motekaitis RJ. NIST Critically selected stability constants of metal complexes data base. Gaithersburg (MD): U.S. Department of Commerce; 2003. NIST Standard Reference Database 46.

Mason RP, Sheu GR. Role of the ocean in the global mercury cycle. Global Biogeochem Cycles 2002;16:1093.

Merritt KA, Amirbahman A. Mercury dynamics in sulfide-rich sediments: geochemical influence on contaminant mobilization within the penobscot river estuary, Maine, USA. Geochim Cosmochim Acta 2007;71:929–941.

Mierle G, Ingram R. The role of humic substances in the mobilization of mercury from watersheds. Water Air Soil Pollut 1991;56:349–357.

Morel FMM, Kraepiel AML, Amyot M. The chemical cycle and bioaccumulation of mercury. Annu Rev Ecol Syst 1998;29:543–566.

Paquette KE, Helz GR. Inorganic speciation of mercury in sulfidic waters: the importance of zero-valent sulfur. Environ Sci Technol 1997;31:2148–2153.

Potter RW, Barnes HL. Phase relations in the binary Hg-S. Am Mineral 1978;63:1143–1152.

Powell KJ, Brown PL, Byrne RH, Gajda T, Hefter G, Sjöberg S, Wanner H. Chemical speciation of Hg(ii) with environmental inorganic ligands. Aust J Chem 2004;57:993–1000.

Qian J, Skyllberg U, Frech W, Bleam WF, Bloom PR, Petit PE. Bonding of methyl mercury to reduced sulfur groups in soil and stream organic matter as determined by X-ray absorption spectroscopy and binding affinity studies. Geochim Cosmochim Acta 2002;66:3873–3885.

Ravichandran M, Aiken GR, Reddy MM, Ryan JN. Enhanced dissolution of cinnabar (mercuric sulfide) by dissolved organic matter isolated from the Florida Everglades. Environ Sci Technol 1998;32:3305–3311.

Ravichandran M, Aiken GR, Ryan JN, Reddy MM. Inhibition of precipitation and aggregation of metacinnabar (mercuric sulfide) by dissolved organic matter isolated from the Florida Everglades. Environ Sci Technol 1999;33:1418–1423.

Regnell O, Hammar T, Helgeé A, Troedsson B. Effects of anoxia and sulfide on concentrations of total and methyl mercury in sediment and water in two Hg-polluted lakes. Can J Fish Aquat Sci 2001;58:506–517.

Rickard D. The solubility of FeS. Geochim Cosmochim Acta 2006;70:5779–5789.

Rickard D, Morse JW. Acid volatile sulfide (AVS). Mar Chem 2005;97:141–197.

Rickard D, Luther GW. Chemistry of iron sulfides. Chem Rev 2007;107:514–562.

Sanemasa I. The solubility of elemental mercury vapour in water. Bull Chem Soc Jpn 1975;48:1795–1798.

Sarkar D, Essington ME, Misra KC. Adsorption of mercury(II) by kaolinite. Soil Sci Soc Am J 2000;64:1968–1975.

Schaefer JK, Morel FMM. High methylation rates of mercury bound to cysteine by geobacter sulfurreducens. Nat Geosci 2009;2:123–126.

Schuster E. The behavior of mercury in the soil with special emphasis on the complexation and adsorption processes –A review of the literature. Water Air Soil Pollut 1991;56:667–680.

Schwarzenbach G, Fischer A. Die acidität der sulfane und die zusammensetzung wässeriger polysulfidlösungen. Helv Chim Acta 1960;43:1365–1390.

Schwarzenbach G, Schellenberg M. Die komplexchemie des methylquecksilber-kations. Helv Chim Acta 1965;48:28–46.

Schwarzenbach G, Widmer M. Die loeslichkeit von metallsulfiden. I. Schwarzes quecksilbersulfid. Helv Chim Acta 1963;46:2613–2628.

Senevirathna WU, Zhang H, Gu B. Effect of carboxylic and thiol ligands (oxalate, cysteine) on the kinetics of desorption of Hg(II) from kaolinite. Water Air Soil Pollut 2011;215:573–584.

Sillén LG, Martell AE. Stability constants of metal-ion complexes. London: Chemical Society; 1971 (Suppl 1). Special Publication No. 25.

Skyllberg U. Competition among thiols and inorganic sulfides and polysulfides for Hg and MeHg in wetland soils and sediments under suboxic conditions: illumination of controversies and implications for MeHg net production. J Geophys Res 2008;113:G00C03. DOI: 10.1029/2008JG000745.

Skyllberg U. Mercury biogeochemistry in soils and sediments. In: Singh B, Gräfe M, editors. Synchrotron-based techniques in soils and sediment. Developments in soil science 34. 2010. p 379–410. Elsevier, Oxford.

Skyllberg U, Bloom PR, Qian J, Lin CM, Bleam WF. Complexation of mercury(II) in soil organic matter: EXAFS evidence for linear two-coordination with reduced sulfur groups. Environ Sci Technol 2006;40:4174–4180.

Skyllberg U, Drott A. Competition between disordered iron sulfide and natural organic matter associated thiols for mercury(II)—An EXAFS study. Environ Sci Technol 2010;44:1254–1259.

Skyllberg U, Xia K, Bloom PR, Nater EA, Bleam WF. Binding of mercury(II) to reduced sulfur in soil organic matter along upland-peat soil transects. J Environ Qual 2000;29:855–865.

Skyllberg U, Qian J, Frech W, Combined XANES and EXAFS study on the bonding of methyl mercury to thiol groups in soil and aquatic organic matter. Phys Scr 2005;T115:894–896.

Slowey AJ. Rate of formation and dissolution of mercury sulfide nanoparticles: the dual role of natural organic matter. Geochim Cosmochim Acta 2010;74:4693–4708.

Slowey AJ, Brown JGE. Transformations of mercury, iron, and sulfur during the reductive dissolution of iron oxyhydroxide by sulfide. Geochim Cosmochim Acta 2007;71:877–894.

Sposito G. Chemical equilibria and kinetics in soils. New York (NY): Oxford University Press; 1994.

Summa D, Spiga O, Bernini A, Venditti V, Priora R, Frosali S, Margaritis A, Giuseppe DD, Niccolai N, Simplicio PD. Protein–thiol substitution or protein dethiolation by thiol/disulfide exchange reactions: the albumin model. Proteins Struct Funct Bioinform 2007;69:369–378.

Tossell JA. Theoretical studies on the formation of mercury complexes in solution and the dissolution and reactions of cinnabar. Am Mineral 1999;84:877–883.

Tossell JA, Vaughan DJ. Relationships between valence orbital binding energies and crystal structures in compounds of copper, silver, gold, zinc, cadmium, and mercury. Inorg Chem 1981;20:3333–3340.

Turner A, Millward GE, Le Roux SM. Sediment-water partitioning of inorganic mercury in estuaries. Environ Sci Technol 2001;35:4648–4654.

Waples JS, Nagy KL, Aiken GR, Ryan JN. Dissolution of cinnabar (HgS) in the presence of natural organic matter. Geochim Cosmochim Acta 2005;69:1575.

Watras CJ, Back RC, Halvorsen S, Hudson RJM, Morrison KA, Wente SP. Bioaccumulation of mercury in pelagic freshwater food webs. Sci Total Environ 1998;219:183–208.

Wilkin RT, Barnes HL. Pyrite formation by reactions of iron monosulfides with dissolved inorganic and organic sulfur species. Geochim Cosmochim Acta 1996;60:4167–4179.

Wolfenden S, Charnock JM, Hilton J, Livens FR, Vaughan DJ. Sulfide species as a sink for mercury in lake sediments. Environ Sci Technol 2005;39:6644–6648.

Xia K, Skyllberg UL, Bleam WF, Bloom PR, Nater EA, Helmke PA. X-ray absorption spectroscopic evidence for the complexation of Hg(II) by reduced sulfur in soil humic substances. Environ Sci Technol 1999;33:257–261.

Yamamoto M. Stimulation of elemental mercury oxidation in the presence of chloride ion in aquatic environments. Chemosphere 1996;32:1217–1224.

Yin Y, Allen HE, Li Y, Huang CP, Sanders PF. Adsorption of mercury(II) by soil: effects of pH, chloride, and organic matter. J Environ Qual 1996;25:837–844.

Yoon S-J, Diener LM, Bloom PR, Nater EA, Bleam WF. X-ray absorption studies of CH_3Hg^+-binding sites in humic substances. Geochim Cosmochim Acta 2005;69:1111–1121.

Zhang J, Wang F, House JD, Page B. Thiols in wetland interstitial waters and their role in mercury and methylmercury speciation. Limnol Oceanogr 2004;49:2276–2286.

CHAPTER 8

THE EFFECTS OF DISSOLVED ORGANIC MATTER ON MERCURY BIOGEOCHEMISTRY

CHASE A. GERBIG, JOSEPH N. RYAN, and **GEORGE R. AIKEN**

8.1 INTRODUCTION

Improved understanding of the geochemistry, fate, and transport of mercury (Hg) in aquatic ecosystems is critical for assessing its ecological and human health effects. In particular, the need to understand factors controlling the bioavailability and reactivity of mercury under environmentally relevant conditions has increased as society strives to manage resources and restore ecosystems while ameliorating the effects of mercury. It has long been recognized that the chemical forms of mercury in the water column and sediments are intimately related to its overall effects on living organisms, but a number of important questions concerning processes that control mercury reactivity, especially with regard to bioavailability for methylation, remain to be addressed. Often, the key questions involve chemistry at the aqueous–geological–microbial interface in environments that are chemically complex, such as the sediment–water interface.

Dissolved organic matter (DOM), which is ubiquitous in water, soil, and sediment environments, frequently controls a number of important environmental processes that are relevant for the cycling of metals, including mercury, in aquatic ecosystems. These processes include mineral dissolution and precipitation (Hoch et al., 2000; Waples et al., 2005), photochemical oxidation and reduction reactions (Moran and Covert, 2003; Stubbins et al., 2008), and the speciation, transport, and fate of metals (Perdue, 1998; Haitzer et al., 2003). The compounds that comprise DOM also indirectly influence the fate of metals in aqueous systems by controlling ecological processes. Some of the indirect effects of DOM include influencing pH, serving as a substrate for microbially mediated reactions (Tranvik, 1998; Findlay, 2003), controlling the depth of the photic zone

Environmental Chemistry and Toxicology of Mercury, First Edition.
Edited by Guangliang Liu, Yong Cai, and Nelson O'Driscoll.
© 2012 John Wiley & Sons, Inc. Published 2012 by John Wiley & Sons, Inc.

(Wetzel, 2001), and influencing the availability of nutrients (Qualls and Richardson, 2003).

The most significant processes to define for understanding the chemistries of organic matter and mercury are (i) the effects of DOM on the chemical speciation and bioavailability of mercury for methylation by microorganisms and (ii) the effects of DOM on the partitioning of mercury and methylmercury (MeHg) between dissolved and particulate phases and the biota in the water column. Until recently, very low mercury concentrations in most ecosystems have masked the strength and mechanisms of mercury–DOM interactions, resulting in a poor understanding of important environmental processes. With advances in experimental design and analytical approaches, however, new insights are beginning to emerge. In this chapter, we describe the effects of DOM on mercury biogeochemistry by addressing field-based observations and fundamental chemical interactions that drive mercury and methylmercury reactivity in the aquatic environment.

8.2 DISSOLVED ORGANIC MATTER

DOM is a complex, heterogeneous continuum of low to high molecular weight organic compounds exhibiting different solubilities and reactivities. Organic compounds can be truly dissolved, aggregated into colloids, associated with inorganic colloids, or bound to filterable particles. Historically, organic matter in natural waters has been arbitrarily divided into dissolved and particulate organic carbon based on filtration, generally through 0.45- or 0.7-μm filters (Fig. 8.1). No natural cutoff exists between DOM and particulate organic matter and the distinction is operational.

The study of the composition and environmental significance of organic matter in natural waters is hampered by its inherent chemical complexity, which poses a number of analytical problems in defining its reactivity (Aiken and Leenheer, 1993). Thousands of molecules are known to contribute to the composition of DOM in a given water sample (Stenson et al., 2003; Sleighter et al., 2010). The distribution of these compounds and, hence, the chemical characteristics of DOM in a water body, are influenced by the nature of source materials and the biogeochemical processes involved in carbon cycling within the entire ecosystem, including the terrestrial watershed (Aiken and Cotsaris, 1995; McKnight and Aiken, 1998; Fellman et al., 2010). In addition, for most rivers and streams, DOM concentration and composition vary as a function of hydrology (Aiken and Cotsaris, 1995; Saraceno et al., 2009; Dittman et al., 2010). The variability in the amount and nature of DOM among ecosystems, especially with respect to differences in polarity and aromatic carbon content, are significant factors in controlling DOM reactivity in a number of important environmental processes relevant to mercury biogeochemistry.

DOM is a complex mixture of molecules, and the various molecules comprising DOM react in different ways with mercury. For instance, studies of mercury binding to DOM have shown that only a small fraction of DOM molecules possess

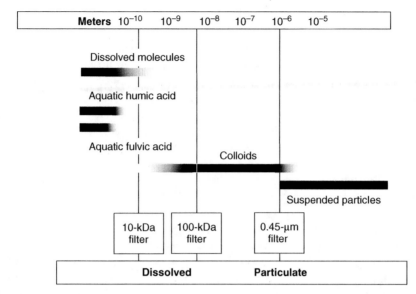

Figure 8.1 Conceptual diagram showing the size distribution of organic matter between particulate and dissolved organic carbon in natural waters.

the necessary functional groups to bind Hg(II) very strongly (Haitzer et al., 2002). Other molecules that bind Hg(II) weakly can nonetheless interact with HgS(s), an important form of mercury in sulfidic environments and cinnabar mining regions, to inhibit HgS(s) precipitation or enhance HgS(s) dissolution (Ravichandran et al., 1998, 1999; Slowey, 2010). Other molecules that may not directly interact with Hg(II) or HgS(s) can influence their fate by controlling photochemical reactions or fueling microbial activity. While certain fractions of DOM react with mercury, a large portion of DOM molecules may be inert with regard to interactions with mercury, especially under the common conditions where the concentration of DOM (milligrams per liter) greatly exceeds that of mercury (nanograms per liter). Complicating the situation is that, for some processes, the pool of compounds comprising DOM may contain compounds that counteract each other with regard to a particular reaction. For instance, the presence of both dissolution-promoting and dissolution-inhibiting compounds has been noted for DOM interactions with bulk (Waples et al., 2005) and colloidal HgS(s) (Slowey, 2010).

Despite advances in methods to characterize DOM, serious challenges remain in defining its reactivity with mercury at the molecular level. A variety of approaches have been employed in the study of DOM in natural systems. The simplest of these, and the most common with regard to field-based studies, is the determination of dissolved organic carbon (DOC) concentration. DOC concentration alone, however, does not provide information on DOM composition. Methods used to learn more about DOM composition in field settings include the measurement of optical properties such as the absorbance of ultraviolet and visible (UV–vis) radiation which is used to calculate parameters such as specific ultraviolet absorbance (SUVA; Weishaar et al., 2003), and spectral slope (Helms et al., 2008) and fluorescence (Fellman et al., 2010). This information is useful for assessing the nature and reactivity of DOM, although it only provides average data about the chromophores and fluorophores within a sample. Utilizing optical data is an attractive approach for studying DOM because data collection is straightforward, the data provide information about both the concentration and composition of DOM (Weishaar et al., 2003; Spencer et al., 2009), and detector systems can be employed for a variety of process-based studies and separation techniques to study DOM composition. In addition, optical data can be obtained *in situ*, allowing for the collection of high frequency environmental data in real time that can be used to better understand the influences of sources and processes occurring within the ecosystem, even at watershed scales (Spencer et al., 2007; Saraceno et al., 2009).

A complementary approach to studying whole water samples is to isolate functionally distinct DOM fractions from whole water samples to determine the fundamental structural and chemical properties of each fraction. The properties of the fractions can be related to the biogenesis and environmental roles of these materials. Many of the methods used to characterize DOM lack sufficient sensitivity to obtain data on DOM samples at concentrations usually encountered in natural ecosystems; thus, isolation or concentration may be required (Aiken and Leenheer, 1993). Fractionation is often accomplished using solid-phase extraction on hydrophobic sorbents such as XAD (Aiken et al., 1992), C_{18} (Green and Blough, 1994), and PPL (Dittmar et al., 2008) resins. Fractionation on XAD resins has been employed to obtain large amounts of isolated organic matter (e.g., aquatic humic and fulvic acids; Fig. 8.1) for subsequent characterization and for use in experiments designed to elucidate chemical processes of interest. Detailed structural information has been obtained on fractionated samples by elemental analyses (Ma et al., 2001), ^{13}C nuclear magnetic resonance (^{13}C-NMR; Lu et al., 2003; Maie et al., 2006), mass spectrometry (Hatcher et al., 2001; Lu et al., 2003; Sleighter et al., 2010), and analyses for specific components of DOM such as lignin, carbohydrates, and phenols (Maie et al., 2006). Synchrotron-based techniques provide information related to chemical-binding environments (i.e., extended X-ray absorption fine structure (EXAFS) spectroscopy; Xia et al. (1999), among others) or information about the redox status of key elements important for metal-binding interactions such as sulfur and nitrogen (i.e., X-ray adsorption near edge spectroscopy (XANES); Vairavamurthy et al., 1997; Vairavamurthy and Wang, 2002; Jokic et al., 2004; Prietzel et al., 2007). Finally, well-characterized, isolated fractions of DOM, such as aquatic humic substances from different environments, have been employed in laboratory experiments designed to provide information on the chemical mechanisms driving DOM interactions with Hg(II) and HgS(s) (Ravichandran et al., 1998, 1999; Haitzer et al., 2002, 2003; Waples et al., 2005; Deonarine and Hsu-Kim, 2009; Slowey, 2010). Application of new analytical approaches is expected to provide additional insights into the chemically complex processes driving interactions of DOM with mercury.

Ultrafiltration is another approach that has been applied to the study of both DOM (Benner et al., 1997) and mercury species in water samples (Cai et al., 1999; Babiarz et al., 2001; Choe and Gill, 2001). In this approach, dissolved samples (Fig. 8.1) are fractionated based on molecular size. The resulting data provide information about the distribution of DOM, mercury, and methylmercury in the dissolved and colloidal size fractions, which is potentially useful in understanding dynamics driving export of mercury species under varying hydrologic and chemical conditions. As with all fractionation approaches, ultrafiltration is subject to potential artifacts and care is required in employing different membrane types, assigning molecular weight sizes without appropriate standardization (Aiken, 1984), and testing for suitability of membranes for mercury studies (Babiarz et al., 2001).

8.3 FIELD OBSERVATIONS

Some of the earliest articles addressing mercury in natural waters noted that DOM and mercury interact strongly to influence mercury behavior (Fitzgerald and Lyons, 1973; Andren and Harriss, 1975). In numerous studies since, strong correlations have been noted between the concentrations of total dissolved mercury and DOM in a variety of environmental settings (Mierle and Ingram, 1991; Grigal, 2002; Balogh et al., 2004; Brigham et al., 2009; Dittman et al., 2010). Elevated fluxes of both mercury and DOM have been observed during high flow events for small catchments, which results in strong relationships between DOM (or DOC) and mercury concentrations (Fig. 8.2). The relationship between mercury and DOM concentrations can vary greatly among different rivers and each system needs to be evaluated separately. Stronger correlations have been observed between mercury and hydrophobic portions of the organic matter pool (typically the fraction of DOM operationally defined as humic and fulvic substances) than between mercury and DOC concentration when hydrophobic fractions have been determined (Mierle and Ingram, 1991; Grigal, 2002; Shanley et al., 2008; Dittman et al., 2010).

For many streams and rivers, hydrologic factors controlling the export of DOM from upper soil horizons and wetlands within a watershed drive the export of mercury, and to a lesser degree, methylmercury. Changes in flow patterns in these systems are significant because upper soil horizons, riparian zones, and wetlands are rich in DOM (Cronan and Aiken, 1985) and also have greater mercury and methylmercury concentrations (Grigal, 2002). Indeed, discharge itself has been noted to be a good predictor of fluvial mercury export in numerous streams and rivers—total dissolved mercury concentrations increase as flow increases (Brigham et al., 2009; Dittman et al., 2010). Increased mercury concentrations during high flow can be attributed to the shift in soil runoff flow patterns to a more horizontal direction when soil is saturated as well as an increase in shallow subsurface and surface runoff. In addition, during periods of high flow, wetlands

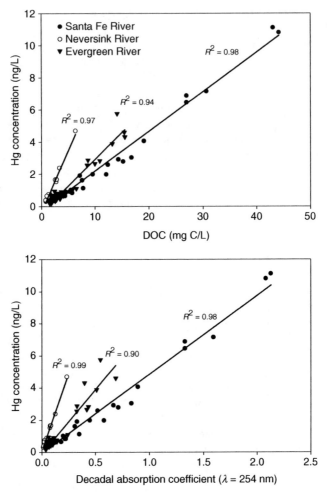

Figure 8.2 The relationship between DOC or UV absorbance ($\lambda = 254$ nm) and filtered mercury concentrations for the Neversink River, NY; Evergreen River, WI; and Santa Fe River, FL. *Source*: Neversink River data is unpublished; Evergreen River and Santa Fe River data from Brigham et al. (2008).

become inundated with water and become hydrologically connected to adjacent rivers and streams, resulting in the export of DOM, mercury, and methylmercury from these systems (Balogh et al., 2006). The importance of connectivity between organic-rich soil horizons, wetlands, and adjacent streams has been noted by Hinton et al. (1998). DOC concentrations increase as higher proportions of runoff are derived from hydrologic flow paths that intersect shallow organic matter-rich soil layers and wetland ecosystems where soluble organic compounds, mercury, and methylmercury have accumulated. The shift in flow paths results in increasing DOC concentrations and compositional changes in the organic matter transported in rivers and streams. Storm events, the onset of the rainy season, or the melting of snowpack can all produce high flow conditions.

Given the strong correlations between DOM optical properties and the presence of aquatic humic substances, these optical properties are potentially useful indicators of mercury in rivers and streams. Mierle and Ingram (1991) first noted the correlation between mercury and color (Hazan units) associated with DOM in brown-water streams and were able to relate mercury export to DOM export. More recently, absorption coefficients determined at a wavelength of 254 nm were shown to be highly correlated to mercury export for a number of stream systems (Fig. 8.2; Dittman et al., 2010). The use of DOM optical data to infer information about mercury concentrations in aquatic ecosystems offers some potentially important advantages. First, acquiring optical data is relatively inexpensive and requires minimal sample handling. Second, the development of optical sensors employing both absorption and fluorescence approaches permit *in situ* measurements of DOM concentrations, and by correlation, mercury, at greater frequency and during all portions of the hydrograph. For those systems where DOM and mercury concentrations are strongly correlated, *in situ* measurements can result in better determination of flux.

The relationship between DOM and mercury concentrations does not always hold. In the Everglades, for instance, correlations between DOM and dissolved mercury concentrations are weaker than those observed in northern riverine ecosystems (Hurley et al., 1998). This difference is likely due to differences in the sources, cycling, and transport of these species in the Everglades compared to other ecosystems. The distribution of total mercury throughout the Everglades is complicated, varying spatially and seasonally (Liu et al., 2008), with concentrations of dissolved mercury generally <5 ng/L throughout the ecosystem (Hurley et al., 1998; Liu et al., 2008). DOM concentrations in the Everglades are generally greater than those found in most aquatic environments and can be generated *in situ* from existing vegetation, detritus, and peat soils or transported from other areas in the Everglades. In addition, correlations between DOM and mercury concentrations are weak-to-nonexistent for urban environments (Mason and Sullivan, 1998; Brigham et al., 2009). In these systems, wastewater discharge and urban runoff strongly influence the export and reactivity of DOM.

8.4 EFFECTS OF DOM ON MERCURY DISTRIBUTIONS BETWEEN SOLUTION AND PARTICLES

A consequence of strong interactions between DOM with Hg(II), HgS(s), and MeHg is that DOM influences the partitioning of mercury species to particles and soil organic matter such that concentrations of dissolved mercury and methylmercury increase in the presence of DOM. A number of studies have demonstrated that DOM is an important factor controlling the dissolution of mercury from soils and sediments (Mierle and Ingram, 1991; Drexel et al., 2002). Factors that influence the concentration of dissolved mercury are significant because many of the processes (both abiotic and biotic) involved in mercury cycling in aquatic environments are hypothesized to be strongly dependent on the concentration of total dissolved mercury. For instance, Skyllberg et al. (2003) showed that concentrations of methylmercury associated with soils and soil solutions correlated positively with the concentration of dissolved mercury in soil waters for a catchment in northern Sweden.

Field-based partitioning coefficients of mercury between the particulate and dissolved phase, described as the partitioning coefficient, are often given by an expression of the form:

$$K_d = \frac{P_{THg}/SS}{F_{THg}}$$

where K_d is the concentration-based partition coefficient (liters per kilogram), P_{THg} is the concentration of total particulate mercury (nanograms per liter), SS is the concentration of suspended sediment (kilograms per liter), and F_{THg} is the concentration of total filterable mercury (nanograms per liter). A similar expression can be written to describe the distribution of methylmercury between dissolved and particulate forms. Reported field-based K_d values generally range from $10^{2.8}$ to $10^{6.6}$ for mercury in natural waters and from $10^{2.6}$ to $10^{5.9}$ for methylmercury (Babiarz et al., 2001; Brigham et al., 2009). The value of K_d depends, in part, on the DOM concentration. For instance, as shown in Fig. 8.3a and 8.3c, K_d is generally weaker with increasing DOC concentration for a suite of rivers as reported by Brigham et al. (2009). It is assumed that at greater DOM concentrations there is less mercury association with suspended sediment.

In form, the field-based K_d is similar to traditional concentration distribution coefficients employed in the chemistry of separation science (Karger et al., 1973). The chemistry-based K_d, which is commonly employed in chromatography and other separation methods, is related to the thermodynamic distribution coefficient. As a consequence, sorption and desorption reactions influencing K_d must be reversible. These constraints do not hold for field-based K_d values, which suffer from a number of complications. First, the nature of the particulate fraction is rarely defined. As a result, the mechanisms of interactions of mercury with the particulate surface are unknown or poorly defined. The organic matter content of the particles, soils, or sediments is a key factor controlling the ability of particles to adsorb mercury (Hammerschmidt and Fitzgerald, 2006; Marvin-DiPasquale et al., 2009); however, this parameter often goes unreported. Second, the particulate fraction, defined as the material retained on a filter (typically 0.45 μm; Fig. 8.1), is a mixture of materials that interact differently with mercury. Liu et al. (2008) demonstrated different degrees of association of mercury with soils, floc, and periphyton in the Florida Everglades, whereas Marvin-DiPasquale et al. (2009) showed that the K_d values for total mercury and methylmercury in riverine sediments were a function of both DOM concentration and the amount

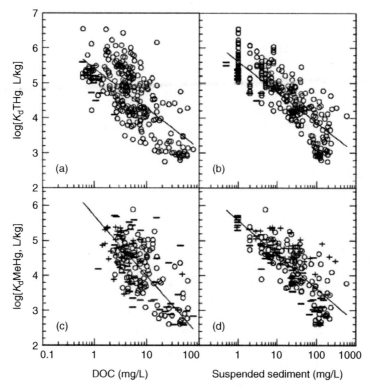

Figure 8.3 The relationship between distribution coefficients (K_d) for total mercury (THg) or methylmercury (MeHg) and DOC or suspended sediment load from a variety of stream ecosystems. *Source*: Reproduced from Figure 5 of Brigham et al. (2009) with permission from the American Chemical Society.

of fine sediment material. Third, what is considered "dissolved" (<0.45 μm; Fig. 8.1) also contains inorganic and organic colloidal materials that interact differently with both mercury and the surfaces of particulate materials compared to dissolved constituents (Babiarz et al., 2001; Choe and Gill, 2001). Babiarz et al. (2001) demonstrated that the colloidal phase exerted a strong control on the distribution of mercury between dissolved and particulate phases for a variety of surface waters resulting in underestimation of field-based K_d values. Lastly, K_d values are often dependent on the concentration of particles in solution, such as suspended sediment—this phenomena is known as the *particle concentration effect* (Fig. 8.3b and 8.3d; Honeyman and Santschi, 1989; Babiarz et al., 2001). Given these factors, nonthermodynamic field-based K_d values—based only on the ratio of filterable versus particulate mercury—are not readily comparable between systems, or within the same system under different hydrologic conditions. In addition, because the reactions driving observed K_d values are not reversible, the usefulness of these data is reduced for modeling purposes.

8.5   MERCURY BINDING STRENGTH

Mercury, a soft B-group metal, exhibits relatively weak interactions with oxygen-containing ligands, moderate strength interactions with nitrogen-containing ligands, and strong interactions with sulfur-containing ligands. Consider the three ligands glycolic acid, glycine, and thioglycolic acid; they only vary in a single functional group (an alcohol, amine, and thiol group, respectively) and serve as an excellent example of the effect of a single functional group on Hg(II) binding strength. The Hg(II) binding constants (β_2; HgL$_2$) are $10^{7.05}$ (Rossotti and Whewell, 1977), $10^{19.3}$ (NIST, 2004), and $10^{43.8}$ (NIST, 2004), respectively (correcting for the slightly different temperatures and ionic strengths at which each constant was measured does not appreciably change the comparison). The oxidation state of the ligand in question is critical in predicting the strength of binding. The electron-dense binding sites created by reduced functionalities create a significantly stronger bond with Hg(II) than a binding site composed of the oxidized version of the same element. An inorganic example is quite telling—sulfate (SO_4^{2-}) is a weak ligand ($K_1 = 10^{1.3}$), whereas sulfide (S^{2-}; $K_1 = 10^{52.4}$) is extremely strong.

The distribution of metal-binding functional groups within DOM is broad. Oxygen-containing functional groups are much more abundant than nitrogen- or sulfur-containing groups. In addition, the functional groups of a single element span a range of possible oxidation states. Sulfur functional groups in organic matter range from highly reduced (e.g., thiols, R-SH) to highly oxidized (e.g., sulfonates, R-SO$_3$H) (Vairavamurthy et al., 1997). Just as the inorganic example of sulfate versus sulfide suggests, the binding of these organic sites with respect to Hg(II) is substantially different—thiol sites exhibit very strong interactions, whereas oxidized sulfur groups are extremely weak. Further, the structural distribution of binding sites in a ligand significantly affects the ligand's ability to bind a metal (and the subsequent strength of that interaction). For this reason, chelating ligands such as ethylenediaminetetraacetic acid (EDTA) bind metals much more effectively than ligands that interact with a metal at a single site. The heteroatom(s) involved in metal binding, the oxidation state of those heteroatoms, and the steric arrangement of the metal complex are important parameters in determining the binding site orientation and strength in DOM.

While model organic ligands and inorganic examples are illustrative, they do not adequately capture the heterogeneity of DOM and the effect of DOM on mercury behavior in the environment. For instance, Ravichandran et al. demonstrated that the effects of DOM on both the dissolution (1998) and inhibition of precipitation (1999) of HgS(s) were poorly replicated by compounds known to interact strongly with mercury. In another example, some model compounds increase Hg(II) methylation because they bind Hg(II) and make it more bioavailable (Schaefer and Morel, 2009). However, increased methylation rates when mercury speciation is controlled by a model compound are inconsistent with the often observed decrease in methylation rates in the presence of DOM (Miskimmin et al., 1992; Barkay et al., 1997).

We begin the discussion of Hg(II)–DOM interactions by first considering the strength of that interaction. The measurement of metal–organic matter binding constants is most frequently quantified with a conditional stability constant. Comparison of constants can be difficult because the constants are specific to the conditions of the experiment, and are not often defined in consistent ways, if they are defined at all. For example, Benoit et al. (2001) defined a conditional stability constant for the reaction:

$$Hg^{2+} + RXH^{n-} = HgX^{(n-1)-} + H^{+}$$

and a corresponding conditional stability constant of log $K = 10.6-11.8$ depending on the DOM isolate. Alternatively, Haitzer et al. (2002) defined a stability constant for the reaction:

$$Hg + DOM = HgDOM$$

and report a corresponding conditional stability constant of log $K = 23.2 \pm 1.0$ L/kg. The Benoit et al. (2001) example assumes some known stoichiometry, a pK_a for the acid functional group, and the ability to calculate a molar concentration of DOM for the calculation of Hg(II) speciation at a given pH. The Haitzer et al. (2002) constant is a mass-based constant (hence the units liters per kilogram), and while free of some assumptions, does not account for pH. When a series of reasonable assumptions are made, and a consistent definition of the constant is used, these conditional stability constants agree, and show very strong binding between Hg(II) and DOM. Only organic thiols exhibit Hg(II) binding strengths comparable in strength to the mercury–DOM interaction observed in these two studies.

The notion that mercury binding to DOM is dominated by thiol-like sites at environmental levels of mercury is well supported in the literature. A number of binding constant studies have measured large conditional stability constants between organic matter and Hg(II) that are consistent with binding by thiols. These studies have used whole water (Hsu and Sedlak, 2003; Lamborg et al., 2003, 2004; Han and Gill, 2005; Black et al., 2007), organic matter isolated from natural waters (Benoit et al., 2001; Haitzer et al., 2002, 2003), organic matter extracted from peats (Drexel et al., 2002; Khwaja et al., 2006), and intact peats (Skyllberg et al., 2000; Drexel et al., 2002). In addition to the variety of organic matter sources and types, a variety of methods were employed including equilibrium dialysis–ligand exchange, reducible mercury titration, octanol–water or toluene–water partitioning, competitive ligand exchange–solid phase extraction, and bromide competition. The consistent conclusions between these significantly different approaches argue for the ubiquity of strong thiol-like binding sites in organic matter.

Although it is clear that some conditions give rise to the measurement of strong binding sites, there are also mercury–organic matter studies that measure weaker carboxyl- and phenol-like interactions between Hg(II) and DOM (Cheam and Gamble, 1974; Lovgren and Sjoberg, 1989; Yin et al., 1997; Haitzer et al., 2002). The predominant difference between these observations and the observations of thiol-like binding sites is the amount of mercury in solution relative to the amount of organic matter. Studies with higher ratios of mercury to DOM measure weaker binding constants. The balance between thiol-like and carboxyl-like binding sites in DOM is driven by the relative abundance of these types of sites. Using one DOM isolate, Haitzer et al. (2002) reported a carboxyl content of DOM of 5.45 mmol/g and a reduced sulfur content of DOM of 0.32 mmol/g. Even if all of the reduced sulfur was in the form of thiols that can interact with metals, there would be an abundance of weaker carboxyl sites in the DOM. However, reduced sulfur in organic matter may be in the form of thiols, dithiols, or polysulfides (with thiophenes also observed in soil humic material; Vairavamurthy et al., 1997; Solomon et al., 2003). Without cleaving sulfur–sulfur bonds, dithiols, and polysulfides in DOM are unlikely to bind with Hg(II) as strongly as thiols (Basinger et al., 1981). Thus, even quantification of reduced sulfur is unlikely to indicate how many strong, thiol-like binding sites may be present in DOM. By measuring the conditional stability constant of Hg(II) with DOM over a wide range of Hg:DOM ratios, Haitzer et al. (2002) was able to quantify the strong binding capacity of a DOM isolate from the Florida Everglades (Fig. 8.4). DOM from different environments may have slightly different strengths and capacities (Haitzer et al., 2003), but the measurements by Haitzer et al. (2002) provide an excellent example of thiol-like versus carboxyl-like binding sites. As indicated in Fig. 8.4, below 1 μg Hg per milligram DOM the stability constant is approximately 10^{23} L/kg, whereas above 10 μg Hg per milligram DOM the stability constant is approximately 10^{10} L/kg. In this study, the stability constant

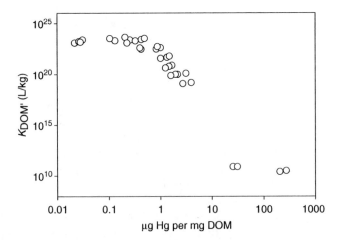

Figure 8.4 Conditional stability constant (K'_{DOM}) for the binding between Hg(II) and a DOM isolate from the F1 site in the Florida Everglades versus the ratio of total mercury to DOM. *Source*: Reproduced from Figure 6 of Haitzer et al. (2002) with permission from the Amercian Chemical Society.

of 10^{23} L/kg is consistent with thiol-like binding sites, whereas the constant of 10^{10} L/kg is consistent with carboxyl-like sites. At approximately 1 μg Hg per milligram DOM, the conditional stability constant begins to decrease, suggesting some carboxyl-like sites are effectively competing for Hg(II), lowering the observed stability constant, and giving an approximate cutoff for the amount of strong binding sites present in the DOM.

Several studies suggest that Hg(II) strong binding sites in soil organic matter are composed of multiple sulfur atoms (Xia et al., 1999; Khwaja et al., 2006; Skyllberg et al., 2006). If we assume that DOM binding sites are similar to soil organic matter binding sites, and two atoms of reduced sulfur are involved in binding a single Hg(II) atom, the strong binding site capacity of DOM reported by Haitzer et al. (2002) represents only 3.1% of the reduced sulfur (1.8% of the total sulfur) in the DOM isolate. Some of the reduced sulfur is likely to be present as weaker binding dithiols and polysulfides, although Xia et al. (1999) interpreted EXAFS data to indicate that there is evidence for the participation of a dithiol-like moiety in Hg(II) binding in concert with strong-binding thiol-like sites. In addition, the multiple-thiol nature of the strong binding sites presents the possibility that lone thiols exist in the DOM but do not strongly interact with Hg(II). Finally, a portion of the reduced sulfur pool may be sterically inaccessible to Hg(II), thus accounting for a portion of reduced organic sulfur that does not participate in Hg(II) binding. Whatever the specific stoichiometry of the Hg(II) binding sites, the Hg(II)–DOM bonds are slow to form, despite the rapid water exchange rate of the Hg(II) ion (Stumm and Morgan, 1996). The highest stability constants for Hg(II)–DOM binding are only measured after approximately 24 h of equilibration time (Gasper et al., 2007; Miller et al., 2007), which gives further evidence for strong DOM binding sites that are highly specific and difficult for Hg(II) to access.

Han and Gill (2005) expand the discussion to a broad set of DOM samples by making their own measurements of conditional stability constants and compiling the Hg(II)–DOM conditional stability constants of multiple studies under one consistent definition of a stability constant (reasonable assumptions were required for some studies). The result shows the variation in ligand concentration (DOM binding sites) as a function of the stability constant (Fig. 8.5). These data depict a continuous distribution of strong Hg(II) binding sites, with the strongest sites also being the least abundant—a phenomenon that is consistent with conclusions for other metals (Town and Filella, 2000) and presents the most robust method for describing the distribution of strength and abundance of Hg(II) complexing sites in DOM observed across multiple studies.

8.6 MERCURY BINDING ENVIRONMENT

The first known direct observations of Hg(II) binding environments in organic matter were reported by Xia et al. (1999) using EXAFS spectroscopy. Using a humic acid extracted from an organic-rich soil horizon and the soil itself, they

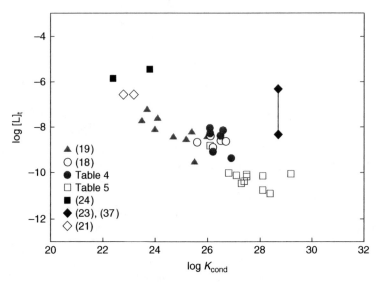

Figure 8.5 The relationship between mercury ligand concentration ($[L]_t$) and the HgL conditional stability constant (K_{cond}) for natural water samples and DOM isolates. *Source*: Reproduced from Figure 4 of Han and Gill (2005) with permission from the Amercian Chemical Society; references are those within Han and Gill (2005).

observed Hg(II) binding environments at mercury to reduced sulfur (S_{red}) molar ratios of 3.1:1 and 0.56:1, respectively, that are composed of oxygen functional groups as well as sulfur functional groups (Fig. 8.6a and 8.6b). Hesterberg et al. (2001) built on this work by using EXAFS to examine Hg(II) binding environments as a function of the Hg:S molar ratio in a different soil humic acid extract (~70% of total sulfur was in a reduced state). In general, as the Hg:S ratio decreased from 1.7 to 0.18, the average number of sulfur atoms coordinating Hg(II) increased, while the average number of oxygen atoms coordinating Hg(II) decreased. At the lowest Hg:S ratio, approximately 90% of the Hg(II) binding by the extracted humic acid was by reduced sulfur functionalities. Further work in soils at Hg:S_{red} ratios as low as 0.01 showed three coordinating sulfur atoms—two sulfur atoms were in a linear S–Hg–S binding arrangement and a third sulfur atom stabilized the complex from a greater distance than the two linear sulfur atoms (Fig. 8.6c; Skyllberg et al., 2006). At Hg:S_{red} ratios greater than 0.1, the complex was similar to what Hesterberg et al. (2001) observed with a Hg(II) complex composed of a sulfur atom as well as coordinating oxygen or nitrogen functional groups (Fig. 8.6d). Overall, the results of X-ray spectroscopy examinations support the conclusions arrived at through binding constant measurements—namely that reduced sulfur functional groups play a dominant role in Hg(II) binding by organic matter when the Hg:DOM ratio is sufficiently low.

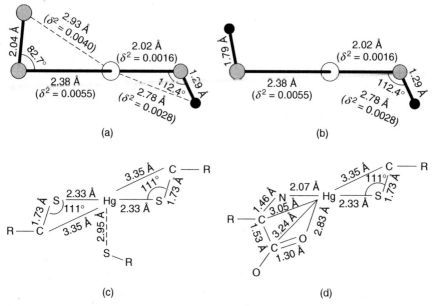

Figure 8.6 Four proposed binding arrangements for Hg(II) in soil organic matter. (a) and (b) are for Hg:S$_{red}$ ratios of 0.56 and 3.1, respectively (open circles represent Hg, hatched represent S, dotted represent O, and closed represent C); each Hg(II) bond is presented with its length in angstroms (Å), and Debye–Waller factor (δ^2), a measure of the dynamic and static disorder of the bond. (c) and (d) represent potential structures from systems with Hg:S$_{red}$ ratios of 0.01–0.05 and 0.10–0.40, respectively. *Source*: (a) and (b) are from Xia et al. (1999), with permission from Amercian Chemical Society; (c) and (d) are from Skyllberg et al. (2006), with permission from Amercian Chemical Society.

The studies that make direct observations of Hg(II) binding by organic matter either use whole soil or organic matter extracted from soil rather than aquatic DOM. One of the primary differences between studying aquatic DOM and soil organic matter is the concentration. While aquatic DOM concentrations are typically on the order of milligrams per liter, these studies with soil and soil organic matter were done between 2.1 and 50 g/L, introducing the potential for intermolecular interactions that are far less likely in DOM solutions. Aggregation, in particular, may be problematic because it could shield binding sites from the bulk solution, preventing Hg(II) interactions. However, the processes that contribute sulfur to organic matter (e.g., abiotic incorporation of inorganic sulfide, biological sources) may be similar in aquatic DOM and soil organic matter from organic horizons and probably lead to similar distributions of sulfur functional groups. Aquatic DOM (Haitzer et al., 2002) and soil humic substances (Skyllberg et al., 2006) both exhibit a capacity for strong Hg(II) binding that includes <5% of all reduced organic sulfur, suggesting that reduced sulfur content of organic matter is a poor proxy for the amount of strong binding sites in both aquatic and soil environments.

8.7 METHYLMERCURY BINDING STRENGTH AND ENVIRONMENT

Studies of methylmercury binding by DOM have followed much the same trajectory as Hg(II) binding studies. Through a combination of binding constant studies at varying ratios of methylmercury to organic matter and the application of spectroscopic methods (particularly in the case of methylmercury interactions with soil organic matter), thermodynamic constants have been developed in concert with a detailed understanding of the methylmercury binding environment in organic matter.

The studies that have measured methylmercury binding by organic matter (dissolved and soil or peat derived) have measured conditional binding constants (under varying conditions, including pH) as high as approximately 10^{17} (based on the reaction $RS + CH3Hg^+ = CH_3HgSR$; Karlsson and Skyllberg, 2003) and have generally concluded that the strength of the MeHg–organic matter interaction is indicative of methylmercury binding by thiol-like binding sites (Hintelmann et al., 1995, 1997; Amirbahman et al., 2002; Khwaja et al., 2010). These studies have noted pH-dependent methylmercury binding by organic matter, particularly at slightly acidic conditions of pH<5. This pH dependence is important because it suggests that thiol groups of varying pK_a values and binding affinities are important at different pH values. For example, Amirbahman et al. (2002) effectively modeled methylmercury binding using a three-site model with the sites having pK_a values of 4, 7, and 10, which are representative pK_a values for disulfane (RSSH), cysteine, and a general thiol, respectively. Alternatively, models that use thiol sites that only have higher pK_a values of 8.50 and 9.95 (Karlsson and Skyllberg, 2003) or only have one low pK_a of 4.0 (Khwaja et al., 2010) have been created. The differences in the conclusions between these studies are more likely the result of experimental parameters, methods, and modeling approaches than structurally different binding environments.

In addition to identifying thiol-like methylmercury binding sites in organic matter, conditional stability constant studies have been used to examine the capacity of organic matter for binding methylmercury. The study with the highest methylmercury concentrations observed the weakest sites, but those weaker sites were still thought to be thiol-like (Amirbahman et al., 2002). The strong binding site content of organic matter for methylmercury has been identified as 0.2–13 ng MeHg per milligram DOM by equilibrium dialysis (Hintelmann et al., 1997) and 14.3–206 ng MeHg per milligram DOM by gel permeation chromatography/hydride generation inductively coupled plasma mass spectrometry (ICP-MS) (O'Driscoll and Evans, 2000). The work of Amirbahman et al. (2002) was carried out between approximately 20 and 215 ng MeHg per milligram DOM, which suggests that the three binding sites they modeled were at least representative of methylmercury binding at more environmentally relevant MeHg:DOM ratios. Studies at lower MeHg:organic matter ratios measure conditional stability constants that are only somewhat higher (Karlsson and Skyllberg, 2003; Khwaja et al., 2010). The range of methylmercury binding constants is much narrower than the range of observed Hg(II) binding constants (e.g.,

10^{10}–10^{23} L/kg as observed by Haitzer et al. (2002) for carboxyl-like and thiol-like DOM sites), likely because the range of MeHg concentrations used to study binding has been narrower and focused on the strong sites. The studies that have examined methylmercury binding constants to organic matter are generally consistent in their conclusions that thiol-like sites dominate binding, although binding constants increase as the ratio of methylmercury to organic matter decreases.

X-ray spectroscopy of MeHg bound to organic matter has confirmed the findings of binding constant studies by directly identifying sulfur-containing binding sites for MeHg in organic matter. At sufficiently low MeHg:organic matter ratios, MeHg binding environments consist of a thiol bond (Hg–S distance of 2.30–2.40 Å) and a Hg–C bond from the methyl group (Qian et al., 2002; Yoon et al., 2005). Increasing the MeHg:S_{red} ratio causes a transition in the average binding environment from sulfur dominated to oxygen dominated (Figure 8.7). Only at MeHg:S_{red} well below 1 does S_{red} dominate MeHg binding. This transition represents the transition from thiol-like sites to carboxyl-like sites, and supports the results of model compound studies where methylmercury is bound by a single ligand site (Schwarzenbach and Schellenberg, 1965). For comparison, a typical environmental ratio of 0.1 ng MeHg per milligram DOM is a MeHg:S_{red} ratio of about 0.002 if the DOM is 1% total sulfur and 70% of that sulfur is reduced. Although other reduced sulfur sites exist in DOM, there is no evidence of anything other than a single thiol-like site coordinating methylmercury at environmentally relevant amounts of methylmercury.

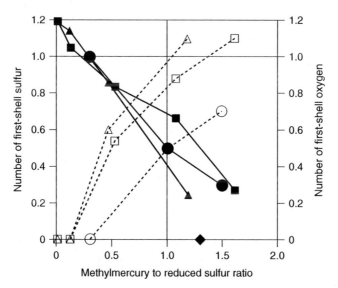

Figure 8.7 The structural variation in methylmercury binding environments with organic matter as a function of the ratio of methylmercury to reduced sulfur. Closed symbols represent the number of sulfur atoms coordinating methylmercury, and open symbols represent the number of oxygen atoms coordinating methylmercury. *Source*: Reproduced from Figure 7 of Yoon et al. (2005) with permission from Elsevier.

8.8   DOM AND MERCURY MINERAL DISSOLUTION

The role of DOM in the dissolution and precipitation reactions of mercury minerals is a critical consideration in some environments. The mercury–sulfide minerals cinnabar (α-HgS) and metacinnabar (β-HgS) make up the majority of mine wastes related to mercury and gold mining (Kim et al., 2000; Lowry et al., 2004), and are also found in environments contaminated by mercury from industrial applications (Barnett et al., 1997; Boszke et al., 2008; Han et al., 2008). Laboratory experiments have demonstrated the potential for metacinnabar to form in natural systems that contain only mercury, sulfide, and DOM (Ravichandran et al., 1999; Deonarine and Hsu-Kim, 2009; Slowey, 2010). Mercury phases other than cinnabar and metacinnabar can be found in the environment (e.g., HgO, $HgCl_2$) and are typically related to mining activities (Rytuba, 2000; Kim et al., 2003), but the sulfide minerals are by far the most thermodynamically stable. It has also been speculated that precipitation of HgS minerals is the dominant mechanism of mercury loss from active mercury pools (Stein et al., 1996). Colloidal forms of HgS minerals may be the dominant transport mechanism for mercury in mining-impacted ecosystems (Slowey et al., 2005). Mercury methylation requires transport of mercury species across microbial membranes, and that process is generally only possible with dissolved species (Morel et al., 1998). Despite the low solubility and slow dissolution of many mercury minerals, methylation has been observed in environments downstream from mercury-bearing mine deposits (Hines et al., 2006; Holloway et al., 2009), which suggests that thermodynamic calculations of solubility may not tell the whole story of dissolution, precipitation, bioavailability, and transport.

The dissolution of cinnabar and metacinnabar in the absence of DOM (and other complicating aspects of natural environments) indicates that dissolution at circumneutral pH is thermodynamically unfavorable (i.e., low mineral solubility), kinetically slow, and similar to minerals generally considered stable (Barnett et al., 2001). In systems designed to simulate acid mine drainage (Burkstaller et al., 1975), or with uncontrolled pH (Holley et al., 2007), the dissolution rates are one to two orders of magnitude higher, but are still relatively slow. Even 14 M HNO_3 is insufficient for rapid dissolution of metacinnabar and cinnabar (Mikac et al., 2003); aqua regia is necessary to completely dissolve the minerals (Bloom et al., 2003; Kim et al., 2003).

Several mechanisms for the slow dissolution of HgS(s) in the absence of organic matter have been proposed, and depend strongly on the conditions of the system. Sulfide (Paquette and Helz, 1995), polysulfide (Jay et al., 2000), and elemental sulfur (Paquette and Helz, 1997) promote dissolution of HgS(s) under anoxic conditions. In contrast to ligand-promoted dissolution under anoxic conditions, oxidative dissolution by Fe(III) (Burkstaller et al., 1975), and dissolved oxygen (Barnett et al., 2001; Holley et al., 2007) has also been documented. The oxidized sulfur species released during oxidative dissolution provide a good measurement of mineral dissolution rates, but measurement of the dissolved mercury concentration has been shown to severely underpredict HgS(s) dissolution

(Burkstaller et al., 1975; Barnett et al., 2001; He et al., 2007; Holley et al., 2007). Voltammetric evidence shows that Hg(II) is adsorbed to the HgS(s) surface after dissolution (Holley et al., 2007). It has been speculated that adsorbed Hg(II) may reduce HgS(s) dissolution rates (Barnett et al., 2001), although the introduction of chloride to complex aqueous Hg(II) did not increase HgS(s) dissolution rates in oxygenated systems at neutral pH (Ravichandran et al., 1998; Barnett et al., 2001). Chloride did increase the rate of cinnabar dissolution in acidic Fe(III) solutions (Burkstaller et al., 1975). The general oxidative dissolution reaction proposed by Barnett et al. (2001):

$$HgS_{(s)} + 2 \equiv S - H + 2O_{2(aq)} \longleftrightarrow (\equiv S-)_2Hg + SO_4{}^{2-} + 2H^+$$

involves the adsorption of released Hg(II) to a sulfhydryl surface site ($\equiv$S–H) and is circumstantially supported by evidence of a $SO_4{}^{2-}$: H^+ ratio of 1:2 in HgS(s) dissolution experiments.

The introduction of DOM to cinnabar dissolution experiments generally results in increased dissolution of the mineral phase (Ravichandran et al., 1998; Waples et al., 2005; He et al., 2007). The data also suggest that not all DOM has the same degree of reactivity. DOM isolates from a range of environments showed mercury release rates from cinnabar dissolution that differed by a factor of 200 (Waples et al., 2005). Because HgS(s) dissolution is not well represented by mercury release rates, the mineral dissolution rate is difficult to compare to studies that used oxidized sulfur species to more accurately measure dissolution rates. However, both studies that measured mercury release from cinnabar dissolution in the presence of DOM isolates note undetectable mercury concentrations in the aqueous solution in the absence of DOM. Increases in DOM concentration resulted in increased dissolution of mercury from cinnabar (Ravichandran et al., 1998), but only up to a threshold after which mercury release was independent of DOM concentration (Waples et al., 2005)—a common characteristic of ligand-promoted dissolution mechanisms characterized by maximum DOM adsorption to the mineral surface. The DOM isolates most effective at dissolving cinnabar were the most aromatic and highest molecular weight (Ravichandran et al., 1998; Waples et al., 2005) as shown in Fig. 8.8. Because the rate of dissolution depended on the aromaticity of DOM, the rate of dissolution was also correlated with the SUVA of the DOM isolates (aromaticity, molecular weight, and SUVA covary in DOM samples). Despite the relationship between SUVA and cinnabar dissolution rate, SUVA was not a good predictor of the amount of DOM adsorbed to the cinnabar surface, unlike what has been observed for oxide minerals (McKnight et al., 1992; Wang et al., 1997). In addition, total sulfur and reduced sulfur contents of the DOM isolates were poor indicators of mercury release from cinnabar (Ravichandran et al., 1998; Waples et al., 2005), even though sulfur functional groups represent the strongest mercury binding sites.

The relationship between aromaticity (and other covarying properties) of DOM and mercury release during cinnabar dissolution does not itself distinguish a mechanism. It is clear from observed sulfate concentrations in excess of released mercury concentrations that oxidative dissolution is taking place and that Hg(II) adsorption to the cinnabar surface is also taking place in the presence of DOM (Ravichandran et al., 1998; He et al., 2007). Mercury release from cinnabar did not change in the absence of oxygen, suggesting that DOM may play a major

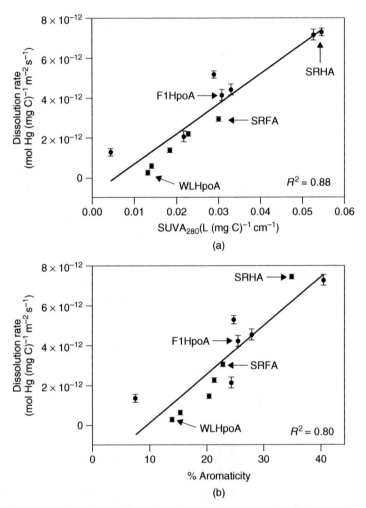

Figure 8.8 The relationship between cinnabar dissolution rate (normalized to DOC exposure and surface area) and three parameters of DOM: specific UV absorbance at 280 nm (SUVA$_{280}$), aromatic carbon, and average molecular weight (next page). WLHPoA is the hydrophobic acid isolate from Williams Lake, MN; F1 HPoA is the hydrophobic acid isolate from the F1 site in the Florida Everglades; Suwannee River fulvic acid (SRFA) and Suwannee River humic acid (SRHA) are the fulvic acid and humic acid isolates, respectively, from the Suwannee River, GA. *Source*: Reproduced from Figure 2 of Waples et al. (2005) with permission from Elsevier.

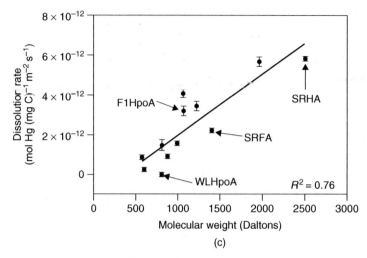

Figure 8.8 (*Continued*)

role in the oxidative process that releases mercury (Ravichandran et al., 1998). Certain portions of the DOM pool, especially quinones, are capable of participating in redox reactions and have been found in wide-ranging environments (Cory and McKnight, 2005). It is unlikely that DOM complexation of mercury plays a major role in increasing mercury release from cinnabar. Dialysis membrane experiments that separated DOM from the cinnabar surface but allowed mercury to pass and complex with the DOM showed mercury release rates that were much lower than when DOM was allowed to contact the cinnabar surface (Waples et al., 2005). Also, the amount of mercury released in solution was well in excess of the strong binding sites of the DOM (Waples et al., 2005). This is not to say that aqueous binding of Hg(II) has no effect on mercury release from cinnabar. Although most ligands proved inadequate for increasing cinnabar dissolution (even strong Hg(II)-chelating agents like EDTA), the thiol ligands cysteine and thioglycolic acid did increase mercury release, just not to the extent of organic matter extracted from natural waters (Ravichandran et al., 1998). It is important to note that the concentration of reduced sulfur functional groups in the experiments with model compounds were typically two orders of magnitude greater than the concentration of reduced sulfur in the DOM experiments, and only a fraction of the reduced sulfur in DOM participates in mercury binding. Although the mechanism for DOM promotion of cinnabar dissolution is uncertain, it is clear that DOM adsorption to the cinnabar surface is a critical component of the dissolution mechanism.

Waples et al. (2005) proposed that the effective rate of DOM-enhanced dissolution of cinnabar is a function of the competitive effects between two distinct pools of DOM—one that promotes dissolution and one that inhibits dissolution. The dissolution-promoting group tends to be more aromatic and readily leaves the cinnabar surface after solubilizing Hg(II) atoms. The dissolution-inhibiting group tends to irreversibly adhere to the surface and block the adsorption of the dissolution-promoting pool to surface sites. When the two pools interact with cinnabar simultaneously, and in equal quantities, dissolution rates were not drastically slower than when only the dissolution-promoting pool had access to the cinnabar. However, when the dissolution-inhibiting pool equilibrated with the cinnabar surface before the dissolution-promoting pool was introduced, the rate of cinnabar dissolution was much slower than when the dissolution-promoting pool alone was allowed access to the cinnabar surface. Organic matter derived from terrestrial origins tends to have more of the dissolution-promoting components than organic matter derived from microbial sources.

The enhanced dissolution of cinnabar and metacinnabar in the presence of unfractionated, natural waters not only supports the role of DOM but also points to the complexities introduced by other constituents of natural waters. In particular, the presence of multivalent cations (e.g., Ca^{2+}, Mg^{2+}, and Al^{3+}) has been shown to drastically change the dissolution of cinnabar in the presence of DOM. Surface water shows mercury release from cinnabar dissolution that is as much as two orders of magnitude lower than the same water after it is passed through a cation exchange resin, which removes multivalent cations (Ravichandran et al., 1998). Some studies have not observed increased cinnabar dissolution rates in the presence of natural waters containing divalent cations (Holley et al., 2007), but other studies have. Specifically, metacinnabar dissolution was higher in low DOC creek water compared to a DOC-free, divalent cation-free NaCl system, and high DOC water from the Florida Everglades increased dissolution to a greater extent than the low DOC creek water (Barnett et al., 2001). Both DOC-containing waters had significant Ca(II) concentrations, suggesting the effect of the DOM in these waters (about an order of magnitude increase in HgS(s) dissolution over the NaCl solution) may not have been fully realized.

8.9 DOM AND MERCURY MINERAL PRECIPITATION

In supersaturated solutions consisting of only mercury and sulfide, the precipitation of HgS(s) takes place within seconds, starting as polysulfide-like Hg–S chains, transitioning to clusters, then less crystalline metacinnabar, and finally forming crystalline metacinnabar particles (Charnock et al., 2003). Cinnabar is the thermodynamically more favorable form of HgS(s) on the earth's surface, but metacinnabar forms first, eventually transforming into cinnabar (Potter and Barnes, 1978). Metacinnabar precipitated *in situ* (as opposed to HgS(s) transported from mining activities) has been observed in relatively few environmental sites, and those sites tend to have higher total mercury concentrations because of local mercury contamination sources (Barnett et al., 1997; Lechler et al., 1997; Beldowski and Pempkowiak, 2003; Han et al., 2008). Transmission electron microscopic images of the metacinnabar formed in the soils near Oak Ridge, TN (a mercury-contaminated site) show particles with diameters of approximately 100 nm. If these particles exist in unimpacted environments, they are likely to go undetected because of their small size (i.e., they will pass 0.2 μm and larger filters and be considered "dissolved") and the difficulty of observing small particles in low abundance in a complex matrix. Thermodynamic speciation of mercury in sulfidic systems focuses on a suite of Hg–S complexes to explain significant amounts of filter-passing mercury (Dyrssen and Wedborg, 1991; Paquette and Helz, 1997; Benoit et al., 1999; Jay et al., 2000; Tossell, 2001; Charnock et al., 2003; Lennie et al., 2003; Bell et al., 2007), but as the Oak Ridge microscopy data show, insoluble inorganic metacinnabar particles can also pass filters and be "dissolved." Generally speaking, membrane filtration is not done consistently and introduces significant artifacts, especially when the distinction between dissolved and particulate is important (Hedberg et al., 2011). In addition, the speciation models tend to discount the effect of DOM because sulfide strongly outcompetes even the strongest DOM binding sites. Uncertainties in the Hg–S thermodynamic constants, which suggests metacinnabar may be a stable form of mercury at environmental concentrations (Deonarine and Hsu-Kim, 2009), inconsistent partitioning of mercury–sulfide species to octanol in the presence of DOM (Miller et al., 2007), and the observation that metacinnabar particles in the presence of DOM partition to octanol (Deonarine and Hsu-Kim, 2009) suggest that DOM is important to mercury speciation in the presence of sulfide and that metacinnabar may be an important form of mercury to consider in natural sulfidic environments.

In the presence of sulfide and DOM, at least some fraction of the mercury takes the form of small metacinnabar particles (Ravichandran et al., 1999; Deonarine and Hsu-Kim, 2009; Slowey, 2010). Stabilization of metal–sulfide particles by organic matter is not a new observation: CuS(s) and ZnS(s) stabilization has been observed in laboratory studies (Horzempa and Helz, 1979), experimental wetlands (Weber et al., 2009), and microbial biofilms (Labrenz et al., 2000; Moreau et al., 2007). The DOM fractions most capable of stabilizing HgS(s) halted nanocolloidal growth at 1–5 nm in diameter (Deonarine and Hsu-Kim, 2009; Slowey, 2010), and stabilized aggregates on the order of 20–200 nm (Ravichandran et al., 1999; Deonarine and Hsu-Kim, 2009; Slowey, 2010). DOC concentrations as low as about 0.5 mg C/L have been shown to effectively slow the aggregation of HgS(s) particles, and increasing DOM concentrations have even stronger negative effects on the growth rate (Deonarine and Hsu-Kim, 2009). Approximately 3 mg C/L has been shown to completely stabilize HgS(s) aggregates <100 nm for at least 24 h (Deonarine and Hsu-Kim, 2009). In sulfidic systems with 10 mg/L DOM and $<10^{-4.3}$ M Hg, all of the mercury passed through a $0.1-\mu m$ filter, but when the mercury concentration was raised to $10^{-2.3}$ M, all of the mercury was retained by the filter (Ravichandran et al., 1999), indicating that size of HgS(s) aggregates depended on total mercury concentration. Considering that environmental concentrations of mercury are on the order of 10^{-10} M, it is not surprising that sampling with 0.2- and 0.45-μm filters have identified an abundance of "dissolved" mercury, even in sulfidic systems. Membrane filtration only provides an operational definition of dissolved species, can be problematic for other metals (Hedberg et al., 2011), and is probably also problematic in distinguishing between dissolved and colloidal forms of mercury.

Similar to the case of HgS(s) dissolution, DOM samples that are more aromatic tend to be most effective in stabilizing HgS(s) precipitates or aggregates (Ravichandran et al., 1999; Deonarine and Hsu-Kim, 2009; Slowey, 2010). The HgS(s) that precipitates in the presence of more aromatic DOM samples is less crystalline than the HgS(s) that precipitates in the presence of less aromatic DOM (Slowey, 2010). Humic and fulvic acids maintain more mercury in solution (as determined by filtration) than other fractions of the DOM pool (Ravichandran et al., 1999). A decrease in the SUVA of DOM that remains in solution after reaction with mercury and sulfide indicates the preferential loss of aromatic carbon as HgS(s) precipitates and DOM adsorbs to the surface (Ravichandran et al., 1999). The adsorption of DOM to HgS(s) surfaces leads to more negatively charged surfaces, which in turn increases electrostatic repulsion and particle stabilization (Ravichandran et al., 1999; Deonarine and Hsu-Kim, 2009). Decreased HgS(s) particle growth in the presence of DOM was observed at lower ionic strength, proving that electrostatic repulsion, which becomes more powerful at lower ionic strength, is the primary mechanism for DOM-coated HgS(s) particle stabilization (Deonarine and Hsu-Kim, 2009).

The exact mechanism for DOM adsorption to HgS(s) is somewhat unclear. Various thiol-containing model ligands have proven to be at least partially effective in preventing HgS(s) aggregation, whereas weaker inorganic and carboxyl ligands were not effective (Ravichandran et al., 1999; Deonarine and Hsu-Kim, 2009). HgS(s) particles are more negatively charged when the thiol ligands thioglycolic acid or cysteine are adsorbed to the surface, much like when DOM is adsorbed. The sulfur content of DOM was not a good predictor of DOM adsorption to cinnabar and metacinnabar (Ravichandran et al., 1998; Waples et al., 2005), although it is clear that total sulfur is not a good predictor of Hg(II) binding capacity, and thus may not be a good predictor of surface activity either. If the mechanism of DOM adsorption to HgS(s) is similar to the adsorption on oxide minerals, the process involves ligand exchange with surface sites, and is not entirely reversible (Gu et al., 1994). A complex relationship exists between DOM binding sites, DOM aromaticity, and HgS(s) surface sites, which promotes the stability of small HgS(s) particles, although the precise mechanism is an area of ongoing study.

Including Ca^{2+} in the solutions satisfied negative surface charges of the DOM-coated HgS(s) by binding with the DOM or adsorbing to the HgS(s) surface, which decreased the electrostatic charge and promoted aggregation to larger particles (Ravichandran et al., 1999). Whole water has not been shown to be especially effective in stabilizing small HgS(s) aggregates (at a mercury concentration of $10^{-4.3}$ M) until the water was run through a cation exchange resin to remove multivalent cations. Following cation exchange, the whole water was more effective than before the cation exchange at stabilizing colloidal HgS(s), but was still less effective than the hydrophobic DOM isolate from the whole water (Ravichandran et al., 1999). The promotion of HgS(s) aggregation by multivalent cations becomes less pronounced (as defined by the amount of $0.1 - \mu m$ filterable mercury) at lower total mercury concentrations (Ravichandran et al. 1999).

At this point, it is clear that DOM can simultaneously stabilize HgS(s) particles and promote the dissolution of HgS(s). These two mechanisms compete with one another in systems supersaturated with mercury and sulfide. The precipitation and redissolution of significant amounts of HgS(s) in the presence of DOM occurs somewhat cyclically over several hundred hours when the initial sulfide concentration is well in excess of the total mercury concentration (Slowey, 2010). DOM can consume excess sulfide and incorporate the sulfide into the organic matter structure (Casagrande et al., 1979; Heitmann and Blodau, 2006). Therefore, ecosystems that have continuous input of sulfide from sulfate-reducing microbes may always have the drivers necessary for dissolution and precipitation. Increasing sulfide concentrations increases the redissolution of DOM-coated HgS(s) (Slowey, 2010). The increased redissolution may be due to the formation of mercury–sulfide complexes (Paquette and Helz, 1995; Benoit et al., 1999; Jay et al., 2000; Lennie et al., 2003; Bell et al., 2007), or it may be due to an interaction with the DOM. At lower sulfide concentrations, more Hg(II) will be bound by the DOM. DOM interacting with Hg(II) may not be available for surface interactions, and thus cannot promote the redissolution of HgS(s). Interacting with all of these processes are multiple pools of DOM that behave differently—some promote dissolution and some inhibit it—and the extent and reversibility of surface adsorption of each pool has not been adequately studied.

The DOM-stabilized HgS(s) observed in laboratory experiments strongly resembles the HgS(s) observed in a mercury-contaminated field site. The HgS(s) formed at the field site was not perfectly crystalline, but resembled metacinnabar, and the size of the HgS(s) particles was on the order of tens of nanometers (Barnett et al., 1997). The fact that the HgS(s) from the field site was more rapidly dissolved than crystalline metacinnabar (Barnett et al., 1997; Han et al., 2008) indicates that special considerations must be made to determine mercury speciation in these environments. The thermodynamic constants for DOM-stabilized metacinnabar-like HgS(s) may not be well represented by the thermodynamic constants of crystalline metacinnabar. The kinetics of dissolution of poorly crystalline, DOM-coated metacinnabar may be significantly different from the kinetics of well-formed metacinnabar. Altered thermodynamic or kinetic properties of naturally formed nanocolloidal sized HgS(s) may also be attributable to their size, as the interfacial energy of a small particle is likely to destabilize the particle and promote dissolution (Gilbert and Banfield, 2005).

The role that nanocolloidal HgS(s) stabilized by DOM plays in uncontaminated environments is not entirely clear. Direct observation of nanocolloidal metacinnabar-like HgS(s) in the laboratory has been limited to concentrations of total mercury that are orders of magnitude higher than typically found in uncontaminated environments. However, ultracentrifugation shows the removal of nanocolloidal mercury species (that are presumably poorly crystalline HgS(s)) when the total mercury concentration is as low as about 1 nM (Slowey, 2010). The only direct observation of nanocolloidal HgS(s) in the environment has thus far been limited to contaminated sites and sites impacted by mining activity. These studies have identified HgS(s) species as small as a few nanometers in diameter, and the aggregates of these particles only reach 200 nm on the top end. Thus, if HgS(s) is present in natural ecosystems, it has always been defined as dissolved when samples are filtered through membranes with pores sizes of 0.2 μm or greater. Low total mercury concentrations are also likely to make it difficult to find HgS(s) species in natural samples that contain significant amounts of other colloidal species. While direct observation of nanocolloidal HgS(s) has not been observed in uncontaminated natural environments, there is strong circumstantial evidence that it exists.

When considering the biogeochemistry of mercury in natural ecosystems, DOM must be considered in almost all processes from the atomic scale to the field scale. Much is known about the binding of mercury and methylmercury by DOM and the positive correlations between mercury and DOM in natural environments. However, other interactions and processes are not as well understood. Data show interesting and potentially important interactions between DOM and HgS(s) minerals, but many of the molecular scale mechanisms are somewhat unclear. Inherent difficulties in studying DOM include the spatial and temporal variability of DOM in natural environments, and isolating the effects of a small but important subset of molecules from a large pool of organic molecules. Continued study of mercury–DOM interactions on all relevant scales will expand our ability to predict and understand mercury biogeochemistry, and will potentially help us assess and mitigate the ecological and health effects of mercury.

ACKNOWLEDGEMENTS

We thank M. Brigham (US Geological Survey), R. Spencer (Woods Hole Research Center), J. Writer (US Geological Survey), and two anonymous reviewers for their critical reviews of the manuscript. Support was provided, in part, by the US Geological Survey's Priority Ecosystem Science Program and National Science Foundation grant #EAR-0447386. The use of trade names in this chapter is for identification purposes only and does not constitute endorsement by the US Geological Survey.

REFERENCES

Aiken GR. Evaluation of ultrafiltration for determining molecular weight of fulvic acid. Environ Sci Technol 1984;18:978–981.

Aiken G, Cotsaris E. Soil and hydrology: their effect on NOM. J Am Water Works Assoc 1995;87:36–45.

Aiken GR, Leenheer JA. Isolation and chemical characterization of dissolved and colloidal organic matter. Chem Ecol 1993;8:135–151.

Aiken GR, McKnight DM, Thorn KA, Thurman EM. Isolation of hydrophilic organic-acids from water using nonionic macroporous resins. Org Geochem 1992;18:567–573.

Amirbahman A, Reid AL, Haines TA, Kahl JS, Arnold C. Association of methylmercury with dissolved humic acids. Environ Sci Technol 2002;36:690–695.

Andren AW, Harriss RC. Observations on the association between mercury and organic matter dissolved in natural waters. Geochim Cosmochim Acta 1975;39:1253–1258.

Babiarz CL, Hurley JP, Hoffmann SR, Andren AW, Shafer MM, Armstrong DE. Partitioning of total mercury and methylmercury to the colloidal phase in freshwaters. Environ Sci Technol 2001;35:4773–4782.

Balogh SJ, Nollet YH, Swain EB. Redox chemistry in Minnesota streams during episodes of increased methylmercury discharge. Environ Sci Technol 2004;38:4921–4927.

Balogh SJ, Swain EB, Nollet YH. Elevated methylmercury concentrations and loadings during flooding in Minnesota rivers. Sci Total Environ 2006;368:138–148.

Barkay T, Gillman M, Turner RR. Effects of dissolved organic carbon and salinity on bioavailability of mercury. Appl Environ Microbiol 1997;63:4267–4271.

Barnett MO, Harris LA, Turner RR, Stevenson RJ, Henson TJ, Melton RC, Hoffman DP. Formation of mercuric sulfide in soil. Environ Sci Technol 1997;31:3037–3043.

Barnett MO, Turner RR, Singer PC. Oxidative dissolution of metacinnabar (β-HgS) by dissolved oxygen. Appl Geochem 2001;16:1499–1512.

Basinger MA, Casas JS, Jones MM, Weaver AD. Structural requirements for Hg(II) antidotes. J Inorg Nucl Chem 1981;43:1419–1425.

Beldowski J, Pempkowiak J. Horizontal and vertical variabilities of mercury concentration and speciation in sediments of the Gdansk Basin, Southern Baltic Sea. Chemosphere 2003;52:645–654.

Bell AMT, Charnock JM, Helz GR, Lennie AR, Livens FR, Mosselmans JFW, Pattrick RAD, Vaughan DJ. Evidence for dissolved polymeric mercury(II)-sulfur complexes? Chem Geol 2007;243:122–127.

Benner R, Biddanda B, Black B, McCarthy M. Abundance, size distribution, and stable carbon and nitrogen isotopic compositions of marine organic matter isolated by tangential-flow ultrafiltration. Mar Chem 1997;57:243–263.

Benoit JM, Mason RP, Gilmour CC. Estimation of mercury-sulfide speciation in sediment pore waters using octanol-water partitioning and implications for availability to methylating bacteria. Environ Toxicol Chem 1999;18:2138–2141.

Benoit JM, Mason RP, Gilmour CC, Aiken GR. Constants for mercury binding by dissolved organic matter isolates from the Florida Everglades. Geochim Cosmochim Acta 2001;65:4445–4451.

Black FJ, Bruland KW, Flegal AR. Competing ligand exchange-solid phase extraction method for the determination of the complexation of dissolved inorganic mercury(II) in natural waters. Anal Chim Acta 2007;598:318–333.

Bloom NS, Preus E, Katon J, Hiltner M. Selective extractions to assess the biogeochemically relevant fractionation of inorganic mercury in sediments and soils. Anal Chim Acta 2003;479:233–248.

Boszke L, Kowalski A, Astel A, Barański A, Gworek B, Siepak J. Mercury mobility and bioavailability in soil from contaminated area. Environ Geol 2008;55:1075–1087.

Brigham ME, Duris JW, Wentz DA, Button DT, Chasar LC. Total mercury, methylmercury, and ancillary water-quality and streamflow data for selected streams in Oregon, Wisconsin, and Florida, 2002–2006, U.S. Geological Survey Data Series 341. 2008. p 11.

Brigham ME, Wentz DA, Aiken GR, Krabbenhoft DP. Mercury cycling in stream ecosystems. 1. Water column chemistry and transport. Environ Sci Technol 2009;43:2720–2725.

Burkstaller JE, McCarty PL, Parks GA. Oxidation of cinnabar by Fe(III) in acid mine waters. Environ Sci Technol 1975;9:676–678.

Cai Y, Jaffe R, Jones RD. Interactions between dissolved organic carbon and mercury species in surface waters of the Florida Everglades. Appl Geochem 1999;14:395–407.

Casagrande DJ, Idowu G, Friedman A, Rickert P, Siefert K, Schlenz D. H_2S incorporation in coal precursors: Origins of organic sulphur in coal. Nature 1979;282:599–600.

Charnock JM, Moyes LN, Pattrick RAD, Mosselmans JFW, Vaughan DJ, Livens FR. The structural evolution of mercury sulfide precipitate: an XAS and XRD study. Am Mineral 2003;88:1197–1203.

Cheam V, Gamble DS. Metal-fulvic acid chelation equilibrium in aqueous $NaNO_3$ solution-Hg(II), Cd(II), and Cu(II) fulvate complexes. Can J Soil Sci 1974;54:413–417.

Choe K-Y, Gill GA. Isolation of colloidal monomethyl mercury in natural waters using cross-flow ultrafiltration techniques. Mar Chem 2001;76:305–318.

Cory RM, McKnight DM. Fluorescence spectroscopy reveals ubiquitous presence of oxidized and reduced quinones in dissolved organic matter. Environ Sci Technol 2005;39:8142–8149.

Cronan CS, Aiken GR. Chemistry and transport of soluble humic substances in forested watersheds of the Adirondack Park, New York. Geochim Cosmochim Acta 1985;49:1697–1705.

Deonarine A, Hsu-Kim H. Precipitation of mercuric sulfide nanoparticles in NOM-containing water: implications for the natural environment. Environ Sci Technol 2009;43:2368–2373.

Dittman JA, Shanley JB, Driscoll CT, Aiken GR, Chalmers AT, Towse JE, Selvendiran P. Mercury dynamics in relation to dissolved organic carbon concentration and quality during high flow events in three northeastern U.S. streams. Water Resour Res 2010;46: W07522.

Dittmar T, Koch B, Hertkorn N, Kattner G. A simple and efficient method for the solid-phase extraction of dissolved organic matter (SPE-DOM) from seawater. Limnol Oceanogr: Methods 2008;6:230–235.

Drexel RT, Haitzer M, Ryan JN, Aiken GR, Nagy KL. Mercury(II) sorption to two Florida Everglades peats: evidence for strong and weak binding and competition by dissolved organic matter released from the peat. Environ Sci Technol 2002;36:4058–4064.

Dyrssen D, Wedborg M. The sulphur-mercury(II) system in natural waters. Water Air Soil Pollut 1991;56:507–519.

Fellman JB, Hood E, Spencer RGM. Fluorescence spectroscopy opens new windows into dissolved organic matter dynamics in freshwater ecosystems: A review. Limnol Oceanogr 2010;55:2452–2462.

Findlay S. Bacterial response to variation in dissolved organic matter. In: Findlay SEG, Sinsabaugh RL, editors. Aquatic ecosystems: interactivity of dissolved organic matter. Burlington: Academic Press; 2003. p 363–379.

Fitzgerald WF, Lyons WB. Organic mercury compounds in coastal waters. Nature 1973;242:452–453.

Gasper JD, Aiken GR, Ryan JN. A critical review of three methods used for the measurement of mercury (Hg^{2+}) -dissolved organic matter stability constants. Appl Geochem 2007;22:1583–1597.

Gilbert B, Banfield JF. Molecular-scale processes involving nanoparticulate minerals in biogeochemical systems. Rev Mineral Geochem 2005;59:109–155.

Green SA, Blough NV. Optical absorption and fluorescence properties of chromophoric dissolved organic matter in natural waters. Limnol Oceanogr 1994;39:1903–1916.

Grigal DF. Inputs and outputs of mercury from terrestrial watersheds: a review. Environ Rev 2002,10.1–39.

Gu BH, Schmitt J, Chen ZH, Liang LY, McCarthy JF. Adsorption and desorption of natural organic-matter on iron-oxide-mechanisms and models. Environ Sci Technol 1994;28:38–46.

Haitzer M, Aiken GR, Ryan JN. Binding of mercury(II) to dissolved organic matter: The role of the mercury-to-DOM concentration ratio. Environ Sci Technol 2002;36:3564–3570.

Haitzer M, Aiken GR, Ryan JN. Binding of mercury(II) to aquatic humic substances: Influence of pH and source of humic substances. Environ Sci Technol 2003;37:2436–2441.

Hammerschmidt CR, Fitzgerald WF. Methylmercury cycling in sediments on the continental shelf of southern New England. Geochim Cosmochim Acta 2006;70:918–930.

Han SH, Gill GA. Determination of mercury complexation in coastal and estuarine waters using competitive ligand exchange method. Environ Sci Technol 2005;39:6607–6615.

Han F, Shiyab S, Chen J, Su Y, Monts D, Waggoner C, Matta F. Extractability and bioavailability of mercury from a mercury sulfide contaminated soil in Oak Ridge, Tennessee, USA. Water Air Soil Pollut 2008;194:67–75.

Hatcher PG, Dria KJ, Kim S, Frazier SW. Modern analytical studies of humic substances. Soil Sci 2001;166:770–794.

He Z, Traina SJ, Weavers LK. Sonochemical dissolution of cinnabar (α-HgS). Environ Sci Technol 2007;41:773–778.

Hedberg Y, Herting G, Wallinder IO. Risks of using membrane filtration for trace metal analysis and assessing the dissolved metal fraction of aqueous media-A study on zinc, copper and nickel. Environ Pollut 2011;159:1144–1150.

Heitmann T, Blodau C. Oxidation and incorporation of hydrogen sulfide by dissolved organic matter. Chem Geol 2006;235:12–20.

Helms JR, Stubbins A, Ritchie JD, Minor EC, Kieber DJ, Mopper K. Absorption spectral slopes and slope ratios as indicators of molecular weight, source, and photobleaching of chromophoric dissolved organic matter. Limnol Oceanogr 2008;53:955–969.

Hesterberg D, Chou JW, Hutchison KJ, Sayers DE. Bonding of Hg(II) to reduced organic, sulfur in humic acid as affected by S/Hg ratio. Environ Sci Technol 2001;35:2741–2745.

Hines ME, Faganeli J, Adatto I, Horvat M. Microbial mercury transformations in marine, estuarine and freshwater sediment downstream of the Idrija Mercury Mine, Slovenia. Appl Geochem 2006;21:1924–1939.

Hintelmann H, Welbourn PM, Evans RD. Binding of methylmercury compounds by humic and fulvic acids. Water Air Soil Pollut 1995;80:1031–1034.

Hintelmann H, Welbourn PM, Evans RD. Measurement of complexation of methylmercury(II) compounds by freshwater humic substances using equilibrium dialysis. Environ Sci Technol 1997;31:489–495.

Hinton MJ, Schiff SL, English MC. Sources and flowpaths of dissolved organic carbon during storms in two forested watersheds of the Precambrian Shield. Biogeochem 1998;41:175–197.

Hoch AR, Reddy MM, Aiken GR. Calcite crystal growth inhibition by humic substances with emphasis on hydrophobic acids from the Florida Everglades. Geochim Cosmochim Acta 2000;64:61–72.

Holley EA, James McQuillan A, Craw D, Kim JP, Sander SG. Mercury mobilization by oxidative dissolution of cinnabar (α-HgS) and metacinnabar (β-HgS). Chem Geol 2007;240:313–325.

Holloway JM, Goldhaber MB, Scow KM, Drenovsky RE. Spatial and seasonal variations in mercury methylation and microbial community structure in a historic mercury mining area, Yolo County, California. Chem Geol 2009;267:85–95.

Honeyman BD, Santschi PH. A Brownian-pumping model for oceanic trace metal scavenging: Evidence from Th isotopes. J Mar Res 1989;47:951–992.

Horzempa LM, Helz GR. Controls on the stability of sulfide sols: colloidal covellite as an example. Geochim Cosmochim Acta 1979;43:1645–1650.

Hsu H, Sedlak DL. Strong Hg(II) complexation in municipal wastewater effluent and surface waters. Environ Sci Technol 2003;37:2743–2749.

Hurley JP, Krabbenhoft DP, Cleckner LB, Olson ML, Aiken GR, Rawlik Jr PS. System controls on the aqueous distribution of mercury in the northern Florida Everglades. Biogeochem 1998;40:293–311.

Jay JA, Morel FMM, Hemond HF. Mercury speciation in the presence of polysulfides. Environ Sci Technol 2000;34:2196–2200.

Jokic A, Cutler JN, Anderson DW, Walley FL. Detection of heterocyclic N compounds in whole soils using N-XANES spectroscopy. Can J Soil Sci 2004;84:291–293.

Karger BL, Snyder LR, Horvath C. An Introduction to Separation Science. 1st ed. New York: Wiley-Interscience; 1973.

Karlsson T, Skyllberg U. Bonding of ppb levels of methyl mercury to reduced sulfur groups in soil organic matter. Environ Sci Technol 2003;37:4912–4918.

Khwaja AR, Bloom PR, Brezonik PL. Binding constants of divalent mercury (Hg^{2+} in soil humic acids and soil organic matter. Environ Sci Technol 2006;40:844–849.

Khwaja AR, Bloom PR, Brezonik PL. Binding strength of methylmercury to aquatic NOM. Environ Sci Technol 2010;44:6151–6156.

Kim CS, Bloom NS, Rytuba JJ, Brown Jr GE. Mercury speciation by X-ray absorption fine structure spectroscopy and sequential chemical extractions: A comparison of speciation methods. Environ Sci Technol 2003;37:5102–5108.

Kim CS, Brown GE, Rytuba JJ. Characterization and speciation of mercury-bearing mine wastes using X-ray absorption spectroscopy. Sci Total Environ 2000;261:157–168.

Labrenz M, Druschel GK, Thomsen-Ebert T, Gilbert B, Welch SA, Kemner KM, Logan GA, Summons RE, Stasio GD, Bond PL, Lai B, Kelly SD, Banfield JF. Formation of sphalerite (ZnS) deposits in natural biofilms of sulfate-reducing bacteria. Science 2000;290:1744–1747.

Lamborg CH, Fitzgerald WF, Skoog A, Visscher PT. The abundance and source of mercury-binding organic ligands in Long Island Sound. Mar Chem 2004;90:151–163.

Lamborg CH, Tseng CM, Fitzgerald WF, Balcom PH, Hammerschmidt CR. Determination of the mercury complexation characteristics of dissolved organic matter in natural waters with "reducible Hg" titrations. Environ Sci Technol 2003;37:3316–3322.

Lechler PJ, Miller JR, Hsu L-C, Desilets MO. Mercury mobility at the Carson River Superfund Site, west-central Nevada, USA: interpretation of mercury speciation data in mill tailings, soils, and sediments. J Geochem Explor 1997;58:259–267.

Lennie AR, Charnock JM, Pattrick RAD. Structure of mercury(II)-sulfur complexes by EXAFS spectroscopic measurements. Chem Geol 2003;199:199–207.

Liu G, Cai Y, Philippi T, Kalla P, Scheidt D, Richards J, Scinto L, Appleby C. Distribution of total and methylmercury in different ecosystem compartments in the Everglades: Implications for mercury bioaccumulation. Environ Pollut 2008;153:257–265.

Lovgren L, Sjoberg S. Equilibrium approaches to natural-water systems-7. Complexation reactions of copper(II), cadmium(II) and mercury(II) with dissolved organic-matter in a concentrated bog-water. Water Res 1989;23:327–332.

Lowry GV, Shaw S, Kim CS, Rytuba JJ, Brown GE. Macroscopic and microscopic observations of particle-facilitated mercury transport from New Idria and Sulphur Bank mercury mine tailings. Environ Sci Technol 2004;38:5101–5111.

Lu XQ, Maie N, Hanna JV, Childers DL, Jaffe R. Molecular characterization of dissolved organic matter in freshwater wetlands of the Florida Everglades. Water Res 2003;37:2599–2606.

Ma H, Allen HE, Yin Y. Characterization of isolated fractions of dissolved organic matter from natural waters and a wastewater effluent. Water Res 2001;35:985–996.

Maie N, Jaffé R, Miyoshi T, Childers D. Quantitative and qualitative aspects of dissolved organic carbon leached from senescent plants in an oligotrophic wetland. Biogeochem 2006;78:285–314.

Marvin-DiPasquale M, Lutz MA, Brigham ME, Krabbenhoft DP, Aiken GR, Orem WH, Hall BD. Mercury cycling in stream ecosystems. 2. Benthic methylmercury production and bed sediment-pore water partitioning. Environ Sci Technol 2009;43:2726–2732.

Mason RP, Sullivan KA. Mercury and methylmercury transport through an urban watershed. Water Res 1998;32:321–330.

McKnight DM, Aiken GR. Sources and age of aquatic humic substances. In: Hessen DO, Tranvik LJ, editors. Aquatic humic substances: ecology and biogeochemistry (ecological studies v. 133). Berlin, Germany: Springer-Verlag; 1998. p 9–40.

McKnight DM, Bencala KE, Zellweger GW, Aiken GR, Feder GL, Thorn KA. Sorption of dissolved organic-carbon by hydrous aluminum and iron-oxides occurring at the confluence of Deer Creek with the Snake River, Summit County, Colorado. Environ Sci Technol 1992;26:1388–1396.

Mierle G, Ingram R. The role of humic substances in the mobilization of mercury from watersheds. Water Air Soil Pollut 1991;56:349–357.

Mikac N, Foucher D, Niessen S, Lojen S, Fischer JC. Influence of chloride and sediment matrix on the extractability of HgS (cinnabar and metacinnabar) by nitric acid. Anal Bioanal Chem 2003;377:1196–1201.

Miller CL, Mason RP, Gilmour CC, Heyes A. Influence of dissolved organic matter on the complexation of mercury under sulfidic conditions. Environ Toxicol Chem 2007;26:624–633.

Miskimmin BM, Rudd JWM, Kelly CA. Influence of dissolved organic carbon, pH, and microbial respiration rates on mercury methylation and demethylation in lake water. Can J Fish Aquat Sci 1992;49:17–22.

Moran MA, Covert JS. Photochemically mediated linkages between dissolved organic matter and bacterioplankton. In: Findlay SEG, Sinsabaugh RL, editors. Aquatic ecosystems: interactivity of dissolved organic matter. Burlington: Academic Press; 2003. p 243–262.

Moreau JW, Weber PK, Martin MC, Gilbert B, Hutcheon ID, Banfield JF. Extracellular proteins limit the dispersal of biogenic nanoparticles. Science 2007;316:1600–1603.

Morel FMM, Kraepiel AML, Amyot M. The chemical cycle and bioaccumulation of mercury. Annu Rev Ecol Syst 1998;29:543–566.

National Institute of Standards and Technology (NIST). NIST Critically selected stability constants of metal complexes database. version 8.0. Gaithersburg (MD): NIST; 2004.

O'Driscoll NJ, Evans RD. Analysis of methyl mercury binding to freshwater humic and fulvic acids by gel permeation chromatography/hydride generation ICP-MS. Environ Sci Technol 2000;34:4039–4043.

Paquette K, Helz G. Solubility of cinnabar (red HgS) and implications for mercury speciation in sulfidic waters. Water Air Soil Pollut 1995;80:1053–1056.

Paquette KE, Helz GR. Inorganic speciation of mercury in sulfidic waters: The importance of zero-valent sulfur. Environ Sci Technol 1997;31:2148–2153.

Perdue EM. Chemical composition, structure and metal binding properties. In: Hessen DO, Tranvik LJ, editors. Aquatic humic substances: ecology and biogeochemistry (Ecological Studies v. 133). Berlin, Germany: Springer-Verlag; 1998. p 41–62.

Potter RW, Barnes HL. Phase relations in the binary Hg-S. Am Mineral 1978;63:1143–1152.

Prietzel J, Thieme J, Salome M, Knicker H. Sulfur K-edge XANES spectroscopy reveals differences in sulfur speciation of bulk soils, humic acid, fulvic acid, and particle size separates. Soil Biol Biochem 2007;39:877–890.

Qian J, Skyllberg U, Frech W, Bleam WF, Bloom PR, Petit PE. Bonding of methyl mercury to reduced sulfur groups in soil and stream organic matter as determined by x-ray absorption spectroscopy and binding affinity studies. Geochim Cosmochim Acta 2002;66:3873–3885.

Qualls RG, Richardson CJ. Factors controlling concentration, export, and decomposition of dissolved organic nutrients in the Everglades of Florida. Biogeochem 2003;62:197–229.

Ravichandran M, Aiken GR, Reddy MM, Ryan JN. Enhanced dissolution of cinnabar (mercuric sulfide) by dissolved organic matter isolated from the Florida Everglades. Environ Sci Technol 1998;32:3305–3311.

Ravichandran M, Aiken GR, Ryan JN, Reddy MM. Inhibition of precipitation and aggregation of metacinnabar (mercuric sulfide) by dissolved organic matter isolated from the Florida Everglades. Environ Sci Technol 1999;33:1418–1423.

Rossotti FJC, Whewell RJ. Structure and stability of carboxylate complexes. Part 16. Stability constants of some mercury(II) carboxylates. J Chem Soc Dalton Trans 1977;12:1223–1229.

Rytuba JJ. Mercury mine drainage and processes that control its environmental impact. Sci Total Environ 2000;260:57–71.

Saraceno JF, Pellerin BA, Downing BD, Boss E, Bachand PAM, Bergamaschi BA. High-frequency in situ optical measurements during a storm event: Assessing relationships between dissolved organic matter, sediment concentrations, and hydrologic processes. J Geophys Res 2009;114: G00F09.

Schaefer JK, Morel FMM. High methylation rates of mercury bound to cysteine by Geobacter sulfurreducens. Nat Geosci 2009;2:123–126.

Schwarzenbach G, Schellenberg M. Die komplexchemie des methylquecksilber-kations. Helv Chim Acta 1965;48:28–46.

Shanley JB, Alisa Mast M, Campbell DH, Aiken GR, Krabbenhoft DP, Hunt RJ, Walker JF, Schuster PF, Chalmers A, Aulenbach BT, Peters NE, Marvin-DiPasquale M, Clow DW, Shafer MM. Comparison of total mercury and methylmercury cycling at five sites using the small watershed approach. Environ Pollut 2008;154:143–154.

Skyllberg U, Bloom PR, Qian J, Lin CM, Bleam WF. Complexation of mercury(II) in soil organic matter: EXAFS evidence for linear two-coordination with reduced sulfur groups. Environ Sci Technol 2006;40:4174–4180.

Skyllberg U, Qian J, Frech W, Xia K, Bleam WF. Distribution of mercury, methyl mercury and organic sulphur species in soil, soil solution and stream of a boreal forest catchment. Biogeochem 2003;64:53–76.

Skyllberg U, Xia K, Bloom PR, Nater EA, Bleam WF. Binding of mercury(II) to reduced sulfur in soil organic matter along upland-peat soil transects. J Environ Qual 2000;29:855–865.

Sleighter RL, Liu Z, Xue J, Hatcher PG. Multivariate statistical approaches for the characterization of dissolved organic matter analyzed by ultrahigh resolution mass spectrometry. Environ Sci Technol 2010;44:7576–7582.

Slowey AJ. Rate of formation and dissolution of mercury sulfide nanoparticles: the dual role of natural organic matter. Geochim Cosmochim Acta 2010;74:4693–4708.

Slowey AJ, Rytuba JJ, Brown GE. Speciation of mercury and mode of transport from placer gold mine tailings. Environ Sci Technol 2005;39:1547–1554.

Solomon D, Lehmann J, Martinez CE. Sulfur K-edge XANES spectroscopy as a tool for understanding sulfur dynamics in soil organic matter. Soil Sci Soc Am J 2003;67:1721–1731.

Spencer RGM, Aiken GR, Butler KD, Dornblaser MM, Striegl RG, Hernes PJ. Utilizing chromophoric dissolved organic matter measurements to derive export and reactivity of dissolved organic carbon exported to the Arctic Ocean: A case study of the Yukon River, Alaska. Geophys Res Lett 2009;36: L06401.

Spencer RGM, Baker A, Ahad JME, Cowie GL, Ganeshram R, Upstill-Goddard RC, Uher G. Discriminatory classification of natural and anthropogenic waters in two U.K. estuaries. Sci Total Environ 2007;373:305–323.

Stein ED, Cohen Y, Winer AM. Environmental distribution and transformation of mercury compounds. Crit Rev Environ Sci Technol 1996;26:1–43.

Stenson AC, Marshall AG, Cooper WT. Exact masses and chemical formulas of individual Suwannee River fulvic acids from ultrahigh resolution electrospray ionization Fourier transform ion cyclotron resonance mass spectra. Anal Chem 2003;75:1275–1284.

Stubbins A, Hubbard V, Uher G, Law CS, Upstill-Goddard RC, Aiken GR, Mopper K. Relating carbon monoxide photoproduction to dissolved organic matter functionality. Environ Sci Technol 2008;42:3271–3276.

Stumm W, Morgan JJ. Aquatic Chemistry. 3rd ed. New York: Wiley-Interscience; 1996.

Tossell JA. Calculation of the structures, stabilities, and properties of mercury sulfide species in aqueous solution. J Phys Chem A 2001;105:935–941.

Town RM, Filella M. Dispelling the myths: Is the existence of L1 and L2 ligands necessary to explain metal ion speciation in natural waters? LimnolOceanogr 2000;45:1341–1357.

Tranvik LJ. Degradation of dissolved organic matter in humic waters by bacteria. In: Hessen DO, Tranvik LJ, editors. Aquatic humic substances: ecology and biogeochemistry (Ecological Studies v. 133). Berlin, Germany: Springer-Verlag; 1998. p 259–283.

Vairavamurthy A, Wang S. Organic nitrogen in geomacromolecules: Insights on speciation and transformation with K-edge XANES spectroscopy. Environ Sci Technol 2002;36:3050–3056.

Vairavamurthy MA, Maletic D, Wang S, Manowitz B, Eglinton T, Lyons T. Characterization of sulfur-containing functional groups in sedimentary humic substances by X-ray absorption near-edge structure spectroscopy. Energy Fuels 1997;11:546–553.

Wang L, Chin Y-P, Traina SJ. Adsorption of (poly)maleic acid and an aquatic fulvic acid by geothite. Geochim Cosmochim Acta 1997;61:5313–5324.

Waples JS, Nagy KL, Aiken GR, Ryan JN. Dissolution of cinnabar (HgS) in the presence of natural organic matter. Geochim Cosmochim Acta 2005;69:1575–1588.

Weber FA, Voegelin A, Kaegi R, Kretzschmar R. Contaminant mobilization by metallic copper and metal sulphide colloids in flooded soil. Nat Geosci 2009;2:267–271.

Weishaar JL, Aiken GR, Bergamaschi BA, Fram MS, Fujii R, Mopper K. Evaluation of specific ultraviolet absorbance as an indicator of the chemical composition and reactivity of dissolved organic carbon. Environ Sci Technol 2003;37:4702–4708.

Wetzel RG. Limnology: lake and river ecosystems. 3rd ed. Orlando (FL): Academic Press; 2001.

Xia K, Skyllberg UL, Bleam WF, Bloom PR, Nater EA, Helmke PA. X-ray absorption spectroscopic evidence for the complexation of Hg(II) by reduced sulfur in soil humic substances. Environ Sci Technol 1999;33:257–261.

Yin YJ, Allen HE, Huang CP, Sanders PF. Interaction of Hg(II) with soil-derived humic substances. Anal Chim Acta 1997;341:73–82.

Yoon SJ, Diener LM, Bloom PR, Nater EA, Bleam WF. X-ray absorption studies of CH_3Hg^+-binding sites in humic substances. Geochim Cosmochim Acta 2005;69:1111–1121.

CHAPTER 9

TRACKING GEOCHEMICAL TRANSFORMATIONS AND TRANSPORT OF MERCURY THROUGH ISOTOPE FRACTIONATION

HOLGER HINTELMANN and WANG ZHENG

9.1 INTRODUCTION

Mercury is a toxic heavy metal and a highly pervasive global pollutant that occurs in the environment in various chemical species of different mobility, bioavailability, and reactivity (Mason et al., 1994; Fitzgerald and Lamborg, 2003). For example, inorganic Hg(II) is considered as the pivotal species in aquatic systems because it is the precursor of both Hg(0), which volatilizes and contributes to the global Hg cycle, and methylmercury, which is highly toxic and can bioaccumulate through the food web. Therefore, the availability and reactivity of Hg(II) to reduction and methylation processes is the critical factor controlling Hg speciation in water. Furthermore, the reactivity of Hg(II) is significantly affected by the complexation of Hg^{2+} cation by various inorganic and organic ligands, such as hydroxide (OH^-), halides (X^-), dissolved organic matter (DOM), and sulfide (Lindqvist et al., 1991; Schuster, 1991; Gabriel and Williamson, 2004). Both natural and anthropogenic sources contribute to the global mercury inventory. Significant anthropogenic emission has resulted in an increase in global Hg fluxes by about a factor of 3 since industrialization (Fitzgerald and Lamborg, 2003). Therefore, it is of urgent need to understand the fundamental mechanisms of Hg speciation and to distinguish between different Hg sources in order to manage Hg in the environment.

Significant knowledge gaps remain in understanding the source and biogeochemical transformation pathways of mercury, which prompted the use of Hg isotope fractionation as an innovative approach to answer some of the remaining

Environmental Chemistry and Toxicology of Mercury, First Edition.
Edited by Guangliang Liu, Yong Cai, and Nelson O'Driscoll.
© 2012 John Wiley & Sons, Inc. Published 2012 by John Wiley & Sons, Inc.

294 TRACKING OF MERCURY THROUGH ISOTOPE FRACTIONATION

questions. In general, stable isotopes fractionate during many biogeochemical processes, imprinting specific isotope compositions in end products, and allowing us to trace sources and pathways of the element of interest. Therefore, the determination of stable isotope fractionation has become one of the most important tools in studying the biogeochemical transformation of various elements. Light elements, such as H, C, O, and S, are the most extensively studied and exhibit the largest degree of isotope fractionation. Heavy metals were thought to fractionate far less because of their high atomic mass and low relative mass difference between isotopes. However, with the development of highly precise analytical technology such as multicollector inductively coupled plasma mass spectrometry (MC-ICPMS), a plethora of studies devoted to the isotope fractionation of heavy elements, such as Fe (Johnson et al., 2008), Cd (Wombacher et al., 2003), Se (Johnson, 2004), and Hg emerged during the past two decades and has significantly magnified the understanding of their biogeochemistry.

The initial studies regarding mercury isotope fractionation focused primarily on refining analytical methods and quantifying isotope compositions of geologic and aquatic specimens, including cinnabar, metacinnabar, sediments, soil, coal, and fish (Lauretta et al., 2001; Hintelmann and Lu, 2003; Hintelmann and Ogrinc, 2003; Smith et al., 2005, 2008; Foucher and Hintelmann, 2006; Bergquist and Blum, 2007; Biswas et al., 2008; Ghosh et al., 2008; Jackson et al., 2008; Carignan et al., 2009; Foucher et al., 2009; Gantner et al., 2009; Gehrke et al., 2009; Laffont et al., 2009; Sherman et al., 2009; Stetson et al., 2009; Zambardi et al., 2009; Feng et al., 2010; Senn et al., 2010). These studies established that the naturally occurring, mass-dependent isotope variations are significant and resolvable for an element as heavy as mercury. More importantly, they constituted the range of isotope variation of mercury in Nature. However, those measured isotope ratios are not fixed, but may be altered by transformation processes, which complicate the tracking of the path from a potential pollution source to receptor sites. Consequently, understanding the mechanisms of Hg isotope fractionation has been recognized as crucial to applying measured isotope data to track Hg sources. Recently, isotope fractionations during several critical transformation processes of mercury species in aquatic systems have been investigated, including volatilization (Zheng et al., 2007), evaporation (Estrade et al., 2009), reduction (Bergquist and Blum, 2007; Kritee et al., 2007, 2008; Zheng and Hintelmann, 2009–2010b), methylation/demethylation (Kritee et al., 2009; Rodriguez-Gonzalez et al., 2009), and complexation (Wiederhold et al., 2010). These laboratory investigations break down the bulk isotope variation observed in natural samples into elementary steps, thereby providing mechanistic insights to the cause of natural isotope variation.

In this chapter, recent reports on isotope fractionation of Hg are summarized and its relationship to the biogeochemical transformation of Hg is discussed. Theoretical and experimental investigation into mass independent fractionation (MIF) mechanisms (magnetic isotope effect (MIE), nuclear field shift (NFS), self-shielding, etc.) and how they can be applied in probing reaction pathways are also addressed in this chapter.

9.1.1 Basics of Isotope Fractionation

On the molecular level, isotopes can be fractionated according to several properties of the nuclei. The nuclear mass affects the frequencies of molecular vibration, which is the most mass-sensitive motion of molecules and determines the mass-dependent thermodynamic and kinetic isotope effects (Criss, 1999). According to Bigeleisen and Mayer (1947), the magnitude of mass-dependent fractionation (MDF) is controlled by the change in vibrational frequencies ($\Delta \nu$) during bond fracture and formation. $\Delta \nu$ is determined by the total force constants (F) and atomic mass:

$$\ln(\alpha_{XA-XB}) \propto \frac{\Delta M}{M^2} \frac{\Delta F_{XA-XB}}{T^2} \tag{9.1}$$

where α_{XA-XB} is the equilibrium isotope fractionation factor between substances XA and XB, ΔM is the difference in the mass of two isotopes, M is the average atomic mass, ΔF_{XA-XB} is the difference in the sum of force constants acting on the atom in substance XA versus XB, and T is the absolute temperature. Using this relationship, one can infer the type of reactions of element X by simply comparing the degree of isotope fractionation. A full description of MDF can be found in Bigeleisen and Mayer (1947) and the generalized mass dependence laws for elements with three or more stable isotopes can be found in Young et al. (2002). Other properties of nuclei, such as nuclear spin and charge distribution may also give rise to isotope fractionation that does not follow the expected mass-dependent relationships. These isotope fractionations are usually termed *mass independent, non-mass-dependent*, or *anomalous* isotope effects. MIF is not a ubiquitous isotope effect and may be only triggered by specific reactions. Such constraints make the MIF a particularly interesting phenomenon that signals a specific reaction mechanism or transformation pathway of elements in their cycles (Thiemens, 2002; Thiemens et al., 2007).

Various degrees and types of MDF and MIF have been determined in a variety of equilibrium and kinetic processes studied for Hg. Most kinetic processes follow a Rayleigh-type fractionation, a unidirectional process that involves the progressive removal of fractional increments of a trace substance from a larger reservoir. A consistent relationship is usually maintained between the reservoir and the instant increments. In the case of isotope fractionation, this consistent relationship can be described by the following Rayleigh equation:

$$\ln \frac{R}{R_i} = (\alpha - 1) \ln f_R \tag{9.2}$$

where R_i is the isotope ratio of the initial reservoir, R is the isotope ratio of the reservoir at a certain instance when the fraction of the original material remaining in the reservoir is defined by f, and α is the isotope fractionation factor. MDF that occurs during Rayleigh processes such as volatilization, reduction, and evaporation, share some common features, but differ distinctly in the degree of fractionation. They all tend to enrich heavier isotopes in the reservoir. For example, during the reduction of Hg(II) in the aqueous phase, lighter isotopes are preferentially reduced to Hg(0) and subsequently removed from water by volatilization, resulting in enrichment of lighter isotopes in the atmosphere. MDF generated by different processes are usually discerned by their magnitudes. For example, the mass-dependent kinetic isotope effects associated with volatilization of Hg(0) may be partly responsible for the $<1‰$ variation in $^{202}Hg/^{198}Hg$ measured in hydrothermal fluids (Sherman et al., 2009), while a $>2‰$ variation in $^{202}Hg/^{198}Hg$ measured in aquatic food webs indicates that processes with stronger isotope fractionation, such as reduction and methylation, are involved in shaping the isotope compositions in aquatic species (Gantner et al., 2009). The fractionation factor is a convenient measure of the degree of MDF. It usually is a constant in most cases, but was also found to vary when the rate-limiting step or the temperature changes. For example, a significant suppression in fractionation was observed in both microbial demethylation (Kritee et al., 2009) and methylation (Rodriguez-Gonzalez et al., 2009) at high cell densities toward the end of Rayleigh processes. One reason for the suppression is the shift of the rate-limiting step from intracellular reactions to diffusion across cell membranes, which generates much smaller isotope fractionation than intracellular reactions that involve Hg–C bond formation and breakage.

By 2007, the MIF of mercury isotopes had been observed by several groups working independently (Bergquist and Blum, 2007; Jackson et al., 2008; Laffont et al., 2009), making the use of stable isotope fractionation in source tracking and mechanism studies even more promising. MIF can be induced by a variety of mechanisms other than differences in vibrational energy levels that dictates MDF, and, therefore, add more variations to the pattern of isotope ratios indicative of certain transformation processes or reaction mechanisms. For example, the first isotope anomalies determined in fish and other aquatic organisms showed distinct enrichment of isotopes with odd mass numbers (^{199}Hg and ^{201}Hg) compared to the even number isotopes (^{198}Hg, ^{200}Hg, ^{202}Hg, and ^{204}Hg) (Bergquist and Blum, 2007; Jackson et al., 2008). These isotope anomalies were soon found to be consistent with the MIF caused by photochemical reduction of Hg(II) by DOM in natural waters (Bergquist and Blum, 2007; Zheng and Hintelmann, 2009), which preferentially reduces even isotopes. On the other hand, the depletion of odd isotopes was determined in samples that track atmospheric Hg, such as lichen (Carignan et al., 2009). These data complement those found in aquatic species, and further underline photochemical reduction as one of the causes of the selective enrichment or depletion of odd isotopes. Until now, photochemical reduction is still the process that generates the highest MIF of Hg isotopes. Another type of MIF was later determined in non-photochemical reduction, evaporation, and Hg–thiol complexation (Estrade et al., 2009; Wiederhold et al., 2010; Zheng and Hintelmann, 2010b). This MIF also produces anomalies for odd isotopes, but in the opposite direction and almost one order of magnitude lower than those produced by photochemical reactions. Recently, another MIF effect occurring during ionization of Hg(0) vapor within compact fluorescence light bulbs was reported, which did not follow the odd–even separation but rather preferentially ionized less abundant isotopes (Mead et al., 2010). This MIF was suggested to be related to photochemical self-shielding, resembling a similar effect observed for oxygen isotopes within nebula (Lyons and Young, 2005). The various MIF effects complicate the application of stable isotope fractionation in source tracking, but also broaden its range by allowing more processes to be identified by specific isotope effects. In-depth understanding of the mechanisms of MIF and sophisticated experimental design and analytical techniques are required to resolve the various MIF effects during natural speciation of Hg.

Despite the emerging popularity of MIF as a powerful tool in tracking Hg transformations, its mechanisms are still not fully uncovered. Most recent data on MIF of Hg isotopes and possibly other heavy elements is primarily explained by two mechanisms: MIE and NFS. The MIE is a spin-selective isotope effect, which separates isotopes with and without unpaired nuclear spins and arises from hyperfine interaction between nuclear and electron spins. All effects of this kind reported so far are based on the radical pair mechanism, which manifests itself via the cage effect (Turro and Kraeutler, 1980; Turro, 1983; Steiner and Ulrich, 1989; Buchachenko, 2001; Buchachenko, 2009), whereby a pair of reactive molecules in solution may be temporarily trapped by the solvent "cage," causing them to remain as colliding neighbors for a short period of time before random motion allows them to escape the cage (Braden et al., 2001; Oelkers and Tyler, 2008). Specifically, the recombination of a radical pair before their escape is spin selective. When a germinate radical pair is generated as a triplet, recombination of this radical pair is spin forbidden unless a triplet to singlet intersystem crossing (ISC) occurs as a result of electron–nuclear hyperfine coupling or spin–orbital coupling. The spin conversion rate can be enhanced by magnetic isotopes (those with unpaired nuclear spins) via hyperfine coupling. Therefore, radical pairs with magnetic isotopes are more likely to undergo cage recombination, which leads to the accumulation of magnetic isotopes in reactants, while nonmagnetic isotopes are more likely to escape the radical cage and become new species (Fig. 9.1). Odd Hg isotopes, ^{199}Hg and ^{201}Hg, have a total nuclear spin angular momentum of $I = 1/2$ and 3/2, respectively, and are thus subject to spin-selective separation from even isotopes during processes generating radical pairs, for example, during

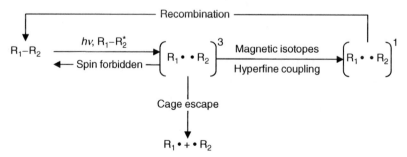

Figure 9.1 A scheme of the magnetic isotope effect operated via a radical pair. The superscript "1" represents singlet excited states, and "3" represents triplet excited states.

photochemical reduction (Buchachenko et al., 2007; Buchachenko, 2009). Consequently, the MIE is a kinetic isotope effect depending on the recombination rate of radical pairs, which is mainly controlled by hyperfine coupling constants. The unique spin-selective feature of the MIE makes it a sensitive probe to reaction mechanisms involving radicals.

NFS is observed as part of isotope shifts in atomic spectra (King, 1984). It originates from the effect of nuclear volume on electrons. Variations in nuclear size and shape change the nuclear charge distribution, which results in a slightly different electrostatic field to interact with electrons having a high density at the nucleus (i.e., s orbital electrons). The ground state electron energy of a lighter/smaller isotope is lower than that of a heavier/larger isotope because of the smaller size and larger nuclear charge distribution of the lighter isotope. Therefore, the lowest energy of a system is found when the larger isotopes occupy sites with lower electron density at the nucleus and smaller isotopes occupy sites with high electron density at the nucleus (i.e., more s electrons). As a result, NFS will lead to preferential enrichment of heavier/larger isotopes in the chemical species with the smallest number of s electrons in the valence orbital (Bigeleisen, 2006; Schauble, 2007). Nuclear volume and mass both increase with the number of neutrons in an isotope, but nuclear volume does not increase linearly. Instead, it shows an odd–even staggering pattern (isotopes with odd neutron numbers tend to be smaller than what is predicted from linearity, e.g., Fig. 9.2). For this reason, isotope fractionation driven by nuclear volume will generally not scale linearly with mass, causing isotope anomalies for odd isotopes. NFS is more pronounced for heavy elements (King, 1984). Schauble (2007) calculated contributions of NFS to isotope fractionation factors for various species of Hg and Tl, and predicted generally higher contributions of NFS to isotope fractionation relative to MDF effects. Compared to MIE, NFS is typically lower in magnitude, but is more easily triggered, and thus affects more reactions.

9.1.2 Mercury Stable Isotope System

This section provides a brief background about mercury stable isotope systems. Mercury has seven stable isotopes: ^{196}Hg (average natural abundance: 0.15%), ^{198}Hg (9.97%), ^{199}Hg (16.87%), ^{200}Hg 23.10%), ^{201}Hg (13.18%), ^{202}Hg (29.86%), and ^{204}Hg (6.87%) (Rosman and Taylor, 1998). The ^{202}Hg/^{198}Hg isotope pair is usually selected to describe MDF because ^{202}Hg has the highest abundance and the large mass difference between ^{202}Hg and ^{198}Hg generates a relatively high fractionation compared to other isotope pairs, minimizing the interference of analytical errors. Hg isotopic compositions of environmental samples are reported in delta values as the deviation from a common reference standard. Currently, the NIST SRM3133 mercury solution serves as the mutually accepted reference point:

$$\delta^x \text{Hg} = 1000 \times \left(\frac{R_{\text{Sample}}^{x/198}}{R_{\text{NIST3133}}^{x/198}} - 1 \right) \tag{9.3}$$

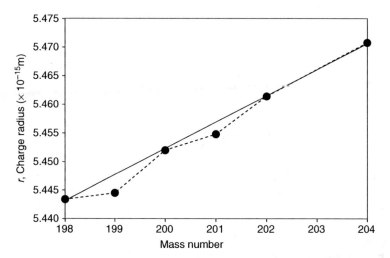

Figure 9.2 Charge radii of the stable Hg isotopes (Nadjakov et al., 1994). The solid line is the linear regression of the charge radii of even isotopes. Odd isotopes are smaller than the linear radii.

where x is the mass number of Hg isotopes. Isotope anomalies (MIF) are characterized using the "capital delta" notation (Δ) as follows:

$$\Delta^x Hg = \delta^x Hg - \beta \times \delta^{202} Hg \tag{9.4}$$

where β is the scale factor of the theoretical mass-dependent fractionation law (Young et al., 2002) for kinetic and equilibrium fractionation, respectively:

$$\beta_{kinetic} = \frac{\ln(m_{198}/m_x)}{\ln(m_{198}/m_{202})} \tag{9.5}$$

$$\beta_{equilibrium} = \frac{1/m_{198} - 1/m_x}{1/m_{198} - 1/m_{202}} \tag{9.6}$$

Often, we are interested in describing the difference in isotopic composition of two (sample) reservoirs, for example, reactants and products. This difference is commonly expressed using the fractionation factor:

$$\alpha^x_{A-B} = R_A^{x/198} / R_B^{x/198} \tag{9.7}$$

Since α is usually close to unity with differences in the fourth or fifth decimal place, it is sometimes more convenient to express differences in per mil by taking the natural log of α and multiplying it by 1000, which is simply written as $1000\ln\alpha$. Or alternatively, one can employ the ε notation:

$$\varepsilon^x_{A-B} = 1000(\alpha^x_{A-B} - 1) \approx 1000 \ln \alpha \tag{9.8}$$

The ε notation has the advantage over using $1000\ln\alpha$ of being a more exact expression of the per mil fractionation. We will, therefore, use the ε notation in the following sections when describing differences in isotopic composition between two sample reservoirs.

High precision stable Hg isotope analysis of environmental samples is achieved by measuring Hg isotope ratios employing MC-ICP-MS together with proper sample–matrix separation and mass bias correction strategies. A number of early publications over the past decade demonstrated and optimized the use of various sample introduction strategies, of which continuous-flow cold vapor generation CV-MC-ICP-MS is most widely applied (Lauretta et al., 2001; Hintelmann and Lu, 2003; Xie et al., 2005; Foucher and Hintelmann, 2006). Various mass bias correction strategies were developed and sample-standard bracketing in combination with simultaneous measurement of $^{205}Tl/^{203}Tl$ ratios (e.g., NIST SRM997 Tl solution) is currently accepted as the most accurate method (Yang and Sturgeon, 2003; Blum and Bergquist, 2007; Meija et al., 2009). Traditionally, CV-MC-ICPMS can only measure samples with relatively high Hg concentrations (>2 ng/mL). Recent developments in matrix separation/preconcentration techniques using ion exchange and gas chromatography enable us to determine Hg isotope ratios in low level samples such as natural water (Chen et al., 2010) and simultaneous measurement of isotope ratios in both inorganic Hg(II) and monomethylmercury (MMHg) (Epov et al., 2008), which permits the measurement of a wider range of natural samples, broadening our view of Hg isotope variations in Nature. Under optimal analytical conditions and including complete separation of Hg from the sample matrix, analysis of matrix-matched bracketing standards of the same concentration, careful monitoring of background signals, and performance of on-peak blank corrections, analytical precision of $\pm 0.08\permil$ (2 SD) for $\delta^{202}Hg$ and $\pm 0.05\permil$ (2 SD) for $\Delta^{199}Hg$ are achievable (Blum and Bergquist, 2007).

9.2 FRACTIONATION OF MERCURY ISOTOPES IN ENVIRONMENTAL PROCESSES

Owing to its unique chemical and physical characteristics, mercury can undergo a variety of environmental reactions and processes, leading to a complex geochemical cycle. There is now also a rapidly expanding literature describing the fractionation of Hg isotopes, while cycling through the environment. The following sections focus on specific processes, which have been studied for isotope fractionation, put the individual studies into context, and discuss the implications of illuminating the fate of Hg in the environment. Table 9.1 summarizes the experimental studies conducted to date, which detected and quantified Hg isotope fractionation factors associated with distinct biogeochemical transformations. In general, the kinetic processes tend to enrich heavier isotopes in the reactants, as long as MDF is the principal driving force ($\varepsilon < 0$). MIF adds more variation to the pattern of isotope fractionation and may even change the direction of isotope enrichment.

TABLE 9.1 Experimental Fractionation Factors (ε) Determined for a Variety of Hg Transformations

Processes	ε^{199}	2SD	ε^{202}	2SD	Isotope Effects	Experimental Conditions	References
Biotic, kinetic							
Microbial reduction of Hg(II)	—	—	$-1.40 \sim -2.00$	0.20	MDF	*Bacteria strain* *Escherichia coli JM109/pPB117*, vary with temperature	Kritee et al. (2007)
	—	—	$-1.20 \sim -1.40$	0.10	MDF	Hg(II) resistant, *Bacillus cereus Strain 5* and *Anoxybacillius sp Strain FB9*	Kritee et al. (2008)
	—	—	-1.80	0.30	MDF	Hg(II) sensitive, *Shewanella oneidensis MR-1*	Kritee et al. (2008)
Microbial methylation	—	—	-2.60	0.40	MDF	*Desulfobulbus propionicus*, dark anaerobic condition, pyruvate as carbon source	Rodriguez-Gonzalez et al. (2009)
Microbial degradation of MeHg	—	—	-0.40	0.20	MDF	*Escherichia coli JM109/pPB117*	Kritee et al. (2009)
Abiotic, photo- chemical, kinetic						*Electron donor and light source*	
Photoreduction of Hg(II)	-0.60	0.	-0.60	20	MDF,(+)MIE	Suwannee River fulvic acid, Hg/DOM = 60,000–100,000 ng/mg, natural sunlight	(Bergquist and Blum, 2007)
	-1.94	0.60	-1.06	0.04	MDF, (+)MIE	Dorset Lake bulk DOM, Hg/DOM = 8330 ng/mg, natural sunlight, and Xe lamp	Zheng and Hintelmann. (2009)

(continued)

TABLE 9.1 (Continued)

Processes	ε^{199}	2SD	ε^{202}	2SD	Isotope Effects	Experimental Conditions	References
	0.69	0.04	−1.32	0.07	MDF, (−)MIE	Cysteine, ligand/Hg = 2000, Xe lamp	Zheng and Hintelmann. (2010a)
	−0.26	0.04	−1.71	0.03	MDF, (+)MIE, NFS	Serine, ligand/Hg = 2000, Xe lamp	Zheng and Hintelmann. (2010a)
	—	—	−0.55	0.10	MDF, NFS	Formic acid, UVC Hg lamp, $\lambda = 254$ nm	(Yang and Sturgeon, 2009)
Photodegradation of MeHg	−3.61	0.70	−1.30	0.20	MDF, (+)MIE	Suwannee River fulvic acid, DOM = 1 mg/L, natural sunlight	(Bergquist and Blum, 2007)
	−8.33	1.30	−1.70	0.30	MDF, (+)MIE	Suwannee River fulvic acid, DOM = 10 mg/L, natural sunlight	(Bergquist and Blum, 2007)
	—	—	−0.13 ~ −0.36	—	MDF, (+)MIE	UVC Hg lamp, $\lambda = 254$ nm, vary with pH, and radical scavengers	(Malinovsky et al., 2010)
Abiotic, non-photochemical, kinetic						*Electron or carbon donors*	
Non-photochemical reduction of Hg(II)	−0.19	0.02	−1.52	0.06	MDF, NFS	Dorset Lake bulk DOM, Hg/DOM = 10, 000 ng/mg	Zheng and Hintelmann. (2010b)

Process						Description	Reference
	−0.22	0.02	−1.56	0.11	MDF, NFS	SnCl$_2$	Zheng and Hintelmann, (2010b)
	—	—	−0.43 ~ −0.49	0.08	MDF, NFS	SnCl$_2$ and NaBH$_4$	(Yang and Sturgeon, 2009)
Abiotic ethylation	—	—	−1.20	0.40	MDF	Abiotic, NaBEt$_4$ as ethylation reagent	(Yang and Sturgeon, 2009)
Volatilization	—	—	−0.47	0.04	MDF	Dissolved Hg(0) in water solution to Hg(0) vapor	Zheng et al. (2007)
Kinetic evaporation	—	—	−6.68	1.10	MDF, NFS	Vacuum evaporation of metallic Hg(0)	(Estrade et al., 2009)
Abiotic, equilibrium							
Complexation between Hg(II) and thiol resins	—	—	−0.53	0.15	MDF, NFS	Hg(II) chloride to Hg(II)–thiol	(Wiederhold et al., 2010)
	—	—	−0.62	0.17	MDF, NFS	Hg(II) nitrate to Hg(II)–thiol	(Wiederhold et al., 2010)
Equilibrium evaporation	—	—	−0.86	0.22	MDF, NFS	Equilibrium between metallic Hg(0) and Hg(0) vapor	(Estrade et al., 2009)

All fractionation factors are defined as isotope ratios of products versus reactants ($R_{product}/R_{reactant}$). ε^{199} are shown for MIF.

9.2.1 Volatilization and Evaporation

Volatilization and evaporation are mass transfer processes, where elemental Hg crosses the gas–liquid interface from a condensed phase to the gaseous phase. Owing to elemental mercury's high vapor pressure and small Henry's Law constant, they are among the most common phase transfer processes of Hg in Nature. Volatilization controls the water/air exchange of Hg in natural waters and is the major pathway of atmospheric Hg input. Evaporation of metallic mercury can take place in a variety of industrial applications such as mining and refining. Both processes are frequently encountered in hydrothermal activities where mantle-derived Hg is transferred to various surface reservoirs. Isotope fractionation during these processes can thus provide critical information about geothermal transport, water/air exchange, and industrial emission of Hg.

During an early study of Hg isotopes in natural hydrothermal systems, Smith et al. (2005) suggested that Hg(0) released from hydrothermal solutions would have lower $\delta^{202}Hg$ compared to Hg remaining in solution, likely due to the boiling and degassing as the fluid ascended. This was demonstrated experimentally by Zheng et al. (2007), who studied the kinetic isotope fractionation of Hg during Hg(0) volatilization from a saturated solution and determined a relatively small, mass-dependent fractionation factor ε^{202} between -0.44 and -0.47. Rayleigh's fractionation law (Eq. 9.2) was followed and lighter isotopes were preferentially enriched in the gaseous phase (Fig. 9.3). Under natural conditions, volatilization could account for as much as $\sim 1\%o$ ($\delta^{202}Hg$) fractionation depending on its degree of completion. Therefore, with proper constraints, this fractionation factor could be used to identify reservoirs where Hg is lost to the atmosphere and quantify the fraction that was removed based on the Rayleigh relationship between isotope ratios and the fraction of reactants. For example, Sherman et al. (2009) found decreasing Hg concentrations and increasing $\delta^{202}Hg$ from a hot spring along its downstream transect. A Rayleigh model was applied to this system and a fractionation factor of -0.59 was determined, which is slightly larger than the value determined for volatilization only, suggesting that the isotope fractionation is primarily driven by volatilization but other mass-dependent processes such as precipitation may also contribute to the final value. The isotope effect of volatilization is also expected to be manifested in surface water, which accounts for the majority of Hg traffic between water and atmosphere. However, fractionation by volatilization is often obscured by processes, which generate much stronger fractionation, such as redox reactions. Evidence for the contribution of volatilization to Hg isotope signatures, especially in atmospheric Hg, is still lacking.

The mass transfer during liquid–vapor evaporation may produce a wide range of isotope fractionation factors depending on whether the process is driven by equilibrium or kinetic processes (Estrade et al., 2009). Kinetic evaporation under vacuum resulted in the largest mass-dependent fractionation factor ($\varepsilon^{202} = -6.7$) among all experimentally studied transformations, being by one order of magnitude larger than the fractionation observed during volatilization and equilibrium evaporation ($\varepsilon^{202} = -0.86$). The large variation in MDF between these mass

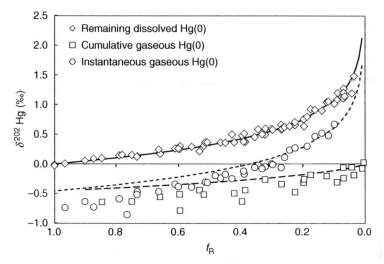

Figure 9.3 Rayleigh fractionation process of Hg isotopes during volatilization. f_R is the fraction of the remaining dissolved Hg(0) in aqueous phase. Solid and dashed lines are theoretical Rayleigh models based on the ε^{202} value of volatilization. Increasing δ^{202}Hg in the remaining reactant suggests lighter isotopes are preferentially volatilized.

transfer processes can be explained by Equation 9.2. Much higher ΔF is expected from the fracture of metallic bonds than from overcoming of van der Waal forces between dissolved Hg(0) and solvent molecules in the case of volatilization. Under equilibrium conditions, MDF is suppressed by strong condensation of Hg vapor. Interestingly, a small degree of negative isotope anomalies (Δ^{199}Hg from -0.12‰ to -0.02‰) was observed in the residual Hg liquid. It was attributed to the NFS effect. In metallic bonds, the 6s valence electrons of mercury are shared; therefore, smaller isotopes with higher nuclear charge density tend to share valence electrons less than larger isotopes, resulting in weaker metallic bonds and higher vapor pressure (hence enrichment in vapor) in smaller isotopes. Potentially, the NFS could be used to identify charge transfer reactions and the presence of highly covalent Hg species (such as metallic Hg and organomercury). However, owing to its relatively low magnitude compared to MIE, its application is still limited to reactions involving very small contributions of other MIF processes (e.g., MIE), such as abiotic non-photochemical reduction (Section 9.2.3.2) or Hg(II)−thiol complexation (Section 9.2.2).

9.2.2 Complexation of Hg(II) by Organic Ligands

Complexation refers to the formation of Hg(II)−ligand complexes such as the Hg(II)−thiol complex. Hg is also known to form strong complexes with DOM in natural water (Ravichandran, 2004). This reaction has a tremendous impact on Hg speciation. For example, strong complexation with DOM can mobilize Hg from soil and sediments and transport it into water bodies, making it more available for photochemical and microbial transformations (Wallschlager et al., 1996). Preference of Hg for reduced sulfur functional groups over carboxyl groups in DOM affects its reactivity during photochemical reduction (Xia et al., 1999). The bioaccumulation of MMHg in biota is also attributed to the high affinity of MMHg to sulfur-containing proteins such as cysteine and glutathione (Ullrich et al., 2001). Isotope fractionation produced by this type of reaction would help track the bonding condition of Hg, which is critical to understand its speciation.

Thus far, only the Hg(II)–thiol complex has been studied. Wiederhold et al. (2010) studied the equilibrium complexation between inorganic Hg(II) and a thiol resin. Thiol-bound Hg was enriched with light Hg isotopes by $-0.53\permil$ and $-0.62\permil$ (δ^{202}Hg) relative to $HgCl_2$ and $Hg(OH)_2$, respectively. Isotope anomalies produced in the Hg–thiol compound are small (Δ^{199}Hg $<0.1\permil$) but vary systematically with the fraction of sorbed Hg(II), suggesting that NFS may be involved, which could be explained by shifts in electron density during ligand exchange. The magnitude of NFS would then reflect the change in the 6s orbital electron density. Therefore, complexes with more electronegative ligands, such as Hg–chloro compounds, tend to have lower 6s orbital electron density and favor the enrichment of larger isotopes, whereas S ligands bind to Hg with more covalent character, resulting in higher 6s electron density and hence enrichment of smaller isotopes (lighter isotope signature).

While Hg–thiol complexation may serve as a general surrogate for Hg binding to the reduced sulfur sites in natural DOM and proteins, the net Hg isotope fractionation during binding to natural DOM is difficult to predict. Different binding sites and variations in the chelating bonding environment within DOM would likely produce a wide range of bond vibrations and charge densities at 6s orbitals, which may lead to various degrees of MDF and NFS. More investigation of this type of processes is definitely necessary considering the dominance of Hg(II)–DOM and Hg(II)–sulfide complexes in natural water, sediment, and biota.

Another study on MMHg binding to the thiol group of cysteine in an enzyme suggested the involvement of MIE (Buchachenko et al., 2004). Strong enrichment of ^{199}Hg and ^{201}Hg in CH_3HgSR was observed and hence, the formation of an intermittent ($CH_3Hg^{\bullet} + {}^{\bullet}SR$) radical pair was proposed. However, the fact that radical intermediates are out of character for ionic reactions, the extremely large fractionation measured, and the scarce provision of analytical procedure cast significant doubts on the validity of this study and the reported data.

9.2.3 Abiotic Reduction of Hg(II) and MMHg to Hg(0)

Redox reactions are pivotal processes in the biogeochemical transformation of mercury in aquatic systems. The reduction of Hg(II) and MMHg to Hg(0) increases the emission of Hg(0) to the atmosphere, and limits the bioavailable Hg(II) pool that may otherwise be methylated. Hg reduction can be initiated by both biotic and abiotic pathways. Biotic reduction is mediated by various microorganisms (Mason et al., 1995; Siciliano et al., 2002; Fantozzi et al., 2009).

Abiotic reduction is usually initiated by DOM via either photochemical (Amyot et al., 1994; Xiao et al., 1995; Amyot et al., 1997b) or non-photochemical pathways (Alberts et al., 1974; Allard and Arsenie, 1991). Reduction reactions are known to generate relatively high isotope fractionation during the natural Hg cycle. The magnitude of ε^{202} ranges from -0.4 (microbial reduction of MMHg; Kritee et al., 2009) to -1.7 (photochemical reduction of Hg(II) by serine and microbial reduction of Hg(II); Kritee et al., 2007; Zheng and Hintelmann, 2010a). A variety of isotope effects may be involved depending on the reduction mechanism. In the presence of MDF, the reduced Hg(0) is enriched with lighter isotopes (smaller δ^{202}Hg) compared to the oxidized Hg(II) and MMHg species. However, reduction is usually accompanied by various MIF effects, which make the isotope fractionation pattern not only more complicated but also more distinct and characteristic for specific reduction pathways.

9.2.3.1 Photochemical Reduction and its Relationship with Hg-DOM Complexation.

A growing number of field studies have demonstrated that sunlight can promote photochemical reduction of Hg(II) and MMHg in various freshwater (Lalonde et al., 2003; O'Driscoll et al., 2004; Poulain et al., 2004; Southworth et al., 2007) and seawater environments (Amyot et al., 1997a; Lanzillotta et al., 2002; Rolfhus and Fitzgerald, 2004). In fact, photochemical reduction is one of the most important mechanisms of elemental Hg(0) production in natural waters, and therefore plays a key role in controlling Hg(0) emission and Hg bioavailability. The most distinct feature of isotope fractionation during photochemical reduction is the often significant MIF. Three types of MIF have been identified during this process. The most common MIF is observed when the reduction is driven by natural DOM, which imparts a positive MIE, that is, $(+)$MIE, enriching odd, magnetic isotopes (^{199}Hg and ^{201}Hg) in oxidized species (Bergquist and Blum, 2007; Zheng and Hintelmann, 2009). A reversed MIE, $(-)$MIE leads to an enrichment of ^{199}Hg and ^{201}Hg in the reduced Hg(0) during photolysis of Hg(II) bound to thiols (Zheng and Hintelmann, 2010a) and reduction of Hg(II) in surface snow (Sherman et al., 2010). NFS is usually less significant than MIE, but still accounts for a fraction of isotope anomalies and becomes more important, when MIE is inhibited. $(+)$MIE was first observed in an experimental study by Bergquist and Blum (2007). Inorganic Hg(II) or MMHg were mixed with Suwannee River fulvic acid (SRFA) at a high Hg/DOC (dissolved organic carbon) ratio of $60-100$ μg/mg and exposed to natural sunlight. Only odd isotopes, ^{199}Hg and ^{201}Hg, showed distinct isotope anomalies (Fig. 9.4). The remaining oxidized Hg in solution was significantly enriched with ^{199}Hg and ^{201}Hg, with a Δ^{199}Hg up to $\sim$2‰. Moreover, Δ^{199}Hg and Δ^{201}Hg seem to be linearly correlated. Empirical slopes Δ^{199}Hg/Δ^{201}Hg of 1.00 for Hg(II) and 1.36 for MMHg were determined. The selective enrichment of ^{199}Hg and ^{201}Hg was considered to be a result of $(+)$MIE caused by the formation of radical pairs involving Hg$^{+\bullet}$ and organic radicals.

DOM plays a critical role in controlling photochemical reduction mechanisms and its resulting isotope fractionation during this process (Garcia et al., 2005).

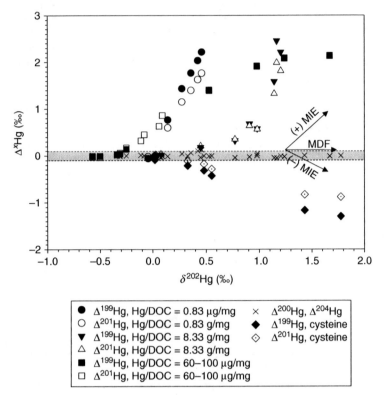

Figure 9.4 Δ^xHg (x = 199, 200, 201, and 204) versus δ^{202}Hg for the remaining oxidized Hg(II) during photochemical reduction of Hg(II) in the presence of dissolved organic matter or cysteine. The shaded band between −0.1 and 0.1‰ represents the general external reproducibility (2 SD) of analysis for isotope compositions. Δ^{200}Hg and Δ^{204}Hg fall within the analytical uncertainty, indicating no isotope anomalies for even isotopes, while Δ^{199}Hg and Δ^{201}Hg show either positive or negative anomalies in the oxidized form. Positive anomalies, such as those produced by natural DOM, are a result of (+)MIE, while negative anomalies, such as those produced by cysteine, indicate the predominance of (−)MIE. *Source*: Data labeled with "cysteine" is from Zheng and Hintelmann (2010a). Data at Hg/DOC = 0.83 and 8.33 µg/mg is from Zheng and Hintelmann (2009), while data at Hg/DOC = 60–100 µg/mg is from Bergquist and Blum (2007).

More detailed experiments focusing on the effect of DOM were conducted by Zheng and Hintelmann (2009) using natural lake water with lower Hg/DOC ratios ranging from 34.6 to 8330 ng/mg, which are more relevant for natural conditions. Similar MIF as by Bergquist and Blum (2007) was obtained, but the degree of MIF varied with Hg/DOC ratios. High Hg/DOC (8.33 µg/mg) generated notably lower MIF than intermediate and low Hg/DOC (<0.83 µg/mg) (Fig. 9.4). This result is not surprising because not all Hg binds to the same sites of DOM. Many studies have demonstrated that Hg preferentially binds to reduced sulfur groups such as thiol and disulfide/disulfane functional groups rather than to oxygen functional groups in organic matter (Xia et al., 1999; Drexel et al., 2002). Reduced sulfur groups are usually much less abundant than oxygen groups (e.g., carboxyl or phenol groups) (Hesterberg et al., 2001). Under natural conditions, where the Hg concentration is lower than the concentration of reduced sulfur in DOM, Hg primarily binds with high stability constants (e.g., $K = 10^{21}$ to 10^{24}) (Haitzer et al., 2002; Ravichandran, 2004) to reduced sulfur. With increasing Hg/DOC ratios, and when Hg concentrations far exceed reduced sulfur concentrations, it is expected that a small fraction of Hg saturates all of the reduced sulfur and the majority of Hg binds to oxygen functional groups, which yield much lower stability constants (e.g., typically $K = 10^{10}$) (Haitzer et al., 2002). Therefore, the apparent isotope fractionation associated with the bulk DOM is actually a combination of various fractionation processes occurring at different Hg–DOM bonds, which differ in bond strength and produce different radical pairs. Also, the "bulk" fractionation factors are likely different from one water body to another because of differences in the composition of DOM.

To investigate the isotope effects produced by specific functional groups, low molecular weight organic compounds (LMWOCs) with and without reduced sulfur were used as surrogates for strong and weak binding sites of DOM (Zheng and Hintelmann, 2010a). These experiments revealed that different ligands generate opposite MIE, depending on the presence or absence of sulfur. (+)MIE is usually observed during photochemical reduction of bulk DOM, and also produced by most ligands with only O/N functional groups, while (−)MIE is produced by ligands with S functional groups, such as cysteine (Fig. 9.4). The reason reduced S ligands tends to generate (−)MIE is not yet clear. A tentative explanation suggests that the photolysis of Hg–O/N bonds generates triplet radical pairs, while singlet radical pairs are favored by Hg–S bonds. Magnetic isotopes (^{199}Hg and ^{201}Hg) will promote an ISC for both type of radical pairs, and thus lead to opposite spin in their cage products, which eventually enriches magnetic isotopes in opposite directions (Fig. 9.5). The implication of the two MIEs is that one can infer the type of ligands Hg is associated with before photolysis. For example, one important difference between the reduction by natural DOM and LMWOC is that no (−)MIE was determined for natural DOM, suggesting that the majority of Hg(0) in natural waters originates from the reduction of Hg(II) species that bind to O/N functional groups in DOM rather than S functional groups.

However, MIE is not always the dominant isotope effect during photochemical reactions. Several conditions such as alkaline pH, presence of radical scavengers, and strong secondary photochemical reduction, may inhibit MIE. Malinovsky et al. (2010) studied UV (254 nm, mercury vapor lamp) photolysis of CH_3HgCl with different pH and solvent matrices. The largest MIE (Δ^{199}Hg up to 1.5‰) was found in solutions with the lowest pH (4.0) and containing only CH_3HgCl (0.05 mM). At alkaline pH (>8.6, adjusted by NH_3), MIE was almost completely suppressed (Δ^{199}Hg <0.2‰). The high OH^- anion concentration in alkaline solution is proposed to act as a free radical scavenger, which inhibits MIE by shortening the lifetime of radical pairs and reducing the "cage effect." This inhibition was also observed with the presence of ascorbic acid, another radical

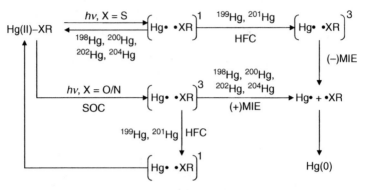

Figure 9.5 The schematic mechanism of (+)MIE and (−)MIE for a generalized Hg(II)–XR complex, where XR represents reduced sulfur or O/N donor groups of LMWOC. The superscript "1" represents singlet excited states, and "3" represents triplet excited states. HFC and SOC stand for hyperfine coupling and spin–orbital coupling, respectively.

scavenger (Malinovsky et al., 2010). Besides direct photolysis, secondary photochemical processes may be initiated, when excessive organic ligands are present, which generate intermediates that are capable of reducing Hg(II). For example, carboxyl groups may produce $HCOO^{\bullet}$ radicals during photolysis, which further reacts with oxygen to produce hydroperoxyl and superoxide radicals ($HO_2^{\bullet}$ and O_2^{-}) (Zhang, 2006):

$$HCOO^{\bullet} + O_2 \rightarrow HO_2^{\bullet} + CO_2 \tag{9.9}$$

$$HO_2^{\bullet} \rightarrow H^+ + O_2 \tag{9.10}$$

Hg(II) can be reduced by these radicals. Unlike direct photolysis, secondary reduction does not generate spin-related radical pairs since these radicals are scavenged once they transfer unpaired electrons to Hg(II). Therefore, this reduction mechanism is not likely to trigger MIE. Instead, the electron transfer process is subject to NFS, which typically produces much less isotope anomalies than MIE. This could explain the very small isotope anomalies ($\Delta^{199}Hg$ <0.1‰) determined in photolysis experiments without radical scavengers (Yang and Sturgeon, 2009). Secondary reduction seems to be more significant when Hg(II) is bound to oxygen functional groups rather than reduced sulfur groups. Zheng and Hintelmann (2010a) studied the reduction of Hg(II) by serine and cysteine with ligand/Hg >2000 under a Xe lamp (300–800 nm). Distinct NFS with $\Delta^{199}Hg$ of up to −0.28‰ in the remaining Hg(II) was observed in the serine solution, indicating that secondary reduction outcompetes direct photolysis. (−)MIE was the dominant isotope effect in the cysteine solution, suggesting that direct photolysis is the main reduction pathway.

Photodegradation of MMHg is usually more sensitive to MIE than reduction of inorganic Hg(II) because the cleavage of the Hg–C bond may produce additional radical pairs (e.g., $CH_3^{\bullet} + {}^{\bullet}HgCl$) other than those produced by MeHg–DOM. For example, the degree of MIE can be approximately assessed by the fractionation factor of odd isotopes. Photodegradation of MMHg produces a much higher ε^{199} of -3.6 compared to inorganic Hg(II), for which a ε^{199} of -0.6 was observed under the same experimental conditions (Bergquist and Blum, 2007).

Owing to its strong MIE, photochemical reduction is the only process known so far that is able to produce significant isotope anomalies in natural reservoirs. It has been proposed that MIF signatures in aquatic food webs are originally generated in the water column by photochemical reactions and subsequently transferred to the organism via food uptake and bioaccumulation (Bergquist and Blum, 2007). More precisely and considering that only MMHg is biomagnified, it would mean that (partial) photodegradation of MMHg is the key process in labeling aquatic food webs. A variety of freshwater and seawater organisms, such as zooplankton and fish, are found to accumulate positive Δ^{199}Hg and Δ^{201}Hg (Bergquist and Blum, 2007; Jackson et al., 2008; Gantner et al., 2009; Laffont et al., 2009; Senn et al., 2010), indicating the influence of (+)MIE. The degree of isotope anomalies is thought to be related to the Hg source. Gantner et al. (2009) studied the food web in arctic lakes, and found that pelagic zooplankton accumulating MMHg directly from water columns showed a pronounced MIF signature with Δ^{199}Hg of up to 3.4‰, while benthic chironomids that are exposed to Hg sediments showed much lower anomalies with Δ^{199}Hg only up to 1.31‰, indicating a larger contribution of sedimentary Hg, which usually shows only a small MIF. Benthic chironomids make up a large proportion of arctic char diet, resulting in lower MIF in char than in zooplankton (Gantner et al., 2009). Senn et al. (2010) compared the MIF signatures in oceanic and coastal fish. Oceanic fish have notably higher Δ^{201}Hg ($\sim$1.5‰) than those of coastal fish ($\sim$0.4‰). This also was explained by isotopically distinct MMHg sources, with oceanic MMHg having undergone substantial photodegradation before entering the base of the food web. An alternative explanation for the isotope anomalies in fish is *in vivo* MIF. Δ^{199}Hg and Δ^{201}Hg in fish were found to correlate positively with δ^{15}N, suggesting that the degree of MIF increases with the trophic level (Das et al., 2009). Das et al. (2009) argued that small fishes at a lower trophic level most likely approximate the isotopic signature of water, but species at higher trophic levels bioaccumulate and biomagnify MMHg, which may induce MIF via metabolic reactions inside fish. However, it is not yet clear which biochemical reaction is responsible for the *in vivo* MIF as all biotic processes experimentally studied so far (microbial reduction and methylation/demethylation) showed no evidence of MIF.

Photochemical reduction is also largely responsible for the MIF signature in atmospheric Hg. Hg(0) produced in the water column by photochemical reduction will be depleted in ^{199}Hg and ^{201}Hg as a result of (+)MIE and it carries negative Δ^{199}Hg and Δ^{201}Hg, when volatilizing into the air. Reservoirs that collect atmospheric Hg deposition, such as ground vegetation, may also pick up these negative atmospheric Hg isotope anomalies. For example, lichen is a biomonitor of atmospheric heavy metals. Lichen samples from three separate locations showed similar odd isotope depletion with Δ^{199}Hg of up to -1‰ (Carignan et al., 2009), suggesting a significant impact of photochemical reduction on the global atmospheric Hg pool. Although (+)MIE is the primary mechanism for MIF signatures observed in most natural samples, (−)MIE is observed in arctic surface snow and the emitted Hg vapor (Sherman et al., 2010). Snow samples are depleted in odd isotopes with Δ^{199}Hg of up to −5.08‰, while the gaseous Hg(0) collected by a flux chamber showed much less odd isotope depletion (Δ^{199}Hg up to −1.87‰). This MIF signature is explained by photochemical reduction during polar atmospheric mercury depletion events (AMDEs). Photochemically initiated reactions involving halogen and halogen oxide radicals oxidize gaseous Hg(0) in the lower atmospheric boundary layer to compounds that are rapidly deposited to the snowpack, resulting in the depletion of atmospheric Hg in polar region (Lindberg et al., 2002). These deposited Hg can undergo photochemical reduction within snow and be reemitted back to the atmosphere. MIF during this process is possible and enriches odd isotopes in emitted Hg(0) as a result of (−)MIE.

9.2.3.2 Abiotic Non-Photochemical Reduction.

Abiotic reduction of Hg(II) in the absence of light is a ubiquitous process in natural water and soil. Organic matter plays a major role in controlling the redox cycle of Hg in the dark (Matthiessen, 1998). The redox properties of organic matter have been attributed to quinones, which function as intermediate electron shuttles during electron transfer (Scott et al., 1998; Bauer et al., 2007). A transfer of two electrons per quinone unit has been postulated, although it may actually take place in successive one-electron steps leading to one-electron radical intermediates known as *semiquinones* (Meisel and Fessenden, 1976; Rosso et al., 2004). Therefore, it was hypothesized that quinone or semiquinone moieties in organic matter are involved in electron transfer, leading to Hg(II) reduction (Alberts et al., 1974).

Isotope fractionation caused by non-photochemical reduction is dominated by MDF and NFS. In fact, the highest experimentally measured NFS is found during a kinetic reduction of $HgCl_2$ by natural DOM or $SnCl_2$ (Zheng and Hintelmann, 2010b). Negative isotope anomalies were produced in oxidized Hg(II) species with Δ^{199}Hg of up to −0.6‰ after 98% of the Hg(II) was reduced (Zheng and Hintelmann, 2010b). Under natural conditions, where the degree of Hg(II) reduction is not likely to reach >90%, the Δ^{199}Hg should be limited to −0.3‰ assuming a maximum reduction of ~70%. The relative contributions of MDF and NFS to the overall fractionation factor depend on the degree of differences in bond strengths and electron densities. For the reduction of $HgCl_2$, the contributions of MDF and NFS were experimentally determined to be ~40% and 60%, respectively (Zheng and Hintelmann, 2010b). The isotope fractionation seems to be independent of the reducing reagents since DOM and $SnCl_2$ generated very similar MDF and NFS.

So far, three processes were identified to induce NFS: evaporation, complexation, and reduction. Reduction generates the highest isotope anomalies, suggesting that it is subject to the strongest NFS. The magnitude of NFS is a measure of the shift in 6s orbital electron density of Hg. The change in electron density caused by gain or loss of electrons during redox reactions is much higher than that associated with evaporation or complexation, which do not change the redox state of Hg. NFS is also affected by the nature of the ligand, since they share electrons with the Hg(II) cation to different degrees. It is possible to model the contribution of NFS to overall fractionation factors using first-principle quantum mechanical theory for simple molecules (Schauble, 2007; Wiederhold et al., 2010). Wiederhold et al. (2010) presented density function theory (DFT) calculations for a variety of Hg(II)–chloro, Hg(II)–hydroxide, and Hg(II)–thiol complexes relative to elemental Hg vapor at 298 K. The contribution of NFS ranged from 46% to 85% with an average of 62%. These calculations are consistent with the experimental estimation in Zheng and Hintelmann (2010b) and an earlier theoretical work by Schauble (2007). In general, complexes with high ionic characteristic have higher NFS when they are reduced to Hg(0) vapor, such as the Hg(II) cation and $HgCl_4^-$, while more covalent complexes, such as Hg–thiol, $Hg(CH_3)_2$, and CH_3HgCl, tend to generate lower NFS.

Non-photochemical reduction can be easily distinguished from photochemical reduction using isotope fractionation. Large, positive isotope anomalies such as those observed in photochemical reduction are not likely expected in non-photochemical reduction since MIE is not induced. Also, the $\Delta^{199}Hg/\Delta^{201}Hg$ slope is different between these two reduction pathways. NFS typically generates a slope of 1.5–1.6, which is observed in both reduction (Zheng and Hintelmann, 2010b) and complexation (Wiederhold et al., 2010) reactions. This slope is substantially higher than that typically found during photochemical reduction (1.0–1.3; Bergquist and Blum, 2007; Zheng and Hintelmann, 2009). However, caution is in order when using $\Delta^{199}Hg/\Delta^{201}Hg$ slopes to differentiate reduction pathways since it is simply an empirical value, lacking any theoretical or mechanistic explanation. Also, photochemical reduction of Hg(II) is usually accompanied by concurrent non-photochemical reduction processes, and thus, the net $\Delta^{199}Hg/\Delta^{201}Hg$ observed during photochemical reduction may actually reflect a combination of MIEs and, to a lesser extent, NFS. Furthermore, the accuracy of this slope is limited by the number of data and the precision of Δ values. More thorough investigations of the origin and mechanisms controlling this slope are necessary before this parameter can be safely used for tracking Hg transformation pathways involving MIF.

9.2.4 Microbial Reduction of Hg(II) and Degradation of MMHg

Biological reduction of Hg(II) to Hg(0) is widespread among bacteria. The most extensively studied process is mediated by Hg-resistant microbes and involves the *mer* pathway, which is found in numerous aerobic Hg-resistant bacteria. Briefly, the *mer* system consists of periplasmatic MerP, which associates with Hg(II) and hands it over to the MerT transporter, which transfers Hg(II) to the cytoplasmatic mercuric reductase MerA. Kritee et al. (2007, 2008) conducted extensive experiments with gram negative bacteria, showing that the reduction by the *mer*-mediated pathway preferentially reduces lighter isotopes of Hg, causing a mass-dependent Rayleigh fractionation with ε^{202} between 1.20 and 2.00. They proposed a model for Hg-resistant bacteria, according to which the reduction of Hg(II) is the rate-limiting and fractionation-inducing step. Only in situations where the Hg(II) substrate is limited and concentrations are small relative to the number of bacterial cells, might the diffusion of Hg(II) toward and uptake by cells become rate limiting. These steps do not prefer one isotope over the other (at least not measurably) and progressively suppress the Hg isotope fractionation observed in the overall reduction process. While different strains show subtle differences in the extent of fractionation, the range is small and the composition of environmental bacterial communities is therefore not expected to affect the degree of Hg isotope fractionation during microbial reduction in Nature. In fact, a similar experiment with a natural microbial community yielded a $\varepsilon^{202} = 1.30$ (Kritee et al., 2007).

The biological degradation of MMHg is differentiated between an oxidative pathway producing Hg(II) and CO_2 and a reductive mechanism leading to CH_4 and Hg(0). The reductive pathway dominates in polluted sediments (Schaefer et al., 2004) and is also induced by enzymes related to the *mer* system. It is considered a detoxification mechanism and is found in "broad-spectrum" resistant bacteria. Similar to the reduction of Hg(II), the degradation of MMHg is a multistep process. The critical step is the cleaving of the Hg–C bond by organomercurial-lyase MerB, leading to the formation of Hg(II), which is subsequently reduced by mercuric reductase MerA to produce Hg(0). The oxidative mechanism seems to dominate at normal, nonelevated MMHg concentrations and is associated with methanogenic and sulfate-reducing bacteria (SRB) (Marvin-Dipasquale and Oremland, 1998; Hines et al., 2006). Unfortunately, very little is known about this pathway and to date, neither the molecular mechanisms nor specific bacterial strains involved in this process have been isolated. Experiments studying the fractionation of Hg isotopes during bacterial degradation of MMHg concentrated on the reductive pathway mediated by the *mer* system. This process consistently induced a mass-dependent Rayleigh fractionation with $\varepsilon^{202} = 0.40$ (Kritee et al., 2009). The authors suggest that the fractionation-inducing step during MMHg degradation is the cleaving of the Hg–C bond by MerB. This was deduced from a comparison of turnover rates, which are significantly higher for MerA compared to MerB and all steps following the catalyzed bond breakage should, therefore, not be rate limiting. As with the reduction process, the diffusion/uptake of MMHg dominates at high cell densities or low MMHg availability, and suppresses the overall Hg isotope fractionation during MMHg degradation.

It is important and critical to note that both biological pathways of Hg(II) reduction and MMHg degradation show no indication whatsoever for MIF, and all fractionation effects can solely be explained by MDF. This is to be expected, considering that the MIE requires a radical reaction pathway. Recent studies have shown a clear involvement of SH groups in the Hg–C bond cleavage with no evidence of radical formation (Melnick and Parkin, 2007) and Kritee et al. (2009)

convincingly explain why MIE effects during biological Hg transformations are highly unlikely. The absence of MIF clearly separates biological from photochemical processes. This distinction may serve as a powerful tool to differentiate between biotic and abiotic Hg transformation pathways in Nature. It may allow us to trace the recent "history" of Hg in the environment by simply monitoring the type of fractionation imprinted onto samples.

9.2.5 Methylation of Hg(II)

Methylation of mercury is a crucial biogeochemical process in the natural mercury cycle. There is a rich literature describing the reaction, which is deemed to be mediated mainly by sulfate-reducing bacteria in anaerobic environments (Hintelmann, 2010). The resulting organic methylmercury is highly toxic, bioaccumulates, and is of greatest concern from a human health point of view. Despite this overriding importance of MMHg spurring most of the research related to the environmental fate of mercury, there are surprisingly few studies that have investigated the fractionation of Hg isotopes during methylation. A possible explanation is the analytical challenge associated with this task. Unlike all the previously discussed studies, such experiments inevitably require the isolation of MMHg from the sample matrix for subsequent measurement of MMHg species, rather than a determination of the isotope ratios of the total Hg present in the sample. One study has tackled this challenge by extracting MMHg, followed by digestion to Hg(II) and conventional Hg isotope ratio determination (Jackson et al., 2008). A more sophisticated and technically more involved approach involves the chromatographic separation of MMHg from other species followed by on-line MC-ICP/MS measurement (Epov et al., 2008; Dzurko et al., 2009). Using the latter strategy, methylation experiments have been conducted with pure bacterial culture and the change in isotope ratios was monitored. By spiking pure cultures of *Desulfobulbus proprionicus* or *Desulfovibrio desulfuricans* with inorganic Hg(II), MMHg created by the SRB was systematically enriched with the light isotopes compared to the inorganic Hg used for the incubation. δ^{202}Hg values varied from $-1.71‰$ to $-0.78‰$ with an average value of $-1.15 \pm 0.26‰$ (Dzurko, 2006). Another study exposed Hg(II) to a different *Desulfobulbus proprionicus* strain under fermentative conditions observed $\varepsilon^{202} = 2.60$ (Rodriguez-Gonzalez et al., 2009). Not unexpectedly, neither of the two studies found any evidence for MIF during bacterial methylation of Hg(II).

9.3   Hg ISOTOPE VARIATIONS IN NATURE

In recent years, an increasing number of studies determined isotope compositions of Hg in natural samples, ranging from the Earth's upper mantle, crust, and surface to the hydrosphere and atmosphere. These studies greatly contributed to establishing a global and historical inventory and systematic of Hg isotopes. However, with the mounting evidence of natural variations in Hg isotope composition, a question remains: how are they related to the biogeochemical transformation of Hg? Enrichment of mercury from natural geogenic sources in the upper crust involves mobilization from mercury-containing source rocks, transport by hydrothermal fluids, deposition in ores, and dispersal into the adjacent and overlying lithosphere, hydrosphere, and atmosphere (Rytuba, 2005). Hg originating from different geogenic or anthropogenic sources may bear different initial isotope compositions. But they may be modified by subsequent processes, such as hydrothermal transport, ore deposition, and cycling in the biosphere, before they are recorded in natural samples. Therefore, it is critical to connect natural isotope compositions and preceding processes in order to establish an isotopic cycle of Hg in parallel to its speciation cycle. To illustrate the range of Hg isotope variation in Nature, Fig. 9.6 summarizes both MDF (δ^{202}Hg) and MIF signatures (Δ^{199}Hg) of Hg in environmental samples published to date.

9.3.1   Geogenic Hg (Mantle- and Crust-Derived Hg)

Geogenic Hg (sample no. 1–6 in Fig. 9.6) is mantle- and crust-derived Hg such as Hg from source rocks, hydrothermal systems, volcanic emission, and Hg minerals. They represent a more primordial and preindustrial source of Hg with less influence of anthropogenic contributions. Data for nonfractionated mantle and crust samples are still scarce since most geogenic Hg undergoes complex geochemical transformations, including equilibrium fluid–solid fractionation, kinetically controlled mass transfer, and redox reactions. Crustal rocks have a relatively narrow range of MDF with the bulk of samples having δ^{202}Hg of $-0.56 \pm 0.51\text{‰}$ (1 SD, $n = 35$) (Smith et al., 2008). Hydrothermal fluids have a slightly larger fractionation and more variation compared to source rocks with δ^{202}Hg = $-0.86 \pm 0.97\text{‰}$ (1 SD, $n = 32$) (Smith et al., 2008; Sherman et al., 2009). Volcanic emission is an important natural Hg source. Gaseous volcanic emissions have an MDF signature in between source rocks and hydrothermal fluids (δ^{202}Hg = $-0.71 \pm 0.30\text{‰}$, 1 SD, $n = 32$), while particulate emissions have a much lower fractionation, which results in lower overall MDF signatures for all volcanic samples (Zambardi et al., 2009). Metallic Hg and the primary mineral, cinnabar, mined worldwide fall well within the range of source rocks and hydrothermal systems. For example, metallic Hg mined from Almadén, Spain, the largest industrial source of Hg, has a δ^{202}Hg of -0.5 to -0.6‰ (Estrade et al., 2010b). A larger variation in MDF was also reported for other Hg minerals (e.g., metacinnabar, calomel, and terlinguaite) (Stetson et al., 2009). The reported Hg minerals are primarily hypogene in origin, formed by hydrothermal mineralization. Hg in crustal source rocks can be liberated by evaporation or leaching by hot fluids in the form of Hg(0), and is then transported in hydrothermal solutions. As the hydrothermal fluids move upward, the changing temperature and pressure cause the solubility of Hg to decrease and Hg can either escape via volatilization, which is proposed to account for the $\sim 1\text{‰}$ (δ^{202}Hg) fractionation between source rocks and hydrothermal system, or

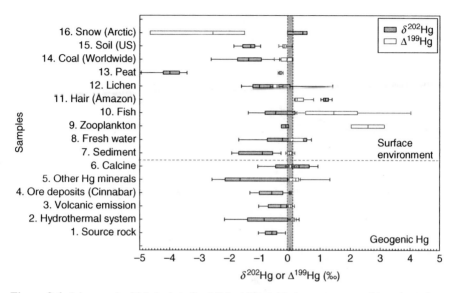

Figure 9.6 A box-and-whisker plot of published Hg stable isotope compositions in various natural samples. The box shows the 25th, 50th, and 75th quartiles and the whisker shows the 10th and 90th quartiles. δ^{202}Hg represents MDF signature, while Δ^{199}Hg represents MIF signature. The shaded band between -0.1 and 0.1‰ represents the general external reproducibility (2 SD) of analysis for isotope compositions. References for samples 1–16 are the following: 1. Smith et al. (2008), 2. Sherman et al. (2009) and Smith et al. (2008), 3. Zambardi et al. (2009), 4. Hintelmann and Lu (2003), Smith et al. (2008) and Stetson et al. (2009), 5. Stetson et al. (2009), 6. Stetson et al. (2009), 7. Feng et al. (2010), Foucher and Hintelmann (2006), Foucher et al. (2009), Gantner et al. (2009) and Gehrke et al. (2009), 8. Chen et al. (2010), 9. Gantner et al. (2009) and Jackson et al. (2008), 10. Bergquist and Blum (2007), Gantner et al. (2009), Jackson et al. (2008), Laffont et al. (2009) and Senn et al. (2010), 11. Laffont et al. (2009), 12. Carignan et al. (2009) and Estrade et al. (2010a), 13. Ghosh et al. (2008), 14. Biswas et al. (2008), 15. Biswas et al. (2008), and 16. Sherman et al. (2010).

can precipitate with sulfides as Hg minerals (e.g., cinnabar, HgS) or as impurities in other minerals (Krupp, 1988). Ore deposition is known to cause significant isotope fractionation for many elements, such as Fe (Butler et al., 2005; Markl et al., 2006b), Cu (Ehrlich et al., 2004; Markl et al., 2006a) and S (Ohmoto and Rye, 1979). For example, the formation of FeS and CuS from Fe(II) and Cu(II) can enrich lighter isotopes in FeS and CuS (Ehrlich et al., 2004; Markl et al., 2006b). Likewise, precipitation of HgS leads to small enrichment of lighter isotopes in HgS. Foucher (2008) found that δ^{202}Hg increased by 0.2‰ in the dissolved phase after >80% of Hg had disappeared from solution. This effect may partially account for the span of negative MDF signature determined in Hg minerals compared to source rocks. It is interesting to note that almost all geogenic Hg shows negative MDF (δ^{202}Hg<0), while calcine, a common retorted ore residue in mining areas, shows positive δ^{202}Hg of up to 1‰. Extraction of Hg during mining is generally carried out in a retort or a rotary furnace by heating Hg ore to $600-700°C$. This process is usually incomplete and therefore preferentially releases lighter isotopes, resulting in heavier $\delta^{202}Hg$ in the calcine compared to the original ore (Stetson et al., 2009).

MIF in geogenic Hg samples is generally very small with $\Delta^{199}Hg$ typically below 0.2‰. Considering the importance of redox reactions in geogenic processes, the lack of MIF suggests that photochemical reactions or other reactions that produce paramagnetic intermediates are not significant during the formation of geogenic Hg samples, as would be expected for processes occurring deep in the Earth.

9.3.2   Hg in Aquatic Systems, Food Webs, and the Atmosphere

Once Hg is exposed to the Earth's surface, it enters the geochemical cycle in land, water, food webs, and atmosphere. In general, Hg isotope compositions in the biosphere show larger variations than geogenic Hg (sample no. 7–16 in Fig. 9.6). Higher mobility of Hg, more involvement of microbial and photochemical processes in solution and gas phase and increased anthropogenic effects may contribute to the larger isotope fractionation. Sediment and fresh water have quite different MDF signatures. Sediment is more influenced by geogenic Hg and tends to retain anthropogenic contributions, while aqueous Hg is more exposed to photochemical and microbial reactions, affected by precipitation and replenished by surface runoff, atmospheric deposition, and resuspension from sediment. However, to date, only one study has reported isotope data in fresh water samples (Chen et al., 2010). With this very limited body of information, it is currently difficult to ascertain the MDF signature of fresh water. Trophic transfer within aquatic food webs is found to induce isotope fractionation. For example, the hair of Amazon indigenous people, who have a daily fish diet, is enriched in heavier isotopes by $\sim 1-2‰$ ($\delta^{202}Hg$) compared to fish (Laffont et al., 2009), suggesting that metabolic process such as excretion of faeces, *in vivo* demethylation, and blood–hair transport may be responsible for the variation of MDF with trophic levels. Samples that act as reservoirs of atmospheric Hg such as lichen, peat, coal, and soil (sample no. 12–15 in Fig. 9.6) have generally lighter MDF signatures compared to aquatic samples, which may indicate that lighter isotopes are preferentially released into the atmosphere by both natural and anthropogenic sources. Arctic snow is subject to strong photochemical reduction, resulting in an enrichment of heavy isotopes relative to other atmospheric reservoirs.

MIF is particularly powerful in tracking Hg cycles in these surface reservoirs. So far, the most pronounced MIF determined in natural samples is (+)MIE, which produces positive $\Delta^{199}Hg$ in aquatic samples (fresh water, zooplankton, fish, and human hair) and negative $\Delta^{199}Hg$ in atmospheric deposition (e.g., lichen, peat, and coal). For example, the Hg isotope signature in coal is a complex combination of atmospheric, terrestrial, aquatic, and hydrothermal inputs in the initial coal-forming environment. It is difficult to discern the contributions of these inputs using $\delta^{202}Hg$. However, depletion of ^{199}Hg and ^{201}Hg with up to $-0.6‰$ of $\Delta^{199}Hg$ was found in coal worldwide, indicating a significant atmospheric input that is likely modified by photochemical reduction of Hg(II) (Biswas et al., 2008). Contrarily, fish and other aquatic organisms showed significant enrichment of ^{199}Hg and ^{201}Hg, which is in accordance with the MIF observed in the remaining Hg(II) reservoir during photochemical reduction. Diverse aquatic species and atmospheric depositions from various locations showed primarily (+)MIE signatures, suggesting that a significant amount of Hg in the global environment is likely to have undergone photochemical transformations. This provides further evidence of the dominance of photochemical reduction of Hg(II) and degassing of Hg(0) as the source of atmospheric Hg. Although less common, (−)MIE can also occur in Nature and has been reported for arctic snow, where negative Δ^{199}Hg of up to −5‰ has been found (Sherman et al., 2010). While the mechanism is not yet clear, it is presumably related to photochemical reactions within the snow pack.

9.4 SUMMARY

The increasing concern of the environmental contamination of Hg calls for a better understanding of its sources and fate in Nature. Research on the fractionation of stable isotope of Hg has come a long way from the early beginnings a decade ago. Studies investigating Hg isotope fractionation during transformation processes and measurements of Hg isotope composition in various natural reservoirs are working hand in hand to provide new insights into factors controlling the biogeochemical cycling of Hg (Fig. 9.7). Nevertheless, most of what we know today about natural Hg isotope variations is limited to sample matrices with Hg concentrations sufficiently high for isotopic measurements. Our map of the Hg isotope systems still shows a large number of blank spots. The Hg isotope composition in natural waters including precipitation, atmospheres, and the lower food web remains largely unknown. Likewise, significant knowledge gaps still exist for Hg isotope fractionation associated with aquatic processes, such as adsorption/desorption, demethylation, and oxidation, and the entire atmospheric Hg cycle has not yet characterized for Hg isotope fractionation at all.

From an Hg management point of view, one question commonly arises when assessing Hg isotope ratios to connect the Hg found in the environment with potential sources. It is tempting to compare the Hg signature found in, for example, sediments or biota with those known for fossil fuels such as coal. But before jumping to conclusions, one must consider if the measured environmental signature reflects the source signatures or if and to which degree the original source signature was altered by geochemical process such as those described in this chapter or even obscured during mixing of atmospheric Hg pools of different composition. These questions can ultimately only be answered by having a sound understanding of the Hg isotope system. More detailed mechanistic studies are still required to complete the theoretical framework of the Hg isotope system. Already, the unique MIF effect observed for Hg isotopes under distinct situations is an effective means helping us connect the dots.

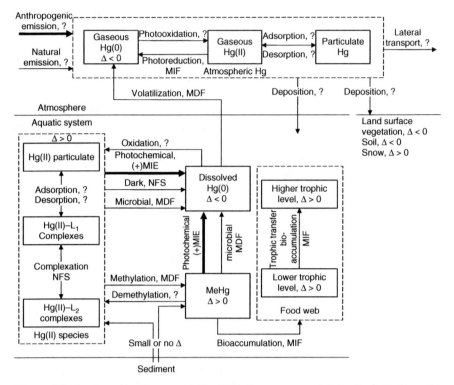

Figure 9.7 A schematic diagram of Hg speciation accompanied by its isotopic cycle. Thicker arrows represent the predominant processes. Isotope fractionation during many transformations is still unknown (denoted as "?").

REFERENCES

Alberts JJ, Schindler JE, Miller RWDEN. Elemental mercury evolution mediated by humic acid. Science 1974;184:895–897.

Allard B, Arsenie I. Abiotic reduction of mercury by humic substances in aquatic system-an important process for the mercury cycle. Water, Air, Soil Pollut 1991;56:457–464.

Amyot M, Gill GA, Morel FMM. Production and loss of dissolved gaseous mercury in coastal seawater. Environ Sci Technol 1997a;31:3606–3611.

Amyot M, Mierle G, Lean D, McQueen DJ. Effect of solar radiation on the formation of dissolved gaseous mercury in temperate lakes. Geochim Cosmochim Acta 1997b;61:975–987.

Amyot M, Mierle G, Lean DRS, Mcqueen DJ. Sunlight-induced formation of dissolved gaseous mercury in lake waters. Environ Sci Technol 1994;28:2366–2371.

Bauer M, Heitmann T, Macalady DL, Blodau C. Electron transfer capacities and reaction kinetics of peat dissolved organic matter. Environ Sci Technol 2007;41:139–145.

Bergquist BA, Blum JD. Mass-dependent and -independent fractionation of Hg isotopes by photoreduction in aquatic systems. Science 2007;318:417–420.

Bigeleisen, J. Theoretical basis of isotope effects from an autobiographical perspective. In: Kohen A, Limbach H-H, editors. Isotope effects in chemistry and biology. Boca Raton (FL): CRC Press, Taylor & Francis Group; 2006. p 1–39.

Bigeleisen J, Mayer MG. Calculation of equilibrium constants for isotopic exchange reactions. J Chem Phys 1947;15:261–267.

Biswas A, Blum JD, Bergquist BA, Keeler GJ, Xie ZQ. Natural mercury isotope variation in coal deposits and organic soils. Environ Sci Technol 2008;42:8303–8309.

Blum JD, Bergquist BA. Reporting of variations in the natural isotopic composition of mercury. Anal Bioanal Chem 2007;388:353–359.

Braden DA, Parrack EE, Tyler DR. Solvent cage effects. I. Effect of radical mass and size on radical cage pair recombination efficiency. II. Is germinate recombination of polar radicals sensitive to solvent polarity? Coord Chem Rev 2001;211:279–294.

Buchachenko AL. Magnetic isotope effect: nuclear spin control of chemical reactions. J Phys Chem A 2001;105:9995–10011.

Buchachenko AL. Mercury isotope effects in the environmental chemistry and biochemistry of mercury-containing compounds. Russ Chem Rev 2009;78:319–328.

Buchachenko AL, Ivanov VL, Roznyatovskii VA, Artamkina GA, Vorob'ev AK, Ustynyuk YA. Magnetic isotope effect for mercury nuclei in photolysis of bis(p-trifluoromethylbenzyl)mercury. Dokl Phys Chem 2007;413:39–41.

Buchachenko AL, Kouznetsov DA, Shishkov AV. Spin biochemistry: magnetic isotope effect in the reaction of creatine kinase with CH_3HgCl. J Phys Chem A 2004;108:707–710.

Butler IB, Archer C, Vance D, Oldroyd A, Rickard D. Fe isotope fractionation on FeS formation in ambient aqueous solution. Earth Planet Sci Lett 2005;236:430–442.

Carignan J, Estrade N, Sonke JE, Donard OFX. Odd isotope deficits in atmospheric Hg measured in Lichens. Environ Sci Technol 2009;43:5660–5664.

Chen JB, Hintelmann H, Dimock B. Chromatographic pre-concentration of Hg from dilute aqueous solutions for isotopic measurement by MC-ICP-MS. J Anal At Spectrom 2010;25:1402–1409.

Criss RE. Principles of stable isotope distribution. Isotopic Exchange and Equilibrium fractionation. New York: Oxford University Press; 1999, p 40–88.

Das R, Salters VJM, Odom AL. A case for *in vivo* mass-independent fractionation of mercury isotopes in fish. Geochem Geophy Geosy 2009;10: Q11012. DOI: 11010.11029/12009GC002617.

Drexel RT, Haitzer M, Ryan JN, Aiken GR, Nagy KL. Mercury(II) sorption to two Florida everglades peats: evidence for strong and weak binding and competition by dissolved organic matter released from the peat. Env iron Sci Technol 2002;36:4058–4064.

Dzurko M, Foucher D, Hintelmann H. Determination of compound-specific Hg isotope ratios from transient signals using gas chromatography coupled to multicollector inductively coupled plasma mass spectrometry (MC-ICP/MS). Anal Bioanal Chem 2009;393:345–355.

Dzurko MS. Fractionation of mercury isotopes during methylation by sulfate-reducing bacteria [MSc Thesis]. Peterborough (ON): Trent University; 2006.

Ehrlich S, Butler I, Halicz L, Rickard D, Oldroyd A, Matthews A. Experimental study of the copper isotope fractionation between aqueous Cu(II) and covellite, CuS. Chem Geol 2004;209:259–269.

Epov VN, Rodriguez-Gonzalez P, Sonke JE, Tessier E, Amouroux D, Bourgoin LM, Donard OFX. Simultaneous determination of species-specific isotopic composition of Hg by gas chromatography coupled to multicollector ICPMS. Anal Chem 2008;80:3530–3538.

Estrade N, Carignan J, Sonke JE, Donard OFX. Mercury isotope fractionation during liquid-vapor evaporation experiments. Geochim Cosmochim Acta 2009;73:2693–2711.

Estrade N, Carignan J, Donard OFX. Isotope tracing of atmospheric mercury sources in an urban area of northeastern France. Environ Sci Technol 2010a;44:6062–6067.

Estrade N, Carignan J, Sonke JE, Donard OFX. Measuring Hg isotopes in bio-geo-environmental reference materials. Geostand Geoanal Res 2010b;34:79–93.

Fantozzi L, Ferrarac R, Frontini FP, Dini F. Dissolved gaseous mercury production in the dark: evidence for the fundamental role of bacteria in different types of Mediterranean water bodies. Sci Total Environ 2009;407:917–924.

Feng X, Foucher D, Hintelmann H, Yan H, He T, Qiu G. Tracing mercury contamination sources in sediments using mercury isotope compositions. Environ Sci Technol 2010;44:3363–3368.

Fitzgerald WF, Lamborg CH. Geochemistry of mercury in the environment. Treatise on Geochemistry 2003;9:107–148.

Foucher D, Hintelmann H. High-precision measurement of mercury isotope ratios in sediments using cold-vapor generation multi-collector inductively coupled plasma mass spectrometry. Anal Bioanal Chem 2006;384:1470–1478.

Foucher D, Trent University, Peterborough (ON). Personal communication. February 29, 2008.

Foucher D, Ogrinc N, Hintelmann H. Tracing mercury contamination from the Idrija mining region (Slovenia) to the gulf of trieste using Hg isotope ratio measurements. Environ Sci Technol 2009;43:33–39.

Gabriel MC, Williamson DG. Principal biogeochemical factors affecting the speciation and transport of mercury through the terrestrial environment. Environ Geochem Health 2004;26:421–434.

Gantner N, Hintelmann H, Zheng W, Muir DC. Variations in stable isotope fractionation of Hg in food webs of Arctic lakes. Environ Sci Technol 2009;43:9148–9154.

Garcia E, Amyot M, Ariya PA. Relationship between DOC photochemistry and mercury redox transformations in temperate lakes and wetlands. Geochim Cosmochim Acta 2005;69:1917–1924.

Gehrke GE, Blum JD, Meyers PA. The geochemical behavior and isotopic composition of Hg in a mid-Pleistocene western Mediterranean sapropel. Geochim Cosmochim Acta 2009;73:1651–1665.

Ghosh S, Xu YF, Humayun M, Odom L. Mass-independent fractionation of mercury isotopes in the environment. Geochem Geophys Geosyst 2008;9: Q03004. DOI: 03010.01029/02007gc001827.

Haitzer M, Aiken GR, Ryan JN. Binding of mercury(II) to dissolved organic matter: The role of the mercury-to-DOM concentration ratio. Environ Sci Technol 2002;36:3564–3570.

Hesterberg D, Chou JW, Hutchison KJ, Sayers DE. Bonding of Hg(II) to reduced organic, sulfur in humic acid as affected by S/Hg ratio. Environ Sci Technol 2001;35:2741–2745.

Hines ME, Faganeli J, Adatto I, Horvat M. Microbial mercury transformations in marine, estuarine and freshwater sediment downstream of the Idrija mercury mine, Slovenia. Appl Geochem 2006;21:1924–1939.

Hintelmann H. Organomercurials. Their formation and pathways in the environment. In: Sigel A, Sigel H, Sigel RKO, editors. Organometallics in environment and toxicology: Volume 7 of Metal Ions in Life Sciences. Cambridge: Royal Society of Chemistry; 2010. p 365–401.

Hintelmann H, Lu SY. High precision isotope ratio measurements of mercury isotopes in cinnabar ores using multi-collector inductively coupled plasma mass spectrometry. Analyst 2003;128:635–639.

Hintelmann H, Ogrinc N. Determination of stable mercury isotopes by ICP/MS and their application in environmental studies. In: Cai Y, Braids OC, editors. Biogeochemistry of environmentally important trace elements. Washington (DC): Amer Chemical Soc; 2003. p 321–338.

Jackson TA, Whittle DM, Evans MS, Muir DCG. Evidence for mass-independent and mass-dependent fractionation of the stable isotopes of mercury by natural processes in aquatic ecosystems. Appl Geochem 2008;23:547–571.

Johnson TM. A review of mass-dependent fractionation of selenium isotopes and implications for other heavy stable isotopes. Chem Geol 2004;204:201–214.

Johnson CM, Beard BL, Roden EE. The iron isotope fingerprints of redox and biogeochemical cycling in the modern and ancient Earth. Annu Rev Earth Planet Sci 2008;36:457–493.

King WH. Isotope shifts in atomic spectra, New York: Plenum Press; 1984.

Kritee K, Barkay T, Blum JD. Mass dependent stable isotope fractionation of mercury during mer mediated microbial degradation of monomethylmercury. Geochim Cosmochim Acta 2009;73:1285–1296.

Kritee K, Blum JD, Barkay T. Mercury stable isotope fractionation during reduction of Hg(II) by different microbial pathways. Environ Sci Technol 2008;42:9171–9177.

Kritee K, Blum JD, Johnson MW, Bergquist BA, Barkay T. Mercury stable isotope fractionation during reduction of Hg(II) to Hg(0) by mercury resistant microorganisms. Environ Sci Technol 2007;41:1889–1895.

Krupp R. Physicochemical aspects of mercury metallogenesis. Chem Geol 1988;69:345–356.

Laffont L, Sonke JE, Maurice L, Hintelmann H, Pouilly M, Sanchez Bacarreza Y, Perez T, Behra P. Anomalous mercury isotopic compositions of fish and human hair in the Bolivian Amazon. Environ Sci Technol 2009;43:8985–8990.

Lalonde JD, Amyot M, Doyon MR, Auclair JC. Photo-induced Hg(II) reduction in snow from the remote and temperate experimental lakes area (Ontario, Canada). J Geophys Res-Atmos 2003;108:4200–4207.

Lanzillotta E, Ceccarini C, Ferrara R. Photo-induced formation of dissolved gaseous mercury in coastal and offshore seawater of the Mediterranean basin. Sci Total Environ 2002;300:179–187.

Lauretta DS, Klaue B, Blum JD, Buseck PR. Mercury abundances and isotopic compositions in the Murchison (CM) and Allende (CV) carbonaceous chondrites. Geochim Cosmochim Acta 2001;65:2807–2818.

Lindberg SE, Brooks S, Lin CJ, Scott KJ, Landis MS, Stevens RK, Goodsite M, Richter A. Dynamic oxidation of gaseous mercury in the Arctic troposphere at polar sunrise. Environ Sci Technol 2002;36:1245–1256.

Lindqvist O, Johansson K, Aastrup M, Andersson A, Bringmark L, Hovsenius G, Hakanson L, Iverfeldt A, Meili M, Timm B. Mercury in the Swedish environment-recent research on causes, consequences and corrective methods. Water, Air, Soil Pollut 1991;55: xi–261.

Lyons JR, Young ED. CO self-shielding as the origin of oxygen isotope anomalies in the early solar nebula. Nature 2005;435:317–320.

Malinovsky D, Latruwe K, Moens L, Vanhaecke F. Experimental study of mass-independence of Hg isotope fractionation during photodecomposition of dissolved methylmercury. J Anal At Spectrom 2010;25:950–956.

Markl G, von Blanckenburg F, Wagner T. Iron isotope fractionation during hydrothermal ore deposition and alteration. Geochim Cosmochim Acta 2006b;70:3011–3030.

Markl G, Lahaye Y, Schwinn G. Copper isotopes as monitors of redox processes in hydrothermal mineralization. Geochim Cosmochim Acta 2006a;70:4215–4228.

Marvin-Dipasquale MC, Oremland RS. Bacterial methylmercury degradation in Florida Everglades peat sediment. Environ Sci Technol 1998;32:2556–2563.

Mason RP, Fitzgerald WF, Morel FMM. The biogeochemical cycling of elemental mercury-anthropogenic influences. Geochim Cosmochim Acta 1994;58:3191–3198.

Mason RP, Morel FMM, Hemond HF. The role of microorganisms in elemental mercury formation in natural-waters. Water, Air, Soil Pollut 1995;80:775–787.

Matthiessen A. Reduction of divalent mercury by humic substances-kinetic and quantitative aspects. Sci Total Environ 1998;213:177–183.

Mead C, Anbar AD, Johnson TM. Mass-independent fractionation of Hg isotopes resulting from photochemical self-shielding. Geochim Cosmochim Acta 2010;74: A649–A743.

Meija J, Yang L, Sturgeon R, Mester Z. Mass bias fractionation laws for multi-collector ICPMS: assumptions and their experimental verification. Anal Chem 2009;81:6774–6778.

Meisel D, Fessenden RW. Electron exchange and electron transfer of semiquinones in aqueous solutions. J Am Chem Soc 1976;98:7505–7510.

Melnick JG, Parkin G. Cleaving mercury-alkyl bonds: a functional model for mercury detoxification by MerB. Science 2007;317:225–227.

Nadjakov EG, Marinova KP, Gangrsky YP. Systematics of nuclear-charge radii. At Data Nucl Data Tables 1994;56:133–157.

O'Driscoll NJ, Lean DRS, Loseto LL, Carignan R, Siciliano SD. Effect of dissolved organic carbon on the photoproduction of dissolved gaseous mercury in lakes: potential impacts of forestry. Environ Sci Technol 2004;38:2664–2672.

Oelkers AB, Tyler DR. Radical cage effects: a method for measuring recombination efficiencies of secondary geminate radical cage pairs using pump-probe transient absorption methods. Photochem Photobiol Sci 2008;7:1386–1390.

Ohmoto H, Rye R. Isotopes of sulfur and carbon. In: Barnes HL, editor. Geochemistry of hydrothermal ore deposits. 2nd ed. New York: John Wiley & Sons; 1979. p 509–567.

Poulain AJ, Amyot M, Findlay D, Telor S, Barkay T, Hintelmann H. Biological and photochemical production of dissolved gaseous mercury in a boreal lake. Limnol Oceanogr 2004;49:2265–2275.

Ravichandran M. Interactions between mercury and dissolved organic matter-a review. Chemosphere 2004;55:319–331.

Rodriguez-Gonzalez P, Epov VN, Bridou R, Tessier E, Guyoneaud R, Monperrus M, Amouroux D. Species-specific stable isotope fractionation of mercury during Hg(II) methylation by an anaerobic bacteria (*Desulfobulbus propionicus*) under dark conditions. Environ Sci Technol 2009;43.9183–9188.

Rolfhus KR, Fitzgerald WF. Mechanisms and temporal variability of dissolved gaseous mercury production in coastal seawater. Mar Chem 2004;90:125–136.

Rosman KJR, Taylor PDP. Isotopic compositions of the elements 1997. Pure Appl Chem 1998;70:217–235.

Rosso KM, Smith DMA, Wang ZM, Ainsworth CC, Fredrickson JK. Self-exchange electron transfer kinetics and reduction potentials for anthraquinone disulfonate. J Phys Chem A 2004;108:3292–3303.

Rytuba JJ. Geogenic and mining sources of mercury to the environment. In: Parsons MB, Percival JB, editors. Mercury: sources, measurement, cycles and effects. Halifax (NS): Mineralogical Association of Canada; 2005. p 21–41.

Schaefer JK, Yagi J, Reinfelder JR, Cardona T, Ellickson KM, Tel-Or S, Barkay T. Role of the bacterial organomercury lyase (MerB) in controlling methylmercury accumulation in mercury-contaminated natural waters. Environ Sci Technol 2004;38:4304–4311.

Schauble EA. Role of nuclear volume in driving equilibrium stable isotope fractionation of mercury, thallium, and other very heavy elements. Geochim Cosmochim Acta 2007;71:2170–2189.

Schuster E. The behavior of mercury in the soil with special emphasis on complexation and adsorption processes-a review of the literature. Water, Air, Soil Pollut 1991;56:667–680.

Scott DT, McKnight DM, Blunt-Harris EL, Kolesar SE, Lovley DR. Quinone moieties act as electron acceptors in the reduction of humic substances by humics-reducing microorganisms. Environ Sci Technol 1998;32:2984–2989.

Senn DB, Chesney EJ, Blum JD, Bank MS, Maage A, Shine JP. Stable isotope (N, C, Hg) study of methylmercury sources and trophic transfer in the northern gulf of Mexico. Environ Sci Technol 2010;44:1630–1637.

Sherman LS, Blum JD, Johnson KP, Keeler GJ, Barres JA, Douglas TA. Mass-independent fractionation of mercury isotopes in Arctic snow driven by sunlight. Nat Geosci 2010;3:173–177.

Sherman LS, Blum JD, Nordstrom DK, McCleskey RB, Barkay T, Vetriani C. Mercury isotopic composition of hydrothermal systems in the Yellowstone Plateau volcanic field and Guaymas Basin sea-floor rift. Earth Planet Sci Lett 2009;279:86–96.

Siciliano SD, O'Driscoll NJ, Lean DRS. Microbial reduction and oxidation of mercury in freshwater lakes. Environ Sci Technol 2002;36:3064–3068.

Smith CN, Kesler SE, Blum JD, Rytuba JJ. Isotope geochemistry of mercury in source rocks, mineral deposits and spring deposits of the California Coast Ranges, USA. Earth Planet Sci Lett 2008;269:398–406.

Smith CN, Kesler SE, Klaue B, Blum JD. Mercury isotope fractionation in fossil hydrothermal systems. Geology 2005;33:825–828.

Southworth G, Lindberg S, Hintelmann H, Amyot M, Poulain A, Bogle M, Peterson M, Rudd J, Harris R, Sandilands K, Krabbenhoft D, Olsen M. Evasion of added isotopic mercury from a northern temperate lake. Environ Toxicol Chem 2007;26:53–60.

Steiner UE, Ulrich T. Magnetic-field effects in chemical-kinetics and related phenomena. Chem Rev 1989;89:51–147.

Stetson SJ, Gray JE, Wanty RB, Macalady DL. Isotopic variability of mercury in ore, mine-waste calcine, and leachates of mine-waste calcine from areas mined for mercury. Environ Sci Technol 2009;43:7331–7336.

Thiemens MH. Mass-independent isotope effects and their use in understanding natural processes. Isr J Chem 2002;42:43–54.

Thiemens MH, Heinrich DH, Karl KT. Non-mass-dependent isotopic fractionation processes: mechanisms and recent observations in terrestrial and extraterrestrial environments. In: Keeling RF, editor. Treatise on Geochemistry. Oxford: Pergamon; 2007. p 1–24.

Turro NJ. Influence of nuclear-spin on chemical-reactions-magnetic isotope and magnetic-field effects (a review). Proc Natl Acad Sci USA 1983;80:609–621.

Turro NJ, Kraeutler B. Magnetic field and magnetic isotope effects in organic photochemical reactions. A novel probe of reaction mechanisms and a method for enrichment of magnetic isotopes. Acc Chem Res 1980;13:369–377.

Ullrich SM, Tanton TW, Abdrashitova SA. Mercury in the aquatic environment: a review of factors affecting methylation. Crit Rev Env Sci Tec 2001;31:241–293.

Wallschlager D, Desai MVM, Wilken RD. The role of humic substances in the aqueous mobilization of mercury from contaminated floodplain soils. Water, Air, and Soil Pollut 1996;90:507–520.

Wiederhold JG, Cramer CJ, Daniel K, Infante I, Bourdon B, Kretzschmar R. Equilibrium mercury isotope fractionation between dissolved Hg(II) species and thiol-bound Hg. Environ Sci Technol 2010;44:4191–4197.

Wombacher F, Rehkamper M, Mezger K, Munker C. Stable isotope compositions of cadmium in geological materials and meteorites determined by multiple-collector ICPMS. Geochim Cosmochim Acta 2003;67:4639–4654.

Xia K, Skyllberg UL, Bleam WF, Bloom PR, Nater EA, Helmke PA. X-ray absorption spectroscopic evidence for the complexation of Hg(II) by reduced sulfur in soil humic substances. Environ Sci Technol 1999;33:257–261.

Xiao ZF, Stromberg D, Lindqvist O. Influence of humic substances on photolysis of divalent mercury in aqueous-solution. Water, Air, Soil Pollut 1995;80:789–798.

Xie QL, Lu SY, Evans D, Dillon P, Hintelmann H. High precision Hg isotope analysis of environmental samples using gold trap-MC-ICP-MS. J Anal At Spectrom 2005;20:515–522.

Yang L, Sturgeon RE. Comparison of mass bias correction models for the examination of isotopic composition of mercury using sector field ICP-MS. J Anal At Spectrom 2003;18:1452–1457.

Yang L, Sturgeon R. Isotopic fractionation of mercury induced by reduction and ethylation. Anal Bioanal Chem 2009;393:377–385.

Young ED, Galy A, Nagahara H. Kinetic and equilibrium mass-dependent isotope fractionation laws in nature and their geochemical and cosmochemical significance. Geochim Cosmochim Acta 2002;66:1095–1104.

Zambardi T, Sonke JE, Toutain JP, Sortino F, Shinohara H. Mercury emissions and stable isotopic compositions at Vulcano Island (Italy). Earth Planet Sci Lett 2009;277:236–243.

Zhang H. Photochemical redox reactions of mercury. In: Atwood DA, editor Recent Developments in Mercury Science. Berlin, Germany: Springer; 2006. p 37–79.

Zheng W, Foucher D, Hintelmann H. Mercury isotope fractionation during volatilization of Hg(0) from solution into the gas phase. J Anal At Spectrom 2007;22:1097–1104.

Zheng W, Hintelmann H. Mercury isotope fractionation during photoreduction in natural water is controlled by its Hg/DOC ratio. Geochim Cosmochim Acta 2009;73:6704–6715.

Zheng W, Hintelmann H. Isotope fractionation of mercury during its photochemical reduction by low-molecular-weight organic compounds. J Phys Chem A 2010a;114:4246–4253.

Zheng W, Hintelmann H. Nuclear field shift effect in isotope fractionation of mercury during abiotic reduction in the absence of light. J Phys Chem 2010b;A 114:4238–4245.

PART III

TRANSPORT AND FATE

CHAPTER 10

ATMOSPHERIC TRANSPORT OF MERCURY

OLEG TRAVNIKOV

10.1 INTRODUCTION

Atmospheric transport plays a central role in the dispersion of Hg in the global environment. Once released into the atmosphere because of natural processes or human activities, Hg is easily transported with air masses over long distances and moves between the continents, reaching even remote regions. In contrast to the cycling in terrestrial and aquatic compartments, Hg dispersion in the atmosphere is global and occurs on much shorter timescales than for oceanic transport owing to the more intensive dynamics of atmospheric circulation. Mercury differs from other atmospheric pollutants (such as tropospheric ozone and dust particles) in that its major exposure routes are not directly related to ambient air concentrations. While Hg is mainly distributed throughout the atmosphere, its primary environmental and health impacts are through deposition to aquatic ecosystems, bioaccumulation in aquatic organisms, and consumption of these by humans and wildlife (Mahaffey et al., 2004; Mason et al., 2010; Sunderland et al., 2010). Therefore, deposition on the Earth's surface is an essential part of the Hg route from an emission source to final exposure. These and other aspects of mercury transport in the atmosphere are discussed below.

10.2 GENERAL CONCEPTS OF MERCURY CYCLING IN THE ATMOSPHERE

The peculiar nature of Hg atmospheric transport is defined by two factors: chemical speciation and a long overall residence time in the atmosphere. Mercury is found in the atmosphere in a number of chemical forms with distinctively

Environmental Chemistry and Toxicology of Mercury, First Edition.
Edited by Guangliang Liu, Yong Cai, and Nelson O'Driscoll.
© 2012 John Wiley & Sons, Inc. Published 2012 by John Wiley & Sons, Inc.

different properties. The bulk species, accounting for more than 95% of total atmospheric Hg, is gaseous elemental mercury (GEM or Hg(0)). Owing to its relatively low solubility, it is poorly removed from the atmosphere by precipitation (wet deposition) or surface uptake (dry deposition). Therefore, the major removal mechanism controlling the residence time of Hg(0) in the atmosphere is oxidation to divalent Hg forms (Hg(II)), which occur in both the gaseous phase and as part of aerosol particles. The former, operationally defined as reactive gaseous mercury (RGM), is a highly soluble gas and therefore is subject to rapid removal from the air by wet or dry deposition. The latter (particulate Hg or HgP) represents a tiny part of aerosol composition and reflects the removal properties of fine atmospheric aerosols.

The average atmospheric residence time of Hg(0) is estimated to be 0.5–1 year (Selin, 2009). However, this parameter can significantly vary throughout the atmosphere because of the heterogeneity of oxidation chemistry, depending on the concentration of major oxidants and the ambient conditions. In particular, fast oxidation reactions with reactive halogens lead to a decrease in the Hg(0) residence time in polar regions, the marine boundary layer (MBL), and probably in the upper troposphere (Lindberg et al., 2007). Oxidized Hg forms (RGM and HgP) are characterized by a much shorter residence time—hours to days for RGM and days to weeks for HgP—owing to their rapid removal from the atmosphere by precipitation or surface uptake. Thus, the different Hg forms play diverse roles in the global Hg atmospheric cycle. Gaseous elemental Hg is largely responsible for long-range transport, whereas short-lived RGM and HgP account for removal to the ground. It should be noted that Hg(0) also contributes to the removal process via direct air–surface exchange with vegetation (Gustin and Lindberg, 2005). However, this bidirectional process is relatively slow and rather affects the long-term Hg environmental cycle than particular atmospheric transport mechanisms.

The list of mercury species in the atmosphere is not complete without mention of the aqueous forms. It is expected that both elemental and oxidized forms can dissolve in cloud water and participate in various redox reactions in the aqueous phase (Lin et al., 2006). In spite of the low solubility of Hg(0), it can make a considerable contribution to aqueous Hg chemistry given that its ambient concentrations in free troposphere are commonly two orders of magnitude higher than those of RGM and HgP (Schroeder and Munthe, 1998). The aqueous chemistry includes both oxidation and reduction pathways in reactions with different reactive species dissolved in cloud water (ozone, reactive radicals, sulfur and chlorine compounds, etc.). Ultimately, all aqueous Hg species are washed out from the atmosphere during precipitation events. Thus, aqueous phase chemistry can be considered an additional removal mechanism contributing to Hg wet deposition.

Mercury species are released into the atmosphere from a variety of emission sources associated with natural processes and human activities (see Chapter 1 for more details). Conceptually, sources can be classified into three types: primary natural, primary anthropogenic, and combined secondary sources (Mason et al., 2010). Primary natural sources include Hg releases from volcanic and geothermal activity and emissions from areas geologically enriched in mercury (Fitzgerald and Lamborg, 2005; Mason, 2009; Selin, 2009). Primary anthropogenic sources involve Hg emissions from human activities associated with combustion of fossil fuels, mining, and industrial processes (Pacyna et al., 2009; Pirrone et al., 2009). Combined secondary sources involve reemission into the atmosphere of previously deposited Hg owing to natural or human-induced processes. Mercury is emitted from anthropogenic sources in both elemental and oxidized forms, while natural and secondary Hg emissions are dominated by Hg(0). The chemical speciation of emissions largely affects further Hg fate in the atmosphere, in particular, the relative contribution of emitted Hg to local/regional deposition versus contribution to long-range atmospheric transport.

Once emitted into the atmosphere, the fate of Hg species differs. Short-lived RGM and HgP are readily removed from the air via wet and dry deposition and mostly contribute to local or regional-scale deposition. Conversely, elemental Hg is largely involved in atmospheric circulation and long-range transport. Atmospheric transport may occur both near the Earth's surface in the planetary boundary layer and in the free troposphere, where winds are usually much stronger. Although Hg, as well as other pollutants, is released into the atmospheric boundary layer, it may be transported upward by a number of mechanisms (including thunderstorms and middle-latitude cyclones) to the free troposphere, where it is moved to great distances by relatively strong and persistent winds and mixed down to the surface afterwards (NRC, 2009).

However, in contrast to other air pollutants, the life cycle of Hg in the atmosphere is not then complete. Given the long atmospheric residence time of Hg(0) (up to one year), a large proportion will continue to circulate in the global atmosphere until it is oxidized and removed by precipitation or taken up by the surface. Long-term circulation is accompanied by essential mixing of Hg from various sources and the formation of an atmospheric "global pool" of Hg(0) with a relatively homogeneous spatial distribution of background concentrations. The typical background surface concentration of Hg(0) in the Northern Hemisphere varies within the range $1.5-1.7$ ng/m^3 and is somewhat lower in the Southern Hemisphere in accordance with the location of major anthropogenic emissions north of the equator (Lindberg et al., 2007).

During its dispersion in the free troposphere, Hg(0) is slowly oxidized by a number of reactive compounds (a detailed discussion of Hg atmospheric chemistry is given in Chapter 4). The major gas-phase oxidation agents include ozone (O_3), hydroxyl radical (OH), and reactive bromine (Br). The relative importance of these reactants for Hg(0) oxidation under ambient atmospheric conditions is still unclear (Lindberg et al., 2007; AMAP/UNEP, 2008). Both O_3 and OH are produced photochemically and exist in abundance in the free troposphere. However, the occurrence and importance of the oxidation reactions with these compounds under atmospheric conditions are in doubt (Calvert and Lindberg, 2005). The kinetics of Hg(0) oxidation by Br is very fast (Ariya et al., 2002; Goodsite et al., 2004) , but the sources and ambient concentrations of Br in the free troposphere are not well known. The lack of identification of the reaction products and exact speciation of RGM and HgP represents an additional uncertainty in our understanding of atmospheric Hg chemistry. In particular, RGM and HgP produced as a result of *in situ* oxidation of Hg(0) in the atmosphere are not necessarily the same mercury compounds as the RGM and HgP in primary anthropogenic emissions (AMAP/UNEP, 2008).

Atmospheric mercury can also be oxidized in the aqueous phase of cloud and rain water by O_3, OH, and dissolved chlorine (HOCl/OCl$^-$) (Lin and Pehkonen, 1999; Gårdfeldt et al., 2001; Lin et al., 2006). Although the relative importance of this pathway for the overall Hg cycle in the global atmosphere is probably not as significant as the gas-phase oxidation pathway, it may be substantial in regions of enhanced clouds and precipitation (e.g., the intertropical convergence zone and areas close to the polar front). In addition, an aqueous-phase reduction pathway was proposed via the reaction of aqueous Hg(II) with dissolved SO_2 and reduction of $Hg-SO_3^{2-}$ complexes (Munthe et al., 1991). However, a more recent reevaluation of the reaction kinetics has shown its limited importance owing to the preferential formation of other complexes (van Loon et al., 2000, 2001).

There are a number of special atmospheric environments in which Hg chemical kinetics principally differs from that described above for the free troposphere because of specific local conditions. These include atmospheric mercury depletion events (AMDEs) in polar regions, intensive Hg dynamics in the MBL, and rapid Hg(0) oxidation in the upper troposphere. AMDEs are observed in the Arctic and Antarctic regions during spring (Ebinghaus et al., 2002; Steffen et al., 2008) when Hg(0) concentrations are episodically depleted to very low values owing to fast oxidation by reactive halogens (primarily Br and BrO) with subsequent deposition to the surface (Lindberg et al., 2002; Aria et al., 2004; Skov et al., 2004). This leads to a considerable increase in total Hg deposition in polar regions. However, a considerable proportion of deposited Hg is rapidly photoreduced in snowpack and reemitted into the atmosphere (Kirk et al., 2006; Ferrari et al., 2008; Johnson et al., 2008).

Hg dynamics in the MBL is also affected by halogen chemistry. In the presence of sunlight, rapid oxidation of Hg(0) by halogen species may occur in the open-sea MBL, leading to the formation of RGM and/or HgP and deposition to the water surface (Laurier et al., 2003; Sprovieri et al., 2010a). In seawater, Hg(II) can be reduced by biotic or abiotic processes to Hg(0) and revolatilized, thereby resulting in dynamic exchange of Hg between the atmosphere and marine waters (Lindberg et al., 2007; Selin, 2009). Similar fast halogen-mediated oxidation kinetics is expected in the upper troposphere. Enhanced concentrations of halogen species, lower temperature, and a lack of removal mechanisms lead to increased concentrations of RGM and HgP and decreased concentrations of Hg(0) reflecting oxidation of Hg(0) at altitude (Murphy et al., 2006; Talbot et al., 2007). These increased concentrations of oxidized Hg species at altitude can affect wet deposition through deep convective activity (Guentzel et al., 2001; Selin and Jacob, 2008).

Oxidized Hg species, and Hg(0) in part, are removed from the atmosphere via the two major mechanisms of wet and dry deposition. Wet deposition occurs during precipitation events (rainfall, drizzle, snowfall, etc.) via below-cloud scavenging of oxidized Hg species and washing out of aqueous Hg forms from the cloud environment. Since direct wet removal of Hg(0) is negligible because of its low solubility, wet Hg deposition is largely controlled by the oxidation chemistry and primary emissions of RGM and HgP. In particular, enhanced wet deposition rates were observed in the vicinity of major emission sources because of direct cloud-droplet uptake of emitted oxidized species (Munthe et al., 2001a; Keeler et al., 2006; Guo et al., 2008). In some cases, increased Hg wet deposition fluxes were also explained by the contribution of the pool of increased RGM at altitude (Selin, 2009; Guentzel et al., 2001).

Dry deposition occurs via pollutant interaction with the Earth's surface (soil, rocks, water, anthropogenic materials, etc.) and vegetation. It removes pollutant mass from the near-surface boundary layer and is generally less intensive than rainfall scavenging. However, owing to its continuous nature, dry deposition makes a significant contribution to total removal and can even predominate, particularly in regions with a lack of precipitation. The mechanisms controlling dry deposition differ for various Hg species (Lindberg et al., 2007). For RGM, which is characterized by high sticking ability, the dry deposition rate is limited by turbulent transport to the surface, which is in turn determined by stability conditions of the atmospheric boundary layer. Dry deposition of HgP is also controlled by turbulent transfer through the boundary layer, as well as by sedimentation velocity and the impaction efficiency. Dry removal of Hg(0) occurs mostly over vegetated areas and is controlled by foliage stomatal uptake (Lindberg et al., 1992; Bash et al., 2007).

Hg(0) exchange with vegetation is essentially a bidirectional process involving both uptake by the plant canopy and Hg evasion back to the atmosphere (Mason, 2009). The direction of the exchange depends on a number of factors, including the air concentration of Hg(0), time of day, presence of solar radiation, air temperature, and so on. (Lindberg, 1996; Gustin, 2003; Gustin and Lindberg, 2005). Similar air–surface exchange of Hg(0) has been identified for background soils, depending on both the air and soil Hg content and the surface conditions (Xin and Gustin, 2007). Another process contributing to air–surface exchange consists of prompt recycling of Hg deposition from terrestrial and aquatic surfaces. On deposition, a proportion of newly deposited RGM or HgP is rapidly reduced in terrestrial ecosystems or surface waters by both biotic and abiotic processes and is revolatilized to the atmosphere (Hintelmann et al., 2002; Mason and Sheu, 2002; Selin, 2009). More information on air–surface exchange with aquatic and terrestrial ecosystems and processes within these media can be found in Chapters 12 and 13, respectively.

Thus, the overall Hg cycle in the atmosphere is as follows (Fig. 10.1). Mercury is released to the lower part of the atmosphere—the planet boundary layer (PBL)—from a variety of anthropogenic and natural sources. Emissions from anthropogenic sources include both Hg(0) and oxidized forms (RGM and HgP), while natural emissions mostly consist of elemental Hg. Direct Hg emission out

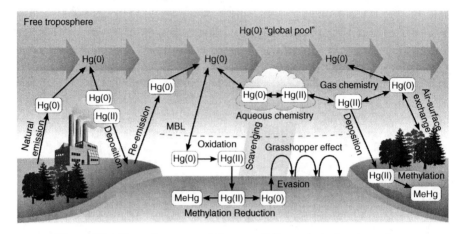

Figure 10.1 General concept of the overall Hg cycle in the atmosphere.

of the PBL to the upper atmosphere is also possible from volcano eruptions (Ferrara et al., 2000). On emission, a large proportion of RGM and HgP is removed through wet or dry deposition, which contributes to local or regional contamination. Some deposited Hg can be reduced to Hg(0) in terrestrial and seawater ecosystems and revolatilized to the atmosphere. Released Hg(0) can be lifted out of the PBL to the free troposphere and becomes diluted in the global Hg(0) pool.

In the free troposphere, Hg(0) is transported over great distances between the continents and to remote regions. Given its long residence time (up to one year), Hg(0) can circle the Earth several times until it is eventually removed from the atmosphere. During atmospheric transport, Hg(0) is chemically transformed to RGM and HgP and removed to the ground via wet deposition or uptake by the surface. Particularly fast Hg oxidation and removal occur in polar regions during AMDEs. Over the oceans, Hg(0) can also be mixed down to the MBL, where it is rapidly oxidized and deposited to the ocean surface. After reduction in seawater, it is reemitted into the atmosphere, contributing to intensive air–seawater exchange that can lead to "grasshopper" dispersion of Hg in the MBL. On deposition to the continents, Hg is partly reemitted back to the atmosphere, which closes the environmental cycle, and partly contributes to the soil and freshwater pools undergoing methylation and biota uptake.

10.3 METHODS FOR STUDYING ATMOSPHERIC MERCURY TRANSPORT

Atmospheric mercury transport and exchange with other media are largely studied by means of in situ monitoring and application of chemical transport models (CTMs). Direct or indirect observations of Hg species under different atmospheric conditions, as well as evaluation of deposition/evasion fluxes, provide realistic data on Hg levels at various locations around the globe and their temporal dynamics, and help in understanding the key processes of Hg atmospheric cycling. Model assessment of Hg fate and transport in the atmosphere gives more complete information on the spatial distribution of Hg levels and transport pathways, and can help in source attribution and predictions of future pollution changes. Model simulations are based in turn on estimates of Hg emissions from both anthropogenic and natural sources. A rational combination of all these assessment components (monitoring, modeling, and emission estimates) constitutes an integrated approach for studying the atmospheric Hg cycle.

Atmospheric monitoring of Hg includes measurements of ambient air concentrations of Hg(0) and other Hg species, evaluation of vertical concentration profiles, and estimates of wet and dry deposition fluxes, as well as air–surface exchange. Observations are made at both ground-based stationary monitoring sites and mobile platforms, including ship- and aircraft-based laboratories. The stationary sites can yield long-term semicontinuous observations at a single location, which are useful for evaluating temporal pollution trends. Mobile platforms provide detailed and miscellaneous measurements of pollution levels and atmospheric processes over larger areas obtained during intensive measurement campaigns.

Measurements of atmospheric concentrations of total gaseous mercury (TGM), mostly composed of Hg(0) and RGM, are carried out using both manual methods (Brosset, 1987; Bloom and Fitzgerald, 1988) and automated analyzers (Urba et al., 1995; Tekran, 1998). These techniques are typically based on gold amalgamation and spectroscopic detection of Hg. The comparability of different methods was assessed in a number of field intercomparisons of atmospheric Hg measurements (Schroeder et al., 1995; Ebinghaus et al., 1999; Munthe et al., 2001b). In particular, there was good agreement of TGM concentrations in air determined using different techniques, which means that combinations of data sets from different regions of the world and different time periods can be used for consistent analysis (Ebinghaus et al., 2009). By contrast, measurements of RGM and HgP concentrations in air are associated with large uncertainties (Ebinghaus et al., 1999; Munthe et al., 2001b). Although neither of the available methods can be considered a routine monitoring technique for these species, they are highly valuable tools for research-based measurements aimed at improving our understanding of the atmospheric behavior of Hg species (Munthe et al., 2001b).

Wet deposition measurements are widely performed by collection of event or weekly precipitation samples, with concomitant recording of rainfall depth for direct estimation of the deposition flux (Mason et al., 2010). Both automated and manual sampling are used (Vermette et al., 1995; Dvonch et al., 1998). Various methods for determining total mercury in precipitation and the wet deposition flux show fairly good agreement in field intercomparisons (Munthe et al., 2001b). When comparing analysis results for the same sample by qualified independent laboratories, the uncertainty is typically <10% (Lindberg et al., 2007).

Measurements of dry Hg deposition are more challenging since surface uptake is a relatively slow and spatially distributed process that strongly depends on the surface type and ambient conditions and differs considerably for different Hg species. A variety of measurement techniques are used to evaluate dry Hg deposition rates (Lindberg et al., 2007; Mason et al., 2010). Direct methods include collection of RGM and HgP on surrogate surfaces (Caldwell et al., 2006; Marsik et al., 2007; Lyman et al., 2009) , use of flux chambers or dynamic flux bags (Kim and Lindberg, 1995; Zhang et al., 2005) , and application of micrometeorological techniques (gradient, modified Bowen ratio, and relaxed eddy accumulation) for estimates of Hg(0) and RGM air–surface exchange (Skov et al., 2006; Lyman et al., 2007). Indirect methods consist of measuring air concentrations of Hg species and meteorological parameters and evaluation of deposition fluxes based on the estimated deposition velocity (Lindberg et al., 1992; Miller et al., 2005). Dry Hg deposition to forests can also be roughly estimated as the sum of litterfall and net throughfall deposition (the latter is defined as the difference between throughfall deposition and open-area wet deposition) (Rea et al., 2001; Munthe et al., 2004) ; however, this method does not take into account Hg accumulated in the remaining foliage and other parts of the plant.

Valuable information on long-term changes in Hg deposition since preindustrial times caused by human activity can be obtained from natural environmental archives, including lake sediments, peat, and glacial ice. It is widely accepted that these historic archives are complex records of atmospheric deposition that provide a means to reconstruct atmospheric Hg load trends (Fitzgerald et al., 1998; Lindberg et al., 2007). Although all these natural records show a significant increase in Hg deposition during the past two centuries, the magnitude of accumulation enhancement differs between the archive types. While a variety of sediment-core records reveal a three- to fivefold increase in deposition rates from preindustrial times (Fitzgerald et al., 2005; Biester et al., 2007) , studies of peat bog and glacial ice cores suggest much greater deposition enhancement (Roos-Barraclough et al., 2006; Schuster et al., 2002). The reasons for the difference may be related to a number of factors, including dating uncertainties, diagenesis, postdepositional migration, and so on (Lindberg et al., 2007). Among other archives, lake sediments, as closed systems, are considered to be internally more consistent and reliable for estimates of historical Hg deposition trends (Biester et al., 2007).

Available measurements of ambient Hg concentrations, deposition, and air–surface exchange fluxes are still very limited and do not provide exhaustive information on Hg dispersion and cycling in the atmosphere. The majority of currently available observational data from both stationary monitoring networks and field campaigns are restricted to Europe and North America, the Arctic, and some other regions of the Northern Hemisphere. Some episodic observations are also available from marine and oceanic cruises, as well as from airborne platforms. Measurement data coverage is very poor for the Southern Hemisphere. Moreover, observations on their own have a limited ability to characterize source–receptor relationships and predict future changes in pollution levels. To fill these gaps, CTMs are widely used and give more comprehensive and detailed information on mercury pollution.

CTMs are universal tools for Hg pollution assessment that link pollutant emissions to ambient distributions (NRC, 2009). In addition to direct application for exploring pollution levels and transport pathways, models can also be used for investigating physical and chemical processes that control the fate of Hg in the atmosphere. In spite of considerable progress in the analytical chemistry of atmospheric Hg and the development of contemporary measurement techniques during the last decade, current knowledge on Hg behavior in the atmosphere is still incomplete. There are significant gaps in our understanding of chemical processes affecting atmospheric Hg transport and deposition, the characteristics of air–surface exchange, and the processes responsible for reemission of mercury into the atmosphere. Therefore, application of self-consistent global and regional-scale models in combination with extensive monitoring data could facilitate a greater understanding of the principal mechanisms governing Hg dispersion and cycling in the environment and improvements in model parameterization. Atmospheric modeling can also be used to evaluate emission inventories. Existing global mercury emission data involve significant uncertainties, in particular, for estimates of natural and secondary emissions from terrestrial and oceanic sources. Application of CTMs using different emission estimates and subsequent comparison of the modeling results with measurements can provide an additional evaluation of the emission inventories (Travnikov et al., 2010).

CTMs used for simulation of atmospheric Hg dispersion vary in their formulation, geographic coverage, and spatial resolution, depending on the case in point (AMAP/UNEP, 2008). For evaluating concentrations and deposition in the immediate vicinity of large emission sources or in the urban environment, local-scale models can be used. These models are typically Gaussian-type or plume models (Constantinou et al., 1995; Lohman et al., 2006) that use a simplified description of pollutant transport and dispersion from a single emission source, but can include a detailed formulation of chemical and removal processes. Application of these models is restricted to short distances from emission sources where the influence of the regional and global mercury background is relatively insignificant. Regional or continent-scale models address atmospheric dispersion and transboundary transport within a continent or a particular region. The models are usually applied for detailed simulations of mercury dispersion over large regions containing numerous emission sources (Europe, North America, East Asia, etc.) (Bullock et al., 2008; Pan et al., 2008; Travnikov and Ilyin, 2009). Mercury depositions over such areas are determined in terms of both regional emissions of short-lived mercury forms and in situ oxidation of Hg(0) transported globally. Therefore, regional simulations largely depend on boundary conditions (concentrations of Hg species imposed on the boundaries of the modeling domain).

To avoid such restrictions and to generate estimates of global mercury dispersion and intercontinental transport, global transport models are applied (Seigneur et al., 2004; Selin et al., 2007; Dastoor and Davignon, 2009). Hemispheric models represent an intermediate case between regional and global models because they cover pollutant dispersion over one of the hemispheres but still have a lateral boundary along the equator (Christensen et al., 2004; Travnikov, 2005). Global and hemispheric CTMs require a spin-up procedure to reach certain initial or steady-state conditions. Therefore, they are commonly applied for relatively long periods (at least one or several years for Hg) but have lower spatial resolution than regional models. Global-scale CTMs offer the advantage of self-consistent simulations constrained by available observational data and can be used for evaluation of scientific hypothesis on critical Hg processes (chemical mechanisms, emissions, removal, etc.) (Lohman et al., 2008; Seigneur et al., 2008).

Multimedia box models represent a special case of mercury environmental modeling. Such models describe the cycling of mercury between different environmental reservoirs (e.g., atmosphere, ocean, soil, and vegetation) in a simplified manner using a mass balance technique based on prescribed exchange rates between media and measurement data (Lamborg et al., 2002; Mason and Sheu, 2002). This simple approach facilitates simulation of the mercury cycle in the environment over very long periods (hundreds of years) and evaluation of global mercury fluxes between media (Sunderland and Mason, 2007). However, there is a tendency among the Hg modeling community to include the multimedia approach into full-scale CTMs to account for Hg cycling between different environmental media (Selin et al., 2008).

Most CTMs consider the full chain of mercury processes in the atmosphere, including emission from anthropogenic and natural sources, atmospheric transport, chemical transformations, and deposition to terrestrial and oceanic surfaces. For a realistic description of atmospheric processes, the models require a variety of meteorological information, including three-dimensional (3D) fields for wind speed components, air density and temperature, precipitation rates, and so on. Depending on the digestion procedure of supporting meteorological information, CTMs are divided into on-line and off-line driven models. The former implies incorporation of pollutant-specific processes (chemistry, removal) into general-purpose weather forecast or atmospheric circulation models. This allows real-time support of simulated dispersion processes with the required meteorological information (Dastoor and Larocque, 2004; Jung et al., 2009). The latter model type is driven by meteorological fields generated by an external preprocessor and assimilated with a certain periodicity (Bullock and Brehme, 2002; Travnikov and Ilyin, 2009).

All mercury CTMs typically use extensive chemical mechanisms describing transformations of Hg species in the atmosphere. As a rule, they consider three gaseous Hg species (Hg(0), RGM, HgP) and a number of mercury species dissolved in cloud water. Owing to the significant knowledge gaps in atmospheric Hg chemistry mentioned above (see also Chapter 4), there is no consensus within the modeling community on the principal chemical mechanisms governing Hg fate in the atmosphere. Limited observational data for constraining mercury CTMs facilitate the application of different chemical mechanisms to account for measured Hg levels and fluxes. It is expected that the primary gas-phase oxidants of Hg(0) include O_3, OH, H_2O_2, and/or reactive halogens (Br, BrO, Br_2, Cl, ClO, Cl_2, etc.). Most contemporary models incorporate oxidation reactions driven by all or some of these substances in their chemical schemes.

For instance, reactions of Hg(0) oxidation by O_3 and OH were considered the major oxidation mechanisms during the past decade and allowed reproduction of observed Hg(0) concentrations and wet deposition fluxes on both global and regional scales (Ryaboshapko et al., 2007a, 2007b). However, these chemical mechanisms failed to simulate fast Hg(0) oxidation during AMDEs and the diurnal cycle of RGM concentrations in the MBL (Selin et al., 2007). Therefore, few models include an explicit treatment of Hg(0) oxidation by reactive halogens as well as air–surface exchange in polar regions during AMDEs (Dastoor et al., 2008; Travnikov and Ilyin, 2010). There has been a successful effort to explain the whole gas-phase Hg oxidation chemistry solely in terms of reaction with Br (Holmes et al., 2010). In the aqueous phase, oxidation reactions with O_3, OH, and HOCl/OCl$^-$ and some reduction pathways (e.g., reduction of Hg–SO$_3^{2-}$ complexes and photoreduction of Hg^{2+}) are considered in models, along with the equilibrium distribution between dissolved Hg(II) species (Lin et al., 2006).

Processes responsible for Hg removal from the atmosphere include scavenging of mercury species by precipitation and deposition through interaction with the surface. In mercury CTMs, wet deposition is commonly distinguished in terms of in-cloud and below-cloud washout and is represented in models using simplified scavenging coefficients (Christensen et al., 2004) or more complicated cloud microphysics techniques (Petersen et al., 2001; Dastoor and Larocque, 2004). Mercury species undergoing wet deposition include RGM, HgP, and Hg species dissolved in cloud water. Gaseous Hg(0) does not undergo direct scavenging by precipitation because of its low solubility, but it can be washed out indirectly through dissolution and oxidation in cloud water.

Dry deposition is represented in contemporary CTMs using either the resistance analogy method (Wesely and Hicks, 2000) or prescribed dry deposition velocities. In the former case, the dry deposition velocity is defined as the inverse sum of successive resistances (aerodynamic resistance, quasi-laminar sublayer resistance, and surface resistance), which describes the dry deposition process more accurately under different atmospheric stability conditions (Cohen et al., 2004; Pan et al., 2008). In the latter case, fixed dry deposition velocities based on measurement data are applied (Syrakov, 1995). All mercury models consider dry deposition of two short-lived mercury species, RGM, and HgP. In addition, some models explicitly simulate dry deposition of Hg(0) to vegetated surfaces using the simple dry deposition velocity technique (Seigneur et al., 2004; Travnikov and Ilyin, 2009). Other models (mainly regional models) do not take this process into account and assume compensation of Hg(0) dry deposition by reemission of previously deposited mercury.

A number of intercomparison studies have been performed during the last decade to analyze model differences and to quantify uncertainties in the results produced by various models. The first, the Intercomparison Study of Numerical Models for Long-Range Atmospheric Transport of Mercury, was organized by the Meteorological Synthesizing Centre-East (MSC-E) and focused on Hg pollution in Europe (Ryaboshapko et al., 2007a,b). The second, the North American Mercury Model Intercomparison Study (NAMMIS), was conducted under the guidance of the US Environmental Protection Agency (EPA) and involved a number of regional and global-scale models for simulation of Hg transport and deposition over North America (Bullock et al., 2008, 2009). The third inter-comparison study was organized within the framework of the Task Force on Hemispheric Transport of Air Pollution (TF HTAP) under the UN Economic Commission for Europe (ECE) Convention on Long-Range Transboundary Air Pollution (CLRTAP) and carried out a multimodel evaluation of intercontinental transport of different air pollutants, including Hg, using mainly global and hemispheric models (Travnikov et al., 2010).

10.4 ASSESSMENTS OF AIRBORNE MERCURY POLLUTION

Particular applications of monitoring and modeling methods for assessment of airborne Hg pollution are discussed below. Evaluation of atmospheric Hg transport and deposition is performed on both regional and global scales and involves observations of Hg concentrations in ambient air and deposition fluxes, as well as application of CTMs. Historically, assessments of Hg pollution levels were initiated for major industrial regions in Europe, North America, and East Asia. However, the global nature of atmospheric Hg dispersion stimulated consideration of the problem on a global scale involving investigation of Hg atmospheric transport between the continents and of the adverse impact on remote terrestrial and marine ecosystems. Particular attention was paid to the Arctic and Antarctic regions owing to the recently discovered AMDE phenomenon and the significant impact of Hg pollution on pristine polar environments.

10.4.1 Europe

Regular observations of background Hg levels in Europe are made at stations of the monitoring network of the European Monitoring and Evaluation Programme (EMEP; http://www.emep.int). Currently, the network includes 26 sites measuring Hg concentrations in air and/or precipitation that are located mainly in the western and northern parts of Europe (Fig. 10.2; Ilyin et al., 2010). Some stations of the network are operated jointly with other regional environmental programs (Oslo and Paris Convention, OSPAR; Helsinki Commission, HELCOM; Arctic Monitoring and Assessment Program, AMAP). Measurements of Hg concentrations in air and precipitation at EMEP/OSPAR sites have been extensively evaluated (Wangberg et al., 2007). A considerable decrease in Hg deposition (10–30%) was found for the period 1995–2002, likely because of emission reductions in Europe. By contrast, no decreasing trend for TGM was observed for the same period, probably because of compensation of European TGM emission reductions with increased emissions in other regions of the Northern Hemisphere. Spatial trends for air concentrations of Hg species in Europe were also studied in a number of research projects, including Mercury Over Europe (MOE), Mediterranean atmospheric mercury cycle system (MAMCS), and An integrated approach to assess the mercury cycling in the Mediterranean basin (EU-MERCYMS) (Sprovieri et al., 2010b and references therein). Air concentrations of TGM, RGM, and HgP

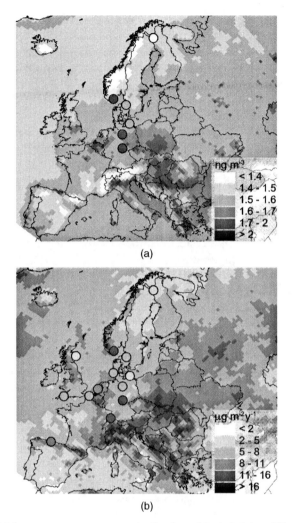

(a)

(b)

Figure 10.2 Total gaseous mercury concentration in ambient air (a) and Hg wet deposition (b) over Europe in 2008 simulated using the MSCE-HM model and measured at stations of the EMEP monitoring network (Ilyin et al., 2010).

were observed during four synchronized seasonal field campaigns in 1998–1999 at five coastal sites in the Mediterranean region and five sites in northern Europe. A slight gradient for TGM and significant gradients for RGM and HgP concentrations that increased from northern Europe to the Mediterranean were observed, probably because of higher emission rates from the Mediterranean Sea coupled with enhanced chemical production of RGM and HgP in the MBL (Sprovieri et al., 2003; Hedgecock et al., 2005).

A number of regional-scale mercury CTMs have been developed and applied for simulation of atmospheric Hg transport and deposition over Europe. One of the first comprehensive Hg modeling systems was elaborated on the basis of the Eulerian reference frame of the Acid Deposition and Oxidant Model (ADOM). It was applied in an investigation of the regional transport and deposition of Hg species within the MOE project and showed adequate performance in comparison to observations (Petersen et al., 2001). A simple Lagrangian-type model was constructed and applied to estimate transport and deposition of Hg across Europe, as well as the overall Hg flux budget for the United Kingdom (Lee et al., 2001). An air–seawater coupled regional model, MECAWEx, was applied for simulation of mercury cycling in the Mediterranean region within the MAMCS project (Hedgecock et al., 2006). The simulation results showed that Hg evasion from the sea surface significantly exceeds total (wet and dry) deposition, making the Mediterranean Sea a net emitter of Hg. The coupled regional/hemispheric Hg modeling system (MSCE-HM) is being applied within EMEP for operational simulations of transboundary pollution in Europe by heavy metals including Hg (Travnikov and Ilyin, 2009). Spatial distributions of model-simulated TGM concentrations in ambient air and wet Hg deposition for 2008 are given in Fig. 10.2, along with observations from the EMEP monitoring network. The increased TGM concentrations (1.6–2 ng/m^3) and wet deposition fluxes (10–20 μg/m^2/year) are characteristic of Central and Southern Europe (Ilyin et al., 2010).

Most of the above-mentioned mercury CTMs were included in the model intercomparison study organized by EMEP/MSC-E (Ryaboshapko et al., 2002; Ryaboshapko et al., 2007a, 2007b). The aim of the study was to evaluate the ability of models to simulate atmospheric transport and transboundary fluxes of Hg in Europe and it was conducted in three phases. The first phase compared simulations of the physicochemical transformation of Hg species in cloud and fog water. The second phase focused on evaluation of simulation results against detailed observations from field measurement campaigns. The third phase involved comparison of the model results with long-term measurements of Hg concentrations and wet deposition. The models considered showed reasonable agreement (within ±20%) between model-predicted and observed concentrations of Hg(0). Simulated wet Hg deposition in Western and Central Europe agreed with observations within ±45%, whereas the variation in model-predicted dry deposition was more significant (Ryaboshapko et al., 2007b).

10.4.2 North America

In North America, the largest and most ambitious Hg monitoring network is the Mercury Deposition Network (MDN), which is part of the National Atmospheric Deposition Program (NADP). The MDN now includes more than 100 monitoring sites across North America and provides a consistent survey of Hg concentrations in precipitation and wet deposition fluxes (NADP/MDN, 2010). Analysis of the monitoring data shows that the spatial pattern of Hg concentrations observed in wet deposition samples at some sites is not well correlated with the spatial distribution of known Hg sources. In particular, there were relatively low Hg concentrations in precipitation collected in Pennsylvania and Ohio, where there are many coal-fired power plants, and high values at locations with fewer Hg sources in Florida (Ebinghaus et al., 2009). This confirms that removal processes (oxidation/scavenging) are important in determining Hg deposition patterns with changing meteorological conditions (Sprovieri et al., 2010b). Although MDN is essential for an understanding of the spatial and temporal patterns of wet Hg deposition, it can hardly explain the processes responsible for enhanced levels and temporal changes of Hg deposition without coherent measurements of Hg species in air. Therefore, in 2009, the NADP established the Atmospheric Mercury Network (AMNet), a subset of the existing MDN sites, which will measure air concentrations of speciated Hg fractions along with wet deposition (http://nadp.sws.uiuc.edu/amn/).

The Canadian Atmospheric Mercury Network (CAMNet) was established in 1996 to provide long-term measurements of TGM concentrations and wet deposition across Canada. Wet deposition is measured at CAMNet sites as part of the MDN. Long-term monitoring data for TGM collected from CAMNet sites between 1995 and 2005 were analyzed for temporal trends, seasonality, and comparability within the network (Temme et al., 2007). TGM concentrations at all the CAMNet sites were similar to or slightly lower than those observed at European background sites. A statistically significant trend for TGM concentrations at rural sites was revealed for this time period. The greatest decreases were observed close to urban areas, probably reflecting changes in local and regional emissions. In addition, long-term atmospheric concentrations of Hg species were measured at some sites within the CAMNet in Quebec, Nova Scotia, and Ontario (Han et al., 2004; Poissant et al., 2005).

Monitoring activities in North America were supplemented by the development and application of a number of regional and global-scale models. A comprehensive Hg regional model was developed by Bullock and Brehme (2002) based on the US EPA Community Multiscale Air Quality (CMAQ) modeling system. This was then further developed and extensively applied by other research groups in a variety of modeling studies for North America and other regions. Lin and Tao (2003) used the CMAQ-Hg model to calculate the regional mass budget of Hg in eastern North America. Another model modification was applied to evaluate the effect of nonanthropogenic emissions on Hg concentrations and deposition levels in North America (Gbor et al., 2006). The authors demonstrated that total natural emission averaged over the region was approximately twice as large as anthropogenic emission. A modified version of CMAQ-Hg was also used to quantify model uncertainties associated with the formulation of various physical and chemical processes in the model, including wet and dry deposition, chemical kinetics, and oxidation reaction products (Lin et al., 2007).

A multiscale modeling system consisting of a global CTM for Hg (CTM-Hg) and a nested regional model (TEAM) was applied to estimate Hg deposition over the contiguous United States (Seigneur et al., 2004). Mercury deposition to the Great Lakes was studied in detail using the Hybrid Single Particle Lagrangian Integrated Trajectory (HYSPLIT) model (Cohen et al., 2004). The global CTM GEOS-Chem adapted for Hg simulations was used to explain spatial patterns and

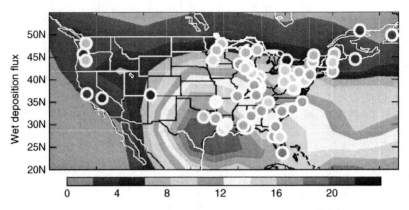

Figure 10.3 Total Hg wet deposition flux over the United States in 2004–2005 ($\mu g/m^2/$ year) simulated using the GEOS-Chem model and measured at stations of the Mercury Deposition Network, National Atmospheric Deposition Program (NADP/MDN, 2010). *Source*: Reprinted from Selin and Jacob (2008) with permission from Elsevier.

seasonal variations in Hg deposition observed over the United States (Fig. 10.3; Selin and Jacob, 2008). In particular, the high wet deposition observed over the Southeast United States was attributed to scavenging of upper-altitude RGM by deep convection, whereas seasonal variation at higher latitudes was explained by a combination of enhanced summertime oxidation of Hg(0) and inefficient scavenging of RGM and HgP by snow.

Both regional and global-scale models were included in a Hg model inter-comparison study with a focus on North America (Bullock, 2008, 2009). The regional models (CMAQ-Hg, REMSAD and TEAM) were compared in a tightly constrained testing environment using the same horizontal and vertical domain structure, emissions data, and meteorological fields. The global models (CTM-Hg, GEOS-Chem, and GRAHM) were used to define three separate sets of initial and boundary conditions for the regional models. The results revealed that the Hg concentration patterns predicted by the regional-scale models differed significantly, even when the same boundary conditions were used. Simulated wet deposition fluxes were strongly influenced by the shared precipitation data, but differences of >50% were still apparent. Simulated dry deposition of mercury varied between the models by a factor of nearly 10 in some locations because of the different parameterizations implemented in the models.

10.4.3 East Asia

There is no coordinated regional-scale Hg monitoring network established in East Asia so far. Nevertheless, numerous observations of ambient Hg concentrations in urban, rural, and remote locations are made among small national networks, at individual monitoring sites, and during field campaigns. In general, regional background Hg concentrations measured in East Asia are considerably higher than those in remote areas of Europe and North America. For instance, high TGM concentrations (3.58 ± 1.78 ng/m^3) have been recorded in 2005–2006 during an intensive field campaign at Mt. Changbai, a remote area in northeastern China (Wan et al., 2009a). Concentrations of oxidized Hg species (65 pg/m^3 for RGM and 77 pg/m^3 for HgP) were also significantly higher than typical background levels in the Northern Hemisphere (Wan et al., 2009b). Long-term observations of TGM were also performed from May 2005 to June 2006 at the Moxi site of the Mt. Gongga alpine ecosystem observation and experiment station in southwestern China (Fu et al., 2008). Average TGM concentrations were ~3.98 ng/m^3 and were affected by local zinc smelting activities and fuel combustion. Comparable regional background concentrations were observed during April 2006–June 2007 in the same mountain area, with a mean annual TGM concentration of 3.90 ± 1.20 ng/m^3 (Fu et al., 2009). Relatively moderate TGM concentrations (2.80 ± 1.51 ng/m^3) that are still higher than global background values were measured at the summit of Mt. Leigong in south China from May 2008 to May 2009 (Fu et al., 2010). These concentrations are lower than those in semirural and industrial/urban areas and are affected by both regional sources and long-range transport from central, south, and southwest China. Similar TGM concentrations (~2.94 ng/m^3) were measured at Wanqingsha, a rural site in southern China in November/December 2008 (Li et al., 2011).

Regional background TGM levels were routinely measured at the coastal global atmospheric watch (GAW) station on An-Myun Island, Korea, for the period December 2004–April 2006 (Nguyen et al., 2007). Relatively high TGM concentrations (4.61 ± 2.21 ng/m^3) were observed, which generally peaked in spring and reached a minimum in summer. Slightly lower TGM concentrations (3.85 ± 1.68 ng/m^3) were measured at another remote area on Jeju Island, Korea, from May 2006 to May 2007, where the seasonal patterns were also characterized by relatively high concentrations in spring and fall. This was attributed to the combined effect of industrial sources, Asian dust, and volcanic activity. The variability of atmospheric Hg species was studied at a remote site (Cape Hedo Observatory) on Okinawa Island, Japan, from March to May 2004, downwind of the major Asian source regions (Chand et al., 2008). Under prevailing meteorological conditions, episodes of higher levels of atmospheric Hg were observed, with mean concentrations of Hg(0), RGM, and HgP of 2.04 ± 0.38 ng/m^3, 4.5 ± 5.4 pg/m^3, and 3.0 ± 2.5 pg/m^3, respectively.

Model research into East Asia Hg pollution was recently initiated using two regional-scale models. Pan et al. (2006) developed a Hg extension of the Sulfur Transport Eulerian Model (STEM-Hg) and applied this for tracking the chemical transport of Hg plumes emitted from large point sources in China. The STEM-Hg model was later used to simulate Hg transport and deposition over East Asia and to calculate the regional Hg budget for this region (Pan et al., 2008, 2010). The model results showed strong seasonal variations in Hg concentration and deposition, with signals from large point sources. More recently, an updated version of CMAQ-Hg was applied for a detailed study of Hg chemical transport and deposition in East Asia and emission outflow from the region (Lin

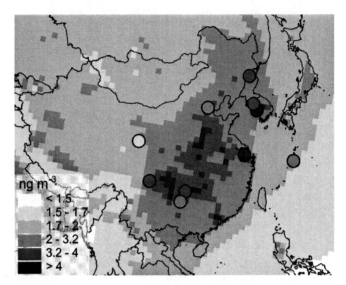

Figure 10.4 Ambient concentrations of Hg(0) over East Asia in 2005 simulated using the CMAQ-Hg model (based on results submitted to the HTAP intercomparison study; Travnikov et al., 2010) and measured at a number of remote and suburban sites (Lin et al., 2010 and references therein).

et al., 2010). The regional Hg mass budget also showed strong seasonal variability, with net removal of RGM and HgP and net export of Hg(0) from the region. The gross emission outflow from the East Asian region was estimated at 1520±150 Mg/year, of which 50–60% was caused by emissions from natural sources. Figure 10.4 shows the spatial distribution of air Hg(0) concentrations over East Asia in 2005 simulated using CMAQ-Hg and available measurements in remote and rural locations.

10.4.4 Polar Regions

The Arctic and Antarctic regions are unique ecosystems owing to their remoteness from major industrial regions and relatively small population, as well as specific climatic conditions and atmospheric circulation. Particular interest in these regions within the Hg research community was accelerated by the discovery of the AMDE phenomenon, which prompted an intensive study of atmospheric Hg processes. This resulted in numerous measurement studies and field experiments performed in various Arctic and Antarctic locations. A comprehensive review of measurements performed in polar regions was carried out by Steffen et al. (2008). The first continuous measurements of surface-level Hg concentrations in the Arctic were performed at Alert, Canada, in 1995 (Schroeder et al., 1998). During this study, it was found that Hg(0) underwent extraordinary fluctuations, decreasing at times to very low values untypical for other locations. This phenomenon was identified afterward as AMDE. The occurrence of AMDEs was subsequently observed throughout the Arctic, in Svalbard, Alaska, Greenland, the coasts of Hudson Bay, and the Kara Sea (Steffen et al., 2008 and references therein). On the basis of these observations, it was suggested and then confirmed through direct measurements that Hg(0) is converted to RGM and HgP during AMDEs (Lu et al., 2001; Lindberg et al., 2001). Moreover, it was demonstrated that only half of the converted Hg(0) remains in the air, with the supposition that the remainder is deposited onto nearby snow and ice surfaces (Steffen et al., 2002).

Soon after the first report on AMDEs by Schroeder et al. (1998), the phenomenon was observed in Coastal Antarctica (Ebinghaus et al., 2002). Dommergue et al. (2010) carried out a comprehensive review of measurements in Antarctica. The first baseline data for the concentration and speciation of atmospheric mercury in Antarctica were reported by De Mora et al. (1993). The measurements of data suggested that TGM concentrations in Antarctica were substantially lower than those observed elsewhere. Continuous highly time-resolved measurements of TGM were carried out at the German Research Station at Neumayer between January 2000 and February 2001 (Ebinghaus et al., 2002). The measured TGM series showed several AMDEs during the Antarctic spring (between August and November 2000). Similar springtime mercury dynamics was observed at two other coastal locations at Terra Nova Bay (Sprovieri et al., 2002) and McMurdo (Brooks et al., 2008a). In contrast to the coastal locations, the elevated altitude Polar Plateau experienced nearly constant oxidized Hg enhancements over the sunlit period, peaking in the summer (Brooks et al., 2008b).

The effect of AMDEs on contamination in the Arctic was investigated in several modeling studies. A significant increase in mercury deposition due to AMDEs has been predicted across the entire Arctic area, as well as in surrounding areas, by the DEHM model (Christensen et al., 2004). Simulations of atmospheric Hg transport and deposition over the Northern Hemisphere were performed for the period from 1999 to 2000. According to the model predictions, total annual Hg deposition to the area north of the Arctic Circle increases because of AMDEs from 89 to 208 t. Ariya et al. (2004) applied a global-scale model (GRAHM) and estimated that ~325 t of Hg are deposited annually to the Arctic north of 60°N, of which 100 t can be attributed to AMDEs. In another study, Travnikov (2005) simulated a 20% increase in total Hg deposition to the Arctic due to AMDEs. However, in coastal regions, the contribution of AMDEs to Hg deposition can exceed 50%.

Dastoor et al. (2008) estimated a total annual Hg deposition of 428 t, Hg reemission of 254 t, and Hg net accumulation of 174 t within the Arctic Circle using an updated version of GRAHM that includes reemission of mercury from snow. The model successfully reproduced both AMDEs and reemission events measured at Alert, Canada (Fig. 10.5). It was found that besides halogen chemistry, some meteorological conditions (such as local atmospheric transport, boundary layer height, solar radiation, cloud cover, and temperature inversion) play an important role in the mechanism of AMDEs in polar regions. The model

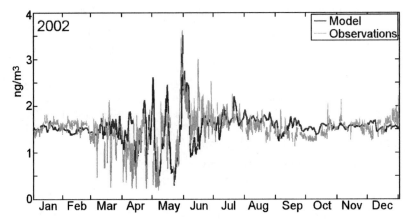

Figure 10.5 Concentrations of Hg(0) measured at Alert, Canada and simulated using the GRAHM model. *Source*: Reprinted with permission from Dastoor et al. (2008). Copyright 2008 American Chemical Society.

was subsequently extensively evaluated against measurements from 6 Arctic and 11 Canadian mid-latitude and sub-Arctic sites (Durnford et al., 2010).

10.4.5 Intercontinental Transport

The global nature of atmospheric Hg dispersion and long-range transport between the continents has been studied using both experimental and modeling methods. For instance, experimental evidence of the trans-Pacific transport of Hg from East Asia to North America has been demonstrated in a number of studies. Episodic events of increased air Hg(0) concentrations have been recorded at the Mt. Bachelor Observatory in central Oregon (Jaffe et al., 2005) and during aircraft measurement campaigns (Friedli et al., 2004; Radke et al., 2007) , and these episodes have been linked to air masses originating from Asia based on correlation with other air pollutants. Jaffe et al. (2005) observed a number of long-range transport episodes for air pollution at Mt. Bachelor (Figure 10.6a). The Hg(0)/CO concentration ratios in these pollution plumes were very similar to the ratio observed in several Asian outflows observed at Hedo Station, Okinawa, Japan, which implies the same origin for the plumes.

In addition, Dastoor and Davignon (2009) investigated the origin of high Hg concentrations at Mt. Bachelor and the transport mechanism during the episode of 23–28 April 2004 (Fig. 10.6a) by performing a series of model simulations. The model was able to reproduce the high Hg(0) concentration episode on 25 April 2004 (day of year 116), simulating transport of Asian emissions across the Pacific over a period of four to five days and descending over western North America through a deep anticyclonic system (Fig. 10.6b). Model simulations suggest that direct anthropogenic emissions in East Asia contribute ~19% of Hg deposition in western North America. The same long-range Hg pollution episode at Mt. Bachelor was studied by Strode et al. (2008) , who used the GEOS-Chem model for

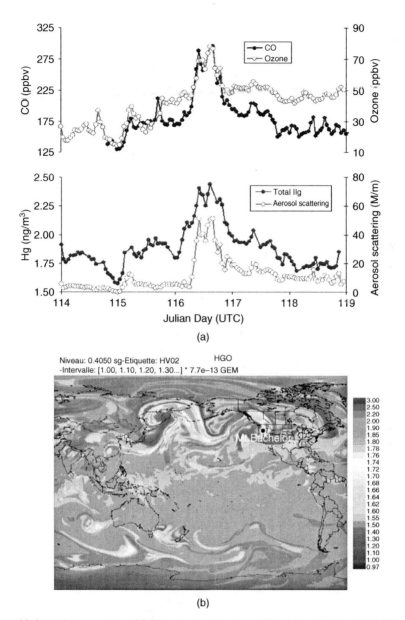

(a)

(b)

Figure 10.6 (a) Observations of TGM along with other pollutants at Mt. Bachelor Observatory from 23 to 28 April 2004 (days of year 114–119). (b) Air concentration of Hg(0) (ng/m^3) at 500 mb simulated using the GRAHM model and showing the Asian Hg outflow episode that reached North America on 25 April 2004. *Source*: (Upper panel) Reprinted from Jaffe et al. (2005) with permission from Elsevier; (lower panel) reprinted from Dastoor and Davignon (2009) with kind permission from Springer Science+Business Media B.V.).

tagged simulations by region of origin and for natural emissions and reemission. The model successfully captured mean Hg(0) concentrations during the episode at Mt. Bachelor, but underestimated the magnitude of observed long-range transport events. The model also underestimated the Hg(0)/CO enhancement ratio, which suggests that Asian emissions in the existing anthropogenic inventory may also be underestimated.

Long-range transport of Hg to the Arctic and sub-Arctic areas of Canada was studied by Durnford et al. (2010). They applied GRAHM to investigate source attribution of Hg observations at 6 Arctic and 11 sub-Arctic and mid-latitude monitoring stations from major source regions of the Northern Hemisphere. They found that Asia, despite having relatively low transport efficiencies, was the dominant source of TGM at all verification stations. Asian sources contributed the greatest Hg mass to the study region and generated the most long-range transport events. However, for the Arctic, transport efficiencies from Russia tended to be the strongest. The springtime preference for trans-Pacific transport of Asian emissions was evident only for mid-latitude stations and was masked in the Arctic by the occurrence of AMDEs. It was also demonstrated that Hg transport from all source regions occurred principally in the mid-troposphere.

Several modeling studies have been conducted to estimate source attribution of Hg deposition and the effect of intercontinental transport. Using a hemispheric model of Hg airborne transport and deposition (MSCE-Hg-Hem), Travnikov (2005) found that ~40% of annual Hg deposition to Europe originated from distant sources, including 15% from Asia and 5% from North America. The study also revealed that North America is particularly affected by emission sources on other continents, with up to 67% of total deposition from foreign anthropogenic and natural sources, including ~24% from Asian and 14% from European sources. By contrast, the total contribution of foreign sources does not exceed 32% in Asia. It was concluded that the contribution of intercontinental atmospheric transport of Hg is comparable to that of regional pollution throughout the Northern Hemisphere. Seigneur et al. (2004) studied the source attribution of Hg deposition over the contiguous United States using a coupled regional/global modeling system (TEAM/CTM-Hg) and found that North American anthropogenic emissions contributed on average 25–30% to Hg deposition in the United States and varied from 10% to 80% in different locations. Asian anthropogenic emissions contributed ~20% and their spatial variation was also significant (5–36%), being higher in the west and declining across the country. They also found large variation in the deposition associated with natural sources (6–59%), with this source being more important in the western United States.

A global land–ocean–atmosphere model (GEOS-Chem) was applied to study the source attribution of Hg deposition over the United States taking into account the legacy of past anthropogenic emissions (Selin and Jacob, 2008). The results agree in general with those mentioned above: present-day Hg deposition in the United States includes 20% from primary anthropogenic emissions in North America, 22% from primary anthropogenic emissions outside North America (mostly East Asia), 26% from recycling through the land and ocean reservoirs, and 38% from natural origins. In the above-mentioned study, Strode et al. (2008) found that the contribution of all North American sources (anthropogenic, natural, and reemission) to deposition in the continental United States was comparable to that of Asian sources and accounted for ∼25% of total deposition. Moreover, the study revealed that the relative importance of Asian and North American sources to deposition over the United States varied significantly across the country. Results from an updated version of the GEOS-Chem model based on bromine as the major oxidant for atmospheric Hg(0) (Holmes et al., 2010) show that domestic anthropogenic sources may contribute up to 60% to total deposition in the eastern United States, where most anthropogenic point sources of RGM and HgP are located. For the western United States, the estimated contribution of domestic anthropogenic sources to deposition is much smaller.

The impact of intercontinental atmospheric transport of Hg on regional contamination levels was systematically studied in the HTAP multimodel experiment (Travnikov et al., 2010). This included both evaluation of source attribution for Hg deposition in various regions of the Northern Hemisphere and forecasts of future Hg contamination changes for a number of emissions reduction scenarios. Five global models and one regional/hemispheric model were included in the study and these differ significantly in their formulation of atmospheric transport and chemistry, natural and secondary emissions, and so on. Therefore, comparison of the simulation results provides a consistent picture of the state of the art and uncertainties in contemporary global-scale Hg modeling. The average global distribution of Hg(0) concentration in ambient air according to the model ensemble is given in Fig. 10.7. It follows from the simulation results that increased Hg(0) concentrations (> 2 ng/m^3) are characteristics of the major industrial regions—East and South Asia, Europe, North America, and South Africa. There is also a pronounced gradient for surface Hg(0) concentrations between the Southern and Northern Hemispheres resulting from the location of major anthropogenic emissions north of the Equator. The simulated pattern generally matches long-term observations of background Hg(0) concentrations.

In spite of considerable difference in deposition estimates because of differences in both model formulation and input data, the models were consistent in evaluation of source attribution. It was concluded that the contribution of Hg intercontinental transport was significant, particularly in regions with few local emission sources. In fact, the contribution of foreign anthropogenic sources to annual Hg deposition fluxes varies from 10% to 30% on average anywhere on the globe. Moreover, 35–70% of total deposition to most regions consists of deposition contributed by global natural and secondary emissions. East Asia is the most dominant source region, with annual contributions from anthropogenic sources of 10–14% to Hg deposition in other regions, followed by contributions from Europe (2–5%), South Asia (2–3%), and North America (1–2%) (Travnikov et al., 2010).

Future changes in Hg pollution levels were simulated on the basis of three emission scenarios for 2020; these represent the *status quo* (SQ) conditions, economic progress, and wide implementation of emission control technologies

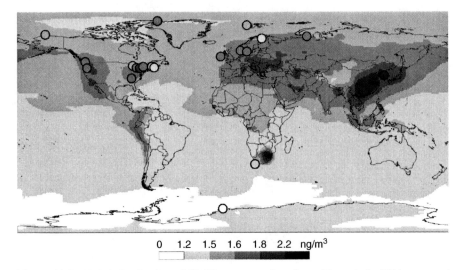

0   1.2   1.5   1.6   1.8   2.2   ng/m³

Figure 10.7 Global distribution of Hg(0) concentrations in ambient air in 2001 averaged over the HTAP model ensemble. Circles represent long-term observations from the AMAP, EMEP, CAMNet networks, and at some other monitoring sites (Travnikov et al., 2010 and references therein).

currently used throughout Europe and North America (extended emission control, EXEC), and implementation of all feasible control technologies, leading to the maximum degree of emissions reduction (maximum feasible technological reduction, MFTR) (AMAP/UNEP, 2008). The model ensemble predicted consistent changes in Hg deposition levels in the future. Depending on the scenario applied, Hg deposition will increase by 2–25% (for SQ) or decrease by 25–35% (for EXEC and MFTR) in different industrial regions. In remote regions, such as the Arctic, the changes are expected to be smaller, ranging from an increase of 1.5–5% (SQ) to a decrease of 15–20% (EXEC, MFTR).

10.5 KNOWLEDGE GAPS

Despite significant progress in the development of Hg measurement and modeling methods during the past decade, numerous uncertainties and knowledge gaps remain for different aspects of Hg fate and transport in the atmosphere. The principal uncertainties are associated with Hg atmospheric chemistry. The key chemical mechanisms responsible for Hg oxidation and reduction in the atmosphere are not well understood. There is increasing evidence that the gas-phase reaction with atomic bromine probably controls Hg oxidation and subsequent deposition under various atmospheric conditions. However, further research is needed to evaluate the relative importance of this mechanism for the atmosphere as a whole and the possibility of other oxidation pathways. Large uncertainties also pertain to the kinetics and reaction rate constants. A lack of knowledge of the reaction products and the chemical composition of operationally defined Hg species—RGM and HgP—impedes a fundamental understanding of the major physicochemical processes and improvements in mercury models. A better understanding of Hg chemistry through laboratory studies and field measurements is needed, in particular, for gaseous and heterogeneous oxidation mechanisms, kinetics, and products under different atmospheric conditions. The chemical mechanisms studied can be evaluated by applying self-consistent global CTMs in combination with extensive observational data.

Atmospheric emissions are a crucial parameter affecting the assessment of Hg dispersion and cycling. Uncertainties associated with emission estimates are discussed in Chapter 1. Here, we briefly note some principal emission characteristics affecting the quality of Hg atmospheric assessment. Reliable model estimates of Hg atmospheric transport and deposition are sensitive to both the magnitude and spatial distribution of anthropogenic emissions. Moreover, the nature of airborne pollution and the relative contribution of local/regional and intercontinental transport are defined by emissions speciation. Evaluation of long-term cycling and accumulation in the environment requires knowledge of historical Hg emission changes since preindustrial times. Natural and biogenic emissions account for a substantial proportion of total Hg input to the atmosphere. Therefore, reliable estimates of Hg emission fluxes from natural surfaces, as well as the factors influencing the emission process, are important for global-scale model simulations.

The development of Hg transport models and evaluations of modeling results are limited by the availability of observational data on air concentrations of Hg species and air–surface exchange fluxes. Currently available measurements of Hg(0) concentrations in ambient air are restricted to several national/regional monitoring networks in the Northern Hemisphere, a few locations in the Southern Hemisphere, and observations from a number of field campaigns. Measurements of other Hg species are very sparse. Therefore, extension of the geographical coverage of observational data, along with increasing duration of measurements, is needed to facilitate model development. In addition, a thorough evaluation of model performance requires information on the vertical distribution of Hg species, which could be obtained from aircraft-based measurement platforms or elevated mountain monitoring sites. These and other requirements for observational data can be satisfied by establishment of a coordinated global monitoring network, which could incorporate existing national and regional monitoring networks but should also include a number of additional ground-based sites to obtain global coverage and should be supported by intensive aircraft- and ship-based measurement campaigns (Sprovieri et al., 2010b).

Atmospheric deposition and air–surface exchange are key processes accounting for Hg cycling between the atmosphere and other environmental media. Wet deposition is relatively well documented in terms of long-term measurements from a number of monitoring networks and field campaigns. However, similar to observations of air concentrations, the coverage for wet deposition measurements is rather limited and can hardly be used for full-scale model evaluation.

The mechanisms for Hg dry deposition and air–surface exchange are poorly understood. The lack of observational data on dry deposition of Hg species to different Earth surfaces leads to large uncertainties in model estimates of total Hg deposition fluxes. Additional complexity is introduced by the bidirectional nature of Hg(0) air–surface exchange and reemission of deposited oxidized forms owing to reduction in terrestrial or aquatic environments. Therefore, extension of regular observations of wet and, in particular, dry deposition of Hg is required for improvements in model formulation and Hg deposition estimates, along with studies for a quantitative and mechanistic understanding of Hg emissions from various surfaces. Furthermore, the development and application of multimedia biogeochemical models that take into account the entire Hg cycle in the environment represent an interesting perspective. This will be particularly relevant for evaluation of long-term trends, future scenarios, and the impact of climate change on Hg pollution.

REFERENCES

AMAP/UNEP. Technical background report to the global atmospheric mercury assessment. Arctic Monitoring and Assessment Programme/UNEP Chemicals Branch. 2008. Available at http://www.unep.org/hazardoussubstances/Mercury/Mercury-Publications/ReportsPublications/tabid/3593/Default.aspx. Accessed 2011 Sep 16.

Ariya PA, Dastoor AP, Amyot M, Schroeder W, Barrie L, Anlauf K, Raofie F, Ryzhkov A, Davignon D, Lalonde J, Steffen A. The Arctic: A sink for mercury. Tellus B 2004;56(5):397–403.

Ariya PA, Khalizov A, Gidas A. Reactions of gaseous mercury with atomic and molecular halogens: kinetics, product studies, and atmospheric implications. J Phys Chem 2002;106:7310–7320.

Bash JO, Bresnahan P, Miller DR. Dynamic surface interface exchanges of mercury: A review and compartmentalized modeling framework. J Appl Meteorol Climatol 2007;46(10):1606–1618.

Biester H, Bindler R, Martínez-Cortizas A, Engstrom DR. Modeling the past atmospheric deposition of mercury using natural archives. Environ Sci Technol 2007;41:4851–4860.

Bloom NS, Fitzgerald WF. Determination of volatile mercury species at the picogram level by low temperature gas chromatography with cold vapor atomic fluorescence detection. Anal Chim Acta 1988;209:151–161.

Brooks S, Arimoto R, Lindberg S, Southworth G. Antarctic polar plateau snow surface conversion of deposited oxidized mercury to gaseous elemental mercury with fractional long-term burial. Atmos Environ 2008a;42:2877–2884.

Brooks S, Lindberg S, Southworth G, Arimoto R. Springtime atmospheric mercury speciation in the McMurdo, Antarctica coastal region. Atmos Environ 2008b;42:2885–2893.

Brosset C. The behaviour of mercury in the physical environment. Water Air Soil Pollut 1987;34:145–166.

Bullock OR, Brehme KA. Atmospheric mercury simulation using the CMAQ model: formulation description and analysis of wet deposition results. Atmos Environ 2002;36:2135–2146.

Bullock OR, Atkinson D, Braverman T, Civerolo K, Dastoor A, Davignon D, Ku J-Y, Lohman K, Myers TC, Park RJ, Seigneur C, Selin NE, Sistla G, Vijayaraghavan K. The North American Mercury Model Intercomparison Study (NAMMIS): Study description and model-to-model comparisons. J Geophys Res 2008;113: D17310.

Bullock OR, Atkinson D, Braverman T, Civerolo K, Dastoor A, Davignon D, Ku J-Y, Lohman K, Myers TC, Park RJ, Seigneur C, Selin NE, Sistla G, Vijayaraghavan K. An analysis of simulated wet deposition of mercury from the North American Mercury Model Intercomparison Study. J Geophys Res 2009;114: D08301.

Caldwell CA, Swartzendruber P, Prestbo E. Concentration and dry deposition of mercury species in arid south central New Mexico (2001–2002). Environ Sci Technol 2006;40:7535–7540.

Calvert JG, Lindberg SE. Mechanisms of mercury removal by O3 and OH in the atmosphere. Atmos Environ 2005;39:3355–3567.

Chand D, Jaffe D, Prestbo E, Swartzendruber PC, Hafner W, Weiss-Penzias P, Kato S, Takami A, Hatakeyama S, Kajii Y. Reactive and particulate mercury in the Asian marine boundary layer. Atmos Environ 2008;42:7988–7996.

Christensen JH, Brandt J, Frohn LM, Skov H. Modelling of mercury in the Arctic with the danish eulerian hemispheric model. Atmos Chem Phys 2004;4:2251–2257.

Cohen M, Artz R, Draxler R, Miller P, Poissant L, Niemi D, Ratte D, Deslauriers M, Duval R, Laurin R, Slotnick J, Nettesheim T, McDonald J. Modelling the atmospheric transport and deposition of mercury to the Great Lakes. Environ Res 2004;95:247–265.

Constantinou E, Wu XA, Seigneur C. Development and application of a reactive plume model for mercury emissions. Water Air Soil Pollut 1995;80:325–335.

Dastoor AP, Davignon D. Global mercury modelling at Environment Canada. In: Pirrone N, Mason RP, editors. Mercury fate and transport in the global atmosphere: emissions, measurements, and models. New York: Springer; 2009. pp. 389–400.

Dastoor AP, Davignon D, Theys N, Roozendael MV, Steffen A, Ariya PA. Modeling dynamic exchange of gaseous elemental mercury at polar sunrise. Environ Sci Technol 2008;42:5183–5188.

Dastoor AP, Larocque Y. Global circulation of atmospheric mercury: a modelling study. Atmos Environ 2004;38:147–161.

De Mora SJ, Patterson JE, Bibby DM. Baseline atmospheric mercury studies at Ross Island, Antarctica. Antarct Sci 1993;5:323–326.

Dommergue A, Sprovieri F, Pirrone N, Ebinghaus R, Brooks S, Courteaud J, Ferrari CP. Overview of mercury measurements in the Antarctic troposphere. Atmos Chem Phys 2010;10:3309–3319.

Durnford D, Dastoor A, Figueras-Nieto D, Ryjkov A. Long range transport of mercury to the Arctic and across Canada. Atmos Chem Phys 2010;10:6063–6086.

Dvonch JT, Graney JR, Marsik FJ, Keeler GJ, Stevens RK. An investigation of source–receptor relationships for mercury in south Florida using event precipitation data. Sci Total Environ 1998;213:95–108.

Ebinghaus R, Jennings SG, Schroeder WH, Berg T, Donaghy T, Guentzel J, Kenny C, Kock HH, Kvietkus K, Schneeberger D, Slemr F, Sommar J, Urba A, Wallschläger D, Xiao Z. International field intercomparison measurements of atmospheric mercury species at Mace Head, Ireland. Atmos Environ 1999;33(18):3063–3073.

Ebinghaus R, Kock HH, Temme C, Einax JW, Löwe AG, Richter A, Burrows JP, Schroeder WH. Antarctic springtime depletion of atmospheric mercury. Environ Sci Technol 2002;36:1238–1244.

Ebinghaus R, Banic C, Beauchamp S, Jaffe D, Kock HH, Pirrone N, Poissant L, Sprovieri F, Weiss-Penzias PS. Spatial coverage and temporal trends of land-based atmospheric mercury measurements in the Northern and Southern Hemispheres. In: Pirrone N, Mason RP, editors. Mercury fate and transport in the global atmosphere: emissions, measurements, and models. New York: Springer; 2009. pp. 223–292.

Ferrari CP, Padova C, Faïn X, Gauchard P-A, Dommergue A, Aspmo K, Berg T, Cairns W, Barbante C, Cescon P, Kaleschke L, Richter A, Wittrock F, Boutron C. Atmospheric mercury depletion event study in Ny-Alesund (Svalbard) in spring 2005. Deposition and transformation of Hg in surface snow during springtime. Sci Total Environ 2008;397:167–177.

Ferrara R, Mazzolai B, Lanzillotta E, Nucaro E, Pirrone N. Volcanoes as emission sources of atmospheric mercury in the Mediterranean basin. Sci Total Environ 2000;259:115–121.

Fitzgerald WF, Engstrom DR, Lamborg CH, Tseng C-M, Balcom PH, Hammerschmidt CR. Modern and historic atmospheric mercury fluxes in northern Alaska: global Sources and Arctic depletion. Environ Sci Technol 2005;39:557–568.

Fitzgerald WF, Engstrom DR, Mason RP, Nater EA. The case for atmospheric mercury contamination in remote areas. Environ Sci Technol 1998;32:1–7.

Fitzgerald WF, Lamborg CH. Geochemistry of mercury in the environment. In: Lollar BS, editor. Treatise on geochemistry. New York: Elsevier; 2005. pp. 107–148.

Friedli HR, Radke LF, Prescott R, Li P, Woo J-H, Carmichael GR. Mercury in the atmosphere around Japan, Korea, and China as observed during the 2001 ACE-Asia field campaign: measurements, distributions, sources, and implications. J Geophys Res 2004;109: D19S25.

Fu XW, Feng X, Dong ZQ, Yin RS, Wang JX, Yang ZR, Zhang H. Atmospheric gaseous elemental mercury (GEM) concentrations and mercury depositions at a high-altitude mountain peak in south China. Atmos Chem Phys 2010;10:2425–2437.

Fu X, Feng X, Zhu W. Temporal and spatial distributions of TGM in Gongga mountain area, Sichuan province, P.R. China: Regional sources and long range atmospheric transport. Sci Total Environ 2009;407:2306–2314.

Fu X, Feng X, Zhu W, Wang S, Lu J. Total gaseous mercury concentrations in ambient air in the eastern slope of Mt. Gongga, South-Eastern fringe of the Tibetan plateau, China. Atmos Environ 2008;42(5):970–979.

Gårdfeldt K, Sommar J, Stroemberg D, Feng X. Oxidation of atomic mercury by hydroxyl radicals and photoinduced decomposition of methylmercury in the aqueous phase. Atmos Environ 2001;35:303–304.

Gbor PK, Wen D, Meng F, Yang F, Sloan JJ. Modeling of mercury emission, transport and deposition in North America. Atmos Environ 2006;41:1135–1149.

Goodsite ME, Plane JM, Skov H. A theoretical study of the oxidation of Hg(0) to HgBr2 in the troposphere. Environ Sci Technol 2004;38:1772–1776.

Guentzel JL, Landing WM, Gill GA, Pollman CD. Processes influencing rainfall deposition of mercury in Florida. Environ Sci Technol 2001;35:863–873.

Guo Y, Feng X, Li Z, He T, Yan H, Meng B, Zhang J, Qiu G. Distribution and wet deposition fluxes of total and methyl mercury in Wujiang River Basin, Guizhou, China. Atmos Environ 2008;42:7096–7103.

Gustin MS. Are mercury emissions from geologic sources significant? A status report. Sci Total Environ 2003;304(1–3):153–167.

Gustin M, Lindberg S. Terrestrial mercury fluxes: is the net exchange up, down or neither? In: Pirrone N, Mahaffey K, editors. Dynamics of mercury pollution on regional and global scales: atmospheric processes, human exposure around the world. Nowell (MA): 2005.

Han YJ, Holsen TM, Lai SO, Hopke PK, Yi SM, Liu W, Pagano J, Falanga L, Milligan M, Andolina C. Atmospheric gaseous mercury concentrations in New York State: Relationships with meteorological data and other pollutants. Atmos Environ 2004;38(37):6431–6446.

Hedgecock IM, Pirrone N, Trunfio GA, Sprovieri F. Integrated mercury cycling, transport, and air-water exchange (MECAWEx) model. J Geophys Res 2006;111: D20302.

Hedgecock IM, Trunfio GA, Pirrone N, Sprovieri F. Mercury chemistry in the MBL: Mediterranean case and sensitivity studies using the AMCOTS (Atmospheric Mercury Chemistry over the Sea) model. Atmos Environ 2005;39:7217–7230.

Hintelmann H, Harris R, Heyes A, Hurley JP, Kelly CA, Krabbenhoft DP, Lindberg S, Rudd JWM, Scott KJ, St.Louis VL. Reactivity and mobility of new and old mercury deposition in a boreal forest ecosystem during the first year of the METAALICUS study. Environ Sci Technol 2002;36:5034–5040.

Holmes CD, Jacob DJ, Corbitt ES, Mao J, Yang X, Talbot R, Slemr F. Global atmospheric model for mercury including oxidation by bromine atoms. Atmos Chem Phys Discuss 2010;10:19845–19900.

Ilyin I, Rozovskaya O, Sokovyh V, Travnikov O, Varygina M, Aas W, Uggerud HT. Heavy metals: transboundary pollution of the environment. EMEP Status Report 2/2010. Moscow, Russia; 2010. Available at http://www.msceast.org/publications.html. Accessed 2011 Sep 16.

Jaffe D, Prestbo E, Swartzendruber P, Weiss-Penzias P, Kato S, Takami A, Hatakeyama S, Yoshizumi K. Export of atmospheric mercury from Asia. Atmos Environ 2005;38:3029–3038.

Johnson KP, Blum JD, Keeler GJ, Douglas T. Investigation of the deposition and emission of mercury in arctic snow during an atmospheric mercury depletion event. J Geophys Res 2008;113: D17304.

Jung G, Hedgecock IM, Pirrone N. ECHMERIT V1.0—a new global fully coupled mercury-chemistry and transport model. Geosci Model Dev 2009;2:175–195.

Keeler GJ, Landis MS, Norris GA, Christianson EM, Dvonch JT. Sources of mercury wet deposition in eastern Ohio, USA. Environ Sci Technol 2006;40(19):5874–5881.

Kim K-H, Lindberg SE. Design and initial tests of a dynamic enclosure chamber for measurements of vapor-phase mercury fluxes over soil. Water Air Soil Pollut 1995;80:1059–1068.

Kirk JL, St. Louis VL, Sharp MJ. Rapid reduction and reemission of mercury deposited to snowpacks during atmospheric mercury depletion events at Churchill, Manitoba, Canada. Environ Sci Technol 2006;40:7590–7596.

Lamborg CH, Fitzgerald WF, O'Donnell J, Torgersen T. A non-steady-state compartment model of global-scale mercury biochemistry with inter-hemispheric atmospheric gradients. Geochim Cosmochim Acta 2002;66:1105–1118.

Laurier FJG, Mason RP, Whalin L, Kato S. Reactive gaseous mercury formation in the North Pacific Ocean's marine boundary layer: a potential role of halogen chemistry. J Geophys Res 2003;108(D17): 4529.

Lee DS, Nemitz E, Fowler D, Kingdon RD. Modelling atmospheric mercury transport and deposition across Europe and the UK. Atmos Environ 2001;35(32):5455–5466.

Li Z, Xia C, Wang X, Xiang Y, Xie Z. Total gaseous mercury in Pearl River Delta region, China during 2008 winter period. Atmos Environ 2011;45:834–838.

Lin C-J, Pehkonen SO. The chemistry of atmospheric mercury: a review. Atmos Environ 1999;33:2067–2079.

Lin C-J, Pongprueksa P, Bullock OR, Linberg SE, Pehkonen SO, Jang C, Braverman T, Ho TC. Scientific uncertainties in atmospheric mercury models II: Sensitivity analysis in the CONUS domain. Atmos Environ 2007;41:6544–6560.

Lin C-J, Pongprueksa P, Linberg SE, Pehkonen SO, Byun D, Jang C. Scientific uncertainties in atmospheric mercury models: Model science evaluation. Atmos Environ 2006;40:2911–2928.

Lin C-J, Pan L, Streets DG, Shetty SK, Jang C, Feng X, Chu H-W, Ho TC. Estimating mercury emission outflow from East Asia using CMAQ-Hg. Atmos Chem Phys 2010;10:1853–1864.

Lin X, Tao Y. A numerical modelling study on regional mercury budget for eastern North America. Atmos Chem Phys 2003;3:535–548.

Lindberg SE, Meyers TP, Taylor GE, Turner RR. Atmospheric/surface exchange of mercury in a forest: Results of modeling and gradient approaches. J Geophys Res 1992;97(D2):2519–2528.

Lindberg S. Forests and the global biogeochemical cycle of mercury. In: Baeyens W, Ebinghaus R, Vasiliev O, editors. Global and regional mercury cycles: sources, fluxes and mass balances. Dordrecht: Kluwer Academic Publishers; 1996. pp. 359–380.

Lindberg SE, Brooks SB, Lin CJ, Scott K, Meyers T, Chambers L, Landis M, Stevens RK. Formation of reactive gaseous mercury in the Arctic: evidence of oxidation of Hg^0 to gas-phase HgII compounds after arctic sunrise. Water Air Soil Pollut 2001;1:295–302.

Lindberg SE, Brooks S, Lin C-J, Scott KJ, Landis MS, Stevens RK, Goodsite M, Richter A. Dynamic oxidation of gaseous mercury in the Arctic troposphere at Polar sunrise. Environ Sci Technol 2002;36:1245–1256.

Lindberg S, Bullock R, Ebinghaus R, Engstrom D, Feng X, Fitzgerald W, Pirrone N, Prestbo E, Seigneur C. A synthesis of progress and uncertainties in attributing the sources of mercury in deposition. Ambio 2007;36(1):19–32.

Lohman K, Seigneur C, Gustin M, Lindberg S. Sensitivity of the global atmospheric cycling of mercury to emissions. Appl Geochem 2008;23:454–466.

Lohman K, Seigneur C, Edgerton E, Jansen J. Modeling mercury in power plant plumes. Environ Sci Technol 2006;40:3848–3854.

Lu JY, Schroeder WH, Barrie LA, Steffen A, Welch HE, Martin K, Lockhar L, Hunt RV, Boila G, Richter A. Magnification of atmospheric mercury deposition to polar regions in springtime: the link to tropospheric ozone depletion chemistry. Geophys Res Lett 2001;28:3219–3222.

Lyman SN, Gustin MS, Prestbo EM, Marsik FJ. Estimation of dry deposition of atmospheric mercury in Nevada by direct and indirect methods. Environ Sci Technol 2007;41:1970–1976.

Lyman SN, Gustin MS, Prestbo EM, Kilner PI, Edgerton E, Hartsell B. Testing and application of surrogate surfaces for understanding potential gaseous oxidized mercury dry deposition. Environ Sci Technol 2009;43:6235–6241.

Mahaffey KR, Clickner RP, Bodurow CC. Blood organic mercury and dietary mercury intake: National Health and Nutrition Examination Survey, 1999 and 2000. Environ Health Perspect 2004;112(5):562–670.

Marsik FJ, Keeler GJ, Landis MS. The dry-deposition of speciated mercury to the Florida Everglades: Measurements and modeling. Atmos Environ 2007;41:136–149.

Mason RP, Sheu GR. Role of the ocean in the global mercury cycle. Global Biogeochem Cycles 2002;16(4): 1093.

Mason RP. Air-sea exchange and marine boundary layer atmospheric transformations of mercury and their importance in the global mercury cycle. In: Pirrone N, Mason RP, editors. Dynamics of mercury pollution on regional and global scales. New York: Springer; 2005. pp. 213–239.

Mason R. Mercury emissions from natural processes and their importance in the global mercury cycle. In: Pirrone N, Mason RP, editors. Mercury fate and transport in the global atmosphere: emissions, measurements, and models. New York: Springer; 2009. pp. 173–191.

Mason R, Pirrone N, Hedgecock I, Suzuki N, Levin L. Conceptual overview. In: HTAP 2010 Assessment Report. Part B, Mercury. Geneva: UN–Economic Commission for Europe; 2010. pp. 1–26.

Miller EK, Vanarsdale A, Keeler GJ, Chalmers A, Poissant L, Kamman NC, Brulotte R. Estimation and mapping of wet and dry mercury deposition across northeastern North America. Ecotoxicology 2005;14:53–70.

Munthe J, Bishop K, Driscoll C, Graydon J, Hultberg H, Lindberg S, Matzner E, Porvari P, Rea A, Schwesig D, St Louis V, Verta M. Input-output of Hg in forested catchments in Europe and North America. RMZ-Mater Geoenviron 2004;51:1243–1246.

Munthe J, Xiao ZF, Lindqvist O. The aqueous reduction of divalent mercury by sulfite. Water Air Soil Pollut 1991;56:621–630.

Munthe J, Kindbom K, Kruger O, Peterson G, Pacyna J, Iverfeldt A. Examining source-receptor relationships for mercury in Scandinavia. Water Air Soil Pollut Focus 2001a;1:99–110.

Munthe J, Wangberg I, Pirrone N, Iverfeld A, Ferrara R, Ebinghaus R, Feng R, Gerdfelt K, Keeler GJ, Lanzillotta E, Lindberg SE, Lu J, Mamane Y, Prestbo E, Schmolke S, Schroder WH, Sommar J, Sprovieri F, Stevens RK, Stratton W, Tuncel G, Urba A. Intercomparison of methods for sampling and analysis of atmospheric mercury species. Atmos Environ 2001b;35:3007–3017.

Murphy DM, Hudson PK, Thomson DS, Sheridan PJ, Wilson JC. Observations of mercury-containing aerosols. Environ Sci Technol 2006;40:3163–3167.

NADP/MDN. National Atmospheric Deposition Program (NRSP-3). Mercury Deposition Network (MDN). NADP Program Office, Illinois State Water Survey, 2204 Griffith Dr., Champaign, IL 61820. 2010. Available at http://nadp.sws.uiuc.edu/MDN/. Accessed 2011 Sep 16.

Nguyen HT, Kim KH, Kim MY, Hong S, Youn YH, Shon ZH, Lee JS. Monitoring of atmospheric mercury at a Global Atmospheric Watch (GAW) site on An-Myun Island, Korea. Water Air Soil Pollut 2007;185:149–164.

Nguyen HT, Kim MY, Kim KH. The influence of long-range transport on atmospheric mercury on Jeju Island, Korea. Sci Total Environ 2010;408:1295–1307.

NRC. Global sources of local pollution: an assessment of long-range transport of key air pollutants to and from the United States committee on the significance of international transport of air pollutants. National Research Council; 2009. p. 248, ISBN: 0-309-14402-7. Available at http://www.nap.edu/catalog/12743.html. Accessed 2011 Sep 16.

Pacyna EG, Pacyna JM, Sundseth K, Munthe J, Kindbom K, Wilson S, Steenhuisen F, Maxson P. Global emission of mercury to the atmosphere from anthropogenic sources in 2005 and projections to 2020. Atmos Environ 2010;44:2487–2499.

Pan L, Woo J-H, Carmichael GR, Tang Y, Friedli HR, Radke LF. Regional distribution and emissions of mercury in east Asia: A modeling analysis of Asian Pacific Regional Aerosol Characterization Experiment (ACE-Asia) observations. J Geophys Res 2006;111: D07109.

Pan L, Carmichael GR, Adhikary B, Tang Y, Streets D, Woo J-H, Friedli HR, Radke LF. A regional analysis of the fate and transport of mercury in East Asia and an assessment of major uncertainties. Atmos Environ 2008;42:1144–1159.

Pan L, Lin C-J, Carmichael GR, Streets DG, Tang Y, Woo J-H, Shetty SK, Chu H-W, Ho TC, Friedli HR, Feng X. Study of atmospheric mercury budget in East Asia using STEM-Hg modeling system. Sci Total Environ 2010;408(16):3277–3291.

Petersen G, Bloxam R, Wong S, Munthe J, Krüger O, Schmolke SR, Kumar AV. A comprehensive Eulerian modelling framework for airborne mercury species: model development and applications in Europe. Atmos Environ 2001;35:3063–3074.

Pirrone N, Cinnirella S, Feng X, Finkelman RB, Friedli HR, Leaner J, Mason R, Mukherjee AB, Stracher G, Streets DG, Telmer K. Global mercury emissions to the atmosphere from natural and anthropogenic sources. In: Pirrone N, Mason RP, editors. Mercury fate and transport in the global atmosphere: emissions, measurements, and models. Springer; 2009. pp. 3–49.

Poissant L, Pilote M, Beauvais C, Constant P, Zhang HH. A year of continuous measurements of three atmospheric mercury species (GEM, RGM and Hgp) in southern Québec, Canada. Atmos Environ 2005;39:1275–1287.

Radke LF, Friedli HR, Heikes BG. Atmospheric mercury over the NE Pacific during spring 2002: Gradients, residence time, upper troposphere lower stratosphere loss, and long-range transport. J Geophys Res 2007;112: D19305.

Rea AW, Lindberg SE, Keeler GJ. Dry deposition and foliar leaching of mercury and selected trace elements in deciduous forest throughfall. Atmos Environ 2001;35:1352–1364.

Roos-Barraclough F, Givelet N, Cheburkin AK, Shotyk W, Norton SA. Use of Br and Se in peat to reconstruct the natural and anthropogenic fluxes of atmospheric Hg: A 10000-year record from caribou bog, Maine. Environ Sci Technol 2006;40:3188–3194.

Ryaboshapko A, Bullock OR, Christensen J, Cohen M, Dastoor A, Ilyin I, Petersen G, Syrakov D, Artz RS, Davignon D, Draxler RR, Munthe J. Intercomparison study of atmospheric mercury models: 1. Comparison of models with short-term measurements. Sci Total Environ 2007a;376:228–240.

Ryaboshapko A, Bullock OR, Christensen J, Cohen M, Dastoor A, Ilyin I, Petersen G, Syrakov D, Travnikov O, Artz RS, Davignon D, Draxler RR, Munthe J, Pacyna J. Intercomparison study of atmospheric mercury models: 2. Modelling results vs. long-term observations and comparison of country deposition budgets. Sci Total Environ 2007b;377:319–333.

Schroeder WH, Anlauf KG, Barrie LA, Lu JY, Steffen A, Schneeberger DR, Berg T. Arctic springtime depletion of mercury. Nature 1998;394:331–332.

Schroeder WH, Keeler G, Kock H, Roussel P, Schneeberger D, Schaedlich F. International field intercomparison of atmospheric mercury measurement methods. Water Air Soil Pollut 1995;80:611–620.

Schroeder WH, Munthe J. Atmospheric Mercury—an overview. Atmos Environ 1998;32:809–822.

Schuster PF, Krabbenhoft DF, Naftz DL, Cecil LD, Olson ML, Dewild JF, Susong DD, Green JR, Abbott ML. Atmospheric mercury deposition during the last 270 years: a glacial ice core record of natural and anthropogenic sources. Environ Sci Technol 2002;36:2303–2310.

Seigneur C, Lohman K. Effect of bromine chemistry on the atmospheric mercury cycle. J Geophys Res 2008;113: D23309.

Seigneur C, Vijayaraghavan K, Lohman K, Karamchandani P, Scott C. Global source attribution for mercury deposition in the United States. Environmental Science and Technology 2004;38:555–569.

Selin NE. Global biogeochemical cycling of mercury: A review. Annu Rev Environ Resour 2009;34:43–63.

Selin NE, Jacob DJ. Seasonal and spatial patterns of mercury wet deposition in the United States: constraints on the contribution from North American anthropogenic sources. Atmos Environ 2008;42:5193–5204.

Selin NE, Jacob DJ, Park RJ, Yantosca RM, Strode S, Jaegle L, Jaffe D. Chemical cycling and deposition of atmospheric mercury: global constraints from observations. J Geophys Res 2007;112: D02308.

Selin NE, Jacob DJ, Yantosca RM, Strode S, Jaegle L, Sunderland EM. Global 3-D land-ocean-atmosphere model for mercury: Present-day versus preindustrial cycles and anthropogenic enrichment factors for deposition. Global Biogeochem Cycles 2008;22: GB2011.

Skov H, Brooks S, Goodsite ME, Lindberg SE, Meyers TP, Landis M, Larsen MRB, Jensen B, McConville G, Chung KH, Christensen J. The fluxes of reactive gaseous mercury measured with a newly developed method using relaxed eddy accumulation. Atmos Environ 2006;40:5452–5463.

Skov H, Christensen JH, Heidam NZ, Jensen B, Wahlin P, Geernaert G. Fate of elemental mercury in the Artic during atmospheric depletion episodes and the load of atmospheric mercury to the Arctic. Environ Sci Technol 2004;38:2373–2382.

Sprovieri F, Hedgecock IM, Pirrone N. An investigation of the origins of reactive gaseous mercury in the Mediterranean marine boundary layer. Atmos Chem Phys 2010a;10:3985–3997.

Sprovieri F, Pirrone N, Ebinghaus R, Kock H, Dommergue A. A review of worldwide atmospheric mercury measurements. Atmos Chem Phys 2010b;10:8245–8265.

Sprovieri F, Pirrone N, Gärdfeldt K, Sommar J. Mercury speciation in the marine boundary layer along a 6000km cruise path around the Mediterranean Sea. Atmos Environ 2003;37: S6371–21–S6371–39.

Sprovieri F, Pirrone N, Hedgecock IM, Landis MS, Stevens RK. Intensive atmospheric mercury measurements at Terra Nova Bay in Antarctica during November and December 2000. J Geophys Res 2002;107: 4722.

Stamenkovic J, Gustin MS. Nonstomatal versus stomatal uptake of atmospheric mercury. Environ Sci Technol 2009;43(5):1367–1372.

Steffen A, Douglas T, Amyot M, Ariya P, Aspmo K, Berg T, Bottenheim J, Brooks S, Cobbett F, Dastoor A, Dommergue A, Ebinghaus R, Ferrari C, Gardfeldt K, Goodsite ME, Lean D, Poulain AJ, Scherz C, Skov H, Sommar J, Temme C. A synthesis of atmospheric mercury depletion event chemistry in the atmosphere and snow. Atmos Chem Phys 2008;8:1445–1482.

Steffen A, Schroeder WH, Bottenheim J, Narayan J, Fuentes JD. Atmospheric mercury concentrations: measurements and profiles near snow and ice surfaces in the Canadian Arctic during Alert 2000. Atmos Environ 2002;36:2653–2661.

Strode SA, Jaeglé L, Jaffe DA, Swartzendruber PC, Selin NE, Holmes C, Yantosca RM. Trans-Pacific transport of mercury. J Geophys Res 2008;113: D15305.

Sunderland EM, Mason RP. Human impacts on open ocean mercury concentrations. Global Biogeochem Cycles 2007;21: GB4022.

Sunderland E, Corbitt E, Cossa D, Evers D, Friedli H, Krabbenhoft D, Levin L, Pirrone N, Rice G. Impacts of intercontinental transport on human & ecological health. In: HTAP 2010 Assessment Report. Part B, Mercury. Geneva: UN–Economic Commission for Europe; 2010. pp. 145–178.

Syrakov D. On a PC-oriented Eulerian multi-level model for long-term calculations of the regional sulphur deposition. In: Gryning SE, Schiermeier FA, editors. Air pollution modelling and its application. XI 21. New York and London: Plenum Press; 1995. pp. 645–646.

Talbot R, Mao H, Scheuer E, Dibb J, Avery M. Total depletion of Hg in the upper troposphere-lower stratosphere. Geophys Res Lett 2007;34: L23804.

Tekran. Model 2357A—principles of operation. Toronto, Canada: Tekran Inc.; 1998.

Temme C, Blanchard P, Steffen A, Banic C, Beauchamp S, Poissant L, Tordon R, Wiens B. Trend, seasonal and multivariate analysis study of total gaseous mercury data from the Canadian atmospheric mercury measurement network (CAMNet). Atmos Environ 2007;41:5423–5441.

Travnikov O. Contribution of the intercontinental atmospheric transport to mercury pollution in the Northern Hemisphere. Atmos Environ 2005;39:7541–7548.

Travnikov O, Ilyin I. The EMEP/MSC-E mercury modeling system. In: Pirrone N, Mason RP, editors. Mercury fate and transport in the global atmosphere: emissions, measurements, and models. New York: Springer; 2009. pp. 571–587.

Travnikov O, Ilyin I. Development and application of the GLEMOS modelling framework—Mercury. In: Jonson JE, Travnikov O, editors. Development of the EMEP global modelling framework: Progress report. EMEP/MSC-W Technical Report 1/2010; Norwegian Meteorological Institute. Oslo, Norway; 2010. Available at http://emep.int/publ/emep2010_publications.html. Accessed 2011 Sep 16.

Travnikov O, Lin C-J, Dastoor A, Bullock OR, Hedgecock IM, Holmes C, Ilyin I, Jaeglé L, Jung G, Pan L, Pongprueksa P, Ryzhkov A, Seigneur C, Skov H. Global and regional modeling. In: HTAP 2010 Assessment Report. Part B, Mercury. Geneva: UN–Economic Commission for Europe; 2010. pp. 97–144.

Urba A, Kvietkus K, Sakalys J, Xiao Z, Lindqvist O. A new sensitive and portable mercury vapor analyzer Gardis-1A. Water Air Soil Pollut 1995;80:1305–1309.

van Loon L, Mader E, Scott SL. Reduction of the aqueous mercuric ion by sulfite: UV spectrum of $HgS\,O_3$ and its intramolecular redox reactions. J Phys Chem 2000;104:1621–1626.

van Loon LL, Mader EA, Scott SL. Sulfite stabilization and reduction of the aqueous mercuric ion: kinetic determination of sequential formation constants. J Phys Chem 2001;105:3190–3195.

Vermette SJ, Lindberg SE, Bloom N. Field tests for a regional mercury deposition network: sampling design and test results. Atmos Environ 1995;29:247–1252.

Wan Q, Feng X, Lu J, Zheng W, Song X, Han S, Xu H. Atmospheric mercury in Changbai Mountain area, northeastern China I. The seasonal distribution pattern of total gaseous mercury and its potential sources. Environ Res 2009a;109:201–206.

Wan Q, Feng X, Lu J, Zheng W, Song X, Li P, Han S, Xu H. Atmospheric mercury in Changbai Mountain area, northeastern China II. The distribution of reactive gaseous mercury and particulate mercury and mercury deposition fluxes. Environ Res 2009b;109:721–727.

Wangberg I, Munthe J, Berg T, Ebinghaus R, Kock HH, Temme C, Bieber E, Spain TG, Stolk A. Trends in air concentration and deposition of mercury in the coastal environment of the North Sea Area. Atmos Environ 2007;41(12):2612–2619.

Wesely ML, Hicks BB. A review of the current status of knowledge on dry deposition. Atmos Environ 2000;34:2261–2222.

Xin M, Gustin MS. Gaseous elemental mercury exchange with low mercury containing soils: investigation of controlling factors. Appl Geochem 2007;22(7):1451–1466.

Zhang HH, Poissant L, Xu X, Pilote M. Explorative and innovative dynamic flux bag method development and testing for mercury air-vegetation gas exchange flux. Atmos Environ 2005;39:7481–7493.

CHAPTER 11

ADSORPTION OF MERCURY ON SOLIDS IN THE AQUATIC ENVIRONMENT

GUANGLIANG LIU, YANBIN LI, and YONG CAI

11.1 INTRODUCTION

There are a number of pathways by which mercury (Hg) can enter the aquatic environment: inorganic Hg(II) and methylmercury (MeHg) from atmospheric deposition (wet and dry) can enter water bodies directly; Hg(II) and methylmercury can be transported to water bodies in the runoff (bound to suspended soil/humus or attached to dissolved organic carbon); or Hg(II) and methylmercury can leach into the water body from groundwater flow in the upper soil layers (USEPA, 1997; Morel et al., 1998; Fitzgerald et al., 2007a,b). In the aquatic system, mercury can undergo a series of complicated biogeochemical processes, including transformation and transport, which determine the speciation of mercury in the aquatic environment and the transport of mercury species between water and solid phases (Morel et al., 1998; Fitzgerald et al., 2007b).

Mercury can exist in three oxidation states: 0, +1, and +2, forming elemental Hg (Hg(0)) at 0 valence and mercurous (Hg(I)) and mercuric (Hg(II)) compounds at +1 and +2 valences. In the aquatic environment (including water, sediment, and biota phases), most of the mercury is in the inorganic and organic forms of divalent mercuric compounds, with Hg(0) being a considerable fraction of dissolved Hg in water phase (USEPA, 1997; Ullrich et al., 2001). The speciation of mercury present in the aquatic environment critically affects the transport processes of mercury species. The following two paragraphs provide a brief overview of mercury speciation in the aquatic environment.

The speciation of inorganic Hg(II) compounds in the aquatic environment is affected by the presence of various inorganic ligands. For example, at high sulfide concentrations (e.g., in sulfidic waters and interstitial waters of bottom

Environmental Chemistry and Toxicology of Mercury, First Edition.
Edited by Guangliang Liu, Yong Cai, and Nelson O'Driscoll.
© 2012 John Wiley & Sons, Inc. Published 2012 by John Wiley & Sons, Inc.

sediments), the chemistry of Hg is primarily controlled by sulfide through the formation of soluble bi- and polysulfide complexes between Hg and sulfide (e.g., $HgSH^+$, $Hg(SH)_2$, $Hg(SH)S^-$, HgS_2^{2-}, $Hg(S_x)_2^{2-}$, and $Hg(S_x)OH^-$), depending on pH and Eh (Ullrich et al., 2001; Wolfenden et al., 2005; Drott et al., 2007; Belzile et al., 2008; Zhong and Wang, 2009a). In the absence of sulfide, the speciation of inorganic Hg is controlled by other ligands such as chloride and hydroxide, with three uncharged complexes ($Hg(OH)_2$, $HgOHCl$, and $HgCl_2$) dominating in freshwaters, whereas complexes of Hg(II)–polychlorides (e.g., $HgCl_3^-$ and $HgCl_4^{2-}$) prevailing in the presence of increasing chloride concentrations and in seawaters (Nriagu, 1979; Morel et al., 1998; Ullrich et al., 2001; Fitzgerald et al., 2007a). Organic Hg(II) species include primarily methylmercury (MeHg) and in some cases dimethylmercury (DMHg) (in marine environments) and ethylmercury (EtHg) (particularly in wetlands) (Mason and Fitzgerald, 1993; Mason et al., 1998; Mason and Benoit, 2003; Fitzgerald et al., 2007a). As with inorganic Hg(II), MeHg can also form highly stable complexes with sulfide and other ligands (such as CH_3HgS^- and CH_3HgCl), depending on the concentrations of various ligands (Morel et al., 1998; Ullrich et al., 2001; Fitzgerald et al., 2007a).

In addition to complexation with inorganic ligands, both inorganic and organic forms of Hg(II) compounds can be bound by natural organic matter (NOM), including dissolved organic matter (DOM), colloidal organic matter (COM), and particulate organic matter (POM), which likely dominates the chemistry of Hg species in many freshwater systems (Ullrich et al., 2001). For example, both laboratory experimental and modeling results have suggested that more than 90% of inorganic Hg(II) and from 70% to 97% of MeHg in water may be associated with DOM (primarily humic substances) in some lakes, although the complexation of Hg species with NOM may be decreased in seawater because of chloride ion competition (USEPA, 1997; Morel et al., 1998; Ullrich et al., 2001; Fitzgerald et al., 2007a,b).

Once entering an aquatic system, mercury can undergo various biogeochemical processes, which include transformation processes, such as association/ dissociation with various ligands, precipitation/dissolution as minerals (e.g., mercury sulfide), oxidation/reduction reactions, and methylation/demethylation, and transport processes, such as volatilization into the atmosphere, adsorption/desorption to suspended particulate matter and sediments, sedimentation/resuspension, leaching and transport to groundwater, and uptake by aquatic biota (Stein et al., 1996; Haitzer et al., 2003; Fitzgerald et al., 2007b). The movement of mercury through each specific watershed may be unique, but adsorption of inorganic Hg(II) and MeHg onto particulate matter and subsequent sedimentation is expected to be the dominant process for determining the fate of mercury in aquatic environments.

The adsorption/desorption of mercury species on suspended and sediment solid particles (including inorganic and organic) is a key factor determining the concentration of dissolved mercury. The partition of mercury between dissolved and solid phases influences mobility, reactivity, and bioavailability of mercury species and subsequently controls the fate and biological uptake of mercury. For instance, through adsorption onto particulate matter and subsequent sedimentation of solid particles, the major fraction of mercury in an aqueous system is expected to be stored in sediments, with limited mobility (USEPA, 1997). Meanwhile, the adsorption of inorganic Hg(II), which is the precursor for the production of MeHg, is likely to reduce the bioavailability of mercury species for bacterial uptake and therefore inhibit mercury methylation, which would reduce the bioaccumulation of mercury in biota (Ullrich et al., 2001).

Considering the complexity of mercury transport in the aquatic environment, this chapter has no intention to address all aspects of aquatic transport processes of mercury. Instead, this chapter focuses on the adsorption of mercury on solid particles, with a special emphasis on the effects of the presence of inorganic and organic colloids on mercury adsorption on particulate matter. The following part of this chapter briefly summarizes and discusses previous studies on the adsorption/desorption processes of mercury in water bodies. A separate section follows to address the role of organic and inorganic colloids in mercury adsorption, which has recently received much attention (Stein et al., 1996; He et al., 2005; Brigham et al., 2009; Liao et al., 2009; Zhong and Wang, 2009a, 2009b; Gondikas et al., 2010; Skyllberg and Drott, 2010; Deonarine et al., 2011; Aiken et al., 2011a, 2011b).

11.2 ADSORPTION OF MERCURY ON SOLIDS

In aquatic systems, adsorption/desorption of mercury plays a dominant role in the distribution of mercury species among the dissolved, colloidal, and particulate phases, controlling the transport, transformation, biological uptake, and toxicity of mercury. Numerous studies have been conducted to examine the adsorption/desorption of mercury species, in particular, inorganic Hg(II), on natural and synthetic particles, including soils, clays, metal (hydr)oxides, and metal sulfides (Lockwood and Chen, 1973; Klusman and Matoske, 1983; Otani et al., 1986; Tiffreau et al., 1995; Yin et al., 1997b; Bonnissel-Gissinger et al., 1999; Walcarius et al., 1999; Hintelmann and Harris, 2004; Brigatti et al., 2005; He et al., 2005; Yang et al., 2008a; Liao et al., 2009). For example, in order to investigate the effects of soil or sediment adsorption on mercury transport, studies have been conducted, by directly using soils or sediments collected from the field, to quantify and characterize mercury adsorption on these complex multicomponent solid matrices (Yin et al., 1996; Yin et al., 1997a, 1997b; Bloom et al., 1998; Biester et al., 2002). For the purpose of better understanding the mechanisms underlying mercury adsorption/desorption processes, a large body of research has been performed employing experimental approaches based on well-defined systems, which include selected (sometimes model) pure solid substrates, such as metal (hydr)oxide and sulfide minerals, clays and related materials, and organic compounds (Lockwood and Chen, 1973; Mac Naughton and James, 1974; Brown et al., 1979; Jean and Bancroft, 1986; Gunneriusson and Sjöberg, 1993; Tiffreau et al., 1995; Singh et al., 1996; Walcarius et al., 1999; Hintelmann and Harris, 2004; Brigatti et al., 2005; Jing et al., 2008; Liao et al., 2009; Zhang et al., 2009). These approaches using well-defined systems provide a better knowledge of the factors controlling the movement and availability of mercury species in aquatic systems (Walcarius et al., 1999).

11.2.1 Mechanisms of Mercury Adsorption on Solids

In suspended particles and sediments, mercury can be adsorbed onto both inorganic minerals (in particular metal oxides) and organic matter (Nriagu, 1979; Stein et al., 1996). The relative importance of inorganic minerals and organic matter in mercury adsorption can vary, depending heavily on the nature of the solid particles and the speciation of mercury species, among many other factors. The role of organic matter in trapping Hg in soils and sediments has been well documented in previous studies, indicating that the organic matter fraction in solids has the capacity to control the Hg enrichment (Skyllberg et al., 2000, 2006; Hissler and Probst, 2006; Skyllberg and Drott, 2010). It is generally thought that much of the mercury in soil is bound to bulk organic matter, with limited mobility (Xia et al., 1999; Qian et al., 2002; Karlsson and Skyllberg, 2003). In heavily polluted areas, mercury is mainly adsorbed onto the mineral fractions of sediments because the organic matter is rapidly saturated by Hg pollution (Hissler and Probst, 2006). In many cases, both the inorganic mineral and organic matter fractions of the solids are important with respect to mercury adsorption and enrichment.

The adsorption of mercury species on organic matter involves the association of mercury with functional groups within organic matter such as S-, O-, and N-containing moieties, in particular reduced S groups (e.g., thiols, sulfides, and disulfides) (Skyllberg et al., 2006; Skyllberg, 2008). Owing to the extremely strong complexation between mercury and reduced S, reduced S groups are suggested to be primarily involved in the complexation of mercury with organic matter, in particular when the ratios of mercury to reduced S are low. When mercury concentration exceeds the concentration of high affinity reduced S sites within organic matter, weaker O- and N-containing ligands may be involved in the complexation. For example, previous spectroscopic studies using extended X-ray absorption fine structure (EXAFS) suggest that about 70% of Hg is complexed by two reduced S groups of humic substances extracted from organic soils at a molar ratio of Hg to reduced organic S of 0.26 (Xia et al., 1999; Hesterberg et al., 2001). However, when the molar ratio between Hg and reduced organic S is 3, the data for first and second shell contributions could be equally fitted by a model with one thiol and one O/N group or by one disulfide and one O/N group, indicating the involvement of O/N group in the complexation of mercury with organic matter (Xia et al., 1999). Further studies, using humic acids extracted from organic soils and intact organic soils, suggest that, at low Hg concentration,

Hg is likely complexed by two thiols at a distance of 2.33 Å in a linear configuration, with a third reduced S (likely an organic sulfide) contributing with a weaker second shell attraction at a distance of 2.92–3.08 Å. At high Hg concentrations when all high affinity S sites are saturated, the association between Hg and organic matter is likely to involve such a structure in which one carbonyl-O or amino-N at 2.07 Å and one carboxyl-O at 2.84 Å are in the first shell and two C atoms at an average distance of 3.14 Å are in the second shell (Skyllberg et al., 2000, 2006; Qian et al., 2002; Skyllberg, 2008; Skyllberg and Drott, 2010).

Inorganic minerals, particularly metal (hydr)oxides, have long been recognized as important surfaces for adsorption of metal species, including mercury species (Walcarius et al., 1999). However, unlike other cation metals for which the adsorption on mineral surfaces can be attributed to ion exchange in the surfaces, the adsorption of mercury is different because above pH 3, aqueous mercury species are present in hydroxylated forms (Posselt et al., 1968; Lockwood and Chen, 1973). The hydrolysis of mercury and the equilibrium solution species play a determining role in the adsorption of mercury on the (hydr)oxide/water interface. In natural waters, mercury may be present in various chemical forms, mainly hydroxo-, chloro-, and hydroxychloro-complexes of Hg(II), which have different affinities for sedimentary minerals (Stein et al., 1996; Bloom et al., 1998; Walcarius et al., 1999; Ullrich et al., 2001; Fitzgerald et al., 2007b). It is thought that mercury hydrolysis is required before adsorption and that only these hydroxylated mercury species can be adsorbed on the mineral surface, while Hg^{2+} cannot (Lockwood and Chen, 1973). The adsorption may occur through the complexation of hydroxylated mercury species with hydroxyls on the mineral surfaces ($\equiv S–OH$). Studies modeling the adsorption of inorganic mercury(II) on (hydr)oxides suggest that, depending on pH and chloride concentration, $HgOH^+$, HgOHCl, and, in particular, the uncharged metal oxide hydrate $Hg(OH)_2$ (which is often the dominant species in natural waters) can be adsorbed at the oxide/water interface, forming, respectively, three chemical forms of stable surface complexes from the reaction between mercury(II) and surface hydroxyls (Eqs 11.1–11.3) (Gunneriusson and Sjöberg, 1993; Gunneriusson et al., 1995; Tiffreau et al., 1995; Walcarius et al., 1999). The adsorption mechanism seems to involve a condensation reaction between a surface hydroxyl group on the mineral surface and a hydroxyl group on mercury, giving the inner-sphere-type complex surface and water as products. Support for this mechanism comes from studies using model metal (hydr)oxides (e.g., quartz) to investigate mercury adsorption on minerals (Walcarius et al., 1999; Brigatti et al., 2005).

$$(\equiv S - OH) + HgOH^+ \Leftrightarrow (\equiv S - O - Hg^+) + H_2O \qquad (11.1)$$

$$(\equiv S - OH) + Hg(OH)_2 \Leftrightarrow (\equiv S - O - Hg - OH) + H_2O \qquad (11.2)$$

$$(\equiv S - OH) + HgOHCl \Leftrightarrow (\equiv S - O - Hg - Cl) + H_2O \qquad (11.3)$$

11.2.2 Rates and Isotherms of Mercury Adsorption

Studies measuring the reaction rates for mercury adsorption on various solids suggest that mercury adsorption is usually a fast reaction (Lockwood and Chen, 1973). In many cases, solution mercury concentrations determined for the shortest reaction times (e.g., minutes to hours after mixing mercury solutions with solids) are similar to the final equilibrium values, especially when low mercury to sorbent ratios are adopted in the experiments. The equilibrium times for adsorption of mercury species, including inorganic Hg(II) and MeHg, vary from a few minutes to hours (even days), but are usually between 30 min and one day (Lockwood and Chen, 1973; Hintelmann and Harris, 2004). It is possible that the adsorption of mercury species involves two steps, as proposed in previous studies. For example, it is speculated that mercury is initially adsorbed onto the surface and subsequently migrates into the solid lattice or is covered by organic biofilms, eventually resulting in the incorporation of mercury into the solid matrix (Mikac et al., 1999; Hintelmann and Harris, 2004). In addition, the colloidal pumping model, in which mercury is initially complexed by colloids (<24 h) and subsequently adsorbed or coagulated onto particles (within days), has been developed to describe the kinetics of mercury adsorption (Stordal et al., 1996b; Babiarz et al., 2001). In these two-step models, the initial adsorption/desorption is fast or even instantaneous (equilibration takes less than 30 min), whereas the second adsorption or migration step may be slow, explaining the large variation in equilibrium times reported in the literature (Lockwood and Chen, 1973; Gagnon and Fisher, 1997; Le Roux et al., 2001; Hintelmann and Harris, 2004).

The adsorption capacity and isotherms of mercury by a variety of natural adsorbents, including minerals such as goethite, illite, kaolinite, silica, and calcite and intact sediment and soil particles (collected from the field or directly from field studies), have been extensively investigated under various experimental conditions (Frenet, 1981; Gagnon and Fisher, 1997; Yin et al., 1997a; Bonnissel-Gissinger et al., 1999; Bilinski et al., 2000; Hintelmann and Harris, 2004; Brigatti et al., 2005). It has been observed that, unlike other divalent cation metals, the adsorption of mercury on solids is relatively low. In fact, complete adsorption of mercury has never been observed, even when using large solid-to-solution ratios and low mercury concentrations (Mac Naughton and James, 1974; Walcarius et al., 1999). In previous studies using silica and other metal oxides as sorbents, only about 60% of the total mercury was present as the adsorbed species (which was similar to the fraction of hydrolyzed mercury species), whereas many other metals are known to be essentially totally adsorbed (Mac Naughton and James, 1974; Brown et al., 1998; Walcarius et al., 1999). The equilibrium data of mercury adsorption (adsorbed mercury vs mercury remaining in solution) can often be best fitted with the Freundlich isotherm rather than with the Langmuir and linear isotherms (Lockwood and Chen, 1973; Hintelmann and Harris, 2004).

When describing mercury adsorption, a distribution (partition) coefficient (K_d, L/kg), which is a fundamental parameter describing in a summarizing way the distribution of a chemical species between the dissolved and solid phases, is often calculated (Stumm, 1992; Ullrich et al., 2001).

$$K_d = \frac{C_s}{C_w} \tag{11.4}$$

where C_s (microgram per kilogram) and C_w (microgram per liter) are the mercury concentrations in the solid and dissolved phases, respectively. C_w is often operationally defined as the concentration of mercury in the filtrate (passing through 0.45- or 0.22-μm filter). In addition to filtration, a chemical fractionation based on differences in chemical reactivity of mercury species is sometimes used to calculate a modified K_d. In these cases, the reactive (or easily reducible, e.g., by stannous chloride) mercury concentration is often used as a substitute for the dissolved fraction (Lindström, 2001). The calculation of the K_d coefficient is widely used, as this parameter is very useful in quantifying mercury adsorption and in developing and applying models to predict quantitatively the transport of Hg in aquatic systems.

Much work has been conducted to determine K_d values for mercury distribution between water and sediments, which includes laboratory experiments using model and natural particles and field studies (Stordal et al., 1996a, 1996b; Coquery et al., 1997; Schluter, 1997; Hurley et al., 1998; Turner et al., 2001; Turner et al., 2004; Brigham et al., 2009). Table 11.1 illustrates selected K_d values reported in the literature. The K_d values vary greatly, with $\log K_d$ ranging approximately from 3 to 6 for total mercury (THg) and from 2 to 6 for MeHg. Many studies suggest that, although the K_d values for THg and MeHg have comparable orders of magnitude, the K_d value for MeHg is slightly lower (Ullrich et al., 2001; Muresan et al., 2007; Brigham et al., 2009). The large disparities in K_d values among these studies may be due to the nature of the solids (including the property and abundance of binding sites present within solids), the method used to determine the dissolved and solid mercury concentrations, and other conditions, such as pH and salinity. Nevertheless, the magnitude of $\log K_d$ values for mercury species exemplifies the strong affinity of inorganic Hg(II) and MeHg for sediment and suspended particles (Muresan et al., 2007).

Mercury adsorption is influenced by a wide variety of environmental factors, such as pH, redox potential, salinity, and the presence of organic and inorganic complexing agents such as organic matter (Driscoll et al., 1995; Ravichandran et al., 1999; Ullrich et al., 2001; Ravichandran, 2004; He et al., 2007; Aiken et al., 2011a). Those factors control the chemical forms of mercury species and surface properties of solid particles and thus influence mercury adsorption. For example, pH has been suggested to play a significant role in controlling Hg(II) adsorption, mobility, and methylation, as it affects both particle surface charge characteristics and mercury speciation (Wang et al., 1991; Barrow and Cox, 1992; Sarkar et al., 1999). In general, intermediate pH ranges (e.g., pH 4–10) favor Hg(II) adsorption, whereas adsorption decreases under strong acidic and basic conditions (e.g., pH <4 or pH >10). The pH effect of mercury adsorption is also dependent on the nature of sorbents and other conditions (Lockwood and Chen, 1973; Stein et al., 1996; Kim et al., 2004a). At increasing concentrations,

TABLE 11.1 Distribution Coefficients (K_d, liters per kilogram) for THg and MeHg Between Water and Sediment (Suspended and Bulk) Reported in the Literature

| Ecosystem Type | log K_d | | Reference |
	THg	MeHg	
Freshwater (lake)[a]	4.6–5.5 (5.0)	3.4–4.9 (4.1)	Watras et al. (2000)
Freshwater (lake)	5.5–5.8	5.7	Mason and Sullivan (1997)
Freshwater (lake)[b]	5.8–6.9 (6.6)	—	Lindström (2001)
Freshwater (wetland)[c]	3.5–5.3 (4.8)	2.2–4.7 (3.4)	Liu et al. (2008, 2009, 2011)
Freshwater (river)	2.8–5.5 (4.9)	2.9–5.8 (4.6)	Babiarz et al. (1998)
Estuary	4.6–5.2	—	Stordal et al. (1996a)
Freshwater (river)	2.8–6.6 (4.8)	2.8–5.9 (4.4)	Brigham et al. (2009)
Freshwater (river)	2.8–5.7 (4.7)	—	Hurley et al. (1995)
Freshwater (river)	5.4–6.0	—	Hurley et al. (1998)
Coast (lagoon)	4.8	3.7	Muresan et al. (2007)
	(Bulk sediment)	(Bulk sediment)	
	6.3	6.4	
	(Fe oxyhydroxides)	(Fe oxyhydroxides)	
	7.6	7.7	
	(Mn oxyhydroxides)	(Mn oxyhydroxides)	

The numbers in parentheses are median values.
[a]Calculated from data reported in the original literature.
[b]In this study, a modified K_d was calculated by substituting the concentration of easily reducible mercury for the dissolved mercury.
[c]The data in this study are actually reported as the distribution ratios of mercury species between the overlying water column and the bulk sediment compartment, as calculated by dividing sediment mercury by mercury concentration in overlying water (filtered through a 100-μm screen).

chloride (Cl^-) may form chlorocomplexes with Hg(II) species, decreasing Hg adsorption on aqueous particulates and sediments (Forbes et al., 1974; Morel et al., 1998; Kim et al., 2004b; Hissler and Probst, 2006; He et al., 2007). The influences of these general factors on Hg adsorption are not further discussed here. Rather, we focus on the effects of organic matter and inorganic colloids on mercury adsorption in the section that follows.

11.3 ROLE OF COLLOIDS IN MERCURY ADSORPTION

There are various colloidal particles (1 nm–1 μm), including organic and inorganic, ubiquitously present in the aquatic environment (Gustafsson and Gschwend, 1997; Hochella, 2002; Aiken et al., 2011a). For example, NOM in waters is often within colloidal size range, representing the major fraction of organic colloids, whereas aquatic metal minerals (e.g., oxides, hydroxides, oxyhydroxides, and sulfides) contribute primarily to inorganic colloids (within nanosized range, 1–100 nm, in many cases) (Gustafsson and Gschwend, 1997;

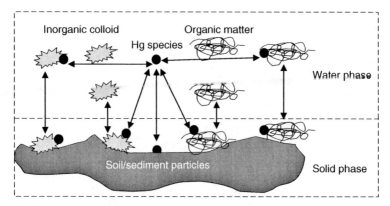

Figure 11.1 A conceptual model of mercury adsorption on solid particles in the presence of organic matter and inorganic colloids.

Waychunas et al., 2005; Waychunas and Zhang, 2008; Aiken et al., 2011a). These organic and inorganic colloids can form complexes with mercury species, influencing mercury speciation and adsorption by solid particles (Fig. 11.1). The formation of the complexes between mercury and colloids could retain mercury species in solutions and thus decrease mercury adsorption onto suspended and sediment solids. In many aquatic systems, colloids (both inorganic and organic) are very likely the dominant factors that control the speciation and mobility of metals (including mercury) (Gustafsson and Gschwend, 1997; Brown, 2001; de Jonge et al., 2004; Hochella and Madden, 2005; Kretzschmar and Schäfer, 2005; Aiken et al., 2011a).

When studying mercury (and other contaminants) adsorption, the conventional method is to separate mercury into dissolved and particle-adsorbed phases, where the dissolved mercury fraction is often determined as the mercury passing through filters with sizes such as 0.45 and 0.22 µm (Mason and Fitzgerald, 1993; Mason et al., 1994; Watras et al., 1995; Babiarz et al., 1998, 2001; Lindström, 2001; Hochella, 2002). However, the so-defined dissolved mercury fraction, which is in fact equated with the filterable fraction, includes the colloidal complexes formed between mercury species and colloids, in addition to truly dissolved mercury species (e.g., free mercuric ions and compounds) (Babiarz et al., 2000, 2003; Lindström, 2001; Haitzer et al., 2003). Considering the presence of colloidal particles in waters, it may be more suitable to differentiate mercury into three phases, namely, particulate (referring to mercury associated with solids >1 µm), colloidal (mercury complexed by NOM and metal minerals within the size range of 1 nm–1 µm), and truly dissolved form (<1 nm, approximately 1 kDa in molecular weight) (Cai et al., 1999; Lead et al., 1999; Babiarz et al., 2001; Haitzer et al., 2002). The differentiation between colloidal and truly dissolved mercury fractions is often operationally defined in practice (e.g., using sequential filtrations to separate these species).

Colloidal and truly dissolved mercury species may exhibit different mobilities, reactivities, and bioavailabilities and thus have different transport routes and transformation pathways. First, colloidal mercury is expected to behave differently than truly dissolved Hg species in terms of mobility and transport. Although dissolved species are traditionally considered to be the most efficient forms for contaminant transport in the aquatic environment, transport of dissolved mercury (particularly in the subsurface) could be significantly retarded because of retention by solids. On the contrary, significant colloid-facilitated transport of a variety of metal contaminants (including mercury) has been demonstrated in a number of recent studies, including both field observations and laboratory column leaching experiments (Choe and Gill, 2003; Choe et al., 2003; Lowry et al., 2004; Slowey et al., 2005a, 2005b). Second, the chemical reactivity and bioavailability of colloidal mercury may be limited, in comparison to truly dissolved mercury species. The published literature generally holds that only the truly dissolved inorganic Hg(II) fraction is available for methylation, whereas mercury associated with colloidal particles may be unable to be taken up by bacteria resulting in inhibition in mercury methylation (Farrell et al., 1998; Benoit et al., 1999–2001b; Cai et al., 1999; Lowry et al., 2004; Brigham et al., 2009).

In consideration of the disparities between colloidal and truly dissolved mercury in mobility and bioavailability, the differentiation between colloidal and truly dissolved species is important in studying the fate and adsorption of mercury. Although many studies have been designed to investigate the role of colloids (in particular NOM) in mercury adsorption, these studies often focus on observing the apparent effects of colloids on mercury adsorption (enhancing or reducing adsorption) by separating mercury into traditionally defined dissolved (typically <0.45 µm) and particulate (often determined by the differences between total and dissolved mercury) phases. It is therefore necessary to further differentiate colloidal and truly dissolved mercury by quantifying these two species and then characterizing mercury adsorption in such a ternary system (particulate, colloidal, and truly dissolved phases) when studying mercury adsorption onto solids in the presence of colloids.

11.3.1 Role of Aquatic Organic Matter in Mercury Adsorption

NOM is known to possess strong affinity for mercury and significantly affect the adsorption and desorption of mercury in natural soils, mineral surfaces, and aquatic ecosystems (Yin et al., 1996; Ravichandran, 2004; Jing et al., 2007). For instance, distribution coefficients of MeHg and Hg(II) were found to be significantly correlated with those for organic carbon in sediments of Long Island Sound, suggesting that adsorption/desorption of Hg species with sediment particles is controlled by partitioning of associated organic ligands (Hammerschmidt et al., 2004).

Binding of mercury to dissolved and colloidal NOM in waters can affect mercury adsorption/desorption in two contrary directions (Schuster, 1991). On one hand, NOM binding with mercury can form stable Hg–DOM complexes and thus hinder or prevent adsorption of mercury to particles. Conversely, NOM can be adsorbed to particles, which can provide additional adsorption sites for mercury and enhance adsorption of mercury. Evidence is increasing for the enhancement of mercury adsorption by particles being related to organic matter. The presence of fulvic acids in water was observed to be able to increase mercury adsorption in the whole pH interval studied (pH 3–10) (Xu and Allard, 1991; Bäckström et al., 2003). In the presence of humic acid previously adsorbed on kaolin in a concentration range of 0–27 mg/g, the Hg(II) adsorption capacity of kaolin at pH 4 was enhanced (Arias et al., 2004). Meanwhile, the presence of humic acid dramatically reduced the desorption ratio of previously adsorbed Hg(II) from >50% to <3% at pH 2.5.

However, contrary results also existed. Effects of DOM (probably including colloidal OM) obtained from different sources on adsorption and desorption of Hg were investigated (Yang et al., 2008b). It was found that the presence of DOM obviously reduced Hg maximum adsorption capacity (to a maximum of 40%). Meanwhile, Hg desorption from the soils was promoted by the addition of DOM (Yang et al., 2008b). Similar inhibitory effects of DOM on the adsorption of Hg(II) were observed in two types of Amazon soils (Miretzky et al., 2005). The adsorption coefficient of mercury (K_d) for sediment obtained from a temporarily drained water infiltration pond was found to be negatively correlated with the concentration of dissolved organic carbon (DOC) (Bengtsson and Picado, 2008). The authors suggest that common DOC concentrations in groundwater and streambeds, 5–20 mg/L, would halve the K_d obtained from standard sorption assays of Hg(II) (Bengtsson and Picado, 2008). In addition, enhancement of Hg(II) desorption by the presence of low molecular weight organic acids or DOM was reported (Yang et al., 2008a).

The type and composition of NOM are important factors controlling the effects of NOM on Hg adsorption. In studies using model organic acids as surrogate for NOM to investigate the influence of NOM on mercury adsorption, it was observed that citric acid had a retarding effect on the adsorption of Hg(II) by kaolinite at pHs of 6.0 and 8.0 and a promoting effect when the pH decreased to 4.0 (Singh et al., 1996). The effects of carboxylic (oxalate) and thiol (cysteine) groups on desorption of Hg(II) from kaolinite were investigated (Senevirathna et al., 2011). Oxalate was found to hardly affect the Hg(II) desorption, but cysteine inhibited the Hg(II) desorption significantly. Jing et al. (2007) investigated the effects of several organic acids on Hg(II) desorption and found that citric acid at high concentrations was the most effective in increasing Hg(II) desorption, followed by tartaric acid and malic acid, and oxalic acid was the least effective. They also found that results obtained at low concentrations of organic ligands could be opposite to that at high concentrations. The presence of organic ligands (tartaric, malic, or oxalic acid) was found to inhibit Hg(II) desorption from one of the studied soils at low concentrations but enhanced Hg(II) desorption at higher concentrations. The authors speculated that most of the added organic acids are adsorbed by organic and inorganic components in the soil when small amounts of organic acids are added, thus Hg(II) may be bound to the organic ligands that are adsorbed on the surfaces of the soil and reduce Hg(II) desorption. At higher organic acid concentrations, most of the added organic ligands remain in solution, and the organic ligands in the solution may compete over particles on binding with Hg(II), resulting in enhanced desorption of Hg(II).

11.3.2 Inorganic Colloids in Mercury Adsorption

There could be two types of inorganic colloids in the aquatic environment affecting the adsorption of mercury species onto solid particles through two different mechanisms. Colloidal metal (especially iron) (oxyhydr)oxides can act as sorbents to complex mercury species on the surface, whereby mercury is retained in the solution and transported as an adsorbed species (Ganguli et al., 2000; Rytuba, 2000; Lowry et al., 2004). In addition, mercury minerals, in particular mercury sulfide (HgS, cinnabar or metacinnabar), can be present in colloidal form in solution (rather than being adsorbed on solids), in which case mercury is transported as discrete colloidal particles (Ganguli et al., 2000; Lowry et al., 2004; Slowey et al., 2005a, 2005b).

Studies designated to directly investigate the effects of inorganic colloids on mercury adsorption on large (noncolloidal) solid particles are rare, probably due to the difficulties in separating and quantifying colloidal species from particulate and truly dissolved species. However, recent research studying the speciation and transport of mercury in anaerobic aquatic environments and in mining tailings sites suggest the prevalence of colloidal mercury species as adsorbed species or as discrete particles and the significance of colloid-facilitated mercury transport relative to dissolved mercury transport (Lowry et al., 2004; Slowey et al., 2005a, 2005b; Lau and Hsu-Kim, 2008; Deonarine and Hsu-Kim, 2009). For example, colloidal HgS (often as nanoscale particles, typically smaller than 30 nm) is observed to exist in a variety of environments such as sediments of mine drainage and porewater of anaerobic sediments and could be the dominant form of mercury transported from mining sites (Lowry et al., 2004; Lau and Hsu-Kim, 2008; Deonarine and Hsu-Kim, 2009; Gondikas et al., 2010). From the colloid-enhanced mercury transport by iron (oxyhydr)oxides and mercury sulfide, one can infer that the presence of these inorganic colloids would decrease or prevent the adsorption of mercury species on solids that can undergo sedimentation. In the adsorption experiments using the filter-passing fraction (e.g., 0.45 or 0.2 µm) as a surrogate for dissolved phase, the mercury species complexed by colloidal iron (oxyhydr)oxides and mercury sulfide colloids could be mistaken for dissolved species, since these particles are small enough to pass through conventional filters (Lindström, 2001; Deonarine and Hsu-Kim, 2009; Gondikas et al., 2010).

11.3.3 Distribution Coefficients of Mercury in the Presence of Colloids

In the presence of organic and/or inorganic colloids, the effect of colloids on the distribution of mercury species between the solution and solid phases need to be accounted for, when calculating distribution coefficients. When mercury species are differentiated into three phases (particulate, colloidal, and dissolved), the following distribution coefficients could be calculated to account for the effects of inorganic or organic colloids (Stumm, 1992; Stordal et al., 1996a; Cai et al., 1999).

$$K_p = \frac{C_s}{C_w^*} \tag{11.5}$$

$$K_{ic} = \frac{C_{ic}}{C_w^*} \tag{11.6}$$

$$K_{oc} = \frac{C_{oc}}{C_w^*} \tag{11.7}$$

$$K_d^{ic*} = \frac{K_p}{1 + K_{ic}M_{ic}} \tag{11.8}$$

$$K_d^{oc*} = \frac{K_p}{1 + K_{oc}M_{oc}} \tag{11.9}$$

Where C_s (microgram per kilogram), C_w^* (microgram per liter), and C_{ic} (or C_{oc}, microgram per milligram) are the concentrations of mercury in solid, truly dissolved, and inorganic (or organic) colloidal phases, respectively. K_p (liter per kilogram) is the distribution coefficient of mercury between the solid and truly dissolved phases. K_{ic} (or K_{oc}, liter per milligram) is the distribution coefficient of mercury between the inorganic (or organic) colloidal and the truly dissolved fraction. M_{ic} (or M_{oc}, milligram per liter) is the concentration of inorganic (or organic) colloids. K_d^{ic*} (or K_d^{oc*}, liter per kilogram) is the apparent distribution coefficient of mercury between the solid and the bulk solution phases.

In the case of coexistence of both inorganic and organic colloids (e.g., iron hydroxides and NOM), the situation becomes more complicated. In such cases, the apparent distribution coefficient of mercury, K_d^{**} (liter per kilogram), can be calculated as follows, to account for the effects from both inorganic and organic colloids.

$$K_d^{**} = \frac{C_s}{C_w^* + C_{ic}M_{ic} + C_{oc}M_{oc}} \tag{11.10}$$

Similarly, this equation can be transformed as

$$K_d^{**} = \frac{K_p}{1 + K_{ic}M_{ic} + K_{oc}M_{oc}} \tag{11.11}$$

The calculations of these distribution coefficients are useful when geochemical models are used to predict the distribution profile of different mercury species. Although in the natural aquatic environments both NOM and iron (oxyhydr)oxides are ubiquitous (Ullrich et al., 2001; Gondikas et al., 2010), previous studies dealing with mercury adsorption did not always calculate all these coefficients, probably due to the lack of a universal definition on how to differentiate truly dissolved, colloidal, and particulate mercury species and the practical difficulties in separating these mercury species. There are, however, a few studies that reported values for both apparent distribution coefficients of mercury between solid and solution and distribution coefficients between truly dissolved phase and NOM (Stordal et al., 1996a, 1996b; Cai et al., 1999).

11.4   CONCLUDING REMARKS

In the aquatic environment, mercury can undergo a series of complicated biogeochemical processes, among which adsorption of inorganic Hg(II) and MeHg onto suspended particles and sediments plays an important role in determining the fate of mercury. The adsorption of mercury on solids and subsequent sedimentation of solid particles would result in mercury accumulation in sediments, decreasing mobility and bioavailability of mercury species.

The two major components of solid particles, inorganic minerals (e.g., metal oxides) and organic matter (e.g., humic substances), are both important for mercury adsorption and enrichment on solids. The adsorption of mercury species on organic matter involves the association of mercury with such S-, O-, and N-containing functional groups within organic matter, in particular, reduced S groups (e.g., thiols, sulfides, and disulfides). Mercury adsorption on inorganic minerals occurs through a condensation reaction between a hydroxyl group on hydroxylated mercury species and a hydroxyl on the mineral surface, forming stable inner-sphere-type surface complexes.

Studies measuring the reaction rates for mercury adsorption on various solids suggest that mercury adsorption is usually a fast reaction or even instantaneous but may involve a slow second step resulting in prolonged equilibration time. The distribution coefficients (K_d) of mercury adsorption, a lump parameter describing mercury distribution between solid and solution phases, suggest the strong affinity of inorganic Hg(II) and MeHg to sediment and suspended particles, although the K_d values vary widely in the literature.

Environmentally ubiquitous aquatic colloidal particles (1 nm–1 μm), including organic (e.g., NOM in waters) and inorganic (e.g., iron oxyhydroxides, often present as nanoscale particles), significantly influence mercury adsorption on large (noncolloidal) solids. Binding of mercury to aquatic NOM (often present in the colloidal size range) may enhance or decrease mercury adsorption, depending on the nature of NOM and solids and other geochemical conditions. The presence of inorganic colloids in waters could form colloidal complexes with mercury species, decreasing mercury adsorption on large solids and enhancing mercury transport in the aquatic environment. Although both truly dissolved and colloidal mercury species are present in solution, the mobility, reactivity, and bioavailability of these mercury fractions may be different, with colloidal mercury probably being subject to aquatic transport but with limited bioavailability. When studying mercury adsorption onto solids in the presence of colloids, it is necessary to differentiate mercury into particulate, colloidal, and truly dissolved phases and then characterize mercury adsorption in such a ternary system (e.g., calculating various distribution coefficients of mercury species between two phases).

REFERENCES

Aiken GR, Hsu-Kim H, Ryan JN. Influence of dissolved organic matter on the environmental fate of metals, nanoparticles, and colloids. Environ Sci Technol 2011a;45:3196–3201.

Aiken G, Hsu-Kim H, Ryan J, Alvarez P. Guest comment: nanoscale metal-organic matter interactions. Environ Sci Technol 2011b;45:3194–3195.

Arias M, Barral MT, Da Silva-Carvalhal J, Mejuto JC, Rubinos D. Interaction of Hg(II) acid with kaolin-humic acid complexes. Clay Miner 2004;39:35–45.

Babiarz CL, Benoit JM, Shafer MM, Andren AW, Hurley JP, Webb DA. Seasonal influences on partitioning and transport of total and methylmercury in rivers from contrasting watersheds. Biogeochemistry 1998;41:237–257.

Babiarz CL, Hoffmann SR, Shafer MM, Hurley JP, Andren AW, Armstrong DE. A critical evaluation of tangential-flow ultrafiltration for trace metal studies in freshwater systems 2 total mercury and methylmercury. Environ Sci Technol 2000;34:3428–3434.

Babiarz CL, Hurley JP, Hoffmann SR, Andren AW, Shafer MM, Armstrong DE. Partitioning of total mercury and methylmercury to the colloidal phase in freshwaters. Environ Sci Technol 2001;35:4773–4782.

Babiarz CL, Hurley JP, Krabbenhoft DP, Gilmour C, Branfireun BA. Application of ultrafiltration and stable isotopic amendments to field studies of mercury partitioning to filterable carbon in lake water and overland runoff. Sci Total Environ 2003;304:295–303.

Bäckström M, Dario M, Karlsson S, Allard B. Effects of a fulvic acid on the adsorption of mercury and cadmium on goethite. Sci Total Environ 2003;304:257–268.

Barrow NJ, Cox VC. The effects of pH and chloride concentration on mercury sorption. I. By goethite. J Soil Sci 1992;43:295–304.

Belzile N, Lang CY, Chen YW, Wang M. The competitive role of organic carbon and dissolved sulfide in controlling the distribution of mercury in freshwater lake sediments. Sci Total Environ 2008;405:226–238.

Bengtsson G, Picado F. Mercury sorption to sediments: dependence on grain size, dissolved organic carbon, and suspended bacteria. Chemosphere 2008;73:526–531.

Benoit JM, Gilmour CC, Mason RP, Heyes A. Sulfide controls on mercury speciation and bioavailability to methylating bacteria in sediment pore waters. Environ Sci Technol 1999;33:1780–1780.

Benoit JM, Gilmour CC, Mason RP. Aspects of bioavailability of mercury for methylation in pure cultures of desulfobulbus propionicus (1pr3). Appl Environ Microbiol 2001a;67:51–58.

Benoit JM, Mason RP, Gilmour CC, Aiken GR. Constants for mercury binding by dissolved organic matter isolates from the Florida Everglades. Geochim Cosmochim Acta 2001b;65:4445–4451.

Biester H, Müller G, Schöler HF. Estimating distribution and retention of mercury in three different soils contaminated by emissions from chlor-alkali plants: part I. Sci Total Environ 2002;284:177–189.

Bilinski H, Kwokal Z, Plavsic M, Wrischer M, Branica M. Mercury distribution in the water column of the stratified Krka river estuary (Croatia): importance of natural organic matter and of strong winds. Water Res 2000;34:2001–2010.

Bloom NS, Gill GA, Cappellino S, Dobbs C, McShea L, Driscoll C, Mason R, Rudd J. Speciation and cycling of mercury in Lavaca Bay, Texas, sediments. Environ Sci Technol 1998;33:7–13.

Bonnissel-Gissinger P, Alnot M, Lickes JP, Ehrhardt JJ, Behra P. Modeling the adsorption of mercury(II) on (Hydr)oxides II: [alpha]-FeOOH (Goethite) and amorphous silica. J Colloid Interface Sci 1999;215:313–322.

Brigatti MF, Colonna S, Malferrari D, Medici L, Poppi L. Mercury adsorption by montmorillonite and vermiculite: a combined XRD, TG-MS, and EXAFS study. Appl Clay Sci 2005;28:1–8.

Brigham ME, Wentz DA, Aiken GR, Krabbenhoft DP. Mercury cycling in stream ecosystems. 1. Water column chemistry and transport. Environ Sci Technol 2009;43:2720–2725.

Brown GE Jr. How minerals react with water. Science 2001;294:67–70.

Brown JR, Bancroft GM, Fyfe WS, McLean RAN. Mercury removal from water by iron sulfide minerals. An electron spectroscopy for chemical analysis (ESCA) study. Environ Sci Technol 1979;13:1142–1144.

Brown GE Jr, Henrich VE, Casey WH, Clark DL, Eggleston C, Felmy A, Goodman DW, Grätzel M, Maciel G, McCarthy MI, Nealson KH, Sverjensky DA, Toney MF, Zachara JM. Metal oxide surfaces and their interactions with aqueous solutions and microbial organisms. Chem Rev 1998;99:77–174.

Cai Y, Jaffé R, Jones RD. Interactions between dissolved organic carbon and mercury species in surface waters of the Florida Everglades. Appl Geochem 1999;14:395–407.

Choe KY, Gill GA. Distribution of particulate, colloidal, and dissolved mercury in San Francisco Bay estuary. 2. Monomethyl mercury. Limnol Oceanogr 2003;48:1547–1556.

Choe KY, Gill GA, Lehman R. Distribution of particulate, colloidal, and dissolved mercury in San Francisco Bay estuary. 1. Total mercury. Limnol Oceanogr 2003;48:1535–1546.

Coquery M, Cossa D, Sanjuan J. Speciation and sorption of mercury in two macro-tidal estuaries. Mar Chem 1997;58:213–227.

Deonarine A, Hsu-Kim H. Precipitation of mercuric sulfide nanoparticles in NOM-containing water: implications for the natural environment. Environ Sci Technol 2009;43:2368–2373.

Deonarine A, Lau BLT, Aiken GR, Ryan JN, Hsu-Kim H. Effects of humic substances on precipitation and aggregation of zinc sulfide nanoparticles. Environ Sci Technol 2011;45:3217–3223.

Driscoll CT, Blette V, Yan C, Schofield CL, Munson R, Holsapple J. The role of dissolved organic carbon in the chemistry and bioavailability of mercury in remote Adirondack lakes. Water Air Soil Pollut 1995;80:499–508.

Drott A, Lambertsson L, Bjorn E, Skyllberg U. Importance of dissolved neutral mercury sulfides for methyl mercury production in contaminated sediments. Environ Sci Technol 2007;41:2270–2276.

Farrell RE, Huang PM, Germida JJ. Biomethylation of mercury(II) adsorbed on mineral colloids common in freshwater sediments. Appl Organomet Chem 1998;12:613–620.

Fitzgerald WF, Lamborg CH, Hammerschmidt CR. Marine biogeochemical cycling of mercury. Chem Rev 2007a;107:641–662.

Fitzgerald WF, Lamborg CH, Heinrich DH, Karl KT. Geochemistry of mercury in the environment, treatise on geochemistry. Oxford: Pergamon; 2007b. p 1–47.

Forbes EA, Posner AM, Quirk JP. The specific adsorption of inorganic Hg(II) species and Co(III) complex ions on goethite. J Colloid Interface Sci 1974;49:403–409.

Frenet M. The distribution of mercury, cadmium and lead between water and suspended matter in the Loire Estuary as a function of the hydrological regime. Water Res 1981;15:1343–1350.

Gagnon C, Fisher NS. Bioavailability of sediment-bound methyl and inorganic mercury to a marine bivalve. Environ Sci Technol 1997;31:993–998.

Ganguli PM, Mason RP, Abu-Saba KE, Anderson RS, Flegal AR. Mercury speciation in drainage from the new idria mercury mine, California. Environ Sci Technol 2000;34:4773–4779.

Gondikas AP, Jang EK, Hsu-Kim H. Influence of amino acids cysteine and serine on aggregation kinetics of zinc and mercury sulfide colloids. J Colloid Interface Sci 2010;347:167–171.

Gunneriusson L, Baxter D, Emteborg H. Complexation at low concentrations of methyl and inorganic mercury(II) to a hydrous goethite ([alpha]-FeOOH) surface. J Colloid Interface Sci 1995;169:262–266.

Gunneriusson L, Sjöberg S. Surface complexation in the H+-goethite ([alpha]-FeOOH)-Hg (II)-chloride system. J Colloid Interface Sci 1993;156:121–128.

Gustafsson O, Gschwend PM. Aquatic colloids: concepts, definitions, and current challenges. Limnol Oceanogr 1997;42:519–528.

Haitzer M, Aiken GR, Ryan JN. Binding of mercury(II) to dissolved organic matter: the role of the mercury-to-DOM concentration ratio. Environ Sci Technol 2002;36:3564–3570.

Haitzer M, Aiken GR, Ryan JN. Binding of mercury(II) to aquatic humic substances: influence of pH and source of humic substances. Environ Sci Technol 2003;37:2436–2441.

Hammerschmidt CR, Fitzgerald WF, Lamborg CH, Balcom PH, Visscher PT. Biogeochemistry of methylmercury in sediments of Long Island Sound. Mar Chem 2004;90:31–52.

He Z, Traina SJ, Bigham JM, Weavers LK. Sonolytic desorption of mercury from aluminum oxide. Environ Sci Technol 2005;39:1037–1044.

He Z, Traina SJ, Weavers LK. Sonolytic desorption of mercury from aluminum oxide: effects of pH, chloride, and organic matter. Environ Sci Technol 2007;41:779–784.

Hesterberg D, Chou JW, Hutchison KJ, Sayers DE. Bonding of Hg(II) to reduced organic sulfur in humic acid as affected by S/Hg ratio. Environ Sci Technol 2001;35:2741–2745.

Hintelmann H, Harris R. Application of multiple stable mercury isotopes to determine the adsorption and desorption dynamics of Hg(II) and MeHg to sediments. Mar Chem 2004;90:165–173.

Hissler C, Probst JL. Chlor-alkali industrial contamination and riverine transport of mercury: distribution and partitioning of mercury between water, suspended matter, and bottom sediment of the Thur River, France. Appl Geochem 2006;21:1837–1854.

Hochella MF. There's plenty of room at the bottom: nanoscience in geochemistry. Geochim Cosmochim Acta 2002;66:735–743.

Hochella MF, Madden AS. Earth's nano-compartment for toxic metals. Elements 2005;1:199–204.

Hurley JP, Benoit JM, Babiarz CL, Shafer MM, Andren AW, Sullivan JR, Hammond R, Webb DA. Influences of watershed characteristics on mercury levels in Wisconsin Rivers. Environ Sci Technol 1995;29:1867–1875.

Hurley JP, Cowell SE, Shafer MM, Hughes PE. Partitioning and transport of total and methyl mercury in the Lower Fox River, Wisconsin. Environ Sci Technol 1998;32:1424–1432.

Jean GE, Bancroft GM. Heavy metal adsorption by sulphide mineral surfaces. Geochim Cosmochim Acta 1986;50:1455–1463.

Jing YD, He ZL, Yang XE. Effects of pH, organic acids, and competitive cations on mercury desorption in soils. Chemosphere 2007;69:1662–1669.

Jing YD, He ZL, Yang XE. Adsorption-desorption characteristics of mercury in paddy soils of China. J Environ Qual 2008;37:680–688.

de Jonge LW, Kjaergaard C, Moldrup P. Colloids and colloid-facilitated transport of contaminants in soils: an introduction. Vadose Zone J 2004;3:321–325.

Karlsson T, Skyllberg U. Bonding of ppb levels of methyl mercury to reduced sulfur groups in soil organic matter. Environ Sci Technol 2003;37:4912–4918.

Kim CS, Rytuba JJ, Brown GE. EXAFS study of mercury(II) sorption to Fe- and Al-(hydr)oxides: I. Effects of pH. J Colloid Interface Sci 2004a;271:1–15.

Kim CS, Rytuba JJ, Brown GE. EXAFS study of mercury(II) sorption to Fe- and Al-(hydr)oxides: II. Effects of chloride and sulfate. J Colloid Interface Sci 2004b;270:9–20.

Klusman RW, Matoske CP. Adsorption of mercury by soils from oil shale development areas in the Piceance Creek basin of Northwestern Colorado. Environ Sci Technol 1983;17:251–256.

Kretzschmar R, Schäfer T. Metal retention and transport on colloidal particles in the environment. Elements 2005;1:205–210.

Lau BLT, Hsu-Kim H. Precipitation and growth of zinc sulfide nanoparticles in the presence of thiol-containing natural organic ligands. Environ Sci Technol 2008;42:7236–7241.

Le Roux SM, Turner A, Millward GE, Ebdon L, Appriou P. Partitioning of mercury onto suspended sediments in estuaries. J Environ Monitor 2001;3:37–42.

Lead JR, Hamilton-Taylor J, Davison W, Harper M. Trace metal sorption by natural particles and coarse colloids. Geochim Cosmochim Acta 1999;63:1661–1670.

Liao L, Selim HM, DeLaune RD. Mercury adsorption-desorption and transport in soils. J Environ Qual 2009;38:1608–1616.

Lindström M. Distribution of particulate and reactive mercury in surface waters of Swedish forest lakes - an empirically based predictive model. Ecol Model 2001;136:81–93.

Liu G, Cai Y, Kalla P, Scheidt D, Richards J, Scinto LJ, Gaiser E, Appleby C. Mercury mass budget estimates and cycling seasonality in the Florida Everglades. Environ Sci Technol 2008;42:1954–1960.

Liu G, Cai Y, Mao Y, Scheidt D, Kalla P, Richards J, Scinto LJ, Tachiev G, Roelant D, Appleby C. Spatial variability in mercury cycling and relevant biogeochemical controls in the Florida Everglades. Environ Sci Technol 2009;43:4361–4366.

Liu G, Naja GM, Kalla P, Scheidt D, Gaiser E, Cai Y. Legacy and fate of mercury and methylmercury in the Florida Everglades. Environ Sci Technol 2011;45:496–501.

Lockwood RA, Chen KY. Adsorption of mercury(II) by hydrous manganese oxides. Environ Sci Technol 1973;7:1028–1034.

Lowry GV, Shaw S, Kim CS, Rytuba JJ, Brown GE. Macroscopic and microscopic observations of particle-facilitated mercury transport from new idria and sulphur bank mercury mine tailings. Environ Sci Technol 2004;38:5101–5111.

Mac Naughton MG, James RO. Adsorption of aqueous mercury (II) complexes at the oxide/water interface. J Colloid Interface Sci 1974;47:431–440.

Mason RP, Benoit JM. Organomercury compounds in the environment. In: Craig PJ, editor. Organometallic compounds in the environment. 2nd ed. West Sussex: John Wiley & Sons, Ltd; 2003.

Mason RP, Fitzgerald WF. The distribution and biogeochemical cycling of mercury in the equatorial Pacific Ocean. Deep Sea Res Part I: Oceanogr Res Pap 1993;40:1897–1924.

Mason RP, Fitzgerald WF, Morel FMM. The biogeochemical cycling of elemental mercury: anthropogenic influences. Geochim Cosmochim Acta 1994;58:3191–3198.

Mason RP, Rolfhus KR, Fitzgerald WF. Mercury in the North Atlantic. Mar Chem 1998;61:37–53.

Mason RP, Sullivan KA. Mercury in Lake Michigan. Environ Sci Technol 1997;31:942–947.

Mikac N, Niessen S, Ouddane B, Wartel M. Speciation of mercury in sediments of the seine estuary (France). Appl Organomet Chem 1999;13:715–725.

Miretzky P, Bisinoti MC, Jardim WE, Rocha JC. Factors affecting Hg (II) adsorption in soils from the Rio Negro basin (Amazon). Quim Nova 2005;28:438–443.

Morel FMM, Kraepiel AML, Amyot M. The chemical cycle and bioaccumulation of mercury. Annu Rev Ecol Syst 1998;29:543–566.

Muresan B, Cossa D, Jézéquel D, Prévot F, Kerbellec S. The biogeochemistry of mercury at the sediment-water interface in the Thau lagoon. 1. Partition and speciation. Estuar Coast Shelf Sci 2007;72:472–484.

Nriagu J. The biogeochemistry of mercury in the environment. New York (NY): Elsevier/North Holland Biomedical Press; 1979. p 696.

Otani Y, Kanaoka C, Usui C, Matsui S, Emi H. Adsorption of mercury vapor on particles. Environ Sci Technol 1986;20:735–738.

Posselt HS, Anderson FJ, Weber WJ. Cation sorption on colloidal hydrous manganese dioxide. Environ Sci Technol 1968;2:1087–1093.

Qian J, Skyllberg U, Frech W, Bleam WF, Bloom PR, Petit PE. Bonding of methyl mercury to reduced sulfur groups in soil and stream organic matter as determined by X-ray absorption spectroscopy and binding affinity studies. Geochim Cosmochim Acta 2002;66:3873–3885.

Ravichandran M. Interactions between mercury and dissolved organic matter - a review. Chemosphere 2004;55:319–331.

Ravichandran M, Aiken GR, Ryan JN, Reddy MM. Inhibition of precipitation and aggregation of metacinnabar (mercuric sulfide) by dissolved organic matter isolated from the Florida Everglades. Environ Sci Technol 1999;33:1418–1423.

Rytuba JJ. Mercury mine drainage and processes that control its environmental impact. Sci Total Environ 2000;260:57–71.

Sarkar D, Essington ME, Misra KC. Adsorption of mercury(II) by variable charge surfaces of quartz and gibbsite. Soil Sci Soc Am J 1999;63:1626–1636.

Schluter K. Sorption of inorganic mercury and monomethyl mercury in an iron-humus podzol soil of southern Norway studied by batch experiments. Environ Geol 1997;30:266–279.

Schuster E. The behavior of mercury in the soil with special emphasis on complexation and adsorption processes-a review of the literature. Water Air Soil Pollut 1991;56:667–680.

Senevirathna WU, Zhang H, Gu BH. Effect of carboxylic and thiol ligands (oxalate, cysteine) on the kinetics of desorption of Hg(II) from kaolinite. Water Air Soil Pollut 2011;215:573–584.

Singh J, Huang PM, Hammer UT, Liaw WK. Influence of citric acid and glycine on the adsorption of mercury(II) by kaolinite under various pH conditions. Clays Clay Miner 1996;44:41–48.

Skyllberg U. Competition among thiols and inorganic sulfides and polysulfides for Hg and MeHg in wetland soils and sediments under suboxic conditions: illumination of controversies and implications for MeHg net production. J Geophys Res 2008;113:G00C03. DOI: 10.1029/2008JG000745.

Skyllberg U, Bloom PR, Qian J, Lin CM, Bleam WF. Complexation of mercury(II) in soil organic matter: EXAFS evidence for linear two-coordination with reduced sulfur groups. Environ Sci Technol 2006;40:4174–4180.

Skyllberg U, Drott A. Competition between disordered iron sulfide and natural organic matter associated thiols for mercury(II)-an EXAFS study. Environ Sci Technol 2010;44:1254–1259.

Skyllberg U, Xia K, Bloom PR, Nater EA, Bleam WF. Binding of mercury(II) to reduced sulfur in soil organic matter along upland-peat soil transects. J Environ Qual 2000;29:855–865.

Slowey AJ, Johnson SB, Rytuba JJ, Brown GE. Role of organic acids in promoting colloidal transport of mercury from mine tailings. Environ Sci Technol 2005a;39:7869–7874.

Slowey AJ, Rytuba JJ, Brown GE. Speciation of mercury and mode of transport from placer gold mine tailings. Environ Sci Technol 2005b;39:1547–1554.

Stein ED, Cohen Y, Winer AM. Environmental distribution and transformation of mercury compounds. Crit Rev Environ Sci Technol 1996;26:1–43.

Stordal MC, Gill GA, Wen LS, Santschi PH. Mercury phase speciation in the surface waters of three Texas estuaries: importance of colloidal forms. Limnol Oceanogr 1996a;41:52–61.

Stordal MC, Santschi PH, Gill GA. Colloidal pumping: evidence for the coagulation process using natural colloids tagged with 203 Hg. Environ Sci Technol 1996b;30:3335–3340.

Stumm W. Chemistry of the solid-water interface. New York (NY): John Wiley & Sons, Inc.; 1992.

Tiffreau C, Lützenkirchen J, Behra P. Modeling the adsorption of mercury(II) on (Hydr)oxides: I. amorphous iron oxide and [alpha]-quartz. J Colloid Interface Sci 1995;172:82–93.

Turner A, Millward GE, Le Roux SM. Sediment-water partitioning of inorganic mercury in estuaries. Environ Sci Technol 2001;35:4648–4654.

Turner A, Millward GE, Le Roux SM. Significance of oxides and particulate organic matter in controlling trace metal partitioning in a contaminated estuary. Mar Chem 2004;88:179–192.

Ullrich SM, Tanton TW, Abdrashitova SA. Mercury in the aquatic environment: a review of factors affecting methylation. Crit Rev Environ Sci Technol 2001;31:241–293.

USEPA. EPA Mercury Study Report to Congress. Washington (DC): Office of Air Quality and Standards and Office of Research and Development, U.S. Environmental Protection Agency; 1997. EPA-452/R-97-009.

Walcarius A, Devoy M Jr, Bessiere J. Electrochemical recognition of selective mercury adsorption on minerals. Environ Sci Technol 1999;33:4278–4284.

Wang J, Huang P, Liaw W, Hammer U. Kinetics of the desorption of mercury from selected freshwater sediments as influenced by chloride. Water Air Soil Pollut 1991;56:533–542.

Watras CJ, Morrison KA, Host JS, Bloom NS. Concentration of mercury species in relationship to other site-specific factors in the surface waters of Northern Wisconsin lakes. Limnol Oceanogr 1995;40:556–565.

Watras CJ, Morrison KA, Hudson RJM, Frost TM, Kratz TK. Decreasing mercury in Northern Wisconsin: temporal patterns in bulk precipitation and a precipitation-dominated lake. Environ Sci Technol 2000;34:4051–4057.

Waychunas GA, Kim CS, Banfield JF. Nanoparticulate iron oxide minerals in soils and sediments: unique properties and contaminant scavenging mechanisms. J Nanopart Res 2005;7:409–433.

Waychunas GA, Zhang H. Structure, chemistry, and properties of mineral nanoparticles. Elements 2008;4:381–387.

Wolfenden S, Charnock JM, Hilton J, Livens FR, Vaughan DJ. Sulfide species as a sink for mercury in lake sediments. Environ Sci Technol 2005;39:6644–6648.

Xia K, Skyllberg UL, Bleam WF, Bloom PR, Nater EA, Helmke PA. X-ray absorption spectroscopic evidence for the complexation of Hg(II) by reduced sulfur in soil humic substances. Environ Sci Technol 1999;33:257–261.

Xu H, Allard B. Effects of a fulvic acid on the speciation and mobility of mercury in aqueous solutions. Water Air Soil Pollut 1991;56:709–717.

Yang YK, Liang L, Wang D. Effect of dissolved organic matter on adsorption and desorption of mercury by soils. J Environ Sci 2008a;20:1097–1102.

Yang YK, Liang L, Wang DY. Effect of dissolved organic matter on adsorption and desorption of mercury by soils. J Environ Sci (China) 2008b;20:1097–1102.

Yin YJ, Allen HE, Huang CP, Sanders PF. Adsorption/desorption isotherms of Hg(II) by soil. Soil Sci 1997a;162:35–45.

Yin YJ, Allen HE, Huang CP, Sparks DL, Sanders PF. Kinetics of mercury(II) adsorption and desorption on soil. Environ Sci Technol 1997b;31:496–503.

Yin YJ, Allen HE, Li YM, Huang CP, Sanders PF. Adsorption of mercury(II) by soil: effects of pH, chloride, and organic matter. J Environ Qual 1996;25:837–844.

Zhang J, Dai J, Wang R, Li F, Wang W. Adsorption and desorption of divalent mercury (Hg2+) on humic acids and fulvic acids extracted from typical soils in China. Colloids Surf, A 2009;335:194–201.

Zhong H, Wang WX. Inorganic mercury binding with different sulfur species in anoxic sediments and their gut juice extractions. Environ Toxicol Chem 2009a;28:1851–1857.

Zhong H, Wang WX. The role of sorption and bacteria in mercury partitioning and bioavailability in artificial sediments. Environ Pollut 2009b;157:981–986.

CHAPTER 12

EXCHANGE OF ELEMENTAL MERCURY BETWEEN THE OCEANS AND THE ATMOSPHERE

ASIF QURESHI, MATTHEW MACLEOD, ELSIE SUNDERLAND, and KONRAD HUNGERBÜHLER

12.1 INTRODUCTION

Oceans are an important reservoir of mercury (Sunderland and Mason, 2007). They contribute up to one-third of the total mercury flux to the atmosphere, in the form of evasion of elemental mercury [Hg(0)]. Quantifying the magnitude and spatial distribution of Hg ocean–air flux is therefore critical for understanding atmospheric concentrations of mercury. In addition, a portion of mercury in oceans may be converted to methylated mercury (MeHg), the bioavailable form that accumulates in fish and poses a risk to human health (Mason and Fitzgerald, 1993; Rolfhus and Fitzgerald, 1995; Sunderland, 2007).

Several competing processes determine the magnitude of ocean–air exchange of mercury (Fig. 12.1). Key factors that are controlled in the oceans are the mass transfer coefficients for mercury transport across the water–air interface and the reduction and oxidation reactions in the surface oceans that determine the amount of Hg(0) available for evasion. In air, reactions in the marine boundary layer above the ocean influence atmospheric concentrations, and consequently the concentration gradient between air and water that determines the actual ocean–air flux.

In this chapter, we focus our attention on factors controlling the water–to–air flux of mercury in the oceans. We review and critically evaluate the theoretical and experimental aspects of mass transfer, flux measurements, and the redox reactions in surface oceans. We also summarize reported rate constants for reduction and oxidation of mercury in surface waters, which can be used in modeling exercises. We finally present results from a model that incorporates the above processes to

Environmental Chemistry and Toxicology of Mercury, First Edition.
Edited by Guangliang Liu, Yong Cai, and Nelson O'Driscoll.
© 2012 John Wiley & Sons, Inc. Published 2012 by John Wiley & Sons, Inc.

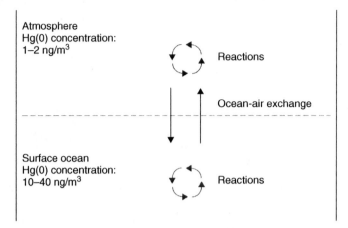

Figure 12.1 Schematic of processes affecting mercury near the ocean–air interface. The ocean–air exchange parameters along with the redox reactions occurring in the surface ocean and the atmosphere determine the direction and net flux of elemental mercury across the interface.

describe the exchange of Hg(0) between oceans and the atmosphere, Goddard Earth Observing System (GEOS)-Chem.

12.2 MODELS OF GAS EXCHANGE OF ELEMENTAL MERCURY AT THE AIR–SEA INTERFACE

The rate and direction of the net flux of elemental mercury between the atmosphere and the oceans at any location and time is dictated by both thermodynamic and kinetic controls. The nature of the kinetic controls depends on the thermodynamic ones; therefore, we first consider the thermodynamic controls.

12.2.1 Thermodynamic Controls

Elemental mercury in the environment seeks to distribute itself between air and water such that free energy is minimized. This phenomenon can be quantified using either of the related concepts of chemical potential (μ) and fugacity (f) (Mackay, 2001). Both μ and f are related to the free energy change associated with mass transfer across an interface between two media such as air and water. Mercury is thus driven to migrate out of media where fugacity or chemical potential are relatively high. Fugacity has the convenient property of being directly proportional to concentration (C), that is,

$$C = Zf \qquad (12.1)$$

The proportionality constant in this relationship, Z, is dependent on characteristics of the pollutant and the environment, and is called a fugacity capacity.

For ideal gasses, fugacity in the gas phase is equal to partial pressure (P), and, from the ideal gas law we can derive the fugacity capacity of the gas phase of the atmosphere (Mackay, 2001):

$$Z_A = \frac{1}{RT} \tag{12.2}$$

The fugacity capacity of the dissolved phase in water can then be deduced from a measurement of the ratio of concentrations of mercury in air and water at equilibrium, which is the Henry's law constant (H). When the Henry's law constant is expressed using the same concentration units in air and water, it is called the air–water partition coefficient, K_{AW}. At equilibrium, the fugacities of mercury in air and water are equal $(f_A = f_W)$ and we can relate K_{AW} to Z_A and Z_W:

$$K_{AW} = \frac{C_A}{C_W} = \frac{Z_A f_A}{Z_W f_W} = \frac{Z_A}{Z_W} \tag{12.3}$$

and

$$Z_W = \frac{Z_A}{K_{AW}} \tag{12.4}$$

Recently, Andersson et al. (2008) applied a gas sparging technique to measure K_{AW} of elemental mercury at temperatures between 5 and 35°C in pure water and artificial sea water. They did not observe a significant difference in K_{AW} between pure water and artificial sea water and recommend the following relationship for calculating K_{AW} of elemental mercury as a function of temperature:

$$K_{AW} = \exp\left(\frac{-2404.3}{T(K)} + 6.92\right) \tag{12.5}$$

This relationship is illustrated in Fig. 12.2 over the temperature range 0–30°C.

It is interesting to compare the ratio of fugacities of elemental mercury derived from measurements in the atmosphere and oceans to assess how close elemental mercury is to equilibrium partitioning and the direction of the fugacity gradient. The concentration of mercury measured at background sites in the atmosphere of the Northern Hemisphere is typically between 1 and 2 ng/m^3. The concentration of elemental mercury in ocean surface water in the Northern Hemisphere is typically between 10 and 40 ng/m^3. If we choose a representative temperature of 10°C, then the fugacity capacity of air (Z_A) is 4.25×10^{-4} mol/m^3/Pa, K_{AW} of elemental mercury is 0.21, and Z_W is 2.05×10^{-3} mol/m^3/Pa. Using these Z values, the fugacity of mercury in air (f_A) is between 12 and 23 nPa, and f_W is between 24 and 97 nPa. Thus, we see that the distribution of elemental mercury between the atmosphere and oceans in the Northern Hemisphere is not far from the expected equilibrium distribution. The ratio (f_W/f_A) has a range of values between approximately 1 and 8, indicating a slight thermodynamic driving force that favors volatilization of elemental mercury from the oceans to the atmosphere.

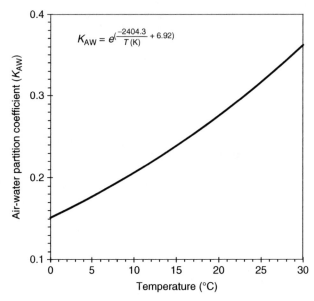

Figure 12.2 Air–water partition coefficient (K_{AW}) of elemental mercury as a function of temperature (Andersson et al., 2008).

12.2.2 Kinetic Controls

Several recent reviews provide a comprehensive discussion of the kinetic controls on exchange of gasses between the atmosphere and water bodies. These include alternative models based on different conceptualizations of transport near the air–water interface (Jaehne and Haussecker, 1998; Frost and Upstill-Goddard, 1999; Schwarzenbach et al., 2003). In general, the rate of diffusive transfer of a substance across the air–water boundary is controlled by an overall mass transfer coefficient, $k_{A/W}$, which has dimensions of velocity. We will use units of meters per hour for mass transfer coefficients, but units of centimeters per second are also common and are provided on the alternate axis of Figs 12.3 and 12.5. The net exchange flux between water and air (N, mol/m²/h) can be calculated as

$$N = k_{A/W} \left(C_W - \frac{C_A}{K_{AW}} \right)$$ (12.6)

where C_A and C_W are expressed in units of mol/m³.

The overall mass transfer coefficient $k_{A/W}$ can be viewed as the net result of mass transfer occurring on the waterside and the air side of the air–water interface, that is, $k_{A/W}$ can be expressed as

$$\frac{1}{k_{A/W}} = \frac{1}{k_W} + \frac{1}{k_A K_{AW}}$$ (12.7)

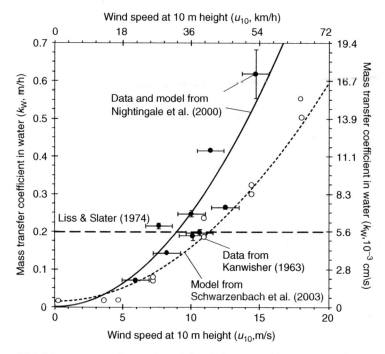

Figure 12.3 Measurement data and models of the waterside mass transfer coefficient (k_W) of a substance with a Schmidt number of 600 as a function of wind speed at 10 m height. Data from Nightingale et al. (2000) were determined from field measurements in the North Sea carried out at a temperatures near $7°C$. Data from Kanwisher (1963) are from a laboratory study of CO_2. The empirical model by Schwarzenbach et al. (2003) was fitted to the data from Kanwisher (1963).

where k_W and k_A are the mass transfer coefficients on the waterside and air side of the boundary. Because air is a much less dense fluid than water, k_A is typically between a factor of 100 and 1000 larger than k_W. Therefore, for substances with $K_{AW} > 10^{-2}$, resistance on the waterside is dominant, and $k_{A/W}$ is approximately equal to k_W. This is the case for mercury, and therefore, the key task to estimate the rate of gas exchange of mercury is to estimate k_W.

The waterside mass transfer coefficient k_W is also a key parameter that is required to constrain models of the biogeochemical cycles of many other gases, including CO_2. Therefore, several laboratory and field experiments have been carried out, some using tracers that can be measured at very low levels, such as sulfur hexafluoride (SF_6) and helium (He) (Nightingale et al., 2000). To extrapolate the results of these experiments to mercury, it is necessary to correct k_W for the tracer to a value that is appropriate for mercury. Under the assumption that the diffusion distance in water is the same for all substances, k_W varies with the diffusion coefficient of the substance (D, cm^2/s). Liss and Slater (1974) further assumed that D is proportional to the square root of the molecular weight

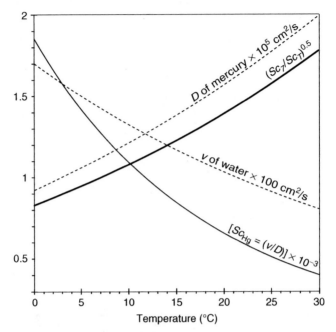

Figure 12.4 Variability in factors controlling the mass transfer coefficient of mercury in water as a function of temperature. D is the diffusion coefficient of mercury (Kuss et al., 2009, Eq. 12.13); v is the kinematic viscosity of water (Schwarzenbach et al., 2003); Sc is the Schmidt number for mercury and is calculated as (v/D). Also shown is the square root of the ratio of Schmidt numbers of mercury at $7°C$ to temperature T, which can be used to extrapolate k_W estimated using Equation 12.11 to temperatures other than $7°C$.

(M) and suggested the following relationship, where the subscript x refers to the tracer:

$$\frac{k_{W,Hg}}{k_{W,x}} = \left(\frac{M_x}{M_{Hg}}\right)^{0.5} \tag{12.8}$$

More recently, it has become common practice to adjust k_W for a tracer to another substance using the square root of the ratio of Schmidt numbers (Sc) (Nightingale et al., 2000; Schwarzenbach et al., 2003):

$$\frac{k_{W,Hg}}{k_{W,x}} = \left(\frac{Sc_{Hg}}{Sc_x}\right)^{0.5} \tag{12.9}$$

The Schmidt number is the dimensionless ratio of the kinematic viscosity of water $(v, cm^2/s)$ and D. Assuming that k_W is related to the Schmidt number rather than to D relaxes the conceptual assumption that the diffusion distance on the waterside of the air–water interface is the same for all substances (Schwarzenbach et al., 2003). The exponent of this relationship has been found empirically to be variable between about 0.3 and 1 (for a review, see Jaehne and Haussecker

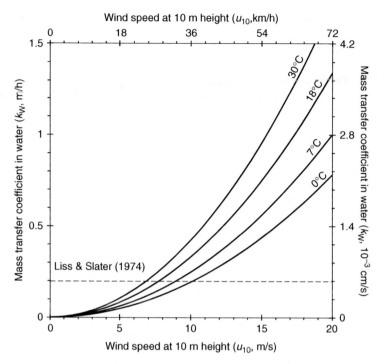

Figure 12.5 Values of the waterside air–water mass transfer coefficient (k_W) for mercury as a function of wind speed and temperature calculated with Equation 12.17.

(1998)), but the value 0.5 is often adopted for calculations of gas exchange in the environment.

Therefore, in summary, estimation of k_W for mercury in environmentally relevant situations requires two steps. First, one must estimate k_W for a volatile tracer based on available laboratory and field data, and second, this estimate must be extrapolated to an estimated k_W for mercury. We deal with each of these steps separately below.

It is empirically observed that k_W increases in a nonlinear way with increasing wind speed above the water surface (Schwarzenbach et al., 2003). This can be attributed to increasing turbulence in the water as a result of shear stress at the air–water interface and to increased effective surface area of the water as a result of formation of ripples and, at higher wind speeds, breaking waves and entrained bubbles. By convention, wind speed at a height of 10 m above the water surface (u_{10}, m/s) is used as a reference value. Wind speed measured at other heights can be converted to u_{10} using the following relationship (Schwarzenbach et al., 2003):

$$u_{10} = \left(\frac{10.4}{\ln(z) + 8.1} \right) u_z \qquad (12.10)$$

where u_z is the wind speed at height z meters above the water surface.

Measured values of k_W from a laboratory study (Kanwisher, 1963) and a field study in the North Sea (Nightingale et al., 2000) as a function of u_{10} are shown in Fig. 12.3. The data from Kanwisher are for CO_2, which has a Schmidt number of 600 at $20°C$, and the data from Nightingale have been adjusted by the authors to represent k_W for a substance with a Schmidt number of 600. The empirical models shown in Fig. 12.3 are (Nightingale et al., 2000)

$$k_W = 0.0025 \times (u_{10})^2 \tag{12.11}$$

and (Schwarzenbach et al., 2003)

$$k_W = 0.0144 + 0.00144 \times (u_{10})^2 \tag{12.12}$$

In both empirical models, k_W has units of meters per hour and u_{10} has units of meters per second. Also shown in Fig. 12.3 is a generic value for k_W suggested by Liss and Slater (1974) for substances with a molecular weight equal to that of CO_2. Several other empirical correlations with different mathematical forms have been suggested by various authors, and some of these are reviewed and illustrated in the text by Schwarzenbach et al. (2003). Most of these provide estimates of k_W that are similar to the model proposed by Schwarzenbach et al. (2003) based on the Kanwisher (1963) data (i.e., Eq. 12.12).

It is evident in Fig. 12.3 that the k_W data from the field experiment of Nightingale et al. (2000) are systematically higher than data from the laboratory experiment of Kanwisher (1963). The discrepancy may be a result of measurement bias between the two methods. However, it may also be a result of factors that differ between the natural and laboratory environment, such as large-scale wave structure. Both the empirical models relate k_W to the square of u_{10}, and the fitting coefficients are within a factor of 2 of each other. The models differ qualitatively at low wind speed (below 4 m/s), but wind speeds in this regime are probably not often relevant in the oceanic environment. In both datasets, there is residual variability in the data that indicates that factors other than those represented by a power-law relationship with wind speed affect k_W. The empirical relationship shown by Nightingale et al. (2000) might be preferred because it is based on k_W determined in the field.

As mentioned above, information about the diffusion coefficient and/or Schmidt number of mercury is needed in order to extrapolate k_W appropriate for CO_2 to a value for mercury. Unfortunately, no direct measurements of D_{Hg} have been made. Adjustment of values of k_W determined for tracer substances to values for mercury have therefore frequently been made using estimates of D_{Hg} derived from correlation equations. The Wilke–Chang method (Wilke and Chang, 1955) and the Othmer and Thakar (1953) equation have both been employed for this purpose. Both these correlations relate D to the molar volume of solutes and were developed based on diffusivity data of mostly organic compounds. When applied to mercury, the Wilke–Chang and Othmer–Thakar correlations both result in estimated values for D_{Hg} of about 3×10^{-5} cm^2/s at $20°C$ (Poissant et al., 2000; Kuss et al., 2009).

Recently, Kuss et al. (2009) applied molecular dynamics simulations to calculate the diffusion coefficient of mercury in fresh water and seawater. They evaluated their simulation estimates against measured diffusion coefficients for xenon and found very good agreement. Kuss et al. (2009) estimated the diffusion coefficient of mercury in seawater (in cm^2/s) as a function of temperature to be

$$D_{Hg} = 0.02293 \exp \left(\frac{-17760}{RT} \right) \tag{12.13}$$

This relationship implies that D_{Hg} is lower by a factor of about 2 than values estimated using the Wilke–Chang (1955) and Othmer–Thakar (1953) relationships. Significantly, the Kuss et al. (2009) relationship for mercury is very similar to the temperature-dependent diffusion coefficient for CO_2 determined experimentally by Jaehne et al. (1987). Kuss et al. (2009) thus point out that only a small error is introduced by using a k_W parameterization for CO_2 directly for Hg.

If we accept the Kuss et al. (2009) approximation that $D_{Hg} = D_{CO2}$, then the Nightingale et al. (2000) relationship (Eq. 12.11) can be applied directly to mercury. However, especially when considering the global mass balance of mercury, it is necessary to estimate the temperature dependence of k_W. This can be accomplished using the square root of the ratio of Schmidt numbers for mercury at different temperatures, that is,

$$\frac{k_{W,T1}}{k_{W,T2}} = \left(\frac{Sc_{T1}}{Sc_{T2}} \right)^{0.5} \tag{12.14}$$

The variability in D_{Hg}, v, and Sc_{Hg} over the temperature range of annual average surface temperatures of the world's oceans is illustrated in Fig. 12.4. Also shown in Fig. 12.4 is the variability in the correction factor $\left(\frac{Sc_7}{Sc_T} \right)^{0.5}$ that can be applied to correct the k_W estimated using Equation 12.11 to temperatures other than 7°C.

As evident in Fig. 12.4, the correction factor $\left(\frac{Sc_7}{Sc_T} \right)^{0.5}$ is very nearly a linear function of temperature over the range 0–30°C. In fact, it can be very well approximated by the following equation:

$$\left(\frac{Sc_7}{Sc_T} \right)^{0.5} = 0.0315T^* + 0.784, \, R^2 = 0.99 \tag{12.15}$$

where T^* is temperature in degrees centigrade.

In summary, a first, generic approximation of k_W for mercury is 0.2 m/h, which is the generic value suggested by Liss and Slater (1974). In applications where k_W for mercury should be estimated as a function of wind speed at 10 m height (u_{10}, m/s) the relationship from Nightingale et al. (2000) can be used:

$$k_W(u_{10}) = 0.0025 \times (u_{10})^2 \tag{12.16}$$

Equation 12.16 is most appropriate at temperatures near $7°C$. When an estimate of k_W as a function of temperatures between 0 and $30°C$ is desired, we recommend the following equation, which includes a linear approximation of the ratio of Schmidt numbers of Hg calculated using the diffusion coefficient from Kuss et al. (2009):

$$k_W(u_{10}, T^*) = (0.0025 \times (u_{10})^2) \times (0.0315T^* + 0.784) \qquad (12.17)$$

This is illustrated in Fig. 12.5.

12.3 FIELD STUDIES OF OCEAN-TO-AIR FLUXES OF MERCURY

The previous section introduced a theoretical description of the parameters required to estimate the water-to-air flux of elemental mercury. In this section, we summarize the experimental methods to determine this flux in the field.

Mercury flux from the ocean surface cannot be directly measured under undisturbed "true" field conditions. Therefore, it is estimated via two methods: (i) Hg(0) concentrations in air and water are determined using experiments and the surface-to-air flux is then estimated using models similar to those in the previous section and (ii) surface-to-air flux is measured using controlled experiments in flux chambers and the results are extrapolated to the ambient environment.

12.3.1 Determination of Elemental Mercury in Air and Water

The most common analytical method to quantify Hg(0) is cold vapor atomic fluorescence spectroscopy (CVAFS) (Bloom and Fitzgerald, 1988). In this method, air containing mercury is passed over gold traps onto which Hg(0) is adsorbed to form an amalgam. In the next step, the flow of purge air is stopped and the gold traps are heated. Mercury adsorbed to the traps desorbs and is transported to the atomic fluorescence unit for quantification. In case of oceans, dissolved gaseous mercury (DGM) from ocean water is purged using nitrogen, argon, or air that contains nondetectable amounts of mercury, and the purged air is quantified for Hg(0) as above. Atomic absorption has also been employed (Urba et al., 1995) instead of atomic fluorescence for DGM quantification. The method of mercury trapping on activated carbon followed by instrumental neutron activation analysis (INAA) has been used for measurement of mercury in ambient air (Munthe et al., 2001) but is not yet reported for the analysis of purged mercury from natural waters.

Commercial instruments for determination of atmospheric Hg(0) or DGM are based on the same spectroscopy principles. The most common instrument is the TEKRAN 2537 analyzer (Bloom and Fitzgerald, 1988). The use of GARDIS-1A analyzer has also been reported (Urba et al., 1995). Both these instruments can make semicontinuous measurements in intervals as small as 5–10 min.

12.3.2 Direct Determination of the Water-to-Air Hg(0) Flux Using Flux Chambers

Flux chambers provide a controlled environment where it is possible to measure the flux of mercury from the ocean surface to the atmosphere within the chamber In a flux chamber experiment, air of a known mercury concentration is pumped through the chamber and flushes the volatilizing mercury. The outlet air then passes through gold traps that adsorb the mercury vapor. The amount of adsorbed mercury is quantified using atomic absorption or fluorescence spectroscopy to estimate the concentration of mercury in the chamber outflow. The surface-to-air flux is then determined as

$$F = \frac{(C_o - C_i)Q}{A} \tag{12.18}$$

where F is the flux (in mass per unit area per unit time), C_o is the concentration of mercury in the chamber outflow, C_i is the concentration of mercury in chamber inflow, Q is the flushing flow rate, and A is the bottom surface area of the chamber.

A typical flux chamber is a rectangular bottomless enclosure made of Teflon-coated stainless steel (Poissant et al., 2004), Plexiglas pastry cover (Wallschläger et al., 1999), Teflon film, polycarbonate, or acrylic (Lindberg et al., 2002). Xiao et al. (1991) have earlier employed stainless steel chambers but apparently had problems with blank contamination (Carpi and Lindberg, 1998). For chambers made of Teflon film, an external frame might be required to maintain the shape of the chamber (Lindberg and Zhang, 2000). Most chambers are rectangular, but Feng et al. (2004) have also used a semicylindrical quartz chamber. This chamber was set up over a partial open-bottom boat made of Plexiglas and wrapped with polystyrene blocks. A flotation arrangement, such as buoyant Styrofoam collars sealed with Teflon, can be used (Lindberg and Zhang, 2000). Typical dimensions of flux chambers are of the order (50–100 cm × 10 cm × 10 cm) (Carpi and Lindberg, 1998; Feng et al., 2002; Lindberg et al., 2002).

When flux chamber measurements are applied to obtain estimates that are consistent with the fluxes over open water, the thermal and aerodynamic conditions inside a chamber should be made as similar as possible to the ambient conditions. Several design variables must be controlled to ensure this, including temperature, incident radiation, and the chamber flushing rate (Wallschläger et al., 1999).

The temperature inside the chambers should be similar to the temperature of ambient air. Constant flushing of chamber air might alleviate this concern; however, the chamber material must not act like a greenhouse. Wavelengths of radiation (visible and ultraviolet, UV) that might stimulate redox reactions in water should be transmitted through the chamber. Plexiglas pastry cover chambers allow wavelengths up to about 380 nm to pass through, and Teflon chambers allow the visible spectrum and most UV radiation to pass through, up to about 250 nm (Wallschläger et al., 1999: Plexiglas material was 3 mm thick and the Teflon foil was 0.2 mm thick; Carpi et al., 2007).

Chamber flushing rate and flow dynamics through the system are critical factors that must be controlled. Very low flow rates may suppress degassing of mercury by building an artificial gradient across the air–water boundary, and very high flow rates may increase the mercury flux by changing the aerodynamic regime at the boundary layer (Zhang et al., 2002). In addition, (i) air flow inside the chamber must sweep over the entire surface to avoid stagnant zones, (ii) opening(s) in the chamber should allow for a uniform airstream to develop at the desired flow rate, and (iii) there should be no air flow perpendicular to the water surface (Gao et al., 1997).

Gao and Yates (1998) and Zhang et al. (2002) made an assessment of the effect of flushing flow rates on the ratio of steady state flux over soil determined by a chamber experiment and a theoretical actual flux across the natural surface. Both have reported that flux chamber measurements underpredict the gaseous flux, and the extent of underprediction was higher at lower flow rates. Higher flow rates give estimates closer to the actual flux, as long as no additional pressure deficit is introduced into the chamber (computed to be insignificant at air flow rates lower than 100 L/min for the considered chamber size of 40 cm $\times$ 40 cm $\times$ 10 cm). In addition, Gao and Yates (1998) report that, for a given flow rate, fluxes estimated using a chamber of smaller dimension are closer to the actual flux. Unfortunately, however, no similar experiments or simulations have been reported for measurement of fluxes over water surfaces.

For fluxes inside the chamber to be equal to the fluxes under ambient conditions, the mass transfer velocity across the air–water interface inside the flux chamber should be equal to the mass transfer velocity (k_W) over the open water surface. Since k_W is dependent on the shear at the surface, shear stress over water surfaces inside and outside the chamber must be equal (Leyris et al., 2005). Experiments or computer simulations are required to evaluate the conditions under which flux chamber measurements, if employed, provide estimates that are most reflective of the actual flux from surface ocean water to the atmosphere.

12.4   RATE CONSTANTS FOR REDUCTION AND OXIDATION OF MERCURY SPECIES IN OCEAN WATERS

While mercury evasion is a physical process, reduction and oxidation of mercury species (Hg(II) and Hg(0), respectively) are two chemical processes that determine the amount of DGM in surface oceans that is available for evasion. Both these groups of processes, physical and chemical, must be adequately determined to understand and predict the overall mass transfer of mercury from surface ocean layers to the atmosphere, on local to global scales.

Reduction and oxidation reactions of mercury occur by both abiotic and biotic pathways. More information on the two processes is summarized in several previously published articles (e.g., Whalin et al. 2007; Qureshi et al. 2010). Not all the divalent mercury present in ocean water is in a reducible form. Only a certain fraction is reducible Hg(II), or $Hg_r(II)$ (e.g., O'Driscoll et al., 2006). The size of this reducible fraction is, in turn, dependent on the incident wavelengths and the intensity of radiation (Qureshi et al., 2010). For example, more reducible mercury is observed under UV-B radiation than under UV-A radiation, and under higher intensities, likely up to an intensity maximum.

The rate of Hg(0) oxidation is also dependent on the intensity and type of radiation. It is currently unclear if the species resulting from mercury oxidation is the divalent mercury species that was initially reduced (Whalin and Mason, 2006; Whalin et al., 2007) or if there is production of a nonreducible form of mercury that must be converted again to a reducible form of divalent mercury for reduction to take place (Qureshi et al., 2010). Presence of such a species would imply that mercury reduction and oxidation process in surface oceans follows a three-species pathway (Qureshi et al., 2010) rather than a two-species pathway as has often been considered (Whalin and Mason, 2006; Whalin et al., 2007). Since the rate constant for oxidation is estimated by fitting observational values with the assumed reaction pathway, it is important to know if two or three mercury species groups are involved.

In assessing the data from literature it is also important to note whether the rate constants that are reported represent net reduction or oxidation, or, gross reduction or oxidation. In a net reaction, both reduction and oxidation occur simultaneously. The observed rate constant is a description of the overall reactions, and it is not possible to determine the rate constants of the individual redox processes. In this chapter, unless otherwise stated, we discuss gross reduction and gross oxidation, which represent the rate constant only for reduction or oxidation of mercury. Rate constants for gross reduction or oxidation must be obtained from experiments in which the electron-transfer process is inhibited (e.g., inhibition of oxidation while determination of reduction rate constant) or its effect is included in calculations of kinetic determination (e.g., information on reduction rate constant is used while determining the rate constant for oxidation).

12.4.1 Techniques for the Estimation of Redox Rate Constants

In a typical experiment to determine rate constants for redox reactions of mercury species in natural waters, a natural or spiked water sample is exposed to radiation, and DGM concentrations in the sample are measured with time (Amyot et al., 1997; O'Driscoll et al., 2006). With a suitably designed experiment, both reduction and oxidation rate constants can be determined (Whalin et al., 2007; Qureshi et al., 2010). Experiments could be conducted in natural sunlight or under light from an artificial source. Effects of various groups of wavelengths, for example, UV-A, UV-B, or visible radiation, can be studied by using radiation filters or, in the case of artificial sources, using lamps that emit the appropriate wavelength ranges (Amyot et al., 1997; Zhang and Lindberg, 2001; O'Driscoll et al., 2006). It is desirable that experiments are conducted in a controlled environment, so that the effects of various contributing factors can be assessed separately.

12.4.2   Rate Constant for Gross Photoreduction

While a water sample is being irradiated in a reaction chamber, reduction and oxidation reactions take place at the same time. However, if elemental mercury is continuously purged out of the water sample, there is no substrate left for the oxidation reaction. In this way, the reduction reaction can be driven to completion.

$$Hg_r(II) \rightarrow Hg(0) \qquad (12.19)$$

Assuming first-order kinetics, the following equation will apply:

$$[Hg(0)(t)] = [Hg_{r \text{ - initial}}(II)] \times (1 - \exp(-kt)) \qquad (12.20)$$

where $[Hg_{r \text{ - initial}}(II)]$ is the amount of reducible divalent mercury present in the sample at the beginning of the experiment.

The changes in elemental mercury concentrations in the purged gas can then be attributed to the reduction process.

12.4.3   Rate Constant for Gross Photooxidation

In a photooxidation experiment, ocean water samples are irradiated in several closed beakers having no headspace. Beakers are then taken out at different times of irradiation and analyzed for DGM concentrations. The DGM concentration measured at any particular time is the net result of both reduction and oxidation reactions. Fitting these results to kinetic equations of the assumed pathway and using the previously determined value of the rate constant for reduction, one can estimate the remaining rate constant (or constants) for oxidation. This calculation depends on the reaction pathway that is assumed; this is currently subject to debate, as explained above.

A list of published rate constants is presented in Table 12.1. Most of the determinations are for freshwater systems. Very few estimates have been made for open ocean water. Gross reduction rate constants determined on a variety of samples, spiked or unspiked, are of order of magnitude 0.2–3/h. Experiments of Mason et al. (1995) report net biotic reduction rate constants of about 10^{-4} to 10^{-3}/h for artificial samples, as well as spiked seawater. This value is 100–1000 times lower than what is observed in other reported experiments. But since reduction and oxidation rate constants for seawater are comparable, it is difficult to say if microbial gross reduction is really orders of magnitude lower than abiotic reduction. Also, since the experiments were conducted under different radiation wavelengths and intensities, it is impossible to make a definitive conclusion. Oxidation rate constants are also of the order of 0.1 to 4.5/h. It is currently unclear if the end product of Hg(0) oxidation is the original reducible mercury or another nonreducible form of mercury that must first be converted to the reducible form again. Qureshi et al. (2010) have reported a rate constant for this conversion, 0.09 to 0.16/h. For oxidation reactions that take place in the dark, presumably after exposure to light, the "dark" oxidation rate constant is of the order of 0.1 to 0.8/h.

TABLE 12.1 Summary of Reduction and Oxidation Rate Constants of Mercury Species

S.No.	Water Sample	Sample Location	Gross or Net	Rate Constant (/h)	Light Source	References
Reduction						
1	Ottawa River	45° 19'N 75° 40'W	Gross	0.23–0.24[a]	UV-A	O'Driscoll et al. (2006)
2	Williams Bay	44° 41'N 72° 02'W	Gross	0.2	UV-A	O'Driscoll et al. (2006)
3	Sharpes Bay	44° 41'N 72° 02'W	Gross	0.21	UV-A	O'Driscoll et al. (2006)
4	Brookes Bay	44° 41'N 72° 02'W	Gross	0.19	UV-A	O'Driscoll et al. (2006)
5	Anstruther Lake	44° 45'N 78° 12'W	Gross	0.27	UV-A	O'Driscoll et al. (2006)
6	North Lake	74° 46'N 95° 06'W	Gross	0.76	UV-A	O'Driscoll et al. (2006)
7	St. Lawrence River	45° 01'N 74° 40'W	Gross	1.1	UV-A	O'Driscoll et al. (2006)
8	Raison River	45° 15'N 74° 45'W	Gross	1.1	UV-A	O'Driscoll et al. (2006)
9	Ottawa River	45° 19'N 75° 40'W	Gross	0.38–0.64	UV-B	O'Driscoll et al. (2006)
10	Williams Bay	44° 41'N 72° 02'W	Gross	0.23	UV-B	O'Driscoll et al. (2006)
11	Sharpes Bay	44° 41'N 72° 02'W	Gross	0.31	UV-B	O'Driscoll et al. (2006)
12	Brookes Bay	44° 41'N 72° 02'W	Gross	0.24	UV-B	O'Driscoll et al. (2006)
13	Anstruther Lake	44° 45'N 78° 12'W	Gross	0.22	UV-B	O'Driscoll et al. (2006)
14	North Lake	74° 46'N 95° 06'W	Gross	0.92	UV-B	O'Driscoll et al. (2006)
15	St. Lawrence River	45° 01'N 74° 40'W	Gross	1.6	UV-B	O'Driscoll et al. (2006)
16	Raison River	45° 15'N 74° 45'W	Gross	0.55	UV-B	O'Driscoll et al. (2006)
17	Isotope amended bay water	Chesapeake Bay	Gross	2.3±0.9[b]	Midday sun	Whalin et al. (2007)
18	Isotope amended fresh water	Patuxent River	Gross	2.5±0.8	Midday sun	Whalin et al. (2007)
19	Isotope amended coastal water	Brigantine Island, New Jersey	Gross	2.3±0.5	Midday sun	Whalin et al. (2007)

(*continued*)

TABLE 12.1 (*Continued*)

S.No.	Water Sample	Sample Location	Gross or Net	Rate Constant (/h)	Light Source	References
20	Isotope amended surface water (<5 m from surface)	Chesapeake Bay and shelf	Gross	$0.002-1^c$	Natural light	Whalin et al. (2007)
21	Isotope amended deep water (<5 m from sediments)	—	Gross	$0.002-0.007^c$	Dark	Whalin et al. (2007)
22	*Pavlova lutherui* culture	—	Gross	0.004	Fluorescent light	Mason et al. (1995)
23	*Thalassiosira weissflogii* culture	—	Gross	0.00017–0.00125	Fluorescent light	Mason et al. (1995)
24	Ocean water	Atlantic Ocean off the Scotian Shelf, 41° 51'N 60° 46'W	Gross	0.15	UV-A	Qureshi et al. (2010)
25	Ocean water	Atlantic Ocean off the Scotian Shelf, 41° 51'N 60° 46'W	Gross	0.4–0.9	UV-B	Qureshi et al. (2010)
26	Lake water, incubated with additional Hg isotopes at natural levels	Experimental Lakes Area (Lake 658), Canada. 49° 43.9' N 93° 44.2'W	Net^d	0.21–0.47	Natural light	Poulain et al. (2004)

#	Description	Location	Type	Value	Light	Reference
27	Wetland near the lake	Experimental Lakes Area (Lake 658), Canada. 49° 43.9′ N 93° 44.2′W	Net[e]	0.76–1.4	Natural light	Poulain et al. (2004)
28	Unspiked river water	Upper St. Lawrence River at Cornwall	Net[f]	2.2±0.2	Visible+UV-A and UV-B	Amyot et al. (2000)
29	Unspiked river water	Upper St. Lawrence River at Cornwall	Net[g]	1.1±0.1	Visible	Amyot et al. (2000)
30	Spiked river water	Upper St. Lawrence River at Cornwall	Net[h]	1.9±0.4–1.7±0.1	UV-A+UV-B	Amyot et al. (2000)
32	Pond water without Fe(III) addition	Oak Ridge National Laboratory, USA	Net	0.05–0.2	Natural light during day	Zhang and Lindberg (2001)
33	Lake water	Whitefish Bay, east end of Lake Superior	Net	0.07–0.3	Natural light during day	Zhang and Lindberg (2001)
34	Distilled water spiked with 0.5 nM Hg	—	Net	0.00046	Fluorescent light	Mason et al. (1995)
36	Artificial seawater with trace metals, nutrients, and vitamins	—	Net	0.0002	Fluorescent light	Mason et al. (1995)
37	Freshwater sample spiked with 0.5 nM Hg	Mystic Lakes, Boston	Net	0.0002	Fluorescent light	Mason et al. (1995)

(continued)

TABLE 12.1 (*Continued*)

S.No.	Water Sample	Sample Location	Gross or Net	Rate Constant (/h)	Light Source	References
38	Coastal seawater spiked with 0.6 nM Hg	Martha's Vineyard, Massachusetts	Net[i]	0.00096	Fluorescent light	Mason et al. (1995)
39	Coastal seawater spiked with 0.6 nM Hg	Martha's Vineyard, Massachusetts	Net[j]	0.00054±0.00025	Fluorescent light	Mason et al. (1995)
40	Coastal seawater spiked with 0.6 nM Hg	Martha's Vineyard, Massachusetts	Net[k]	0.00096	Fluorescent light	Mason et al. (1995)
41	Coastal seawater spiked with 0.6 nM Hg	Martha's Vineyard, Massachusetts	Net[l]	0.0005	Fluorescent light	Mason et al. (1995)
Oxidation						
42	Isotope amended bay water	Chesapeake Bay	Gross[b]	2.6±1	Midday sun	Whalin et al. (2007)
43	Isotope amended fresh water	Patuxent River	Gross	4.3±1.5	Midday sun	Whalin et al. (2007)
44	Isotope amended coastal water	Brigantine Island, New Jersey	Gross	1.5±0.3	Midday sun	Whalin et al. (2007)
45	Ocean water	Atlantic Ocean off the Scotian Shelf, 41° 51'N 60° 46'W	Gross	0.4–1.5	UV-A	Qureshi et al. (2010)

#	Sample	Location		Value	Light	Reference
46	Ocean water	Atlantic Ocean off the Scotian Shelf, 41° 51'N 60° 46'W	Gross	0.7–2.5	UV-B	Qureshi et al. (2010)
47	Spiked—Cap Rouge	~46'N 73'W	Net^{m,n}	0.23	UV-B	Lalonde et al. (2001)
48	Spiked—Escoumins River	48'N 70'W	Net^m	0.26	UV-B	Lalonde et al. (2001)
49	Spiked—Gouffre River	47'N 71'W	Net^m	0.26	UV-B	Lalonde et al. (2001)
50	Spiked—Baie Saint-Paul	47'N 71'W	Net^{m,o}	0.54–0.86	UV-B	Lalonde et al. (2001)
51	Spiked—Baie Escoumins	48'N 70'W	Net^m	0.58	UV-B	Lalonde et al. (2001)
52	Spiked—Gouffre River	47'N 71'W	Net^m	0.56	UV-B	Lalonde et al. (2001)
53	Spiked river water	Upper St. Lawrence River at Cornwall	Net	0.09±0.03	Natural light	Amyot et al. (2000)
54	Spiked natural estuarine water	Baise Saint-Paul Estuary. 46 49'N	Net^{p,q}	0.09	Visible light only	Lalonde et al. (2004)
55	Spiked natural estuarine water	Baise Saint-Paul Estuary. 46 49'N	Net^{p,r}	0.59	Visible+UV-A	Lalonde et al. (2004)
56	Spiked natural estuarine water	Baise Saint-Paul Estuary. 46 49'N	Net^{p,s}	0.67	Visible+UV-A and UV-B	Lalonde et al. (2004)

(*continued*)

TABLE 12.1 (*Continued*)

S.No.	Water Sample	Sample Location	Gross or Net	Rate Constant (/h)	Light Source	References
57	Coastal waters	Galveston Island, Gulf of Mexico	Net[t]	0.09–0.1	Natural light	Amyot et al. (1997)
Dark Oxidation						
58	Ocean water	Atlantic Ocean off the Scotian Shelf. 41° 51′N 60° 46′W	Gross	0.2–0.8	Determined from a graphical analysis of results	Qureshi et al. (2010)
59	Lake water	Lake Croche—45° 56′N 74° 00′W	Net[u, v]	0.02–0.07	Sunlight followed by darkness.	Garcia et al. (2005)
60	Coastal water	Galveston Island, Gulf of Mexico	Net[t]	0.09–0.12	Dark, but after sunlight exposure of 1 h.	Amyot et al. (1997)
61	Spiked river water and coastal water	Choptank River and Seaside Park. New Jersey	Net[w]	0.1–0.4	Dark	Amyot et al. (1997)
62	Pond water with Fe(III) addition	Oak Ridge National Laboratory, USA	Net	0.2	Dark	Zhang and Lindberg (2001)
63	Pond water without Fe(III) addition	Oak Ridge National Laboratory, USA	Net	0.3	Dark	Zhang and Lindberg (2001)
Conversion of nonreducible Hg(II) to reducible Hg(II)						
64	Ocean water	Atlantic Ocean off the Scotian Shelf. 41° 51′N 60° 46′W	Gross	$0.09-0.13^{x(i)}$; $0.11-0.16^{x(ii)}$		Qureshi et al. (2010)

[a] It was found that rate constants were not correlated to the DOC content. DOC concentrations remained the same, but fluorescence decreased on exposure to UV-A; no decrease in fluorescence was observed for UV-B.

[b] Reduction and oxidation rate constants were determined assuming a two-species reversible pathway (as against the three species proposed by Qureshi et al. (2010); however, as Whalin et al. (2007) fitted the rate constant values for the initial 1–2 h, assumption of either two- or three-species pathways lead to similar results; samples were taken at midday. Reduction and oxidation rate constants were below detection for samples taken at 6 a.m. or 10 p.m. Pathway assumed by Whalin et al. (2007): $Hg(II) \rightarrow Hg(0)$, $Hg(0) \rightarrow Hg(II)$.

[c] Lower value taken as 0.5 times the detection limit.

[d] Measured as formation rates, which were in a separate experiment found to be similar in filtered and unfiltered samples. According to O'Driscoll et al. (2006), the oxidation rate constants in lake water are much lower than the reduction rate constants. So, in this lake, the values might be closer to the real gross rate constant.

[e] Measured as formation rates.

[f] The determined values assume a two-species pathway. It is further assumed that all initial Hg(II) was readily reducible, and that the product of oxidation is the initially readily reducible Hg(II).

[g] No difference was observed between filtered and unfiltered samples.

[h] Different spike amounts gave similar rate constants, leading the authors to imply that first-order kinetics were adequate to describe the reactions. Additionally, it was suggested that only mercury substrate and light were the determining factors for reactions and that the amount of reductants present in the sample was probably not a limiting factor.

[i] Unfiltered samples incubated overnight. Formation rates were corrected for abiotic production of 0.00017 ± 0.00008.

[j] Nutrients were added.

[k] 3-μm filtered samples.

[l] 1-μm filtered samples.

[m] Likely to represent gross values under the assumption that reduction does not take place in the absence of any organic matter.

[n] Experiments with artificial water (ultrapure water at pH 8; buffered with NaH_2PO_4 and Na_2HPO_4) showed that no oxidation takes place in pure water with or without HCl. But oxidation takes place when benzoquinone—that produces semiquinone radicals—is added in the presence of chloride. No such change was observed with fulvic acid, which authors attribute to simultaneous oxidation.

[o] Increase in values from ~ 0.2/h in freshwater to greater than 0.5/h in saline waters also corresponded to an increase in chloride concentration (from $\sim 10^{-4}$ to $\sim 10^{-1}$ M).

[p] Spiked water had Hg(0) concentrations in the nanomolar range (0.2–2 nM), as against natural total mercury concentrations of picomolar range. So, the reaction can perhaps be approximated to represent gross rate constants.

TABLE 12.1 (Continued)

[q] Higher oxidation rates were observed after filtration, leading the authors to hypothesize that filtration decreased the photoreduction reactions that depended on heterogeneous processes. However, Poulain et al. (2004) and Qureshi et al. (2010) did not see any appreciable difference in reaction rate constants on filtered or unfiltered waters.

[r] Role of $O_2^{\bullet-}$ was said to be minor, but $^{\bullet}OH$ was stated to likely play a role in oxidation.

[s] Samples irradiated with UV, spiked, and then kept in the dark showed dark oxidation rate constant of about 0.03/h. In another set of experiments, samples were spiked with methanol, an $^{\bullet}OH$ scavenger, and the observed rate constant decreased from 0.43 to 0.32/h. They also mention that methanol can scavenge other reactive species such as $Cl^{\bullet}$ and HO_2 as well.

[t] Could be considered as a gross rate constant if reduction is approximated as zero in the absence of light. Authors also mention that oxidation is probably induced by sunlight.

[u] But likely to represent gross values since reduction will probably not take place in the absence of light.

[v] Samples put in the dark after exposure to sunlight at various times of day. Observed dark oxidation rate constants showed a diel pattern. This can perhaps be attributed to different photoradical productions at different times of the day.

[w] River water was amended with 0.5 M chloride. Volatilization was also a factor. Authors report a loss constant of 0.07–0.1/h for volatilization. Furthermore, in the reduction experiments, addition of Hg(II) increases the DGM produced. The authors inferred that organomercurial compounds are probably not the only substrate for reduction. But they did not consider the possibility of complexing of Hg(II) with organic matter or the role of organic matter as an electron donor.

[x] Qureshi et al. (2010) proposed a three-species pathway for reduction and oxidation of mercury in ocean water: either (i) $Hg_r(II) \rightarrow Hg(0)$, $Hg(0) \rightarrow Hg^*$, and $Hg^* \rightarrow Hg_r(II)$ or (ii) $Hg_r(II) \rightarrow Hg(0)$, $Hg(0) \rightarrow Hg^*$, and $Hg^* \rightarrow Hg_r(II)$ or $Hg^* \rightarrow Hg(0)$. The rate constant for conversion is the rate constant for reaction $Hg^* \rightarrow Hg_r(II)$ or $Hg^* \rightarrow Hg(0)$, as indicated by (i) and (ii), respectively.

12.5   MODELING STUDIES ESTIMATING OCEANIC AIR–SEA EXCHANGE

The theoretical and experimental approaches described above can be used to estimate the ocean–air flux at different spatial and temporal scales. In this section, we present a model, GEOS-Chem, which has been used to estimate this flux at the global scale.

12.5.1   Global Air–Sea Exchange Estimates

Several studies (Mason et al., 1994; Lamborg et al., 2002; Sunderland and Mason, 2007) have used box-modeling approaches to estimate a global flux of mercury from oceans to the atmosphere between 4 and 14 million moles per year (Mmol/year). Sunderland and Mason (2007) used Monte Carlo simulations, given the uncertainty in observed aqueous and atmospheric Hg(0) concentrations, to estimate the 95% confidence intervals in mercury evasion of 9.7–20.7 Mmol/year. Evasion estimates from box-modeling studies generally agree (Table 12.2) with simulations performed using the GEOS-Chem global chemical transport model (CTM) (Strode et al., 2007; Selin et al., 2008; Soerensen et al., 2010).

12.5.2   The Original GEOS-Chem Global Modeling Framework

The original surface slab ocean model in GEOS-Chem was developed by Strode et al. (2007) to represent global air–sea exchange coupled to the original atmospheric Hg simulation developed by Selin et al. (2007). Model versions developed by Selin et al. (2007, 2008) used OH radical and O_3 as the main atmospheric oxidants for Hg(0). Both atmosphere and surface oceans have horizontal resolutions of $4°$ latitude by $5°$ longitude and are driven by assimilated meteorological data from the NASA GEOS. The ocean slab model's vertical depth varies depending on the monthly resolved mixed layer depth of the surface ocean (Kara et al., 2003). The model tracks three inorganic Hg species in the surface ocean: Hg(II), Hg(0), and particle-associated Hg (Hg-p).

TABLE 12.2   Summary of Global Hg(0) Oceanic Evasion Estimates from Different Modeling Studies

Study	Description	Global Net Hg(0) Evasion (Mmol/year)
Mason et al. (1994)	One-compartment box model	10
Lamborg et al. (2002)	Six-compartment box model	4
Mason and Sheu (2002)	Two-compartment box model	13
Strode et al. (2007)	GEOS-Chem	14.1
Sunderland and Mason (2007)	14-Compartment box model	13.1 (9.7–20.7)
Selin et al. (2008)	GEOS-Chem	14.0
Soerensen et al. (2010)	GEOS-Chem	14.7

The original slab ocean model in GEOS-Chem represented oceanic Hg cycling in a simplified manner using three main rate constants that describe net reduction of atmospherically deposited Hg(II) to Hg(0), conversion to nonreactive Hg, and sinking of nonreactive (particulate) Hg. Each rate constant was adjusted to match observations. Air–sea exchange was calculated based on the scheme developed by Nightingale et al. (2000), with diffusivity of aqueous Hg(0) calculated using the Wilke–Chang method (Wilke and Chang, 1955) and the temperature-dependent Henry's law constant for Hg(0) from Wängberg et al. (2001). The model neglected horizontal transport and inputs from rivers but included vertical exchange with subsurface waters through entrainment/detrainment of the mixed layer, Ekman pumping, and vertical diffusion.

A major limitation of the original GEOS-Chem slab ocean model was the assumption of globally uniform subsurface ocean concentrations (1.5 picomol, pM), resulting in virtually all evaded Hg(0) being supplied by recent atmospherically deposited Hg. Mean Hg concentrations are known to vary across ocean regions with the Atlantic Ocean being generally enriched relative to the Pacific Ocean (Gill and Fitzgerald, 1988; Laurier et al., 2004) and equal to or lower than the Mediterranean Sea (Horvat et al., 2003; Cossa et al., 2004; Kotnik et al., 2007; Cossa et al., 2009).

12.5.3 Recent Mechanistic Enhancements to GEOS-Chem Air–Sea Exchange Model

Soerensen et al. (2010) recently developed an improved global simulation of Hg air–sea exchange within the GEOS-Chem model. A major update to the model simulation was the implementation of discrete subsurface ocean concentrations based on observations compiled by Sunderland and Mason (2007) (Fig. 12.6). The new model also replaced the net reduction rate constant implemented in the original GEOS-Chem slab ocean simulation (Strode et al., 2007) by gross terms describing photolytic and biotic reduction, and photo- and dark oxidation (Fig. 12.6). Photoreduction and oxidation rates are parameterized as a function of light intensity in the euphotic zone. Biotic reduction is modeled based on global net primary productivity (NPP) distributions from MODIS satellite data (Behrenfeld and Falkowski, 1997). The model includes a term for dark oxidation in all surface and subsurface model compartments based on Lalonde et al. (2001). The fraction of the dissolved phase Hg(II) pool subject to reduction is based on studies showing that colloidal Hg species can account for up to 50% of the Hg(II) in open ocean environments (Guentzel et al., 1996; Mason and Sullivan, 1999) and that stable chloride complexes abundant at high salinities are more resistant to reduction processes (Stumm and Morgan, 1996; Whalin et al., 2007). The model calculates an average radiation (RAD) for each surface model compartment by using the local shortwave radiation flux at the surface from GEOS-5 and light attenuation based on spectral light absorption/scattering coefficients for seawater, dissolved organic carbon (DOC) and pigments, and their respective concentrations (Wozniak and Dera, 2007). Pigment concentrations are derived from MODIS satellite data, while DOC is based on a global

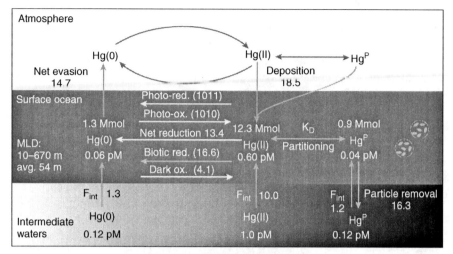

Intermediate water Hg concentrations

(a)

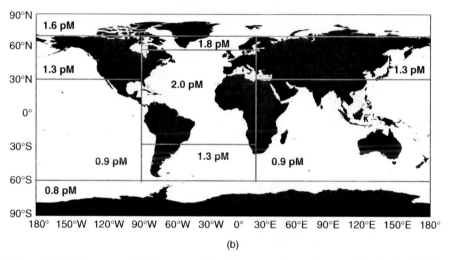

(b)

Figure 12.6 Schematic of the improved surface ocean Hg cycling module in the GEOS-Chem CTM from Soerensen et al. (2010): (a) Global budget for inorganic Hg species in the surface ocean, (b) Intermediate water Hg concentrations used in the model based on observations compiled by Sunderland and Mason (2007), with updates for the North Pacific (Sunderland et al., 2009) and Arctic Oceans (Kirk et al., 2008). Note: Fluxes in (a) in Mmol/year.

mean of 1.5 mg/L in the surface mixed layer (Chester, 2003) and scaled by the distribution of global NPP (also derived from MODIS data) to account for productivity-related concentration differences.

In the new model, settling of Hg(II) sorbed to suspended particulate matter (SPM) is described by linking sorption and removal from the surface layer to organic carbon export fluxes (the ocean biological pump). The affinity of aqueous Hg(II) for the solid phase is described using empirically measured partition coefficients from the Pacific and Atlantic Oceans (Mason and Fitzgerald, 1993; Mason et al., 1998) and SPM concentrations estimated from algal biomass. Settling fluxes of Hg-p are based on the parameterization described in Sunderland and Mason (2007) for export of organic carbon with depth (Antoine et al., 1996; Antia et al., 2001; Schlitzer, 2004; Behrenfeld et al., 2005) and Hg to carbon (Hg:C) ratios. These Hg:C ratios are calculated from the standing stock of organic carbon in the mixed layer based on MODIS satellite *Chl a* measurements (Uitz et al., 2006; Wetzel et al., 2006).

The new GEOS-Chem simulation models fluxes of Hg(0) at the air–sea interface using the parameterization developed by Nightingale et al. (2000), the dimensionless Henry's law coefficient for Hg(0) recently measured by Andersson et al. (2008), a temperature-corrected Schmidt number for CO_2 (Poissant et al., 2000), and the Wilke–Chang method for estimating temperature- and salinity-corrected Hg(0) diffusivity in different ocean regions (Wilke and Chang, 1955).

Globally, the new model showed that 35% of the Hg inputs to the ocean mixed layer on a global basis are from the subsurface ocean, with the remaining 65% from atmospheric Hg deposition (Fig. 12.6). Particle-associated transport of Hg accounts for the majority of removal to subsurface waters. Photolytic redox reactions dominate dark and biotic processes, which are mainly important in niche environments where light penetration is limited. Although globally the ocean is a sink for 3.8 Mmol Hg/year, areas like the North Atlantic are a net source to the atmosphere. In the North Atlantic, large inputs of Hg from Hg-enriched subsurface waters through seasonal entrainment of the mixed layer and elevated Ekman pumping due to high winter winds replenish Hg concentrations in the surface ocean. Ultimately, this causes the pronounced seasonal cycling in Hg(0) evasion shown in Fig. 12.7.

12.5.4   Key Uncertainties and Data Requirements for Future Modeling Research

Sensitivity analyses performed with the GEOS-Chem global model provide an indication of new research directions. The reducible Hg(II) pool is rarely measured in studies collecting data on gross reaction kinetics (Qureshi et al., 2010) and should be a priority for future research because Hg(0) evasion increases/decreases proportionally to this pool in the GEOS-Chem simulation.

Other studies (Loux, 2004, Kuss et al., 2009) have suggested that the diffusivity of Hg(0) in seawater is overestimated by standard calculation methods such as Wilke–Chang (Wilke and Chang, 1955), which could lead to modeled retention of Hg(0) in the surface waters being too low. However, implementing the theoretically derived diffusivity term for Hg(0) proposed by Kuss et al. (2009) in the GEOS-Chem model simulation only increases aqueous Hg(0) concentrations by 5% and results in a decrease in global net evasion of 14%.

As discussed in previous sections, different parameterizations of the air–sea transfer velocity as a function of wind speed can lead to large differences in

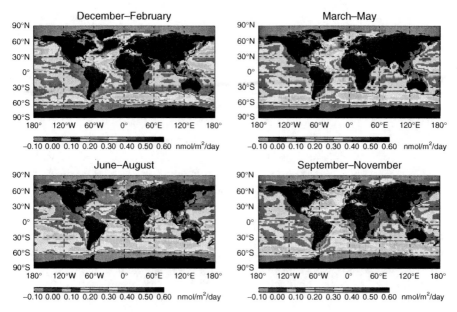

Figure 12.7 Seasonal variability in air–sea exchange of Hg(0) for 2008 using the GEOS-Chem global CTM. Figure from Soerensen et al. (2010).

computed fluxes (Rolfhus and Fitzgerald, 2004; Andersson et al., 2007). Using the gas transfer scheme developed by Liss and Merlivat (1986), generally accepted as a low end estimate, in the GEOS-Chem model results in a 30% reduction in modeled global evasion compared to the standard simulation based on Nightingale et al. (2000) but does not substantially change aqueous Hg(0) concentrations. These results suggest that the Nightingale parameterization (Nightingale et al., 2000) that uses a quadratic relationship between evasion and wind speed is most appropriate because the linear dependence of evasion on wind speed in the Liss and Merlivat (1986) model diminishes the modeled seasonal cycle of Hg concentrations in the marine boundary layer that is observed in the Northern Hemisphere (Soerensen et al., 2010).

12.6 CONCLUSIONS AND FUTURE DIRECTIONS

In this chapter, we have reviewed the theoretical and experimental aspects of the mass transfer of elemental mercury from oceans to the atmosphere. It is shown that globally, thermodynamic controls of ocean–air exchange slightly favor a flux of Hg(0) from oceans to the atmosphere. The waterside air–water mass transfer coefficient dominates resistance to mass transfer of mercury, and we present a review of the literature and recommend relationships (e.g. Eq. 12.17) for estimating this parameter. This information can be used to estimate the flux when the concentrations of mercury in air and water are known. Alternatively, estimates of Hg(0) flux in the field can be estimated from controlled flux chamber experiments. However, the design material, chamber size and flushing rates must be chosen carefully.

Since ocean-to-air flux is also dependent on the concentration of elemental mercury in water, it is important to consider the redox reactions occurring in the surface ocean water that replenish or deplete the Hg(0) pool. Photoreduction rate constants are reported to be in the range 0.2–3/h, photooxidation rate constants in the range 0.1–4.5/h and "dark" oxidation rate constants in the range 0.1–0.8/h. When considering the pathway proposed by Qureshi et al. (2010), a rate constant for conversion of nonreducible Hg(II) to reducible Hg(II) must be considered (range 0.09–0.16/h). In addition, a biotic reduction rate constant could be used (Mason et al., 1995; 10^{-4} to 10^{-3}/h); however, this number represents a net value.

Model simulations show that on a global average, the evasion of elemental mercury is in the range 9.7–20.7 Mmol/year. Simulations from the most recent version of GEOS-Chem indicate that the size of the available pool of reducible Hg(II) in surface ocean water is a key uncertainty in global calculations of air–water flux. Model results were relatively insensitive to changing assumptions about the diffusivity of elemental mercury. Further simulations have shown that the parameterization of Nightingale et al. (2000) incorporated in the current version of the model is suitable for estimating mass transfer coefficient for air–water exchange. The temperature-dependent modification of Nightingale et al. (2000) presented in Equation (12.17) of this chapter can also be used in such calculations.

Ocean–air exchange of mercury is a key process that constrains the global cycling of mercury. Currently, the key uncertainties about this process likely arise from lack of understanding of the rates and pathways of redox reactions of Hg in ocean water (Pirrone et al., 2008). Studies that quantify these processes are very limited. More research is needed on the kinetic processes that occur in surface ocean waters and on the methods that estimate Hg(0) fluxes using flux chambers. Models are needed to integrate the results of these research efforts into an overall mass balance of mercury. Therefore, a continuous development and creation of simple yet robust models is required.

REFERENCES

Amyot M, Gill GA, Morel FMM. Production and loss of dissolved gaseous mercury in coastal seawater. Environ Sci Technol 1997;31:3606–3611.

Amyot M, Lean DRS, Poissant L, Doyon M-R. Distribution and transformation of elemental mercury in the St. Lawrence River and Lake Ontario. Can J Fish Aquat Sci 2000;57(S1):155–163.

Andersson ME, Gardfeldt K, Wängberg I, Sprovieri F, Pirrone N, Lindqvist O. Seasonal and daily variation of mercury evasion at coastal and off shore sites from the Mediterranean Sea. Mar Chem 2007;104:214–226.

Andersson ME, Gaerdfeldt K, Wängberg I, Stroemberg D. Determination of Henry's law constant for elemental mercury. Chemosphere 2008;73:587–592.

Antia AN, Koeve W, Fischer G, Blanz T, Schulz-Bull D, Schölten J, Neuer S, Kremling K, Kuss J, Peinert R, Hebbeln D, Bathmann U, Conte M, Fehner U, Zeitzschel B. Basin-wide particulate organic carbon flux in the Atlantic Ocean, regional export patterns and potential for CO2 sequestration. Global Biogeochem Cycles 2001;15:845–862.

Antoine D, Andre J-M, Morel A. Oceanic primary production 2. Estimation at global scale from satellite (coastal zone color scammer) chlorophyll. Global Biogeochem Cycles 1996;10:57–69.

Behrenfeld M, Boss E, Siegel D, Shea D. Carbon-based ocean productivity and phytoplankton physiology from space. Global Biogeochem Cycles 2005;19. DOI: 10.1029/2004 GB002299.

Behrenfeld MJ, Falkowski PG. Photosynthetic rates derived from satellite-based chlorophyll concentration. Limnol Oceanogr 1997;42:1–20.

Bloom N, Fitzgerald WF. Determination of volatile mercury species at the picogram level by low-temperature gas chromatography with cold-vapour atomic fluorescence detection. Anal Chim Acta 1988;208:151–161.

Carpi A, Frei A, Cocris D, McCloskey R, Contreras E, Ferguson K. Analytical artifacts produced by a polycarbonate chamber compared to a Teflon chamber for measuring surface mercury fluxes. Anal Bioanal Chem 2007;388:361–365.

Carpi A, Lindberg SE. Application of a teflon™ dynamic flux chamber for quantifying soil mercury flux, tests and results over background soil. Atmos Environ 1998;32:872–882.

Chester R. Marine Geochemistry. 2nd ed. Berlin: Blackwell Science Ltd.; 2003.

Cossa D, Averty B, Pirrone N. The origin of methylmercury in open Mediterranean waters. Limnol Oceanogr 2009;54:837–844.

Cossa D, Cotte-Krief MH, Mason R, Bretaudeau-Sanjuan J. Total mercury in the water column near the shelf edge of the European continental margin. Mar Chem 2004;90:21–29.

Feng X, Sommar J, Gardfeldt K, Lindqvist O. Exchange flux of total mercury between air and water surfaces in summer season. Sci China Ser D 2002;45:211–220.

Feng X, Yan H, Wang S, Qiu G, Tang S, Shang L, Dai Q, Hou Y. Seasonal variation of gaseous mercury exchange rate between air and water surface over Baihua reservoir, Guizhou, China. Atmos Environ 2004;38:4721–4732.

Frost T, Upstill-Goddard RC. Air-sea gas exchange into the millennium, progress and uncertainties. Oceanogr Mar Biol 1999;37:1–45.

Gao F, Yates SR. Simulation of enclosure-based methods for measuring gas emissions from soil to the atmosphere. J Geophys Res 1998;103(D20):26127–26136. DOI: 10.1029/98JD01345.

Gao F, Yates SR, Yates MV, Gan J, Ernst FF. Design, fabrication, and application of a dynamic chamber for measuring gas emissions from soil. Environ Sci Technol 1997;31:148–153.

Garcia E, Poulain AJ, Amyot M, Ariya PA. Diel variations in photoinduced oxidation of Hg^0 in freshwater. Chemosphere 2005;59:977–981.

Gill G, Fitzgerald WF. Vertical mercury distributions in the oceans. Geochim Cosmochim Acta 1988;52:1719–1728.

Guentzel JL, Powell RT, Landing WM, Mason RP. Mercury associated with colloidal material in an estuarine and open-ocean environment. Mar Chem 1996;55:177–188.

Horvat M, Kotnik J, Logar M, Fajon V, Zvonaric T, Pirrone N. Speciation of mercury in surface and deep-sea waters in the Mediterranean Sea. Atmos Environ 2003;37(S1): S93–S108.

Jaehne B, Haussecker H. Air-sea gas exchange. Annu Rev Fluid Mech 1998;30:443–468.

Jaehne B, Hinz G, Dietrich W. Measurement of the diffusion coefficients of sparingly soluble gases in water. J Geophys Res 1987;10:767–776.

Kanwisher L. Effect of wind on CO_2 exchange across the sea surface. J Geophys Res 1963;68:3921–3927.

Kara AB, Rochford PA, Hurlburt HE. Mixed layer depth variability over the global ocean. J Geophys Res, Oceans 2003;108. DOI: 10.1029/2000JC000736.

Kirk JL, St. Louis VL, Hintelmann H, Lehnherr I, Else B, Poissant L. Methylated mercury species in marine waters of the Canadian High and Sub Arctic. Environ Sci Technol 2008;42:8367–8373.

Kotnik J, Horvat M, Tessier E, Ogrinc N, Monperrus M, Amouroux D, Fajon V, Gibicar D, Zizek S, Sprovieri F, Pirrone N. Mercury speciation in surface and deep waters of the Mediterranean Sea. Mar Chem 2007;107:13–30.

Kuss J, Holzmann J, Ludwig R. An elemental mercury diffusion coefficient for natural waters determined by molecular dynamics simulation. Environ Sci Technol 2009;43:3183–3186.

Lalonde JD, Amyot M, Kraepiel AML, Morel FMM. Photooxidation of Hg(0) in artificial and natural waters. Environ Sci Technol 2001;35:1367–1372.

Lalonde JD, Amyot M, Orvoine J, Morel FMM, Auclair J-C, Ariya PA. Photoinduced oxidation of $Hg^0(aq)$ in the waters from the St. Lawrence estuary. Environ Sci Technol 2004;38:508–514.

Lamborg C, Fitzgerald W, O'Donnell J, Torgensen T. A non-steady-state compartmental model of global scale mercury biogeochemistry with interhemispheric atmospheric gradients. Geochim Cosmochim Acta 2002;66:1105–1118.

Laurier F, Mason R, Gill G, Whalin L. Mercury distribution in the North Pacific Ocean–20 years of observations. Mar Chem 2004;90:3–19.

Leyris C, Guillot J-M, Fanlo JL, Pourtier L. Comparison and development of dynamic flux chambers to determine odorous compound emission rates from area sources. Chemosphere 2005;59:415–421.

Lindberg SE, Zhang H. Air/water exchange of mercury in the Everglades II, measuring and modeling evasion of mercury from surface waters in the Everglades Nutrient Removal Project. Sci Total Environ 2000;259:135–143.

Lindberg SE, Zhang H, Vette AF, Gustin MS, Barnett MO, Kuiken T. Dynamic flux chamber measurement of gaseous mercury emission fluxes over soils, part 2–effect of flushing flow rate and verification of a two-resistance exchange interface simulation model. Atmos Environ 2002;36:847–859.

Liss PS, Merlivat L. Air-sea exchange rates, introduction and synthesis. In: Buat-Menard P, editor. The role of air-sea exchange in geochemical cycling. Dordrecht: D Reidel Publishing Company; 1986. pp 113–127.

Liss PS, Slater PG. Flux of gases across the air-sea interface. Nature 1974;274:181–184.

Loux NT. A critical assessment of elemental mercury air/water exchange parameters. Chem Spec Bioavailab 2004;16:127–138.

Mackay D. Multimedia environmental models. 2nd ed. Boca Raton (FL): Lewis Publishers, CRC Press LLC; 2001.

Mason RP, Fitzgerald W. The distribution and cycling of mercury in the equatorial Pacific Ocean. Deep-Sea Res Part I 1993;40:1897–1924.

Mason RP, Fitzgerald WF, Morel FMM. The biogeochemical cycling of elemental mercury, Anthropogenic influences. Geochim Cosmochim Acta 1994;58:3191–3198.

Mason RP, Rolfhus K, Fitzgerald W. Mercury in the North Atlantic. Mar Chem 1998;61:37–53.

Mason RP, Sheu G-R. Role of the ocean in the global mercury cycle. Global Biogeochem Cycles 2002;16:1093–1107.

Mason RP, Sullivan KA. The distribution and speciaiton of mercury in the South and equatorial Atlantic. Deep-Sea Res Part II 1999;46:937–956.

Mason RP, Morel FMM, Hemond HF. The role of microorganisms in elemental mercury formation in natural waters. Water Soil Air Pollut 1995;80:775–787.

Munthe J, Wängberg I, Pirrone N, Iverfeldt A, Ferrara R, Ebinghaus R, Feng X, Gardfeldt K, Keeler G, Lanzillotta E, Lindberg SE, Lu J, Mamane Y, Prestbo E, Schmolke S, Schroeder WH, Sommar J, Sprovieri F, Stevens RK, Stratton W, Tuncel G, Urba A. Intercomparison of methods for sampling and analysis of atmospheric mercury species. Atmos Environ 2001;25:3007–3017.

Nightingale PD, Malin G, Law CS, Watson AJ, Liss PS, Liddicoat MI, Boutin J, Upstill-Goddard RC. In situ evaluation of air-sea gas exchange parameterizations using novel conservative and volatile tracers. Global Biogeochem Cycles 2000;14:373–387.

O'Driscoll NJ, Siciliano SD, Lean DRS, Amyot M. Gross photoreduction kinetics of mercury in temperate freshwater lakes and rivers: application to a general model of DGM dynamics. Environ Sci Technol 2006;40:837–843.

Othmer DF, Thakar MS. Correlating diffusion coefficients in liquids. Ind Eng Chem 1953;45:589–593.

Pirrone N, Hedgecock IM, Sprovieri F. New directions: atmospheric mercury, easy to spot and hard to pin down: impasse? Atmos Environ 2008;42:8549–8551.

Poissant L, Amyot M, Pilote M, Lean D. Mercury air-water exchange over the upper St. Lawrence River and Lake Ontario. Environ Sci Technol 2000;34:3069–3078.

Poissant L, Pilote M, Constant P, Beauvais C, Zhang HH, Xu X. Mercury gas exchange over selected bare and flooded sites in the bay St. Fracois wetlands (Quebec, Canada). Atmos Environ 2004;38:4205–4214.

Poulain AJ, Amyot M, Findlay D, Telor S, Barkay T, Hintelmann H. Biological and photochemical production of dissolved gaseous mercury in a boreal lake. Limnol Oceanogr 2004;49:2265–2275.

Qureshi A, O'Driscoll NJ, MacLeod M, Neuhold Y-M, Hungerbühler K. Photoreactions of mercury in surface ocean water, gross reaction kinetics and possible pathways. Environ Sci Technol 2010;44:644–649.

Rolfhus KR, Fitzgerald WF. Linkages between atmospheric mercury deposition and the methylmercury content of marine fish. Water Air Soil Pollut 1995;80:291–297.

Rolfhus KR, Fitzgerald WF. Mechanisms and temporal variability of dissolved gaseous mercury production in coastal seawater. Mar Chem 2004;90:125–136.

Schlitzer R. Export production in the equatorial and north pacific derived from dissolved oxygen, nutrient and carbon data. J Oceanogr 2004;60:53–62.

Schwarzenbach RP, Gschwend P, Imboden DM. Environmental organic chemistry. 2nd ed. Hoboken (NJ): Wiley-Interscience, John Wiley and Sons, Inc.; 2003.

Selin NE, Jacob DJ, Park RJ, Yantosca RM, Strode S, Jaegle L, Jaffe D. Chemical cycling and deposition of atmospheric mercury, global constraints from observations. J Geophys Res, Atmos 2007;112. DOI: 10.1029/2006JD007450.

Selin NE, Jacob DJ, Yantosca R, Strode S, Jaegle L, Sunderland E. Global 3-D land-ocean-atmosphere model for mercury, present-day versus preindustrial cycles and anthropogenic enrichment factors for deposition. Global Biogeochem Cycles 2008;22. DOI: 10.1029/2007 GB003040.

Soerensen A, Sunderland E, Holmes C, Jacob DJ, Yantosca R, Strode S, Skov H, Christensen J, Mason RP. A new global simulation of mercury air-sea exchange for evaluating impacts on marine boundary layer concentrations. Environ Sci Technol 2010;44:8574–8580.

Strode SA, Jaegle L, Selin N, Jacob D, Park R, Yantosca R, Mason R, Slemr F. Air-sea exchange in the global mercury cycle. Global Biogeochem Cycles 2007;21. DOI: 10.1029/2006 GB002766.

Stumm W, Morgan JJ. Aquatic chemistry, chemical equilibria and rates in natural waters. 3rd ed. New York (NY): John Wiley & Sons, Inc.; 1996.

Sunderland EM. Mercury exposure from domestic and imported estuarine and marine fish in the U.S. seafood market. Environ Health Perspect 2007;115:235–242.

Sunderland EM, Krabbenhoft DP, Moreau JW, Strode SA, Landing WM. Mercury sources, distribution, and bioavailability in the North Pacific Ocean, insights from data and models. Global Biogeochem Cycles 2009;23. DOI: 10.1029/2008 GB003425.

Sunderland EM, Mason RP. Human impacts on open ocean mercury concentrations. Global Biogeochem Cycles 2007:21. DOI: 10.1029/2006 GB002876.

Uitz J, Claustre H, Morel A, Hooker SB. Vertical distribution of phytoplankton communities in open ocean, an assessment based on surface chlorophyll. J Geophys Res, Oceans 2006;111. DOI: 10.1029/2005JC003207.

Urba A, Kvietkus K, Sakalys J, Xiao Z, Lindqvist O. A new sensitive and portable mercury vapor analyzer GARDIS-1A. Water Air Soil Pollut 1995;80:1305–1309.

Wallschläger D, Turner RR, London J, Ebinghaus R, Kock HH, Sommar J, Xiao Z. Factors affecting the measurement of mercury emissions from soils with flux chambers. J Geophys Res 1999;D17(104):21859–21871. DOI: 10.1029/1999JD900314.

Wängberg I, Schmolke S, Schager P, Munthe J, Ebinghaus R, Iverfeldt A. Estimates of air-sea exchange of mercury in the Baltic Sea. Atmos Environ 2001;35:5477–5484.

Wetzel P, Maier-Reimer E, Botzet M, Jungclaus J, Keenlyside N, Latif M. Effects of ocean biology on the penetrative radiation in a coupled climate model. J Climate 2006;19:3973–3987.

Whalin LM, Kim E-H, Mason RP. Factors influencing the oxidation, reduction, methylation and demethylation of mercury species in coastal waters. Mar Chem 2007;107:278–294.

Whalin LM, Mason RP. A new method for the investigation of mercury redox chemistry in natural waters utilizing deflatable Teflon® bags and additions of isotopically labeled mercury. Anal Chim Acta 2006;558:211–221.

Wilke CR, Chang P. Correlation of diffusion coefficients in dilute solutions. AIChE J 1955;1:264–270.

Wozniak B, Dera J. Light absorption in sea water. New York (NY): Springer; 2007.

Xiao ZF, Schroeder MH, Lindqvist O. Vertical fluxes of volatile mercury over forest soil and lake surfaces in Sweden. Tellus B 1991;43:267–279.

Zhang H, Lindberg SE. Sunlight and iron(III)-induced photochemical production of dissolved gaseous mercury in freshwater. Environ Sci Technol 2001;35:928–935.

Zhang H, Lindberg SE, Barnett MO, Vette AF, Gustin MS. Dynamic flux chamber measurement of gaseous mercury emission fluxes over soils. Part 1: simulation of gaseous mercury emissions from soils using a two-resistance exchange interface model. Atmos Environ 2002;36.835–846.

CHAPTER 13

EXCHANGE OF MERCURY BETWEEN THE ATMOSPHERE AND TERRESTRIAL ECOSYSTEMS

MAE SEXAUER GUSTIN

13.1 GENERAL OVERVIEW

Once elemental mercury (Hg) enters the atmosphere, it may be globally distributed because this form is relatively inert and recycled between terrestrial and aquatic surfaces. Terrestrial ecosystems may be sources, as well as short- and long-term sinks, for atmospheric Hg. Understanding whether an ecosystem is a source or sink and the magnitude of associated flux is critical for determining the ultimate fate and environmental impacts of anthropogenic releases of this contaminant into the environment. This general overview provides a synthesis of current paradigms explaining terrestrial ecosystem–atmospheric Hg exchange and is then followed by more detailed discussion and citations for relevant work. The latter, however, is not all inclusive, and apologies to those whose work was not included in this review. Methods applied to measure flux, as well as factors controlling air–soil, plant and whole ecosystem exchange are considered.

Currently, Hg in the atmosphere is measured as three operationally defined forms—gaseous elemental Hg (GEM), gaseous oxidized forms of Hg (GOM), and Hg that is particulate bound (PHg). GEM is predominant in the air ($\sim$95–99%), with concentrations in the surface boundary layer ranging from 1 to 5 ng/m^3, while GOM and PHg concentrations are typically two orders of magnitude lower (0–50 pg/m^3) (Valente et al., 2007). GOM is thought to be compounds such as $HgCl_2$, $HgBr_2$, $Hg(OH)_2$ (Lin and Pehkonen, 1999); however, the exact identity is unknown. Owing to the low concentrations in air, quantifying air–surface Hg exchange for most ecosystems entails measurement of small concentration

Environmental Chemistry and Toxicology of Mercury, First Edition.
Edited by Guangliang Liu, Yong Cai, and Nelson O'Driscoll.
© 2012 John Wiley & Sons, Inc. Published 2012 by John Wiley & Sons, Inc.

differentials, application of clean handling protocols and careful assessment of system blanks.

All operationally defined forms of Hg are emitted by anthropogenic sources (Pacyna et al., 2006), while that released from soil and plant surfaces is thought to be predominantly GEM. Some component of GEM emitted from soils may be indigenous since geologic substrates have measureable concentrations of Hg (Hans Wedepohl, 1995). Some rock types (i.e., carbonaceous shale, mineralized materials) and geologic settings (plate tectonic boundaries) are Hg enriched because of geologic processes (Rasmussen, 1994; Gustin, 2003; Rytuba, 2005). Direct emission of GOM has been reported for soils in one controlled laboratory study (Engle et al., 2005). Relatively high concentrations have been observed in air above (10 cm) substrates enriched in Hg (70–1500 pg/m^3) (Giglini, 2003; Nacht et al., 2004). However, it is not known whether the GOM was released from the soil, formed above the soil surface, or was an allocthonous atmospheric input.

Substrates enriched in Hg by geologic processes are estimated to contribute 500–1500 Mg/year to the global atmosphere (Lindqvist et al., 1991; Gustin et al., 2008b). Hg is also released into the air from terrestrial ecosystems where anthropogenic contamination and disturbance has occurred (i.e., mining, industrial spills, landfills, chlor-alkali facilities) (Ferrara et al., 1997; Grönlund et al., 2005; Eckley et al., 2011). For all surfaces a component of the Hg emitted is considered "legacy" or that emitted from any source in the past remaining in the active pool (NRC, 2010). It has been suggested that Hg emitted from ecosystems with low Hg containing soils, which cover most of the earth's terrestrial surface area, is predominantly "legacy" in origin (Gustin et al., 2008a,b).

All forms of atmospheric Hg may be deposited on surfaces by way of wet and dry processes. These may be sequestered within terrestrial compartments or emitted back to the atmosphere, with the relative importance of these processes dependent on the form of Hg, the chemistry of the surface, and environmental conditions. Many models assume that net GEM exchange with soil surfaces is zero; however, as discussed below, some component is assimilated into foliage over the growing season and accumulated in soils. GEM deposited on plant surfaces can also be emitted back into the air. GOM is thought to be more strongly adsorbed by soil components than GEM (Schluter, 2000; Xin et al., 2007). GOM once deposited on foliage surfaces is removed by wash off or volatilization (Graydon et al., 2009). Foliar Hg uptake and subsequent transfer to the soils via through fall and litter fall are important pathways by which atmospheric Hg is transferred to terrestrial ecosystems (Lindberg et al., 2009). Eventually, through soil processes (Schluter, 2000; Obrist et al., 2010) or disturbance, such as fire (Wiedinmyer and Friedli, 2007), Hg input to soils may be converted to GEM and released back to the atmosphere.

Because Hg is a global pollutant, modeling is an important tool for investigating the biogeochemical cycle and the relative importance of sources and sinks. Models are also useful for the development and fine tuning of our understanding of processes controlling the transfer of Hg between air and ecosystems. They are limited by assumptions, available data, and applied reaction and flux rates, with the last derived using theoretical calculations and empirical data. Global Hg models estimate that primary emissions from land-based natural sources, excluding volcanic and geothermal systems, are on the order of 800–1600 Mg/year, with additional legacy emissions from terrestrial ecosystems ranging from 700 to 1200 Mg/year (see summary in Selin, 2009). Together these contribute ~25% of estimated global emissions on an annual basis. In the model scenarios summarized by Selin (2009), the land surface is a greater sink than a source. Two model estimates suggest that the ultimate sink for Hg is deposition and burial in marine sediments and that the lifetime of Hg in the combined atmosphere–ocean–terrestrial system is on the order of 3000 or 10,000 years (Mason and Sheu, 2002; Selin and Jacob, 2008; Selin et al., 2008).

Global models indicate that the atmospheric burden has increased threefold since the beginning of the industrial revolution (Selin, 2009). This correlates with archives of Hg deposition (i.e., lake sediment and peat bog cores) that show a threefold or more increase since the industrial revolution from ~3 to 10–20 $\mu g/m^2$/year (Biester et al., 2007). Continued release of Hg, removed from geologic storage by human activity during energy production, resource extraction, and commodity production, will increase the amount in the active global pool available for long-range transport and recycling between reservoirs (NRC, 2010).

13.2 METHODS AND TOOLS APPLIED FOR MEASUREMENT AND UNDERSTANDING OF AIR–TERRESTRIAL SURFACE EXCHANGE

13.2.1 Measurement of Air Concentrations

GEM, GOM, and PHg in air are determined using operationally defined methods that each involves collection of the individual form on a specific surface from which it is desorbed and quantified as GEM using cold vapor atomic fluorescence or atomic absorption spectroscopy (Ebinghaus et al., 1999; Gustin and Jaffe, 2010). GEM is typically preconcentrated on a gold surface at a time resolution of >1.5 minutes (Tekran Corporation, 2010), or it may be directly measured at a lower time resolution (seconds) and slightly higher detection limit using Zeeman Arc Atomic Absorption (Ohio Lumex Co., 2010). The current method for collection of GOM is the use of KCl-coated denuders (Landis et al., 2002); however, recent work suggests that this method has interferences with ozone and has not been adequately tested (Lyman et al., 2010a,b). A variety of filters have been applied for the collection of PHg (Keeler et al., 1995; Engle et al., 2008). Different automated instruments (i.e., Tekran, Gardius, or Lumex) as well as manual methods have been applied to measure air Hg concentrations for calculation of flux (Carpi and Lindberg, 1998; Gustin et al., 1999; Ericksen et al., 2005; Engle et al., 2006a).

For analytical systems that capture gaseous Hg without prior removal of GOM and PHg, there is some debate as to whether the Hg captured is GEM or total gaseous Hg (TGM = GEM + GOM). This is difficult to ascertain since

GOM concentrations are typically a small percentage of TGM ($<5\%$) and often within the analytical uncertainty of data collected using two colocated instruments ($\sim10\%$). Temme et al. (2002) suggested, based on comparison of data collected in Antarctica using two Tekran systems, one configured to measure TGM and the other to measure GEM, GOM, and PHg, that both GOM and GEM are collected as TGM. A similar 7-month comparison was done in Nevada, United States, at Mercury Deposition Network site MDN 98. During periods when GOM concentrations were $>5\%$ of total gas-phase atmospheric Hg, TGM and GEM concentrations were found to diverge and the sum of the GEM and GOM were more similar to TGM concentrations than GEM alone (Table 13.1). These limited studies suggest that GOM is collected in the TGM measurement; however, this is likely influenced by environmental conditions (both of the above comparisons were done in cases with relatively dry air) and inlet configuration (Gustin and Jaffe, 2010). Lyman et al. (2010a,b) suggested that GOM on inert surfaces can be converted to GEM and released, providing a possible mechanism for the observations in Antarctica and Nevada.

13.2.2 Measurement of Flux

Since environmental conditions significantly influence flux (see discussion below), collection of data over 24 hours and as a function of seasons is necessary to evaluate air–ecosystem exchange on an annual time step. Net flux associated with ecosystem compartments (i.e., soils, plants, litter-covered soils, aquatic surfaces) is often measured with flow through or dynamic gas exchange chambers. Chambers have also been applied to measure flux at the whole ecosystem level, but more often this is done using micrometeorological methods.

TABLE 13.1 Comparison of Data Collected with a Tekran 2537/1130/1135 System Configured to Measure GEM, GOM, and PHg with that Collected with a Tekran 2537 Thought to Quantify TGM

	Entire Dataset		Jun–Jul all Data		Jun–Jul %GOM >5		Jun–Jul %GOM <2	
RPD comparing	TGM vs GEM	TGM vs GEM + GOM	TGM vs GEM	TGM vs GEM + GOM	TGM vs GEM	TGM vs GEM + GOM	TGM vs GEM	TGM vs GEM + GOM
Mean RPD	2.8%	1.4%	8.1%	4.7%	11.4%	2.8%	7.7%	6.8%
Standard deviation RPD	7.9%	7.5%	8.5%	8.6%	6.8%	7.2%	7.8%	7.9%
Count	490	490	124	124	27	27	57	57

RPD indicates relative percent difference between measured TGM and GEM and TGM and GEM + GOM. Note: "TGM" means data output from the TGM Tekran. vs indicates versus with one measurement being compared with another. Count indicates number of data comparisons.

Indirect methods of evaluating flux include application of a specific stable isotope spike to track the movement of Hg through an ecosystem (Harris et al., 2007); whole watershed level mass balance models using litter fall, through fall, and runoff; and archives of net deposition such as lake sediment cores (Biester et al., 2007). Measurements and estimates of wet and dry deposition provide important information on ecosystem inputs; however, these are not an indicator of net flux since Hg deposited may be emitted back to the atmosphere.

Unidirectional or Deposition Fluxes. Wet Hg deposition is measured weekly at ~80 sites as part of the National Atmospheric Deposition Program Mercury Deposition Network in the United States and Canada (Prestbo and Gay, 2009). One important aspect of this data to consider is the efficiency of the wet deposition collector. Reported collection efficiency of the MDN sampler, based on comparison of data collected with colocated Belfort rain gauges, was $98.8 \pm 4.3\%$ in the summer and $87.1 \pm 6.5\%$ in the winter (Prestbo and Gay, 2009). Another factor to consider when estimating wet deposition is that multiple studies have shown a "wash out" effect for Hg collected in precipitation, with concentration decreasing as the volume increased (Lamborg et al., 1995; Landis et al., 2002; Lyman and Gustin, 2009; Prestbo and Gay, 2009).

Dry deposition has been measured and/or estimated using surrogate surfaces for GOM and GOM + PHg; direct leaf washes for GOM + PHg; comparison of precipitation and through fall data collected side by side for GOM + PHg, and litter fall for TGM. Models are also applied to estimate dry deposition, and these are either resistance based or entail application of deposition velocities developed using empirical or theoretical data (Zhang et al., 2009).

Surrogate surfaces applied include cation exchange membranes (Rea et al., 2000; Caldwell et al., 2006; Lyman et al., 2007, 2009; Peterson et al., 2009), Teflon membranes (Rea et al., 2000; Ericksen et al., 2003; Lyman et al., 2009), KCl-impregnated membranes (Lyman et al., 2009), and water surfaces (Sakata and Marumoto, 2005; Marsik et al., 2007). Surrogate surfaces allow for estimation of "potential" deposition since the depositional behavior of a gas to these surfaces may not replicate that occurring to chemically and physically heterogeneous natural surfaces (Wesely and Hicks, 2000). In addition, since Hg flux is bidirectional, some surrogate surfaces may measure only net Hg accumulation on that surface as opposed to gross deposition (Eckley and Branfireun, 2008). Of those described in the literature, both the cation exchange and Teflon membranes performed reasonably well, whereas Lyman et al. (2009) found that KCl-impregnated quartz fiber filters did not retain Hg.

Concentrations of Hg measured in solutions used to wash leaf surfaces and in through fall versus precipitation collected in open areas have been applied to assess potential dry deposition. In several studies, Hg collected in leaf washes was compared to that obtained using Teflon surfaces (Rea et al., 2000; Ericksen et al., 2003). Studies have shown that the leaf wash data may be impacted by the chemistry of the water used as well as the overall washing method and by the plant species (Rasmussen et al., 1991; Rea et al., 2000; Millhollen et al., 2006b; Fay and Gustin, 2007b).

In models, dry deposition is calculated using the equation

$$F = V_d\ C,$$

where F is flux, C is the concentration of the species of interest, and V_d is the dry deposition velocity. Some studies have applied the V_d for nitric acid vapor as a surrogate for GOM (Lindberg et al., 2009), while others have applied values derived during flux measurements (Zhang et al., 2009). The latter may not adequately represent the dry deposition alone since other process may be in operation during net flux measurements. Deposition velocity may also be estimated using the equation

$$V_d = 1/(R_a + R_b + R_c),$$

where R_a is the is the aerodynamic resistance, R_b is the near-surface boundary-layer resistance or quasi-laminar subsurface resistance, and R_c is a surface resistance term that is applied for leaf and soil surfaces (Lyman et al., 2007; Marsik et al., 2007). Lyman et al. (2007) in a sensitivity analyses found that model results were significantly impacted by assumptions regarding the chemical and physical properties of the gas phase. Lin et al. (2006) using the dry deposition scheme of Wesely (1989) found that dry deposition could vary by a factor of 2 depending on the assumed form of GOM.

Dry deposition of GEM to soils and plant surfaces has been observed in the field and laboratory using chambers and micrometeorological methods (see discussion below). Air Hg concentrations, as well as soil and atmospheric chemistry and specific environmental conditions will influence this process. PHg dry deposition is related to particle size (Zhang et al., 2009).

Chamber measurements. Flux chambers are typically placed on top of a soil or water surface and enclose the branch of a tree or leaves of a plant. There is no standard shape, size, or turnover time (volume of air in chamber/flow rate of air through chamber) that has been applied for field chambers (see summary in Eckley et al., 2010). Chamber volumes have ranged from 1 to ~30 l and turnover time from 0.1 to ~15 minutes.

Flux is calculated by dividing the difference in air concentrations exiting (C_o) and entering (C_i) the chamber (ΔC), by the covered surface area (A), which is then multiplied by the total flow (Q) through the chamber

$$F = \Delta C/A \times Q,$$

where F is flux as mass of Hg per area and time. If the measured flux is positive, it means that emission occurs, whereas if it is negative, the surface is a sink.

The calculation of flux often relies on the assumption that the inlet values (C_i) represent the air concentration flowing into the chamber while the outlet (C_o) concentration is measured. Eckley et al. (2010) suggested the following method to ensure that this assumption is valid. First ΔC_{oi}, which represents the difference between C_o and the mean of the C_i measured before and after C_o, and ΔC_{ii}, the difference between the two C_i observations, are calculated. Then, if $|\Delta C_{oi}| > |\Delta C_{ii}|$ the flux may be calculated but if otherwise it may not.

In order to calculate a flux, the concentration differential used in the flux calculation must be greater than the system blank, determined based on the ΔC measured while the chamber is situated on a clean surface. These are often ~ 0.2 ng/m^3 (Gustin et al., 1999; Kuiken et al., 2008a,b; Eckley et al., 2010). The system blank should be characterized during conditions occurring during flux measurements, for temperature and light exposure can promote release of Hg from chamber surfaces. Recent work (Carpi et al., 2007; Eckley et al., 2010) showed that Teflon chambers have better blanks than those constructed from polycarbonate, as well as less carry over between samples.

The material of which the chamber is constructed may influence the flux calculated since the wavelength of light interacting with a surface has been shown to affect flux (Rasmussen et al., 2005; Carpi et al., 2007; Xin et al., 2007; Eckley et al., 2010). Comparison of fluxes measured using Teflon versus polycarbonate chambers from the same material showed that the latter blocks ultraviolet radiation, resulting in values $\sim 30\%$ lower.

Laboratory studies using plants and soils (Zhang et al., 2005; Stamenkovic and Gustin, 2009) have shown greater emission or lower deposition and more variable fluxes when using ambient air versus cleaned air. These observations and work by others (Engle et al., 2005; Zhang et al., 2008; Watras et al., 2009) suggest that atmospheric oxidants play a role in facilitating Hg release from a surface. Because of the potential for air chemistry to influence air–surface exchange, it is recommended that ambient air be used to obtain environmentally relevant flux values. Static chambers have not been applied for measurement of Hg flux. This method would not produce realistic values since air Hg concentration significantly influences flux (Xin et al., 2007; Gustin and Ladwig, 2010).

The lack of a standard protocol for chamber flux measurements brings into question the comparability of data collected using different methods. For example, during the Nevada STORMS mercury method intercomparison, diel patterns in flux obtained varied by an order of magnitude (Gustin et al., 1999; Wallschläger et al., 1999). At the time, it was hypothesized that this was due to different chamber turnover times. Other experimental design factors that could have influenced observed fluxeas include the wavelength of light passing through the chamber, chamber dimensions, air flow path through the chamber, and the height of the inlet measurement. Because of the observed discrepancies, subsequent work has focused on assessing the influence of chamber design on Hg flux (Wallschläger et al., 1999; Gillis and Miller, 2000; Lindberg et al., 2002; Zhang et al., 2002; Engle et al., 2006a; Carpi et al., 2007), with several recommending application of high flushing flow rates and short turnover times (see Table 2 in Eckley et al., 2010).

More recently Eckley et al. (2010) revisited the uncertainties regarding the effects of chamber flow rate and turnover time. They found, as suggested by Zhang et al. (2002), that a smaller diffusion resistance at the surface with higher chamber flows would result in calculation of artificially elevated fluxes. Additionally, at some point, Hg release from the soil cannot keep pace with the increasing turbulence within the chamber as the flow rate increases, and the calculated flux would decrease. Eckley et al. (2010) suggested that chambers be operated at conditions that best simulate *in situ* surface conditions and ambient air concentrations. To do this, air Hg concentrations in the chamber should be similar to those in the air above the surface but such that the outlet concentration allows for calculation of a ΔC value and is greater than the chamber blank. Flow through the chamber should be set to generate an airstream over the surface that is reasonable given the field setting.

Several flux chamber designs have been applied to measure flux associated with plant surfaces that try to maintain ambient conditions within the chamber. These included Teflon bags (Zhang et al., 2005; Graydon et al., 2006) as well as a tall polycarbonate chamber (Fay and Gustin, 2007a).

Chambers are often the method preferred for the measurement of *in situ* flux because they are portable, simple to deploy, and not subject to strict meteorological and site requirements of micrometeorological methods. However, most field chambers cover a small surface area, raising concern with respect to the representativeness of these spot measurements. Additionally, chambers alter the natural surface by imposing a turbulence field that may not be representative of the natural setting and affect the microclimate, including parameters such as light, temperature, and relative humidity.

Large naturally lit laboratory mesocosms ($7.3 \times 5.5 \times 4.5$ m ($l \times w \times d$) or 180×10^3 L) that enclose tons of soil and associated vegetation have been used to measure whole ecosystem Hg flux. This type of setting was found to work well for a system containing Hg-contaminated soils; however, it was not adequate for the measurement of flux for that with low levels of Hg in the soil because of the inability to distinguish flux from the blank (Gustin et al., 2004; Stamenkovic and Gustin, 2007).

Micrometeorological methods. Micrometeorological techniques applied to determine Hg flux include gradient methods (Edwards et al., 2001; Rasmussen et al., 2005; Cobbett and Van Heyst, 2007; Marsik et al., 2007), the modified Bowen ratio method (MBR) (Lindberg et al., 1995; Poissant et al., 2004; Fritsche et al., 2008), and relaxed eddy accumulation (Cobos et al., 2002; Skov et al., 2006). For these, it is assumed that the turbulence field is spatially and temporally homogenous and vertical fluxes of conservative quantities are constant (Wesely and Hicks, 2000). The time resolution for these measurements is typically ≥ 1 h, and the surface area for which flux is characterized is ≥ 50 m^2. Specific environmental conditions are needed to calculate flux (i.e., wind velocity, turbulence conditions) and for the systems to be deployed (often no precipitation, stable power supply). Because of these requirements locations where this method can be applied are limited, and long periods of data collection are often needed (greater than a week) to obtain a robust data set.

Micrometeorological methods have been applied over vegetated surfaces such as agricultural fields (Cobbett et al., 2007), wetlands (Lindberg et al., 2002;

Poissant et al., 2004; Marsik et al., 2007), grasslands (Fritsche et al., 2008), and forests (Lindberg et al., 1998; Bash and Miller, 2009). In these settings, the flux measured reflects that associated with both the vegetation and soil/litter (and in some cases water) surfaces. Measurements have also been made in terrains with little vegetation (Gustin et al., 1995, 1999; Rasmussen et al., 2005) and over snow-covered surfaces (Skov et al., 2006; Brooks et al., 2008).

All but the relaxed eddy accumulation method require measurement of air Hg concentrations at two or more heights, and this is often done by sequentially measuring the concentration at each location. The MBR method requires measurement of gradients of at least one scalar with fast response sensors at the same heights as the Hg measurements. The concentration differential for the former is used to compute an eddy transfer coefficient that is then applied to estimate Hg flux assuming similar behavior. The relaxed eddy accumulation method assumes flux to be proportional to the concentration difference measured in air during upward and downward moving eddies. Flux is calculated using this difference, the standard deviation of vertical wind velocity, and a relaxation coefficient (Skov et al., 2006).

Most fluxes measured using micrometeorological methods are TGM or GEM, with limited work being done for GOM (Lindberg and Stratton, 1998; Lindberg et al., 2002; Poissant et al., 2004; Skov et al., 2006). Measurement of GOM flux is difficult given the low concentrations and analytical precision of current methods (Gustin and Jaffe, 2010).

Limited work has been done comparing fluxes obtained using colocated micrometeorological sampling systems. During the Nevada STORMS project a threefold variation in daytime emissions was recorded using four micrometeorological methods, and temporal correlation of fluxes measured simultaneously was poor. This was suggested to be due to site heterogeneity and different fetch areas being sampled by the systems that were 40–70 m apart. Additionally, micrometeorological methods yielded fluxes that were three times higher than those obtained using field chambers deployed simultaneously and were significantly more variable (Gustin et al., 1999). More recently, Fritsche et al. (2008) applied data collected in a grassland setting with one sampling system to calculate flux using two methods (gradient and modified Bowen ratio) and found a threefold difference in the resulting deposition velocities for Hg ($V_d = 0.09$ and 0.03 cm/s, respectively).

One hypothesis proposed to explain the discrepancy between the chamber and micrometeorological-method-derived fluxes during the NV STORMS project was that the chamber turnover time applied (1–24 min) was too low and surface flux was suppressed (Gustin et al., 1999). Eckley et al. (2010) demonstrated that a lower flux is calculated at the lower turnover times (TOT). Follow-up work at the NV STORMS site showed that fluxes measured with a 1-L polycarbonate field chamber at a flow rate of 5 L/min (TOT of 0.2 min) were not significantly different ($p > 0.05$) from those derived simultaneously and within the footprint of the MBR during wet and dry conditions (Fig. 13.1). Similar to the NV STORMS results, the fluxes measured with the micrometeorological

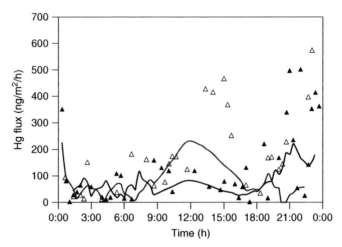

Figure 13.1 Hg flux measured at the Steamboat Springs Nevada, NV STORMS site, in October 1998 over 24 hours when dry (black line closed symbol) and after a precipitation event (light line open symbol) for chamber (lines) and micrometeorological method (triangle). The chamber was 1 L polycarbonate, and the modified Bowen ratio micrometeorological method was applied. Variable night time data is due to advection. For a discussion of the Micrometeorological method see Gustin et al., 1999, and for chamber method, see Engle et al., 2001.

method were much more variable. Rasmussen et al. (2005) compared chamber and micrometeorological-method-derived fluxes and found that the latter were higher; however, the chamber turnover time applied was significantly greater (4–5 min) than the range recommended by Eckley et al. (2010) of 0.3–0.8 min.

Other methods. Use of field chambers and micrometeorological methods does not allow for differentiating whether Hg emitted is old or newly deposited. Addition of stable Hg isotope spikes have been used to understand the potential for "new" Hg to contribute to that measured in fish and to be volatilized back to the atmosphere. In the Mercury Experiment to Assess Atmospheric Loading in Canada and the United States (METAALICUS), Hg was added in precipitation as a $HgCl_2$ isotope spike to three boreal ecosystem compartments (lake, wetland, upland) (Hintelmann et al., 2002; Harris et al., 2007). In another study, the potential for reemission of a stable isotope spike of $HgCl_2$ was investigated after addition to a small plot of semiarid desert soils (Ericksen et al., 2005).

Deposition archives such as lake sediment, peat bog, and ice cores may be used to understand potential ecosystem accumulation. A recent review by Biester et al. (2007) suggested that sediment cores are the most reliable of these tools. Since Hg in snow has been shown to be rapidly reemitted after deposition (see discussion below) with light influencing release, ice core data is not a reliable archive of total Hg input but only of accumulation.

13.3 MEASURED FLUXES

13.3.1 Wet Deposition

Wet deposition data collected across the United States and Canada show annual deposition amounts ranging from 25 $\mu g/m^2$/year in south Florida to less than 3 $\mu g/m^2$/ year in California (see NADP, 2011) with deposition amounts generally correlated with area precipitation volume (Prestbo and Gay, 2009). Precipitation inputs may be absorbed by the soil, transferred to surface water in runoff, or emitted back to the atmosphere. Hg added in precipitation as snow may have a different fate; for example, Lalonde et al. (2001) showed that 50% of the Hg deposited in a snow event was released back to the air over the first 24 h. The amount emitted from snow is also likely to vary as a function of the ecosystem type. For example, Nelson et al. (2008) found that forest covered sites retained more Hg in snow than open areas.

The METAALICUS study found that <1% of isotope added in solution to the watershed was observed in the fish tissue approximately three years after the application; however, that added directly to the lake ecosystem appeared within tissue after two months (Harris et al., 2007). On the basis of intermittently measured soil fluxes, Hintelmann et al. (2002) suggested that <10% of the isotope deposited was released into the air during the first year of the experiment. Also, using intermittent flux measurements, Ericksen et al. (2005) estimated that ~8% of Hg input in precipitation as a $HgCl_2$ isotope spike to desert soils would be released over a year. However, in the latter study, the measured concentration of the spike in the soil 60 days after application was 50% of the initial value. They suggested that this was due to movement downward in the soil column since precipitation events had occurred during this time. An alternate explanation is that rain facilitated reduction of Hg (II) and release of GEM into the air and the isotope was released during a period when flux was not measured. For the METAALICUS work, it is not clear if the exact amount reaching the ground in the precipitation application was measured, and although a component of the applied isotope was measured in the soils, the total stored in the ecosystem soils versus that lost to the air over time has not been reported in the literature.

13.3.2 Dry Deposition

Dry deposition rates for TGM of up to 100 ng/m^2/h have been reported for vegetated and barren soils interacting with Hg-enriched air advected into the area of the flux measurement (cf Lindberg et al., 1998; Eckley et al., 2010). Low rates of dry TGM deposition have been reported for foliar surfaces and low Hg containing soils not impacted by contaminated air masses. For soils, deposition is most often measured for soils that are dry, and during dark or cold conditions (Engle et al., 2001; Gustin et al., 2006; Xin et al., 2007; Lyman and Gustin, 2008; Gustin et al., 2008a; Kuiken et al., 2008a,b; Stamenkovic and Gustin, 2009).

Hg dry deposited on foliage may loosely adhere to the leaf surface and thus be washed off or emitted back to the atmosphere or accumulate within the leaf. In the latter case, foliage is essentially a passive sampler for GEM. Munthe et al. (2004) summarized the results of through fall–litter fall studies done in a variety of forest types on an annual time step. They showed that through fall contributed 5–50% more Hg to the ground surface than precipitation, while litter fall inputs ranged up to −50 to 50% greater than through fall inputs depending on the system. More recent work found no difference in precipitation inputs and through fall for a deciduous forest (Choi et al., 2008); however, for an evergreen boreal system, through fall inputs were 2–4 times that in precipitation (Graydon et al., 2009). These results show that dry deposition on leaf surfaces is an important means by which Hg is transferred from the air to ecosystems; however, the magnitude will vary within and between ecosystems. For example, Graydon et al. (2008) found that Hg fluxes in through fall within a boreal forest ecosystem significantly varied between types of forest canopy within a single catchment. To determine the input by litter fall, it is necessary to measure the concentrations in leaves right after senescence since litter Hg concentration has been found to increase after deposition (Giglini, 2003) most likely because of loss of mass due to carbon respiration.

Zhang et al. (2009) found, using empirical data obtained from the literature, that deposition velocities for GEM were 0.01–0.4 cm/s over vegetated surfaces, with those calculated for forested ecosystems being highest at $\sim$0.4 cm/s and lower estimates obtained for agricultural fields (0.2–0.3 cm/s), wetlands (0.2 cm/s), and grasslands (0.1 cm/s). The values they reported for barren soils were $\leq$0.02 cm/s (flux of $\sim$1.4 ng/m^2/h), which is slightly higher than the typical resolution of flux measurements ($\pm$0.5 ng/m^2/h) given the system blanks and analytical uncertainties. Lower deposition velocities are calculated for litter-covered soils of 0.002 cm/s using the data of Kuiken et al. (2008a,b) and for semiarid desert soils of 0.0015–0.002 cm/s using data of Lyman et al. (2007) and Ericksen et al. (2006). Several studies have demonstrated that as air concentrations increase above typical values ($>$2 ng/m^3), emission rates decrease and deposition increases (Xin et al., 2007; Gustin and Ladwig, 2010; Miller, 2010). Xin et al. (2007) suggested that at $>$5 ng/m^3, air concentrations are an important factor controlling exchange, and deposition becomes an important process. Miller (2010) found GEM deposition velocities up to 0.19 cm/s at exposure concentrations of 100 ng/m^3. On the basis of limited data, Xin et al. (2007) suggested that adsorption of GEM by soil does not follow a Langmuir isotherm and that some GEM is incorporated into the soil. Laboratory work investigating the potential for GEM to be released immediately after a period of deposition also suggested that a component is sequestered (Xin et al., 2007; Miller, 2010). Recent studies of Hg flux associated with bare soils showed that after periods of deposition associated with passing plumes of enriched air, fluxes were elevated but not sufficient to account for all the Hg deposited (Eckley et al., 2010; Miller, 2010). GEM sorption by soils is likely influenced by the overall chemistry, with constituents such as clay minerals, organic material or carbon, iron oxides, and sulfur compounds being important (Fang, 1978; Landa, 1978; Xin et al., 2007; Gustin et al., 2008a).

In contrast, deposition velocities estimated by Zhang et al. (2009) for GOM ranged from 0.4 to 7.6 cm/s. GOM deposition velocities applied in chemical transport models typically range from 0.5 to 4 cm/s (Lin et al., 2006). PHg deposition measurements are very limited and dependent on particle size (0.002–0.2 cm/s; Zhang et al., 2009).

Lyman et al. 2009 found that deposition velocities for GOM measured for surrogate surfaces (1.1 ± 0.6 cm/s) were higher than modeled values (0.4 ± 0.2 cm/s) based on data collected at four field sites, two in the western and two in the eastern United States. The higher uptake by the surface was attributed to lack of surface resistance. Marsik et al. (2007) applied a water surrogate surface and found deposition to water surfaces averaged 13±4 ng/m^2/d, while model estimated values for the same time periods were 3±2 ng/m^2/d. They suggested that the discrepancy was due to either particulate Hg being collected by the water surface or evaporative and wind-based loss.

Lyman et al. (2007) applied surrogate surface measurements, leaf washes, and field chamber flux chamber measurements, along with a resistance model to investigate the potential variability in dry deposition estimates that could be obtained using different techniques at three sites in Nevada, United States. GOM deposition velocities estimated using leaf washes were ~0.1 cm/s, while those for surrogate surfaces and models were 1.5–1.7 cm/s and 0.3–0.8, respectively. They found that estimated dry deposition could be 50–90% of the total deposition based on the method applied. On a seasonal and annual time step, GEM deposition was found to be greater than GOM deposition when a modeled deposition velocity of 0.01 cm/s for the former was applied; however, if limited flux chamber data (accounting for net exchange) was applied, GEM deposition was comparable to or less than GOM deposition. As expected intuitively, GOM deposition was greatest in the summer when concentrations were highest. Interestingly, surrogate surface measured and modeled GOM dry deposition were greater than chamber measured soil emission, suggesting that deposition of GOM could be significantly contributing to GEM being released over time.

Net deposition to terrestrial systems, as shown by lake sediment core records, has increased more than threefold over the past 150 years (cf Biester 2007 and references there in). Numerous studies have reported that the Hg concentration in surface soils are typically greater than that measured at depth (thought to represent geologic background), and several suggested that this is the result of atmospheric deposition and retention (Grigal, 2003; Gustin and Lindberg, 2006), although reduction and movement of Hg up within the soil column cannot be ruled out. For example, Engle et al. (2006b) reported concentrations of 10 ng/g higher in the top 20 cm of soil for three remote semiarid ecosystems in the western United States, while Wiener et al. (2006) reported a sevenfold higher Hg concentration in the O horizon and a threefold higher concentration in the A horizon relative to the C horizon at Voyageurs National Park, MN, United States. For the latter, the concentration difference between the C and A horizon was 100 ng/g, a value similar to that reported for other Midwestern sites (cf Grigal, 2003).

13.3.3 Barren and Litter-Covered Soil Flux

Research that has focused on characterizing Hg emissions from barren Hg-enriched and low Hg containing or background substrates is described in many articles (see summaries in Schluter, 2000; Zhang et al., 2001; Rasmussen et al., 2005; Ericksen et al., 2006; Gustin et al., 2006; Kuiken et al., 2008b). Soil Hg concentration has been shown to impact the magnitude of emissions, while environmental parameters such as temperature, light, precipitation events, percent soil moisture, and atmospheric oxidants influence diel and seasonal patterns (Gustin et al., 2008a,b).

For enriched surfaces, apparent diel patterns in flux occur and most often covary positively with light and temperature and negatively with relative humidity, whereas the pattern and correlations for fluxes measured in association with low Hg containing substrates relationships are not always as clear (Ericksen et al., 2005; Gustin et al., 2008b) (Figure 13.2). For the latter, the observed lack of clarity is due to the low overall flux with respect to our current analytical capabilities, to multiple competing parameters impacting the low flux, as well as intermittent periods of exacerbated Hg emission and deposition affecting the pool of Hg available at the surface. Engle et al. (2001), Song and Van Heyst (2005), and Eckley et al. (2010) found that less Hg was released with sequential watering events, indicating that this process facilitates release of GEM from the surface. The fact that less Hg is released with repeated wetting indicates that Hg released after periods of dryness may differ from areas with more regular precipitation. This also suggests that during dry periods, the surface Hg may be "recharged"

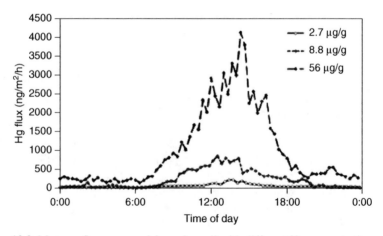

Figure 13.2 Mercury flux measured from dry soil with different Hg concentrations under similar exposure conditions using a 2-L Teflon chamber (see Eckley et al., 2010).

with GEM. This recharging process could occur as elemental Hg deposition from the air, or as Hg(II) within the soil being reduced to elemental Hg and moving to the soil surface (Gustin and Stamenkovic, 2005). Thus, the response of flux to wetting events will vary depending on how long an area has been dry, with desert regions likely showing a greater exacerbation of flux because of a rain event than that exhibited in regions where precipitation is fairly regular.

Because fluxes are strongly influenced by environmental conditions, data collected during a specific time of day and season may not accurately reflect that occurring over a 24-h period or within a longer time frame (Engle et al., 2001; Stamenkovic and Gustin, 2007). One method that has been applied to circumvent the need to collect 24-h flux data has been to assume that a Gaussian distribution for flux over a diel period (Engle et al., 2001). Assessment of long-term data sets have shown that the strength of the correlations for flux and environmental conditions may differ from season to season (Gustin et al., 2008a; Stamenkovic et al., 2008). This is most likely due to synergistic and antagonistic effects between environmental conditions that influence flux (cf Lin et al., 2010). Additionally, how the data is averaged (hourly, daily, and monthly) will affect correlation results. For example, Stamenkovic et al. (2008) showed that coefficients for the relationship of flux versus light were more significant when monthly average values were used relative to those obtained using daily or hourly data.

Using monthly averaged diel data collected intermittently over two years in a controlled setting where soil moisture was fairly constant, Stamenkovic et al. (2008) found that bare soil flux was best correlated with air temperature. In contrast, Eckley et al. (2010) found that solar radiation was the parameter best correlated with flux obtained over 24-h periods on a seasonal time step over a year from a variety of naturally enriched dry substrates. In the latter study, a Teflon chamber was applied, whereas in the former, a polycarbonate chamber was used. The difference in the correlation results could be due to the experimental design since Teflon has been shown to pass a wider range of light wavelengths than polycarbonate. Xin et al. (2007) based on laboratory work with dry substrate suggested that photosynthetic active radiation, the addition of water, and UV-A exposure promoted desorption and reemission of elemental Hg, while UV-B promoted photoreduction of Hg (II) forms in soils. The latter would generate elemental Hg that then could be released into the air. Ericksen et al. (2006) ranked the variables correlated with Hg flux measured at 46 individual locations for a range of soil types with low Hg concentrations in the spring across western and midwestern United States. They suggested the following hierarchy of environmental parameters influencing flux: soil moisture > light > air concentration > relative humidity > temperature. Other work has suggested that atmospheric oxidants may also be important in influencing substrate Hg release (Engle et al., 2005; Zhang et al., 2008; Watras et al., 2009), and this parameter is not often characterized in field studies.

Lin et al. (2010) explored the combined effects of several environmental parameters on flux using a controlled laboratory chamber and a two-level factorial experimental design. Results showed that individually irradiation, soil moisture content, and temperature all significantly enhanced mercury fluxes (by 90–140%), and synergistic effects were observed for all two-factor interactions (20 to 30% of additional flux). They suggested that a quadratic model may be the more precise way to model soil Hg flux.

Net flux reported in the literature for Hg-enriched soils varies from 10 to 1000s of ng/m^2/h, while those reported for low Hg containing soils typically ranges from -10 to 10 ng/m^2/h (cf Schluter, 2000; Engle et al., 2001; Zhang et al., 2001; Ericksen et al., 2006; Stamenkovic et al., 2008; Kuiken et al., 2008a,b). Zhang et al. (2009) noted most fluxes measured from low Hg containing soils reported in the literature are emission. This could be due to the timing of the data collection, operating conditions of the chamber, and/or the fact that there is a large soil pool available. Because continuous measurements of flux are extremely limited, observations should be placed within the context of previous environmental conditions that might have depleted the pool of Hg at the surface or replenished it. Several studies have suggested that over a year inputs by way of deposition and outputs by way of emission may result in net soil exchange associated with low Hg containing soils being close to zero (Ericksen et al., 2006; Gustin et al., 2006; Stamenkovic and Gustin, 2009). Low rates of accumulation over many years could explain the higher concentration in surface soils, but this may not be resolvable with flux data that is collected intermittently or current analytical capabilities.

Kuiken et al. (2008b) found fluxes reported for litter cover soils at forested sites to range from -0.9 to 7 ng/m^2/h. They showed, using data collected over a day on a monthly time step, an annual daytime flux of 0.4 ± 0.5 ng/m^2/h. Twenty percent of their daytime values were deposition. Lowest measured flux values in general were observed in the spring and summer during the time of closed canopy. In another work, Kuiken et al. (2008a) reported on fluxes measured from litter-covered forest soils along the eastern United States seaboard obtained during the spring and found a mean daytime flux of 0.2 ± 0.9 ng/m^2/h with low rates of deposition observed at night and little overall variation. For both these field studies Hg exchange was not well correlated with environmental conditions. Similarly, Stamenkovic and Gustin (2009) found mean flux from litter-covered grassland soils over a year to be -2 to $+2$ ng/m^2/h with little variation as a function of environmental conditions. Cobbett and Van Heyst (2007) reported values of 0.1 ± 0.2 ng/m^2/h over a stubble-covered agricultural field in the fall. Several studies have compared Hg flux associated with litter-covered and barren soils (Zhang et al., 2001; Stamenkovic and Gustin, 2009), with the general result being that the bare soil flux was higher.

13.3.4 Air–Plant Exchange

Plants are a net sink for atmospheric GEM that is assimilated by foliage over the growing season (Ericksen et al., 2003; Grigal, 2003). Graydon et al. (2006) reported a loss of 50% HgCl$_2$ applied as a stable isotope spike in wet deposition to tree foliage and a 20–50% loss from ground vegetation within several days after addition. In follow-up work, Graydon et al. (2009) estimated that the half-life of the Hg spike on ground vegetation was on the order of 700 days. The ultimate fate of the observed GOM lost from vegetation is not known, that is, whether it is emitted into the air or sequestered in the underlying soil.

Factors shown to influence measured foliar concentrations of GEM include air concentration with uptake increasing as a function of exposure concentration; leaf age, with older leaves having higher concentrations; position within the canopy, with those closer to the ground surface having higher concentrations; and environmental conditions such as temperature and CO_2 concentrations (Lindberg et al., 1995; Taylor et al., 1998; Frescholtz et al., 2003; Millhollen et al., 2006a; Fay and Gustin, 2007b and b; Bushey et al., 2008; Stamenkovic and Gustin, 2009). Foliar fluxes measured for vegetation using chambers typically range from -10 to 10 ng/m^2/hr fluctuating between deposition and emission despite the apparent gradual uptake by foliage over time (Graydon et al., 2006; Millhollen et al., 2006b). This has been suggested to be due to the fact that the chamber system measures net flux, and multiple processes are operating at the leaf surface during the short-term flux measurements. Stamenkovic and Gustin (2009) found daily average flux associated with tall grass prairie vegetation to range from -3.3 to 0.5 ng/m^2/h for forbs with no exchange observed for grass species. Graydon et al. (2006) measured fluxes of -10 to 10 ng/m^2/h for tree species. Zhang et al. (2005) reported net deposition rates of $1-0.33$ ng/m^2/h for wetland plants, while Fay and Gustin (2007a) reported values of -5 to 5 ng/m^2/h. Millhollen et al. (2006a) and Fay and Gustin (2007b) observed exchange rates that varied between -20 to $+4$ ng/m^2/h for six tree species at air concentrations of $3-5$ ng/m^3.

Stamenkovic and Gustin (2009) using a controlled laboratory chamber found GEM uptake to occur in the dark and under high CO_2 conditions. On the basis of these observations they suggested that assimilation was not limited to the stomata pathway as is the current paradigm (Lindberg et al., 2009). Additionally, less deposition was observed in ambient air relative to that occurring in cleaned oxidant free air, indicating that air chemistry was also influencing observed short-term exchange.

Foliar uptake rates based on measured tissue concentrations range from 0.2 to 2.8 ng/m^2/h and depend on the plant species (Frescholtz et al., 2003; Bushey et al., 2008; Stamenkovic et al., 2008). In general, grassland plant species have lower uptake rates than evergreen trees, which are less than deciduous trees at similar air exposure concentrations (Millhollen et al., 2006a; Fay and Gustin, 2007b). Laboratory experiments have suggested that a small component of Hg in the foliage of deciduous trees could be derived from the soil, but for evergreen, grass, and forb species soil Hg exposures did not influence observed concentrations (see Frescholtz et al., 2003; Millhollen et al., 2006a; Fay and Gustin, 2007b). Owing to the variability in measured short-term fluxes, it is best to determine total atmospheric accumulation over time using leaf concentrations, and as such, fresh litter fall is a good surrogate for atmospheric Hg input to terrestrial systems by passive foliar uptake.

Accumulation will also vary depending on air concentration. Hartman et al. (2009) showed using a controlled chamber an increase of Hg deposition to foliage by 0.5 ng/m^2/h for every 1 ng/m^3 increase in air concentration, whereas Frescholtz et al. (2003) who investigated uptake by aspen at different air concentrations over 12 weeks found a 0.25 ng/m^2/h increase for every 1 ng/m^3 increase in air concentrations based on foliar concentrations.

13.3.5 Whole Ecosystem Estimates

13.3.5.1 Measuring Net Ecosystem Exchange. Whole ecosystem estimates of flux have been made directly using micrometeorological methods and chambers, by combining fluxes measured for individual ecosystem compartments, and through models.

Micrometeorological-method-derived fluxes reported in the literature are often quite variable ($+100$ to -100 ng m^2/h (Lindberg et al., 1995; Cobos et al., 2002; Poissant et al., 2004; Fritsche et al., 2008; Bash and Miller, 2009)), most likely because the observed values reflect a multitude of processes influencing exchange with different surfaces. Data available often represents limited snapshots in time, and only a few studies have collected seasonal or annual measurements (i.e., Cobbett and Van Heyst, 2007; Fritsche et al., 2008). Since the data collected using these methods represents gas flux, to determine total flux, precipitation inputs need to be considered. Fritsche et al. (2008) measured flux over a grassland for a year and reported an annual flux (not including wet deposition) of -2 to -4 ng/m^2/h. Bash and Miller (2009) reported on flux measured over the growing season for a forest canopy and suggested that, despite significant variability in the magnitude and direction of flux, net deposition was the dominant process in the beginning of the growing season, whereas emission was the primary flux later in the growing season. Cobbett and Van Heyst (2007) reported that fluxes measured intermittently over an agriculture field were -0.4 to 18 ng/m^2/h.

Munthe et al. (2004) summarized the results of numerous studies that estimated net ecosystem flux through use of Hg concentrations in through fall, litter fall, and exported by way of surface waters. In general, depending on the water shed, exports by surface waters were 5–25% of inputs, suggesting that forested ecosystems are a net sink. However, without some estimate of volatile Hg release from these systems, true net ecosystem cannot be calculated. Additionally, as suggested by the METAALICUS results (Harris et al., 2007), Hg transported out of an ecosystem in runoff does not necessarily reflect that input during the year of study.

Whole mesocosm experiments have shown the need for incorporating plants into ecosystem flux models not only because they act as a sink for atmospheric Hg but also because their physical presence can change the observed soil flux. Gustin et al. (2004) summarized the results of using large mesocosms for quantifying Hg flux associated with stands of aspen growing in mercury-contaminated soils. As the plants leafed out, the whole system flux declined, and the decrease in flux could not be accounted for by the uptake of plants alone (0.5%). They suggested that shading of the soils as the plants leafed out was responsible for the significant difference in flux measured for a planted and unplanted replicate mesocosm (40% at midday). Zhang et al. (2001) and Carpi et al. (1997) showed that Hg flux from shaded bare soils was less than that occurring from in full sunlight. Additionally, Kuiken et al. (2008a,b) showed a reduction of flux from litter-covered soil with development of a plant canopy. Thus, flux from bare soils cannot be applied to model that occurring from within the forest canopy.

13.3.5.2 *Modeling Ecosystem Exchange.* Models have been developed to estimate Hg release from areas enriched in Hg by natural and anthropogenic processes that incorporate relationships established between measured fluxes and soil Hg concentrations and environmental conditions. The relationships were then placed within the context of the geologic setting to develop area emission estimates (Ferrara et al., 1997; Gustin, 2003; Kotnik et al., 2005; Rasmussen et al., 2005). Gustin et al. (2003, 2008b) reported a range in area average flux of 2–440 ng/m^2/h across areas of 1–900 km^2 resulting in annual contributions of 2–110 kg/year. They noted that these estimates vary significantly depending on the area applied in the scaling and the distribution and degree of natural enrichment. While providing an estimate of emissions, these models simplify the whole system flux, for only net air–surface exchange was quantified and inputs by way of precipitation and vegetation are not considered. Additionally, flux measurements applied in these models are snapshots in time.

Stamenkovic et al. (2008) studied Hg exchange for a tall grass prairie ecosystem, housed within the same mesocosms as applied by Gustin et al. (2004), using dynamic flux chambers. They found that individual component fluxes could not be combined to give a whole system flux. They developed a model to predict flux using an index of plant canopy development (canopy greenness). Using modeled fluxes and that measured as input by way of watering and litter, they found that the tall grass prairie ecosystem was a net annual sink of atmospheric Hg.

More recently, Hartman et al. (2009) estimated net exchange for three ecosystems types across the contiguous United States—deciduous forest, semiarid desert, and grassland. They applied empirical data to develop a rule-based model for soil Hg exchange. Using a classification and regression tree data analyses method, factors then used to model soil flux were found to be, in decreasing order of importance, soil temperature, biome, solar radiation, and percentage of soil moisture. The developed soil flux model was incorporated into a GIS framework along with environmental conditions on a monthly time step. A layer that accounted for annual mercury inputs by way of precipitation and vegetation was added. These layers were then combined to estimate whether these ecosystems are a net source or sink for atmospheric Hg. Overall soil was a small source of atmospheric Hg, with flux being higher in the winter for all three ecosystem types because of increased soil moisture and lack of plant cover. Taking into consideration wet deposition and foliar inputs, all ecosystems were a net sink for atmospheric Hg. The modeled area included 45% of the surface area of the contiguous United States, and these biomes were a sink for 5–12 Mg of Hg over a year.

13.4   CONCLUSIONS

Terrestrial land areas enriched in Hg by geologic processes are sources of new Hg to the air. However, most of the earth's terrestrial surface is covered by areas with low concentrations in soil. Global models when balancing projected source emissions and the known atmospheric burden have indicated that terrestrial areas are sinks for atmospheric Hg. Hg concentrations in surface soils and sediment cores support this model output. Hg is input to these ecosystems by way of wet deposition (likely as Hg (II); direct dry deposition as GOM, GEM, and PHg; and by way of litter fall. Background soils contain a large pool of Hg with a significant component ($\sim$50% depending on the area) at the surface likely derived from the atmosphere. Dry and wet deposition of atmospheric Hg continues to replenish this pool, and although net gas emission is the major flux observed for soils, inputs are greater than that being released over time.

Hg fluxes measured using chambers and micrometeorological methods directly over plant and soil surfaces vary over space and time and represent records of exchange responding to multiple synergistic and competing factors. Measurement of short-term flux has allowed us to better understand the transitory nature of Hg exchange with terrestrial systems as well as the factors controlling surface Hg exchange. However, because of the variability from hour to hour, day to day, month to month, and likely from year to year, long-term data sets are necessary for developing an understanding of net ecosystem exchange. This is a difficult charge in many respects, and as such, developing a sound understanding of factors controlling air–terrestrial system exchange should be the emphasis so that process-based model estimates may be developed.

Quantifying mercury inputs in litter fall (GEM assimilated) and through fall (dry deposition of GOM and PHg) are good indicators of input (Johnson and Lindberg, 1995) to vegetated systems; however, for those areas with barren or sparsely vegetated soils, dry deposition as GEM and GOM and wet inputs need to be quantified. Of these, the measurement of dry deposition of Hg continues to be a challenge. Developing annual estimates of output are difficult since empirical data collected at one time is a response to a variety of previously occurring and co-occurring parameters. Variability in empirical ecosystem flux data appears to increase with the complexity of the system from which flux is being measured as demonstrated by the high range in values obtained over forested ecosystems (Fig. 13.3).

In considering ecosystem level fluxes the complexity of the system must be considered. For barren soils, GEM dry deposition as well as GOM wet and dry deposition are important sources of Hg generating a surface pool available for release over time. Processes within the soil will also be important in promoting formation of GEM, while those acting on the surface will affect release. Adding a vegetation layer to an ecosystem will not only create a sink for atmospheric Hg but the plant cover will also reduce the capacity of the soil to act as a source. Through fall and litter fall inputs will vary significantly as a function of ecosystem type and as a function of location within the system. Other influences

Complexities to consider with respect to terrestrial system flux

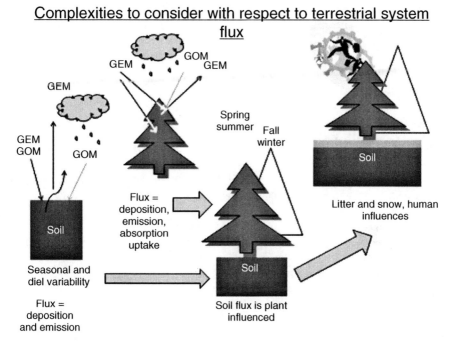

Figure 13.3 Schematic diagram showing the factors to consider in terms of terrestrial ecosystem Hg exchange. Wet and dry deposition are important inputs to soils and plants, with GEM and GOM being input as dry deposition and GOM the likely form input by precipitation. Plants assimilate GEM and plant canopies affect soil Hg exchange by shading and providing a litter cover. Snow may also cover the soil reducing inputs in precipitation. Direct human disturbance and indirect effects as a function of environmental conditions will also influence Hg released from soils.

such as microbial community impact on flux are not known and may need to be considered. Owing to volatile loss of Hg and surface cover, snow will reduce the amount of Hg input to soils by way of precipitation. Lastly, the human element needs to be considered since we alter ecosystem structure, land use, environmental conditions, and ultimately the rate at which Hg is transferred from geologic repositories to the globally active pool. Thus, terrestrial ecosystems are as a whole a sink for atmospheric Hg; however, whether they are short-term or long-term repositories will depend on the future environmental and soil conditions and potential disturbance of these reservoirs over time.

ACKNOWLEDGEMENTS

The author gratefully acknowledges the hard work of many graduate and under-graduate student researchers, as well as several postdoctoral researchers, who have worked with me in the diligent pursuit of good Hg data. Without their work, this chapter could not have been written. The author thanks especially Chris Eckley, Seth Lyman, and Alan Vette for collection of data presented in Table 13.1 and Figures 13.1 and 13.2 and the agencies that have supported research summarized here on Hg in the environment, including US EPA, EPRI, NSF, NvDEP, and USDA.

REFERENCES

Bash JO, Miller DR. Growing season total gaseous mercury (TGM) flux measurements over an Acer rubrum L. stand. Atmos Environ 2009;43:5953–5961.

Biester H, Bindler R, Martinez-Cortizas A, Engstrom DR. Modeling the past atmospheric deposition of mercury using natural archives. Environ Sci Technol 2007;41:4851–4860.

Brooks S, Arimoto R, Lindberg S, Southworth G. Antarctic polar plateau snow surface conversion of deposited oxidized mercury to gaseous elemental mercury with fractional long-term burial. Atmos Environ 2008;42:2877–2884.

Bushey JT, Nallana AG, Montesdeoca MR, Driscoll CT. Mercury dynamics of a northern hardwood canopy. Atmos Environ 2008;42:6905–6914.

Caldwell CA, Swartzendruber P, Prestbo E. Concentration and dry deposition of mercury species in arid south central New Mexico (2001–2002). Environ Sci Technol 2006;40:7535–7540.

Carpi A, Frei A, Cocris D, McCloskey R, Contreras E, Ferguson K. Analytical artifacts produced by a polycarbonate chamber compared to a Teflon chamber for measuring surface mercury fluxes. Anal Bioanal Chem 2007;388:361–365.

Carpi A, Lindberg SE. Sunlight-mediated emission of elemental mercury from soil amended with municipal sewage sludge. Environ Sci Technol 1997;31:2085–2091.

Carpi A, Lindberg SE. Application of a teflon(TM) dynamic flux chamber for quantifying soil mercury flux: tests and results over background soil. Atmos Environ 1998;32:873–882.

Choi H-D, Sharac TJ, Holsen TM. Mercury deposition in the Adirondacks: a comparison between precipitation and throughfall. Atmos Environ 2008;42:1818–1827.

Cobbett FD, Steffen A, Lawson G, Van Heyst BJ. GEM fluxes and atmospheric mercury concentrations (GEM, RGM and Hgp) in the Canadian Arctic at Alert, Nunavut, Canada (February-June 2005). Atmos Environ 2007;41:6527–6543.

Cobbett FD, Van Heyst BJ. Measurements of GEM fluxes and atmospheric mercury concentrations (GEM, RGM and Hgp) from an agricultural field amended with biosolids in Southern Ont., Canada (October 2004-November 2004). Atmos Environ 2007;41:2270–2282.

Cobos DR, Baker JM, Nater EA. Conditional sampling for measuring mercury vapor fluxes. Atmos Environ 2002;36:4309–4321.

Ebinghaus R, Jennings SG, Schroeder WH, Berg T, Donaghy T, Guentzel J, et al. International field intercomparison measurements of atmospheric mercury species at Mace Head, Ireland. Atmos Environ 1999;33:3063–3073.

Eckley CS, Branfireun B. Gaseous mercury emissions from urban surfaces: controls and spatiotemporal trends. Appl Geochem 2008;23:369–383.

Eckley CS, Gustin M, Lin CJ, Li X, Miller MB. The influence of dynamic chamber design and operating parameters on calculated surface-to-air mercury fluxes. Atmos Environ 2010;44:194–203.

Eckley CS, Gustin M, Miller MB, Marsik F. Measurement of surface mercury fluxes at active industrial gold mines in Nevada (USA). Sci Total Environ 2011;409.514–522.

Edwards GC, Rasmussen PE, Schroeder WH, Kemp RJ, Dias GM, Fitzgerald-Hubble CR, et al. Sources of variability in mercury flux measurements. J Geophys Res 2001;106:5421–5435.

Engle MA, Gustin MS, Goff F, Counce DA, Janik CJ, Bergfeld D, et al. Atmospheric mercury emissions from substrates and fumaroles associated with three hydrothermal systems in the western United States. J Geophys Res 2006a;111:D17304.

Engle MA, Gustin MS, Johnson DW, Murphy JF, Miller WW, Walker RF, et al. Mercury distribution in two Sierran forest and one desert sagebrush steppe ecosystems and the effects of fire. Sci Total Environ 2006b;367:222–233.

Engle MA, Gustin MS, Lindberg SE, Gertler AW, Ariya PA. The influence of ozone on atmospheric emissions of gaseous elemental mercury and reactive gaseous mercury from substrates. Atmos Environ 2005;39:7506–7517.

Engle MA, Gustin MS, Zhang H. Quantifying natural source mercury emissions from the Ivanhoe Mining District, north-central Nevada, USA. Atmos Environ 2001;35:3987–3997.

Engle MA, Tate MT, Krabbenhoft DP, Kolker A, Olson ML, Edgerton ES, et al. Characterization and cycling of atmospheric mercury along the central US Gulf Coast. Appl Geochem 2008;23:419–437.

Ericksen JA, Gustin MS, Lindberg SE, Olund SD, Krabbenhoft DP. Assessing the potential for re-emission of mercury deposited in precipitation from arid soils using a stable isotope. Environ Sci Technol 2005;39:8001–8007.

Ericksen JA, Gustin MS, Schorran DE, Johnson DW, Lindberg SE, Coleman JS. Accumulation of atmospheric mercury in forest foliage. Atmos Environ 2003;37:1613–1622.

Ericksen JA, Gustin MS, Xin M, Weisberg PJ, Fernandez GCJ. Air-soil exchange of mercury from background soils in the United States. Sci Total Environ 2006;366:851–863.

Fang SC. Sorption and transformation of mercury vapor by dry soil. Environ Sci Technol 1978;12:285–288.

Fay L, Gustin M. Assessing the influence of different atmospheric and soil mercury concentrations on foliar mercury concentrations in a controlled environment. Water Air Soil Pollut 2007b;181:373–384.

Fay L, Gustin MS. Investigation of mercury accumulation in cattails growing in constructed wetland mesocosms. Wetlands 2007a;27:1056–1065.

Ferrara R, Maserti BE, Andersson M, Edner H, Ragnarson P, Svanberg S. Mercury degassing rate from mineralized areas in the mediterranean basin. Water Air Soil Pollut 1997;93:59–66.

Frescholtz TF, Gustin MS, Schorran DE, Fernandez GCJ. Assessing the source of mercury in foliar tissue of quaking aspen. Environ Toxicol Chem 2003;22:2114–2119.

Fritsche J, Obrist D, Zeeman MJ, Conen F, Eugster W, Alewell C. Elemental mercury fluxes over a sub-alpine grassland determined with two micrometeorological methods. Atmos Environ 2008;42:2922–2933.

Giglini AD. Reactive gaseous mercury concentrations and mercury flux from natural, anthropogenic, and background settings in Northwestern Nevada. Reno (NV): Natural Resources & Environmental Science. Master of Science in Environmental Science and Health, University of Nevada-Reno; 2003. p 99.

Gillis A, Miller DR. Some potential errors in the measurement of mercury gas exchange at the soil surface using a dynamic flux chamber. Sci Total Environ 2000;260:181–189.

Graydon JA, St. Louis VL, Hintelmann H, Lindberg SE, Sandilands KA, Rudd JWM, et al. Long-term wet and dry deposition of total and methyl mercury in the remote boreal ecoregion of Canada. Environ Sci Technol 2008;42:8345–8351.

Graydon JA, St. Louis VL, Hintelmann H, Lindberg SE, Sandilands KA, Rudd JWM, et al. Investigation of uptake and retention of atmospheric Hg(II) by Boreal forest plants using stable Hg isotopes. Environ Sci Technol 2009;43:4960–4966.

Graydon JA, St. Louis VL, Lindberg SE, Hintelmann H, Krabbenhoft DP. Investigation of mercury exchange between forest canopy vegetation and the atmosphere using a new dynamic chamber. Environ Sci Technol 2006;40:4680–4688.

Grigal DF. Mercury sequestration in forests and peatlands: a review. J Environ Qual 2003;32:393–405.

Grönlund R, Edner H, Svanberg S, Kotnik J, Horvat M. Mercury emissions from the Idrija mercury mine measured by differential absorption lidar techniques and a point monitoring absorption spectrometer. Atmos Environ 2005;39:4067–4074.

Gustin MS. Are mercury emissions from geologic sources significant? A status report. Sci Total Environ 2003;304:153–167.

Gustin MS, Engle M, Ericksen J, Lyman S, Stamenkovic J, Xin M. Mercury exchange between the atmosphere and low mercury containing substrates. Appl Geochem 2006;21:1913–1923.

Gustin MS, Ericksen J, Fernandez GC. Determination of the potential for release of mercury from combustion product amended soils, part 1–simulations of beneficial use. J Air Waste Manag Assoc 2008a;58:673–683.

Gustin MS, Ericksen JA, Schorran DE, Johnson DW, Lindberg SE, Coleman JS. Application of controlled mesocosms for understanding mercury air-soil-plant exchange. Environ Sci Technol 2004;38:6044–6050.

Gustin M, Jaffe D. Reducing the uncertainty in measurement and understanding of mercury in the atmosphere. Environ Sci Technol 2010;44:2222–2227.

Gustin M, Ladwig K. Laboratory investigation of Hg release from flue gas desulfurization products. Environ Sci Technol 2010;44:4012–4018.

Gustin MS, Lindberg SE. Terrestrial mercury fluxes, is the net exchange up, down, or neither? In: Pirrone N, Mahaffey KR, editors. Dynamics of mercury pollution on regional and global scales. Volume 1, Atmospheric processes and human exposures around the world. New York: Springer Science+Business Media, LLC; 2006. p 744.

Gustin MS, Lindberg S, Marsik F, Casimir A, Ebinghaus R, Edwards G, et al. Nevada STORMS project: measurement of mercury emissions from naturally enriched surfaces. J Geophys Res 1999;104:21831–21844.

Gustin MS, Lindberg SE, Weisberg PJ. An update on the natural sources and sinks of atmospheric mercury. Appl Geochem 2008b;23:482–493.

Gustin M, Stamenkovic J. Effect of watering and soil moisture on mercury emissions from soils. Biogeochemistry 2005;76:215–232.

Gustin MS, Taylor GE, Leonard Jr TL. Atmospheric mercury concentrations above mercury contaminated mill tailings in the Carson River Drainage Basin, NV. Water Air Soil Pollut 1995;80:217–220.

Hans Wedepohl K. The composition of the continental crust. Geochim Cosmochim Acta 1995;59:1217–1232.

Harris RC, Rudd JWM, Amyot M, Babiarz CL, Beaty KG, Blanchfield PJ, et al. Whole-ecosystem study shows rapis fish-mercury response to changes in mercury deposition. Proc Natl Acad Sci 2007;104:16586–16591.

Hartman JS, Weisberg PJ, Pillai R, Ericksen JA, Kuiken T, Lindberg SE, et al. Application of a rule-based model to estimate mercury exchange for three background biomes in the continental United States. Environ Sci Technol 2009;43:4989–4994.

Hintelmann H, Harris R, Heyes A, Hurley JP, Kelly CA, Krabbenhoft DP, et al. Reactivity and mobility of new and old mercury deposition in a Boreal forest ecosystem during the first year of the METAALICUS study. Environ Sci Technol 2002;36:5034–5040.

Johnson DW, Lindberg SE. The biogeochemical cycling of Hg in forests: alternative methods for quantifying total deposition and soil emission. Water Air Soil Pollut 1995;80:1069–1077.

Keeler G, Glinsorn G, Pirrone N. Particulate mercury in the atmosphere: its significance, transport, transformation and sources. Water Air Soil Pollut 1995;80:159–168.

Kotnik J, Horvat M, Dizdarevic T. Current and past mercury distribution in air over the Idrija Hg mine region, Slovenia. Atmos Environ 2005;39:7570–7579.

Kuiken T, Gustin M, Zhang H, Lindberg S, Sedinger B. Mercury emission from terrestrial background surfaces in the eastern USA. II: air/surface exchange of mercury within forests from South Carolina to New England. Appl Geochem 2008a;23:356–368.

Kuiken T, Zhang H, Gustin M, Lindberg S. Mercury emission from terrestrial background surfaces in the eastern USA. part I: air/surface exchange of mercury within a southeastern deciduous forest (Tennessee) over one year. Appl Geochem 2008b;23:345–355.

Lalonde JD, Poulain AJ, Amyot M. The role of mercury redox reactions in snow on snow-to-air mercury transfer. Environ Sci Technol 2001;36:174–178.

Lamborg CH, Fitzgerald WF, Vandal GM, Rolfhus KR. Atmospheric mercury in northern Wisconsin, Sources and species. Water Air Soil Pollut 1995;80:189–198.

Landa ER. The retention of metallic mercury vapor by soils. Geochim Cosmochim Acta 1978;42:1407–1411.

Landis MS, Stevens RK, Schaedlich F, Prestbo EM. Development and characterization of an annular denuder methodology for the measurement of divalent inorganic reactive gaseous mercury in ambient air. Environ Sci Technol 2002;36:3000–3009.

Lin CJ, Gustin MS, Singhasuk P, Eckley C, Miller M. Measurement-based models for estimating mercury flux from soils. Environ Sci Technol 2010;44:8522–8588.

Lin CJ, Pehkonen SO. Aqueous phase reactions of mercury with free radicals and chlorine: implications for atmospheric mercury chemistry. Chemosphere 1999;38:1253–1263.

Lin CJ, Pongprueksa P, Lindberg SE, Pehkonen SO, Byun D, Jang C. Scientific uncertainties in atmospheric mercury models I: model science evaluation. Atmos Environ 2006;40:2911–2928.

Lindberg S, Bullock R, Ebinghaus R, Engstrom D, Feng X, Fitzgerald W, et al. A synthesis of progress and uncertainties in attributing the sources of mercury in deposition. Ambio J Hum Environ 2009;36:19–33.

Lindberg SE, Dong W, Meyers T. Transpiration of gaseous elemental mercury through vegetation in a subtropical wetland in Florida. Atmos Environ 2002;36:5207–5219.

Lindberg SE, Hanson PJ, Meyers TP, Kim KH. Air/surface exchange of mercury vapor over forests—the need for a reassessment of continental biogenic emissions. Atmos Environ 1998;32:895–908.

Lindberg SE, Kim K-H, Meyers TP, Owens JG. Micrometeorological gradient approach for quantifying air/surface exchange of mercury vapor: tests over contaminated soils. Environ Sci Technol 1995;29:126–135.

Lindberg SE, Stratton WJ. Atmospheric mercury speciation: concentrations and behavior of reactive gaseous mercury in ambient air. Environ Sci Technol 1998;32:49–57.

Lindqvist O, Johansson K, Bringmark L, Timm B, Aastrup M, Andersson A, Hovsenius G, Håkanson L, Iverfeldt Å, Meili M. Mercury in the Swedish environment—recent research on causes, consequences and corrective methods. Water Air Soil Pollut 1991;55: xi–261.

Lyman SN, Gustin MS. Speciation of atmospheric mercury at two sites in northern Nevada, USA. Atmos Environ 2008;42:927–939.

Lyman SN, Gustin MS. Determinants of atmospheric mercury concentrations in Reno, Nevada, U.S.A. Sci Total Environ 2009;408:431–438.

Lyman SN, Gustin MS, Prestbo EM, Kilner PI, Edgerton E, Hartsell B. Testing and application of surrogate surfaces for understanding potential gaseous oxidized mercury dry deposition. Environ Sci Technol 2009;43:6235–6241.

Lyman SN, Gustin MS, Prestbo EM, Marsik FJ. Estimation of dry deposition of atmospheric mercury in Nevada by direct and indirect methods. Environ Sci Technol 2007;41:1970–1976.

Lyman SN, Jaffe DA, Gustin MS. Release of mercury halides from KCl denuders in the presence of ozone. Atmos Chem Phys 2010a;10:8197–8204.

Lyman SN, Jaffe DA, Gustin MS. Technical Note, Release of mercury halides from KCl denuders in the presence of ozone. Atmos. Chem. Phys. 2010;10:8197–8204.

Marsik FJ, Keeler GJ, Landis MS. The dry-deposition of speciated mercury to the Florida Everglades: measurements and modeling. Atmos Environ 2007;41:136–149.

Mason RP, Sheu GR. Role of the ocean in the global mercury cycle. Global Biogeochem Cycles 2002;16:1093.

Miller MB. Characterization of mercury concentration, form, and air-surface exchange associated with the area surrounding and within two Nevada gold mines. Reno: Department of Natural Resources & Environmental Science, Master of Science in Hydrology, University of Nevada-Reno; 2010. p 141.

Millhollen AG, Gustin MS, Obrist D. Foliar mercury accumulation and exchange for three tree species. Environ Sci Technol 2006a;40:6001–6006.

Millhollen AG, Obrist D, Gustin MS. Mercury accumulation in grass and forb species as a function of atmospheric carbon dioxide concentrations and mercury exposures in air and soil. Chemosphere 2006b;65:889–897.

Munthe J, Bishop K, Driscoll C, Graydon J, Hultberg H, Lindberg SE, et al. Input-output of Hg in forested catchments in Europe and North America. Mater Geoenviron 2004;51:1243–1246.

Nacht DM, Gustin MS, Engle MA, Zehner RE, Giglini AD. Atmospheric mercury emissions and speciation at the sulphur bank mercury mine superfund site, Northern California. Environ Sci Technol 2004;38:1977–1983.

NADP, 2011, National Atmospheric Deposition Program, http://nadp.sws.uiuc.edu/ site visited 8-27-2011.

Nelson SJ, Johnson KB, Weathers KC, Loftin CS, Fernandez IJ, Kahl JS, et al. A comparison of winter mercury accumulation at forested and no-canopy sites measured with different snow sampling techniques. Appl Geochem 2008;23:384–398.

NRC. Global sources of local pollution: an assessment of long-range transport of key air pollutants to and from the United States. Washington (DC): The National Academies Press: 2010.

Obrist D, Faïn X, Berger C. Gaseous elemental mercury emissions and CO_2 respiration rates in terrestrial soils under controlled aerobic and anaerobic laboratory conditions. Sci Total Environ 2010;408:1691–1700.

Ohio Lumex Co. 2010. Portable mercury analyzer information. Available at www.ohiolumex.com. Twinsburg (OH). 2006 pp.

Pacyna EG, Pacyna JM, Steenhuisen F, Wilson S. Global anthropogenic mercury emission inventory for 2000. Atmos Environ 2006;40:4048–4063.

Peterson C, Gustin M, Lyman S. Atmospheric mercury concentrations and speciation measured from 2004 to 2007 in Reno, Nevada, USA. Atmos Environ 2009;43:4646–4654.

Poissant L, Pilote M, Constant P, Beauvais C, Zhang HH, Xu X. Mercury gas exchanges over selected bare soil and flooded sites in the bay St. François wetlands (Québec, Canada). Atmos Environ 2004;38:4205–4214.

Prestbo EM, Gay DA. Wet deposition of mercury in the U.S. and Canada, 1996–2005: results and analysis of the NADP mercury deposition network (MDN). Atmos Environ 2009;43:4223–4233.

Rasmussen PE. Current methods of estimating atmospheric mercury fluxes in remote areas. Environ Sci Technol 1994;28:2233–2241.

Rasmussen PE, Edwards G, Schroeder W, Ausma S, Steffen A, Kemp J, et al. Measurement of gaseous mercury fluxes in the terrestrial environment. In: Parsons MB, Percival JB, editors. Mercury, sources, measurements, cycles and effects. Halifax: Mineralogical Association of Canada; 2005. p 123–138.

Rasmussen P, Mierle G, Nriagu J. The analysis of vegetation for total mercury. Water Air Soil Pollut 1991;56:379–390.

Rea AW, Lindberg SE, Keeler GJ. Assessment of dry deposition and foliar leaching of mercury and selected trace elements based on washed foliar and surrogate surfaces. Environ Sci Technol 2000;34:2418–2425.

Rytuba JJ. Geogenic and mining sources of mercury to the environment. In Parsons MB, Percival JB, editors. Mercury, sources, measurements, cycles, and effects. Halifax: Mineralogical Association of Canada; 2005. p 21–36.

Sakata M, Marumoto K. Wet and dry deposition fluxes of mercury in Japan. Atmos Environ 2005;39:3139–3146.

Schluter K. Review: evaporation of mercury from soils. An integration and synthesis of current knowledge. Environ Geol 2000;39:249–271.

Selin NE. Global biogeochemical cycling of mercury: a review. Annu Rev Environ Resour 2009;34:43–63.

Selin NE, Jacob DJ. Seasonal and spatial patterns of mercury wet deposition in the United States: constraints on the contribution from North American anthropogenic sources. Atmos Environ 2008;42:5193–5204.

Selin NE, Jacob DJ, Yantosca RM, Strode S, Jaeglé L, Sunderland EM. Global 3-D land-ocean-atmosphere model for mercury, present-day versus preindustrial cycles and anthropogenic enrichment factors for deposition. Global Biogeochem Cycles 2008;22:GB2011.

Skov H, Brooks SB, Goodsite ME, Lindberg SE, Meyers TP, Landis MS, et al. Fluxes of reactive gaseous mercury measured with a newly developed method using relaxed eddy accumulation. Atmos Environ 2006;40:5452–5463.

Song X, Van Heyst B. Volatilization of mercury from soils in response to simulated precipitation. Atmos Environ 2005;39:7494–7505.

Stamenkovic J, Gustin MS. Evaluation of use of EcoCELL technology for quantifying total gaseous mercury fluxes over background substrates. Atmos Environ 2007;41:3702–3712.

Stamenkovic J, Gustin MS. Nonstomatal versus stomatal uptake of atmospheric mercury. Environ Sci Technol 2009;43:1367–1372.

Stamenkovic J, Gustin MS, Arnone Iii JA, Johnson DW, Larsen JD, Verburg PSJ. Atmospheric mercury exchange with a tallgrass prairie ecosystem housed in mesocosms. Sci Total Environ 2008;406:227–238.

Taylor JGE, Leonard TL, Fernandez GCJ, Gustin MS. Mercury and plants in contaminated soils: 2. Environmental and physiological factors governing mercury flux to the atmosphere. Environ Toxicol Chem 1998;17:2072.

Tekran Corporation. 2010. Available at www.tekran.com (last accessed, Sep 2010).

Temme C, Einax W Jr, Ebinghaus R, Schroeder WH. Measurements of atmospheric mercury species at a coastal site in the Antarctic and over the south Atlantic Ocean during polar summer. Environ Sci Technol 2002;37:22–31.

Valente RJ, Shea C, Lynn Humes K, Tanner RL. Atmospheric mercury in the Great Smoky Mountains compared to regional and global levels. Atmos Environ 2007;41:1861–1873.

Wallschläger D, Turner RR, London J, Ebinghaus R, Kock HH, Sommar J, et al. Factors affecting the measurement of mercury emissions from soils with flux chambers. J Geophys Res 1999;104:21859–21871.

Watras CJ, Morrison KA, Rubsam JL, Rodger B. Atmospheric mercury cycles in northern Wisconsin. Atmos Environ 2009;43:4070–4077.

Wesely ML. Parameterization of surface resistances to gaseous dry deposition in regional-scale numerical models. Atmos Environ 1989;23:1293–1304.

Wesely ML, Hicks BB. A review of the current status of knowledge on dry deposition. Atmos Environ 2000;34:2261–2282.

Wiedinmyer C, Friedli H. Mercury emission estimates from fires: an initial inventory for the United States. Environ Sci Technol 2007;41:8092–8098.

Wiener JG, Knights BC, Sandheinrich MB, Jeremiason JD, Brigham ME, Engstrom DR, et al. Mercury in soils, lakes, and fish in Voyageurs National Park (Minnesota): importance of atmospheric deposition and ecosystem factors. Environ Sci Technol 2006;40:6261–6268.

Xin M, Gustin M, Johnson D. Laboratory investigation of the potential for re-emission of atmospherically derived Hg from soils. Environ Sci Technol 2007;41:4946–4951.

Zhang H, Lindberg SE, Barnett MO, Vette AF, Gustin MS. Dynamic flux chamber measurement of gaseous mercury emission fluxes over soils. Part 1: simulation of gaseous mercury emissions from soils using a two-resistance exchange interface model. Atmos Environ 2002;36:835–846.

Zhang H, Lindberg SE, Kuiken T. Mysterious diel cycles of mercury emission from soils held in the dark at constant temperature. Atmos Environ 2008;42:5424–5433.

Zhang H, Lindberg SE, Marsik FJ, Keeler GJ. Mercury air/surface exchange kinetics of background soils of the Tahquamenon River watershed in the Michigan Upper Peninsula. Water Air Soil Pollut 2001;126:151–169.

Zhang HH, Poissant L, Xu X, Pilote M. Explorative and innovative dynamic flux bag method development and testing for mercury air-vegetation gas exchange fluxes. Atmos Environ 2005;39:7481–7493.

Zhang L, Wright LP, Blanchard P. A review of current knowledge concerning dry deposition of atmospheric mercury. Atmos Environ 2009;43:5853–5864.

PART IV

BIOACCUMULATION, TOXICITY, AND METALLOMICS

CHAPTER 14

BIOACCUMULATION AND BIOMAGNIFICATION OF MERCURY THROUGH FOOD WEBS

KAREN KIDD, MEREDITH CLAYDEN, and TIM JARDINE

14.1 INTRODUCTION

Mercury (Hg) is one of the few metals known to accumulate through food webs to concentrations that are much higher in upper trophic level organisms than those in primary producers or consumers. There are two main forms of Hg that dominate in studies of aquatic or terrestrial ecosystems—inorganic Hg (Hg^{2+}) and methylmercury (CH_3Hg^+). While both have been intensively studied since the 1950s, more of the recent focus has been on CH_3Hg^+ because analytical techniques now allow for measures of low parts per trillion concentrations in waters (Babiarz et al., 2001). It is also the form that dominates in fish tissues (Bloom, 1992), and remains a threat to the health of vertebrates because of its toxicity to the nervous and endocrine systems of fishes, birds, and mammals, including humans (e.g., Grandjean et al., 1999, Burgess, 2005, Crump and Trudeau, 2009).

The abiotic cycling of Hg in aquatic ecosystems is not completely understood and remains an active area of research. Despite the unknowns, it is well established that the physical and chemical characteristics of the river, lake, estuary, or ocean as well as its degree of impact from human activities (i.e., logging, hydroelectrical development, metal mining drainage, industrial discharges) will influence the formation of CH_3Hg^+ from Hg^{2+} and the relative proportions of these two forms of Hg in waters. Some of the key factors affecting their concentrations and fate include water chemistry (e.g., pH, ligands, sulfates, nutrients) and catchment characteristics (e.g., percentage of wetlands). These parameters are often predictive of Hg concentrations in organisms at the base of food webs as well as in upper trophic level consumers (Driscoll et al., 1994). Indeed, concentrations of Hg in one fish species can vary considerably from one

Environmental Chemistry and Toxicology of Mercury, First Edition.
Edited by Guangliang Liu, Yong Cai, and Nelson O'Driscoll.
© 2012 John Wiley & Sons, Inc. Published 2012 by John Wiley & Sons, Inc.

lake to another because of among-system differences in water chemistry, and watershed characteristics and usage (Chen et al., 2005; Kamman et al., 2005), and understanding and explaining this variability has been the focus of much of the Hg research over the past four decades.

As for fish and other aquatic organisms, birds and mammals have variable Hg concentrations within and among regions, and contain high tissue Hg concentrations in areas with point (e.g., metal mines) or geological sources (Anderson et al., 2008). Mercury exposure in terrestrial-dwelling biota comes mainly from their prey and, thus, concentrations of Hg in wildlife are determined by the Hg in their diets. For fish-eating species such as loons, osprey, and mink, high Hg is found in individuals living in ecosystems where fish Hg is also elevated (Burgess, 2005). Some evidence of Hg toxicity exists for wildlife because CH_3Hg^+ affects the nervous and endocrine systems, in turn impacting the animal's ability to forage, reproduce, and thrive (Burgess and Meyer, 2008). Although reasonable knowledge exists about concentrations of Hg in birds and mammals (especially fish eaters) and its effects on their health, much less of the focus of Hg research has been on cycling of this element in terrestrial ecosystems.

In aquatic environments, Hg is taken up directly from the water into organisms and their exposure is affected by the bioavailability of this element. More specifically, the bioavailability of Hg^{2+} and CH_3Hg^+ is determined by the presence of ligands such as dissolved organic carbon (DOC), sulfides, Cl^- and OH^-, and some of these Hg–ligand complexes are more readily adsorbed or absorbed than others through membranes. When concentrations of either Hg^{2+} or CH_3Hg^+ in an organism exceed those in the water, this process is called *bioconcentration*. At steady state, the ratio of the concentration in an organism to what is in the water is called a *bioconcentration factor* (BCF) and is typically determined through controlled laboratory studies. For aquatic organisms, these ratios are an average of ~5000 and ~9000 for Hg^{2+} and CH_3Hg^+, respectively (McGeer et al., 2003).

Although bioconcentration is the main route of uptake at the base of an aquatic food web, primary through tertiary consumers are exposed to Hg^{2+} and CH_3Hg^+ from both the water and their diet, with the relative importance of dietary exposure increasing with an organism's trophic level. As in BCFs, *bioaccumulation factors* (BAFs) are calculated as the ratio of either total Hg (both inorganic and organic forms; THg) or CH_3Hg^+ in an organism versus the concentration of the same form in water; in contrast to BCFs, however, BAFs are interpreted as including uptake from both water and food for organisms above primary producers in the food web and are typically calculated from field measurements. Field studies show that BAFs are lower in short-lived, small-bodied primary consumers (10^5 to 10^6) and higher in long-lived, larger bodied organisms such as fishes (up to 10^7), and are inversely related to concentrations of DOC in the water (Watras et al., 1998).

Mercury is one of the few elements known to biomagnify through food webs, and this happens only for the organic form CH_3Hg^+. *Biomagnification* occurs when the concentration of Hg in a consumer is higher than that of its prey; typical *biomagnification factors* (BMFs)—the ratio of what is in a predator versus its diet—are between $\sim$2 and 10 in aquatic food webs (Watras et al., 1998). Numerous studies have demonstrated that Hg is effectively biomagnified through freshwater (Cabana and Rasmussen, 1994; Cabana et al., 1994) and marine (Campbell et al., 2005) food webs from tropical (Kidd et al., 2003) to arctic (Swanson and Kidd, 2010) latitudes. Because CH_3Hg^+ is more efficiently retained than Hg^{2+} in fishes, >85% of the total Hg (THg) in these organisms is the potent neurotoxin CH_3Hg^+ (Bloom, 1992; Wyn et al., 2009). Methylmercury accumulates more in fish tissues and biomagnifies in food webs because its excretion is much slower ($\sim$2.8 times) than that of Hg^{2+}; in addition, excretion rates are slower in larger animals and at colder water temperatures (Trudel and Rasmussen, 1997).

A number of human activities have increased the concentrations of Hg in the environment since the industrial revolution, including generating electricity from coal, burning of municipal and hospital wastes, and mining and smelting metals (Pacyna et al., 2006). There is a direct link between Hg emissions and deposition and fish concentrations (Harris et al., 2007) and considerable attention has been paid to the temporal increases and/or decreases in biotic concentrations of Hg associated with human activities. Yellow perch (*Perca flavescens*) from 19 of 25 lakes in the Adirondacks of northeastern United States showed decreases or no change in Hg between 1992/1993 and 2005/2006 Dittman and Driscoll, 2009). However, some remote regions in eastern Canada are showing increases in fish Hg (Wyn et al., 2010). Despite some efforts to reduce Hg releases and regional evidence of declines in abiotic and biotic concentrations, many systems still contain fish or fish-eating wildlife with concentrations that are known to threaten their health and that of humans.

This chapter describes the current understanding of how organisms are exposed to and store Hg; the properties of organisms, food webs, and systems that favor the accumulation of Hg in biota; biomagnification and how to assess and contrast this process across ecosystems; and new approaches to assessing sources and movement of Hg through food webs. The chapter is heavily weighted toward aquatic food webs following the relative focus in the scientific literature; surprisingly little is known about the movement of Hg in terrestrial food webs.

14.2   MERCURY IN AQUATIC AND TERRESTRIAL ORGANISMS

14.2.1   Bioavailability in Aqueous Environments

In aqueous environments, Hg is taken up into organisms either through passive diffusion or via active uptake mechanisms (e.g., through Na^+ and Ca^{2+} channels) (Pickhardt et al., 2006) and the rate and magnitude of its uptake depends on its chemical form. There are many organic and inorganic ligands in natural waters that can form complexes with Hg, some of which will sequester it and prevent its passage across biological membranes, and others that will promote its availability to and uptake by biota. In marine systems, chloride ions are important ligands for inorganic Hg. Neutral complexes of $HgCl_2$ cross biological membranes more rapidly than ionic Hg^{2+} (Gutknecht, 1981) and uptake of the former into cells and tissues will be higher in waters with high concentrations of Cl^- ligands (Klinck et al., 2005). Recent evidence also suggests that Hg bound to small thiol compounds such as cysteine is more readily taken up and methylated by sulfur-reducing bacteria (Schaefer and Morel, 2009). Two dominant inorganic ligands for CH_3Hg^+ are Cl^- and OH^-; CH_3HgCl, rather than CH_3HgOH, is more readily taken up into organisms and the former occurs more commonly in waters with lower pH and higher Cl^- (Block et al., 1997). As such, chemical factors that affect the form and availability of Hg in aqueous environments will have considerable influence over what is measured in lower trophic level biota and their consumers.

Dissolved organic matter (DOM), commonly measured as DOC, also plays an important and complex role in Hg bioavailability. Inorganic Hg binds preferentially to thiols and other sulfur-containing functional groups such that in systems containing relatively sulfur- and thiol-rich organic matter, more Hg may be sequestered and rendered unavailable to biota (Ravichandran, 2004). However, under acidic conditions, H^+ may compete with Hg^{2+} for binding sites on DOM and limit its sequestration, leaving more inorganic Hg available for uptake or methylation by organisms. The presence of ions such as Na^+ and K^+ may also compete with Hg^{2+} for binding to negatively charged functional groups on DOM. In addition to affecting Hg complexation, organic matter influences the penetration of light in water bodies and may thereby diminish sunlight-induced demethylation and reduction of Hg^{2+} to $Hg(0)$ (Amyot et al., 1994; Sellers et al., 1996). Thus, there may be less volatilization of Hg in systems with higher DOC, and therefore more Hg retained and available to aquatic organisms (Amyot et al., 1997). Sunlight may also cause photolysis of organic matter and produce radical species such as $^{\bullet}OH$, which in turn can oxidize elemental Hg to Hg^{2+} and make it available to biota (Zhang and Lindberg, 2001). Conversely, some studies have demonstrated enhanced reduction of Hg^{2+} and volatilization in the presence of DOM (e.g., Allard and Arsenie, 1991, Costa and Liss, 2000), which would decrease the pool of bioavailable Hg. Thus, it seems that DOM plays conflicting roles in Hg speciation depending on its form and the redox conditions of different aquatic systems. This conflict is reflected in a number of studies of Hg bioaccumulation through food webs, where some studies have found a positive correlation between DOC and Hg concentrations in biota (Carter et al., 2001; Rencz et al., 2003), and others have found the opposite effect (Snodgrass et al., 2000; Benoit et al., 2001). Pickhardt et al. (2006) also found that uptake of Hg^{2+} into algae is not affected by DOC but that CH_3Hg^+ concentrations in algae are higher in DOC-enriched waters. Despite varying evidence of the role of DOM or DOC in Hg bioavailability and uptake, it is clear that understanding its form and behavior in individual systems will help predict whether it might promote or limit the formation of bioavailable Hg species in aquatic systems. Hg photochemistry and interactions with DOM are discussed in detail in Chapters 6 and 8, and these areas of research will continue to improve our understanding of Hg speciation and bioavailability across different systems.

Along with DOM, other water chemistry variables are important in determining Hg bioavailability. The problem of acid rain and the acidification of lakes and rivers in recent decades has focused attention on the interaction of pH and Hg in organisms, and many studies of freshwater ecosystems show a strong negative relationship between biotic Hg and pH (Scheuhammer, 1991; Spry and Wiener, 1991; Kamman et al., 2005). Despite contradictory evidence on the effect of pH on inorganic Hg solubility, it is clear that CH_3Hg^+ is more soluble under low pH conditions, and decreasing pH is associated with net increases in CH_3Hg^+ production. This may result from a variety of other conditions in sediments and the water column, which are also dependant on pH, such as decreased reduction and volatilization of Hg, decreased availability of binding sites on organic matter, and redox conditions (Ullrich et al., 2001). When oxygen is limited, inorganic Hg may be released from binding with oxyhydroxide compounds of iron and manganese and thereby increase the pool of Hg^{2+} available to methylating bacteria (Chadwick et al., 2006), which may in turn be more abundant in anoxic conditions (Morel et al., 1998; Ullrich et al., 2001; Fleming et al., 2006). A few studies have demonstrated a positive relationship between dissolved iron and Hg in fish such as yellow perch (Gabriel et al., 2009), northern pike (*Esox lucius*), and walleye (*Sander vitreus*; Wren et al., 1991). However, it is not clear whether this is due to similar biogeochemical transport and cycling of Hg and iron, or a greater abundance of iron-reducing, Hg-methylating bacteria in water with high dissolved iron content.

Another critical component of Hg cycling in aquatic systems is its conversion to CH_3Hg^+, as this form is the one that biomagnifies and is toxic to vertebrates. Methylation of inorganic Hg by sulfate- and iron-reducing bacteria in anoxic layers of sediment has been documented in a variety of marine, estuarine, and freshwater environments (Compeau and Bartha, 1985; Ullrich et al., 2001; Fleming et al., 2006). The presence of sulfate also stimulates the production of CH_3Hg^+ (Gilmour et al., 1992), and sulfate deposition and cycling affects concentrations of Hg in fish (Drevnick et al., 2007). Among the thiol (SH) compounds, the amino acid cysteine is particularly effective in promoting the uptake and enzyme-mediated methylation of Hg by bacteria (Schaefer and Morel, 2009). Furthermore, cysteine and other thiols can be present naturally in sediment pore waters in sufficient concentrations as to possibly make cysteine-mediated Hg methylation by bacteria an important contributor to overall Hg methylation (Zhang et al., 2004). In addition, as described in more detail in Chapters 5 and 6, CH_3Hg^+ may also be demethylated by bacteria (and by abiotic processes such as photolysis), thereby reducing the concentrations available for uptake into aquatic organisms. The bioavailability and methylation or demethylation of Hg depends on a multitude of interdependent geochemical factors, and further research is needed to distinguish which of these factors will best predict biotic Hg accumulation in different ecosystems.

14.2.2 Algae and Macrophytes

Given that primary producers like algae and other primary producers are the dominant underlying food source for many aquatic organisms, it is important to understand factors that increase or inhibit Hg storage in this group. Concentrations of THg, Hg^{2+}, and CH_3Hg^+ in algae and macrophytes are typically lower than other components of the food web (<100 ppb dw; Watras et al., 1998). Although fewer studies have examined Hg in aquatic primary producers, likely due to difficulties in isolating algae from bacteria or detritus, certain species of algae may accumulate more CH_3Hg^+ than others, and augment trophic transfer to their consumers. For example, periphyton, *Cladophora* and *Nostoc* were collected from a productive California river; whereas all taxa had similar THg concentrations (up to 0.2 µg/g dw), their proportions of THg as CH_3Hg^+ varied from 8% to 100% (Tsui et al., 2009; see also Table 14.1). The authors speculated that algae such as *Cladophora* with a larger surface area allowed for greater colonization by methylating bacteria (Tsui et al., 2009). Other research has shown that epiphytes have higher Hg concentrations than the macrophytes upon which they grow (Cremona et al., 2009). While primary producers typically have low concentrations of Hg, certain biogeochemical conditions, including point sources and water chemistry, can lead to high concentrations in this compartment at the base of the food web (Hill et al., 1996; Mason et al., 1996; Zizek et al., 2007).

Although all organisms have some uptake of Hg from water, the greatest bioconcentration of both Hg^{2+} and CH_3Hg^+ is found in the lowest trophic levels of the food web, and concentrations of Hg in algae (or seston) can be up to 10^6 times higher than the surrounding waters (Watras et al., 1998). Bioconcentration of Hg^{2+} into algal cells is lower (3- to 88-fold, depending on species) than CH_3Hg^+ and higher in smaller than larger algal species for CH_3Hg^+ but not Hg^{2+} (Pickhardt and Fisher, 2007).

14.2.3 Aquatic Invertebrates

Aquatic invertebrates are exposed to both forms of Hg in water and on the sediments for benthic-dwelling taxa. Uptake of Hg^{2+} and CH_3Hg^+ into the zooplankton genus *Daphnia* is proportional to the concentrations in water, but modeling shows that water uptake was much more important for Hg^{2+} (up to 96%) than for CH_3Hg^+ (2–53%)(Tsui and Wang, 2004). As described above, water chemistry will also affect partitioning of Hg into invertebrates. Higher CH_3Hg^+ concentrations are found in zooplankton from lakes with lower pH and higher DOC (Watras et al., 1998). Sediment-dwelling invertebrates are also exposed to Hg bound to particulates, most of which is inorganic (Kannan et al., 1998; Mikac et al., 1999).

Diet is also an important route of exposure for these primary and secondary consumers. Concentrations of Hg in aquatic invertebrates are affected by both their feeding ecology and the form of Hg in their prey. Although the diet of invertebrates contains both Hg^{2+} and CH_3Hg^+ (Watras et al., 1998; Mason et al., 2000), CH_3Hg^+ is much more efficiently retained in the consumer than

TABLE 14.1 Percent CH₃Hg⁺ in Various Components of Food Webs from Select Studies in the Literature

Group	Tissue	Percentage CH_3Hg^+	Reference
Primary producers			
Terrestrial plants	Whole	0.2 to 2	Gnamus et al. (2000)
Terrestrial plants	Whole	9 ± 2	Regine et al. (2006)
Aquatic macrophytes	Whole	<1	Bowles et al. (2001)
Aquatic macrophytes	Whole	10 ± 3	Regine et al. (2006)
Aquatic macrophytes	Whole	6 to >100	Cremona et al. (2009)
Epiphyton	Whole	2 to 8	Roulet et al. (2000)
Epiphyton	Whole	2 to 24	Cremona et al. (2009)
Periphyton	Whole	0.5 to 8	Hill et al. (1996)
Periphyton	Whole	0.4 to 8.8	Zizek et al. (2007)
Periphyton	Whole	8	Tsui et al. (2009)
Biofilm	Whole	0.9 to 4.1	Desrosiers et al. (2006)
Biofilm	Whole	28 ± 4	Regine et al. (2006)
Cyanobacteria (*Nostoc pruniforme*)	Whole	29 to 44	Tsui et al. (2009)
Filamentous algae (*Cladophora glomerata*)	Whole	50 to >100	Tsui et al. (2009)
Phytoplankton	Whole	13, 31	Watras and Bloom (1992)
Phytoplankton	Whole	15	Roulet et al. (2000)
Invertebrates			
Bivalves (freshwater mussels)	Whole	22 ± 7	Jardine & Kidd (unpublished)
Bivalves (marine mussels)	Whole	7 to 93	Mzoughi et al. (2002)
Zooplankton (freshwater)	Whole	29, 91	Watras and Bloom (1992)
Zooplankton (freshwater)	Whole	11 to 83	Watras et al. (1998)
Zooplankton (freshwater)	Whole	44	Roulet et al. (2000)
Zooplankton (marine)	Whole	1 to 19	Al-Reasi et al. (2007)
Benthic insects	Whole	35 to 52	Regine et al. (2006)
Chaoborus/Chironomidae	Whole	9 to 82	Watras et al. (1998)
Water mites (Hydracarina)	Whole	56 to 88	Watras et al. (1998)
Diptera/Ephemeroptera	Whole	20 to 25	Tremblay et al. (1996)
Trichoptera	Whole	30 to 40	Tremblay et al. (1996)
Hemiptera/Coleoptera	Whole	60 to 85	Tremblay et al. (1996)
Hemiptera	Whole	87 ± 15	Jardine et al. (2009b)
Odonata	Whole	95	Tremblay et al. (1996)
Odonata/Megaloptera/ Perlidae	Whole	78 ± 12	Jardine and Kidd (unpublished)
Spiders (terrestrial)	Whole	49 ± 21	Cristol et al. (2008)
Orthoptera (terrestrial)	Whole	38 ± 24	Cristol et al. (2008)
Lepidoptera (terrestrial)	Whole	24 ± 20	Cristol et al. (2008)
Fish			
Myleus rubripinnus (herbivore)	Muscle	78 ± 5	Regine et al. (2006)

(continued)

TABLE 14.1 (*Continued*)

Group	Tissue	Percentage CH_3Hg^+	Reference
Semaprochilodis varii (benthivore)	Muscle	73 ± 6	Regine et al. (2006)
Leporinus friderici (omnivore)	Muscle	87 ± 7	Regine et al. (2006)
Ageneiosus brevifilis (piscivore)	Muscle	90 ± 8	Regine et al. (2006)
Yellow perch, golden shiners	Whole	95	Watras et al. (1998)
Various (13 marine species)	Muscle	35 to 100	Al-Reasi et al. (2007)
Various (five marine species)	Muscle	88 to 98	Freije and Awadh (2009)
Planktivores (two species)	Whole	54 to 56	Bowles et al. (2001)
Brook trout, blacknose dace	Muscle	~100	Jardine and Kidd (unpublished)
Omnivores (two species)	Whole	75 to 80	Bowles et al. (2001)
Piscivores (three species)	Muscle	79 to 94	Bowles et al. (2001)
Amphibians			
Red-backed salamander (*Plethodon cinereus*)	Whole	46 to 47	Bergeron et al. (2010)
Southern two-lined salamander (*Eurycea bislineata*)	Whole	57 to 62	Bergeron et al. (2010)
American toad (*Bufo americanus*)	Blood	71	Bergeron et al. (2010)
American toad (*Bufo americanus*)	Eggs	48	Bergeron et al. (2010)
American toad (*Bufo americanus*)	Whole	53	Bergeron et al. (2010)
Turtles (four species)	Blood	70 to 100	Bergeron et al. (2007)
Birds			
Passerines (insectivorous, three species)	Liver	79 to 83	Wolfe and Norman (1998)
Passerines (insectivorous, three species)	Brain	81 to 90	Wolfe and Norman (1998)
Mammals			
Marine mammals (three species)	Muscle	~100	Wagemann et al. (1997)
Marine mammals (three species)	Liver	15 to 31	Wagemann et al. (1997)
Roe deer (*Capreolis capreolus*)	Muscle	36 to 46	Gnamus et al. (2000)
Roe deer (*Capreolis capreolus*)	Liver	4 to 11	Gnamus et al. (2000)
Roe deer (*Capreolis capreolus*)	Kidney	0.2 to 0.7	Gnamus et al. (2000)

Hg^{2+} (Tsui and Wang, 2004), possibly because of cellular partitioning whereby CH_3Hg^+ is located in the cytoplasm, while Hg^{2+} is affiliated with cell membranes making the latter less available for retention (Mason et al., 1996). Diet is considered to be the most important route of exposure to CH_3Hg^+ for many invertebrate taxa (e.g., 47–98% of CH_3Hg^+ in *Daphnia* is from their diet, Tsui and Wang, 2004). In rivers and lakes, scrapers, shredders, and collectors that consume little to no animal material often have low concentrations and a low proportion of THg as CH_3Hg^+ (Watras and Bloom, 1992; Tremblay et al., 1996; Watras et al., 1998). Herbivorous and predaceous invertebrates have concentrations of CH_3Hg^+ that are 3–10 and 2–5 times higher, respectively, than their diet and there is an increase in the concentrations and proportions of CH_3Hg^+ from primary to secondary invertebrate consumers (Mason et al., 2000). For example, stream invertebrates that consume mainly terrestrial detritus (shredders) or epilithic algae (grazers) had much lower (twofold to sixfold) concentrations than collectors or predatory taxa (Mason et al., 2000; Tsui et al., 2009; see also Table 14.1). It has been suggested that percentage CH_3Hg^+ in invertebrates can be used as an indicator of their relative trophic position (Mason et al., 2000).

As described above, invertebrates that reside low on the food chain and serve as food for many fishes and birds in aquatic food webs, can have highly variable Hg concentrations among and within species (Chételat and Amyot, 2009). While some taxa can have very high concentrations, these are normally found in contaminated environments (Zizek et al., 2007), and concentrations in uncontaminated habitats typically range from 10 ng/g to 1 μg/g ww (Mason et al., 2000). The highly variable Hg concentrations are a result of varying aqueous and dietary exposures (herbivory vs predatory), and assimilation efficiencies and excretion rates (Tsui and Wang, 2004). The concentration of CH_3Hg^+ in several functional feeding groups of invertebrates is positively related to drainage area and presumed productivity in streams (Tsui et al., 2009). Also, within individual taxa, the lifestage of the invertebrate can affect its concentration of Hg; for example, Chételat et al. (2008) showed that adult chironomids had almost three times higher concentrations than the younger larval stages from High Arctic lakes.

14.2.3.1 Fishes.
For fishes, the skin and gills can be important sites of accumulation of waterborne Hg^{2+}. Inorganic Hg has a strong affinity for mucus (Part and Lock, 1983), although it is not well understood whether this is protective or whether there is further uptake into the fish through the skin. The gills are believed to be the main site of uptake of Hg^{2+} into nonfeeding fishes (Olson and Fromm, 1973) and the mechanism of uptake is thought to be mainly passive diffusion. As with other organisms, water chemistry and complexation of Hg^{2+} to ligands affect its uptake into gills, with more rapid uptake of the $HgCl_2$ complex when compared to ionic Hg (Klinck et al., 2005) and reduced uptake in high DOC waters (Playle, 1998).

Fish obtain most (>90%) of their Hg from their food (Hall et al., 1997; Rodgers, 1994; Harris and Snodgrass, 1993). Therefore, THg in fish is strongly influenced by Hg concentrations in their diet (Borgmann and Whittle, 1992;

Harris and Snodgrass, 1993; Harris and Bodaly, 1998). Top predators such as lake trout (*Salvelinus namaycush*) contain the highest concentrations of Hg in part because they tend to feed upon prey with high Hg concentrations and also because they tend to be longer lived than forage fishes (Kamman et al., 2005; Swanson and Kidd, 2010). It is only recently that we have begun to understand that the biomagnification and bioaccumulation of CH_3Hg^+ in fishes can result in concentrations that can be toxic to the fish themselves. Indeed, several recent and comprehensive reviews show that environmentally relevant exposures to CH_3Hg^+ in laboratory studies can affect behavior and reproduction, and there is increasing suggestion that wild fishes are also affected by this pollutant (Crump and Trudeau, 2009; Weis, 2009; Sandheinrich and Wiener, 2010).

Fish typically have the highest concentrations of Hg in aquatic food webs when compared to primary producers and consumers. Furthermore, most or all of this Hg is in the more toxic methylated form (Bloom, 1992; Table 14.1); as a result many of the upper trophic level species are above the recommended human consumption guidelines in a given jurisdiction. For example, 57% of piscivorous fish in western United States streams and rivers exceed the threshold for consumption (Peterson et al., 2007).

14.2.3.2   *Terrestrial-Dwelling Wildlife.* Diet is also the main route of exposure to Hg for terrestrial wildlife and, as for fishes, the concentrations in a particular species within a region will depend on the presence of human activities (flooding, DesGranges et al., 1998), local conditions (i.e., geology, water chemistry; Evers et al., 1998), and ecology of the species (e.g., fish-eating vs insect-eating; Evers et al., 2005). A number of synopses have been done on concentrations of Hg in wildlife and these show some trends both across and within regions (Evers et al., 1998, 2005; Rimmer et al., 2005); for example, higher Hg is found in common loons from eastern than western North America, reflecting higher atmospheric deposition in the former area, and in loons from acidic systems because of the higher Hg in the fishes from lower pH lakes (Evers et al., 1998).

14.3   MERCURY WITHIN ORGANISMS

Methylmercury is typically found in association with proteinaceous tissues, having an affinity for sulfur-bearing proteins and amino acids such as cysteine (Harris et al., 2003). For this reason, concentrations of Hg, particularly the methylated form, are normally highest in muscle tissues (Bloom, 1992).

The partitioning of Hg within tissues of lower trophic level organisms is not well understood. Storage within an algal cell is known to vary with the form of Hg; whereas the majority of CH_3Hg^+ is found in the algal cytoplasm (up to 64%), most (84–91%) Hg^{2+} adsorbs to the cell wall (Pickhardt et al., 2006).

White muscle is the tissue most often sampled for Hg in fishes because it is high in protein (and as a result high in Hg) but also because it is the most often consumed portion of the fish, making it most relevant in attempting to understand human exposure owing to consumption. Other tissues, however, can be used as surrogates for muscle. Mercury concentrations in fin tissues are highly correlated with those of muscle, but levels are much lower overall (Rolfhus et al., 2008), suggesting low affinity of Hg for the major constituents of fin tissue (i.e., bone). The high correlation, however, is promising for future studies that seek to reduce the lethal sampling of animals.

Kidneys are storage areas for Hg (Celechovska et al., 2008) and other contaminants. Liver and kidney tissues tend to have lower percentage CH_3Hg^+ when compared to muscle (Wagemann et al., 1997; Gnamus et al., 2000; Dominique et al., 2007), although THg concentrations can be higher in these organs compared to muscle (Regine et al., 2006). The lower percentage CH_3Hg^+ may be due to the high amount of fat in these tissues (Jardine et al., 2009a) and the weakly lipophilic nature of Hg (Mason et al., 1996) or due to Hg demethylation processes that occur in the liver (Gonzalez et al., 2005; Eagles-Smith et al., 2009).

In birds and mammals, inert, keratinized structures such as feathers, hair, and claws can be sampled nonlethally from individuals and these tissues store large amounts of Hg that are higher than corresponding soft tissues such as muscle or brain (Wolfe and Norman, 1998). Because keratinous tissues are shed periodically during molting (feathers) or continuously through abrasion (claws), they represent potentially important mechanisms for loss of CH_3Hg^+ by the animal (Furness et al., 1986; Braune and Gaskin, 1987).

From the above observations, some general rules can be crafted for Hg storage in biota. First, concentrations of both THg and CH_3Hg^+ increase with increasing trophic level, but concentrations of CH_3Hg^+ increase more readily. Second, water quality and species composition can greatly influence the concentrations of Hg and the proportion of THg as CH_3Hg^+ at lower trophic levels. Finally, there is considerable variation in the percentage of Hg as CH_3Hg^+ in different tissues of organisms, with liver, kidney, and fish fin tissues having the lowest values; muscle and blood having intermediate values; and hair and feathers having the highest percentages. Whole bodies (e.g., of fish) will, therefore, typically have concentrations and percentage CH_3Hg^+ that represent the proportional contribution of each of these different tissues to the total mass of the animal.

14.4 FACTORS AFFECTING MERCURY IN BIOTA

14.4.1 Growth Rates and Lifespan of Organisms

The accumulation of Hg in organisms is affected by bioavailability (described previously) as well as the organism's bioenergetics. Growth rates are often negatively correlated with Hg concentrations; thus, fast-growing organisms with high food conversion efficiencies (i.e., greater accumulations of mass over the same time period) and lower activity levels will have more dilute Hg in their tissues (Trudel and Rasmussen, 2006), a process known as *growth dilution*. The effect of growth rates on Hg bioaccumulation has been documented in water striders (Hemiptera: Gerridae; Jardine et al., 2009b) and in several species of fish, including lake trout (Borgmann and Whittle, 1992), yellow perch (Essington and Houser, 2003; Dittman and Driscoll, 2009), walleye (Simoneau et al., 2005; McClain et al., 2006) and rainbow trout (*Oncorhynchus mykiss*; Ciardullo et al., 2008), dolphinfish (*Coryphaena hippurus*; Adams, 2009), and catfish (*Clarias gariepinus*; Desta et al., 2007). Intensive fishing has been suggested as a way of decreasing Hg bioaccumulation in aquatic food webs (Schindler et al., 1995), since removal of fish has been shown to diminish competition and increase food availability, which in turn has led to higher fish growth rates and greater dilution of Hg (Verta, 1990; Therien et al., 2003; Mailman et al., 2006; Lepak et al., 2009). Similarly, rapid growth of algal colonies and greater densities of algal cells have been associated with dilution of their Hg concentrations (Pickhardt et al., 2002; Hill and Larsen, 2005; Gorski et al., 2006). Conversely, in areas of low primary productivity and poor nutrient quality, slow rates of growth are correlated with higher concentrations of Hg in algae, which are transferred to higher trophic level organisms such as zooplankton (Pickhardt et al., 2005; Karimi et al., 2007). Following from this, the growth of all organisms depends on the amount and quality of available food. Thus, in areas where primary productivity is low, bioaccumulation of Hg in food webs may be exacerbated and lead to particularly high Hg burdens in top predators. In a study of organisms from an eutrophic and an oligotrophic lake, Kidd et al. (1999) found two to six times higher Hg concentrations in fishes and zooplankton from the less productive system, most likely due to the dilution of Hg by primary producers at the base of the eutrophic food web and the higher growth rates of upper trophic level consumers (Hill and Larsen, 2005).

Closely related to growth rates is the effect of age on Hg concentrations in organisms. Because of the affinity of CH_3Hg^+ for proteins and its tendency to bioaccumulate in muscle tissue, concentrations typically increase in organisms as they age (Ullrich et al., 2001). Thus, long-lived, high trophic level species of fish, birds, and mammals are particularly susceptible to CH_3Hg^+ bioaccumulation (Scheuhammer et al., 2007), especially if they grow slowly. The relationship between age and Hg concentration has been well documented in fish (e.g., lake whitefish, walleye, northern pike, and lake trout; Jackson, 1991; Evans et al., 2005). Stafford and Haines (1997) found that in particular, age and Hg concentrations were strongly positively correlated in non-salmonid fish species. There are, however, instances where concentrations do not change or actually decrease with age/size, likely due to dietary shifts to herbivory (e.g., some tropical fishes; da Silva et al., 2005). For birds, Evers et al. (1998) showed that adult loons (*Gavia immer*) had a Hg burden 10 times greater than that of juveniles; in addition, they found increasing levels of Hg in the feathers of adult loons recaptured after periods of one to four years, which suggests bioaccumulation over their life span. Similar results in other bird species are documented by Scheuhammer et al. (2007). Despite the large number of studies that have demonstrated a relationship between life span and Hg concentrations in organisms, Trudel and Rasmussen, (2006) suggest that in fish, bioenergetics and properties of prey must not be overlooked when considering the causes of increased bioaccumulation with age.

14.4.2 Dietary Habits

The diet of a particular species can vary over time because of changes in prey availability, habitat use, or ontogenetic shifts in feeding. Understanding and quantifying dietary habits of individuals and the relative importance of different prey to a predator's Hg burden is challenging because of the inherent temporal variability and short-term nature of gut contents. However, some generalities exist with respect to how diet influences Hg in food webs. In general, Hg concentrations tend to increase with increasing trophic level such that Hg in detritivores< herbivores< omnivores< piscivores. This has been shown in a number of studies (e.g., Campbell et al., 2003; da Silva et al., 2009).

Diet shifts are a good indicator of the dependence of biotic Hg concentrations on food sources. These often occur on a seasonal basis, as the availability of different food varies. Using stable isotopes of C (δ^{13}C) and N (δ^{15}N) to track diet shifts (see Section 14.5.1), Rimmer et al. (2010) found lower Hg in the blood of Bicknell's thrush (*Catharus bicknelli*) in the summer than spring, which corresponded to a shift from a diet of insect prey toward a more herbivorous diet later in the summer. Similarly, Morrissey et al. (2010) demonstrated that during egg laying, females of the dipper species *Cinclus mexicanus* consumed a more piscivorous diet, which resulted in a transfer of Hg to eggs; this was evident from the δ^{15}N signature in eggs, where those with higher δ^{15}N had higher total Hg concentrations. Correlations between diet shifts and Hg concentrations have also been documented in people who become vegetarians (Srikumar et al., 1992), and in areas where human diet is particularly dependent on seasonal food availability (Lebel et al., 1997; Donkor et al., 2006).

Habitat use is also known to affect Hg concentrations in organisms, and this has been most widely studied in pelagic versus littoral zones of lakes. A recent study by Chételat et al. (2011) has shown that pelagic zooplankton in mid-latitude lakes have higher CH_3Hg^+ concentrations than littoral organisms at a comparable trophic level. Conversely, Eagles-Smith et al. (2008) reported that fish that fed more on pelagic organisms had lower concentrations of Hg than those that fed on benthic organisms. The differences in Hg concentrations between pelagic and littoral components of lake food webs may reflect spatial variation in sources of Hg, particularly in contaminated sites. Eagles-Smith et al. (2008) also showed that pelagic feeding decreased with increasing body size in several fish species. However, this relationship may be obscured when fish feed more equally between pelagic and littoral zones (Swanson et al., 2006). Anadromous fish (those that spawn in freshwater but feed and grow in the sea) often grow faster and are in better condition than individuals of the same species that do not migrate and this life history strategy appears to affect their Hg concentrations. For example, anadromous individuals from an Arctic lake trout population had 40% less Hg than those that remained in the lake, and this appeared to be due to a higher size-at-age for anadromous fish (Swanson and Kidd, 2010). Different habitat use in the Arctic may also affect levels of CH_3Hg^+ in polar bears, where those in pelagic food webs had higher concentrations than those that fed more in sympagic, ice-edge areas (Horton et al., 2009).

The presence of migratory species in an ecosystem can influence Hg in a variety of ways. They can act as a source of nutrients (e.g., marine nutrients into freshwater or terrestrial habitats) and increase productivity, and they can also transport contaminants from one habitat to another (Blais et al., 2005; Swanson and Kidd, 2009; Swanson et al., 2010). This biotransport of nutrients and contaminants has been examined in systems with anadromous fish species such as salmon (Sarica et al., 2004) and migratory birds (Blais et al., 2005), and its effects appear to be greater in systems where species have mass mortalities after spawning (e.g., Pacific salmon) or in systems with very low inherent productivity (e.g., High Arctic systems).

14.4.3 System Properties

Mercury concentrations in ecosystems can vary widely across small and large geographic scales. As we have seen, the properties of organisms within these ecosystems, as well as the characteristics of the food webs they occupy, have important implications for the degree to which Hg accumulates in biota. However, any discussion of the processes that affect Hg bioaccumulation, biomagnification, and bioconcentration would be incomplete without a thorough consideration of the properties of the ecosystems in which these processes are occurring.

14.4.3.1 Watershed Characteristics and Human Activities. A number of characteristics of watersheds are of particular importance in determining the availability and accumulation of Hg in biota. These include both natural attributes, such as the proportion of wetland area in a lake or river catchment, as well as anthropogenic activities such as the presence of hydroelectric developments within a watershed.

Wetlands play an important role in the biogeochemical cycle of Hg and represent significant sites of bacterial Hg methylation (Hall et al., 2008). They are also sources of weakly acidic DOM, and thereby contribute to lower lake pH (O'Driscoll et al., 2005). The percentage of wetland area within a catchment has been positively correlated with levels of CH_3Hg^+ in downstream waters, suggesting that wetlands export this form of Hg to lakes and rivers (St. Louis et al., 1994; Hurley et al., 1995; Rudd, 1995). Percentage wetland area is also positively correlated to concentrations of THg in fish and to CH_3Hg^+ in invertebrates and zooplankton (Westcott and Kalff, 1996; Chasar et al., 2009). Factors that influence the gain or loss of wetlands can therefore be important in determining the amount of CH_3Hg^+ in downstream receiving environments and its uptake into food webs. For example, in many boreal forest ecosystems beavers construct dams that restrict water flow and flood riparian areas, enhancing microbial activity and creating sites for Hg methylation (Driscoll et al., 1998; Roy et al., 2009). Conversely, the draining of wetlands for agricultural or urban development may limit the seasonal wetting and drying of soils and thereby reduce Hg methylation.

Flooding of upland soil and wetlands can release Hg into the water column and increase its concentrations in biota. This is especially apparent in reservoirs and impoundments created by hydroelectric damming (Hecky et al., 1991; Bodaly et al., 1997). In fact, creating reservoirs increases CH_3Hg^+ production in peatlands by up to 40-fold in the period immediately after inundation, and then sustains elevated CH_3Hg^+ concentrations in aquatic biota of all trophic levels over the longer term (Kelly et al., 1997; St. Louis et al., 2004). Marked differences have also been observed in biotic Hg concentrations throughout the food webs of natural lakes versus artificial reservoirs (Surma-Aho et al., 1986; Kamman et al., 2005).

Forestry and logging activities may also affect Hg concentrations in many ecosystems, although this has been especially well studied in boreal forests in Canada and Scandinavia. Removal of forest cover may cause localized increases in the level of the water table, thereby inundating soil and drawing Hg into solution, similar to the effect of flooding associated with hydroelectric dams. Forestry activities and especially clear-cutting also tend to cause siltation into watercourses and thereby increase loading of organic matter (Lamontagne et al., 2000), which itself may affect bioavailability of Hg in aquatic systems (Ravichandran, 2004). Elevated levels of THg and CH_3Hg^+ have been recorded in runoff and lake sediments near forested areas that are clear-cut (Roulet et al., 2000; Porvari et al., 2003). Increases in Hg in water are transferred into the food web, such that higher Hg concentrations have been seen in zooplankton (Garcia and Carignan, 1999) and periphyton from lakes in logged watersheds (Desrosiers et al., 2006). This effect is propagated through the food web because fish such as northern pike also show elevated Hg concentrations compared to fish from watersheds where forestry is not occurring (Garcia and Carignan, 2000, 2005).

Another factor that affects Hg in ecosystems is proximity to point source emissions such as mines, metal smelters, and coal-fired generating stations. Perhaps the most well-known example of a point source of Hg was in the Japanese City of Minamata, where in the 1950s residents developed severe neurologic symptoms as a result of ingesting fish and shellfish contaminated with Hg from a nearby chemical plant producing acetaldehyde (Kurland et al., 1962; Gochfeld, 2003). Other extreme examples of Hg contamination in food webs are seen in areas of mining activity because the waste contains highly soluble forms of this contaminant, which may be readily methylated by microbial activity, especially in the presence of other waste compounds such as iron hydroxides and various thiol-based compounds. Thus, mine waste can represent a significant source of Hg to downstream sediments, which in turn can function as a continuous source of Hg to aquatic biota (Rytuba, 2005). Indeed, high concentrations of Hg have been found in sediments (Hines et al., 2000; Johnson et al., 2009), and across trophic levels, in mine-impacted areas compared to reference sites (Weech et al., 2004; Jardine et al., 2005; Lasut et al., 2010). However, Hg concentrations in fish from relatively pristine areas can be comparable to those from highly contaminated areas, and this is sometimes referred to as the *Hg accumulation paradox*. Schaefer et al. (2004) demonstrated that bacteria from contaminated sites can develop resistance to Hg by demethylating it through the action of the enzyme organomercury lyase (MerB), leading to lower CH_3Hg^+ concentrations in food webs than might be expected for contaminated sites.

Point sources of Hg can influence the proportion of THg as CH_3Hg^+ in tissues of organisms. Plants and animals that are near to point sources such as mines tend to have high concentrations of Hg^{2+} but similar concentrations of CH_3Hg^+ as plants and animals from reference sites, thereby reducing the CH_3Hg^+:THg ratio. For example, periphyton and fish (Family Cyprinidae) in streams draining an industrial site in Tennessee showed an increasing CH_3Hg^+: THg ratio with distance from the site (Hill et al., 1996), and this may also be due in part to the demethylation activity of bacteria in the most contaminated areas.

Many variables related to wind patterns and landscape characteristics appear to affect Hg deposition and accumulation in environments around point sources. Areas downwind of coal-fired generating stations can be affected by local deposition of Hg; for example, Jardine et al. (2009b) found declining concentrations of Hg in lichen from sites increasing in distance from a generating station in New Brunswick, Canada. However, the proximity of habitats to point sources of airborne Hg cannot explain all the variability observed in Hg concentrations among amphibians, fish, and freshwater invertebrates (Pinkney et al., 1997; Jardine et al., 2009b; Weir et al., 2010). Thus, it seems that while some systems will receive elevated inputs of Hg from nearby point sources, bacterial demethylation and localized factors such as wind patterns and the sensitivity of ecosystems are also important determinants of the concentrations of Hg that accumulate in food webs.

Not only do point sources contaminate local environments but they also contribute to widespread global contamination by Hg. Point sources of pollution produce collectively significant deposition of atmospheric Hg into remote and otherwise pristine ecosystems (Fitzgerald et al., 1998; Schuster et al., 2002). For example, concentrations of Hg in Arctic marine and freshwater food webs are relatively high for such remote areas, with no local sources of anthropogenic Hg (Atwell et al., 1998; Campbell et al., 2005; Gantner et al., 2010). Biomagnification in Arctic lake food webs can produce Hg concentrations in Arctic char and other fishes that exceed Health Canada's fish consumption guideline of 0.5 ppm THg (ww); human diets in the Arctic are particularly dependent on fish (marine mammals), and Arctic residents therefore tend to have especially high concentrations of CH_3Hg^+ in their bodies (Van Oostdam et al., 1999). Aquatic systems in the Arctic may be especially sensitive to Hg deposition because of factors such as low primary productivity and the lengthening of the food chain caused by cannibalism within a fish species (Gantner et al., 2010). Another contributing factor in polar systems is the occurrence of depletion events, in which large amounts of Hg are deposited from the atmosphere onto snowpack in the springtime (Ariya et al., 2004). Although it now seems that much of this Hg is photochemically reduced and reemitted to the atmosphere shortly after deposition, depletion events still represent a unique and important source of Hg to Arctic ecosystems (Lalonde et al., 2002). Atmospheric transport and deposition of Hg has also been problematic in sensitive areas of eastern North America, where biological hotspots have been identified in systems with low pH and low primary productivity (Evers et al., 2007; Wyn et al., 2010). In these food webs, Hg concentrations are impacting the reproductive success of top predators such as the common loon (*Gavia immer*) (Burgess et al., 2005).

14.4.3.2 Temperature and Climate. Another factor determining Hg availability and bioaccumulation through food webs is climate. To begin with, Hg-methylation rates increase at warmer temperatures and therefore often peak during the summer, probably as a result of enhanced microbial activity (Bisogni and Lawrence, 1975; Wright and Hamilton, 1982). Hg concentrations in fish have also been shown to peak with summer high temperatures (Bodaly et al., 1993), presumably corresponding to a greater input of CH_3Hg^+ at the base of the food web. Thus, it follows that higher rates of Hg methylation in warmer climates would ultimately produce higher levels of CH_3Hg^+ in top trophic levels because of biomagnification.

However, the level of primary productivity, or trophic status, of an ecosystem is also an important determinant of Hg accumulation in food webs, so it is important to consider this as a possible counteragent to the enhanced bacterial methylation that may occur in hotter climates. Generally, warmer ecosystems have a greater degree of primary productivity (are more eutrophic) and, consequently, most organisms have higher growth rates in these than in colder climates. Thus, dilution of Hg occurs in the relatively high amount of algal biomass at the base of eutrophic food webs; this, in turn, leads to lower concentrations of Hg accumulating in biota of higher trophic levels (Pickhardt et al., 2002, 2005). This is supported by Kidd et al. (1999) and Larsson et al. (2007), who found higher biotic Hg concentrations in oligotrophic compared to eutrophic systems. Other studies have found similar effects for persistent organic pollutants (Larsson et al., 1992).

Considerable discussion and debate is occurring about the effects of climate change on Hg in organisms given that the increases in temperature and changes in precipitation patterns will impact a number of abiotic and biotic processes known to affect Hg cycling. With respect to Hg accumulation in food webs, it is not known whether warmer temperatures will increase or decrease Hg concentrations in upper trophic level biota because the overall trend will be affected by whether concentrations are decreased at the base of the food web and whether biomagnification declines or increases because of changes in the efficiency of Hg and/or energy transfer up the food chain. One current way to examine the effects of climate on Hg in food webs is to contrast studies done in tropical, temperate, and arctic regions. Some of the studies that have used $\delta^{15}N$ to quantify food web magnification of Hg are compiled in Table 14.2. Although data for some system types are limited, a cursory examination does not reveal any general increases or decreases in the log Hg versus $\delta^{15}N$ slope from tropical to Arctic latitudes.

14.4.3.3 Presence of Other Elements. The geology of an area or the pollution of systems with metals or nonmetals from human activities can affect the availability and accumulation of Hg in organisms. One better-known example is

TABLE 14.2 Mercury Biomagnification Slopes (log Hg vs δ^{15}N) Measured in Different Ecosystems (Number of Systems Shown in Brackets)

System Type	Location	Taxa Analyzed	log Hg versus ^{15}N	log Hg versus TL	TMF	Type
Arctic marine[a]	Baffin Bay	Algae, zooplankton, fishes, birds, and mammals	0.20	0.67	4.7	T
Arctic marine[b]	Lancaster Sound	POM, invertebrates, fishes, birds, and mammals	0.20	0.68	4.8	T
Temperate marine[c]	Gulf of Farallones	Invertebrates, fishes, birds, and mammals	0.32	1.09	12.2	U
Temperate marine[d]	Baltic Sea	Plankton, invertebrates, and fish	0.17	—	—	T
Tropical marine[e]	Gulf of Oman	Invertebrates and fishes	0.13	0.44	2.8	T
Temperate estuary[f]	NB, Canada	Invertebrates and fishes	0.04	0.15	1.4	U
Arctic lakes (6 lakes)[g]	Nunavut, Canada	Invertebrates and fishes	0.16–0.26	0.54–0.88	3.4–7.5	M
Arctic lake[h]	Nunavut, Canada	Fishes	0.19	0.65	4.5	T
Temperate lake[i]	WA, USA	Invertebrates and fishes	0.26	0.87	7.4	M
Temperate lakes (14 lakes)[j]	ON, SK, AB, Canada	Invertebrates and fishes	0.14–0.23	—	—	M and T[k]
Temperate river[l]	Potomac basin, USA	Algae, invertebrates, and fishes	0.19	—	—	M
Temperate rivers (21 sites)[m]	NB, Canada	Biofilm, invertebrates and fishes	0.06–0.20	0.22–1.16	1.7–14.5	T
Temperate rivers (21 sites)[m]	NB, Canada	Biofilm, invertebrates and fishes	0.22–0.39	0.32–1.64	2.1–43.6	M

Temperate rivers (8)[n]	OR, WI, FL, USA	Invertebrates and fishes	0.15–0.27	—	—	M and T[o]
Tropical lake[p]	Papua New Guinea	Fishes	0.28	0.95	9.0	M
Tropical lake[o]	Malawi	Invertebrates and fishes	0.20	0.68	4.8	T

[a] Campbell et al. (2005).
[b] Atwell et al. (1998).
[c] Jarman et al. (1996).
[d] Nfon et al. (2009).
[e] Al-Reasi et al. (2007).
[f] Pastershank (2001).
[g] Swanson and Kidd (2010).
[h] Power et al. (2002).
[i] McIntyre and Beauchamp (2007).
[j] Kidd et al., unpublished data.
[k] Methyl Hg for invertebrates and total Hg for fishes.
[l] Tom et al. (2010).
[m] Jardine and Kidd, unpublished data.
[n] Chasar et al. (2009).
[o] Kidd et al. (2003).
[p] Bowles et al. (2001).
TL, trophic level; TMF, trophic magnification factor; Type: M, methyl Hg; T, total Hg; or U, unknown.

for selenium (Se), a nonmetal, or metalloid present in aquatic systems as inorganic selenate or selenite or as organic Se. For decades, researchers have studied whether the presence of selenium (Se; in its inorganic or organic forms) can affect the uptake, toxicity, and storage of Hg in aquatic organisms. However, controversy remains about whether, how, and why these metals interact in the environment and within organisms, and our understanding of how these interactions affect bioaccumulation and toxicity of Hg remains incomplete. For example, some studies have found a negative correlation between Se in water and Hg concentrations in fish, invertebrates, or primary producers, while others have found no relationship between these two metals (see review by Stewart et al., 2010).

14.5   BIOMAGNIFICATION OF MERCURY THROUGH FOOD WEBS

Biomagnification of Hg through aquatic food webs has been studied since the late 1960s when it became evident that fish was the main source of CH_3Hg^+ in the diet of humans and poisoning occurred in areas where CH_3Hg^+ exposure from fish was high (e.g., Minamata Bay, Japan). The trophic transfer of Hg, mainly CH_3Hg^+, has been well studied in a variety of aquatic systems that range in their physical, chemical, and biological characteristics, and it is clear that Hg biomagnification is common across various types of aquatic food webs (Fig. 14.1). CH_3Hg^+ is biomagnified from prey to predator because it is much more efficiently absorbed and accumulated than excreted, especially in larger bodied fishes (Mason et al., 1996; Trudel and Rasmussen, 1997). It is interesting that most of our understanding of Hg in aquatic food webs is based on studies of freshwaters, mainly lakes; this process in marine and estuarine food webs has been comparatively ignored.

The proportion of THg as CH_3Hg^+ increases with increasing trophic level in an aquatic food web (Table 14.1; Mason et al., 1996; Bowles et al., 2001; Zizek et al., 2007). Field studies show that this proportion is normally <20% in primary producers, increasing to almost 100% in top predators such as fish. This is due to the more efficient trophic transfer of CH_3Hg^+ relative to inorganic species with each successive step in the food chain (Mason et al., 1996; Pickhardt et al., 2002). Thus, a herbivorous fish can have low percentage CH_3Hg^+ while a predatory invertebrate can have a high percentage CH_3Hg^+ (Hill et al., 1996; Tremblay et al., 1996; Bowles et al., 2001; Jardine et al., 2009b).

Initially, our understanding of the movement of Hg through aquatic food webs was based on traditional, discrete trophic level (TL) assignments of organisms (i.e., primary producers had TL = 1, primary consumers had TL = 2), and interrelationships between prey and predators that were inferred from gut content analyses or from the literature. Some species can vary in their dietary habits from one system to the next or from one lifestage to another, and, for this reason, it is sometimes unwise to generalize across individuals and populations. In addition, the use of discrete trophic levels ignored the presence of omnivory within a food web. More recently, $\delta^{15}N$ (and occasionally $\delta^{13}C$) have been used to delineate

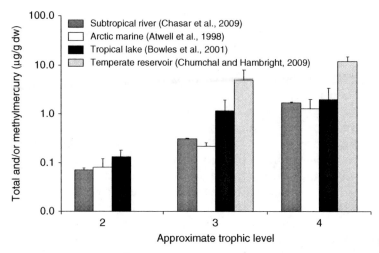

Figure 14.1 Mercury biomagnification in various example aquatic ecosystems. Trophic levels were coarsely assigned using stable nitrogen isotopes. Taxa include benthic insects (trophic level (TL) = 2), forage fish (TL = 3), and piscivorous fish (TL = 4) for the river site (CH_3Hg^+ for TL2, THg for TL3 and 4; Chasar et al., 2009); invertebrates (TL = 2), fish (TL = 3), and birds/mammals (TL = 4) for the marine site (all data THg; Atwell et al., 1998); planktivorous fish (TL = 2), omnivorous fish (TL = 3), and piscivorous fish (TL = 4) from the lake site (all data CH_3Hg^+; Bowles et al., 2001); i. Insectivorous (TL3) and piscivorous (TL4) fishes from a temperate reservoir (all data THg; Chumchal and Hambright, 2009).

feeding habits in aquatic systems (see Section 14.5.1) and better understand Hg biomagnification.

14.5.1 Use of Stable Isotopes to Understand Food Web Structure

Understanding rates of contaminant biomagnification in food webs was greatly enhanced with the introduction of techniques employing natural abundances of stable isotopes of the light elements (Broman et al., 1992). Stable isotopes of nitrogen, carbon, and more recently sulfur have added considerably to our understanding because they act as tracers of organic matter and associated Hg into and through food webs (Jardine et al., 2006). Although stable isotopes are advancing our understanding of how contaminants such as Hg cycle through ecosystems, there remain some limitations of this approach and a number of considerations for experimental design (Jardine et al., 2006, Borgå et al., 2011).

Stable isotopes of nitrogen are the most popular tools for quantifying biomagnification of contaminants including Hg (Jarman et al., 1996). This stems from the observation that the ratio $^{15}N/^{14}N$ (expressed as $\delta^{15}N$) increases in a predictable manner with increasing trophic level, thereby providing a continuous measure of food chain position for consumers (Post, 2002). By exploiting this natural phenomenon we can understand the mechanisms for high Hg concentrations in top predators. In addition, it can now be used to compare Hg biomagnification across systems either as the slope of the regression of log Hg versus $\delta^{15}N$ or trophic level (TL; calculated from $\delta^{15}N$); the former is a measure of the average increase in Hg per mil of $\delta^{15}N$, whereas the latter describes the average increase in Hg per TL. In addition, the antilog of the slope of log Hg versus TL is being used as a trophic magnification factor (TMF) for an entire food web, similar to the BMF described earlier for a predator–prey combination (Table 14.2).

There are three ways in which top predators can achieve different concentrations across sites. In the first, baseline concentrations of Hg in food webs differ (Fig. 14.2a) because of the availability of Hg to primary producers/consumers, as governed by environmental or physiological factors (Watras et al., 1998, Hill and Larsen, 2005). As a result, even though biomagnification rates may be equivalent, the higher Hg at the base of the food web is transferred to top predators. In the second (Fig. 14.2b), although concentrations at the base of the food web may be similar, biomagnification rates through the food web may differ because of the presence of species that accumulate Hg at different rates despite a similar trophic level, or through effects on growth rates and feeding efficiency owing to differences in productivity or environmental stressors (Greenfield et al., 2001; Pickhardt et al., 2002; Trudel and Rasmussen, 2006). In the final scenario (Fig. 14.2c), both baseline concentrations and biomagnification rates are similar, but a longer food chain leading to the top predator results in higher concentrations (Cabana and Rasmussen, 1994; Cabana et al., 1994).

Examples of these three pathways can be found. First, fish from lakes with logging in the catchment had higher Hg concentrations than fish from burnt or reference lakes because baseline Hg concentrations were highest in the former (Garcia and Carignan, 2005). Second, a high biomagnification slope (0.28 for log CH_3Hg^+ vs $\delta^{15}N$, approximately a ninefold change with each trophic level) led to high Hg concentrations in a Neotropical fish in Papua New Guinea (barramundi *Lates calcarifer*; Bowles et al., 2001) despite concentrations in water and sediments being low to average (Bowles et al., 2002). Third, lake trout from lakes with longer food chains have higher Hg concentrations than those from lakes with short food chains (Cabana and Rasmussen, 1994; Cabana et al., 1994). It is also important to note that fish-eating birds and mammals often sit atop these food chains and, as endotherms with higher energy requirements, have far higher food consumption rates and mercury intake than ectotherms. These differences likely affect the biomagnification potential of endotherms, with higher Hg concentrations than expected based on their $\delta^{15}N$ alone, as has been observed for other contaminants (Fisk et al., 2001; Borgå et al., 2011).

Stable isotopes of carbon ($^{13}C/^{12}C$ or $\delta^{13}C$), while used less often than $\delta^{15}N$ to measure Hg in food webs, have nonetheless proven useful as indicators of habitat use and foraging patterns that can inform Hg studies (Power et al., 2002; Kidd et al., 2003). For example, recent investigations have found $\delta^{13}C$ to be a strong predictor of Hg in polar bears, likely reflecting an east–west gradient in $\delta^{13}C$ and Hg (Cardona-Marek et al., 2009), but $\delta^{13}C$ does not always add explanatory power to models describing Hg concentrations (e.g. Senn et al.,

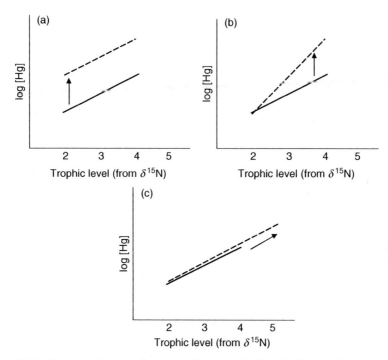

Figure 14.2 Conceptual view of mercury biomagnification in food webs as measured with stable nitrogen isotopes (δ^{15}N). Top predators (trophic levels 4 and 5) can have elevated Hg concentrations as a result of higher baseline Hg concentrations (a), a steeper biomagnification slope (b), or a longer food chain (c).

2010). Interestingly, most studies have found that animals relying on pelagic carbon sources have higher Hg concentrations than those using littoral or benthic carbon sources (Power et al., 2002; Kidd et al., 2003; Ethier et al., 2008; Stewart et al., 2008). Only Eagles-Smith et al. (2008) found the opposite, with higher Hg concentrations in benthic-associated organisms. However, the study site was historically impacted by mining, leading to contaminated sediment that may have influenced Hg concentrations in the benthos (Suchanek et al., 2008).

Given the analytical challenges and resultant cost associated with their determination, stable isotopes of sulfur (^{34}S/^{32}S or δ^{34}S) are used rarely in ecology and less so in contaminant studies. Yet, given the clear role for sulfur-reducing bacteria in Hg methylation, there is an obvious linkage between Hg and S cycling in aquatic ecosystems (Gilmour et al., 1992; Jeremiason et al., 2006). Because many of the same factors (abundance and chemical form) control both S isotope fractionation (Habicht and Canfield, 1997) and the prevalence of methylating activity by microbes (Gilmour et al., 1992), we can hypothesize that relationships between δ^{34}S and Hg concentrations could be observed in aquatic consumers. Indeed, Ethier et al. (2008) report correlations between δ^{34}S and Hg concentrations in pumpkinseed sunfish from lakes in Ontario, Canada, suggesting a link between the cycling of these two elements. Another recent Canadian study of boreal lakes found that analysis of $\delta^{34}S$ can distinguish between planktonic (sulfate in the water column) and benthic (sedimentary) sources of sulfur (Croisetière et al., 2009); thus, S isotopes may complement studies of N and C isotopes by adding greater resolution to our understanding of food web structure and Hg and nutrient sources.

14.5.2 Biomagnification in Freshwater Systems

The majority of our understanding of Hg biomagnification in aquatic food webs comes from studies done in freshwaters. More specifically, lake food webs have been intensively studied (Wiener et al., 2003), whereas stream and river food webs have not (e.g. Tom et al., 2010). With few exceptions (e.g. Chasar et al., 2009), there is a very predictable increase in CH_3Hg^+ concentrations from primary producers to primary consumers, from primary to secondary consumers, and from secondary to tertiary consumers, with the largest increases typically in the lowest trophic levels. As an example, in the pelagic food web of Lake Michigan, CH_3Hg^+ concentrations increase from 10 µg/g dw in zooplankton, to 210 µg/g dw in an insectivorous fish such as the bloater, to 590 µg/g dw in the top predator lake trout (Mason and Sullivan, 1997).

This pattern of increasing CH_3Hg^+ from primary producers to top predators is well established across numerous systems and appears to be independent of the chemical and biological characteristics of the systems (Wiener et al., 2003). Although water chemistry characteristics such as DOC, pH, sulfur, and iron affect the amount and bioavailability of Hg, they do not appear to affect the processes of biomagnification as such. In other words, the extent of these processes is a function of the available pool of Hg at the base of the food web, rather than a product of enhanced biomagnification between trophic levels caused by chemical conditions. Interestingly, this appears to be the case for all environmental variables examined to date, although extensive comparisons are still needed. One potential way to make such comparisons is through the more recent use of $\delta^{15}N$ to quantify Hg biomagnification in food webs, as described in Section 14.5.1 and shown in Table 14.2.

Several studies have now successfully used $\delta^{15}N$ to determine relative trophic positions of organisms within a food web and quantify the rate at which Hg is transferred up through the aquatic food web. Rates of Hg biomagnification (as determined from the slope of the log Hg vs $\delta^{15}N$ relationship) fall within a similar range across varying climates (Campbell et al., 2003, 2005), Houde et al. and levels of acidity (Wyn et al., 2009). These slopes can also be calculated for log Hg versus trophic level (TL; using $\delta^{15}N$ and an enrichment or fractionation factor, see Jardine et al. (2006)). Table 14.2 shows the log THg or CH_3Hg^+ versus $\delta^{15}N$ slopes from a number of biomagnification studies that included primary through tertiary consumers. Although the number of studies is limited, some among-system differences in log Hg versus $\delta^{15}N$ slopes (e.g., 0.16–0.39 for CH_3Hg^+) occur for reasons that are not yet well understood. Similarly, among-system or among-site differences in the log Hg versus $\delta^{15}N$ intercepts occur, likely due to differences in inputs to the base of the food webs but also potentially from variable trophic magnification rates, but their broader utility is not yet appreciated. Interestingly, Tom et al. (2010) found similar slopes across sites within a river but higher regression intercepts at downstream than upstream sites.

14.5.3   Biomagnification in Marine Systems

Mercury biomagnification in marine food webs bears many similarities to what has been observed in freshwaters. There is a progressive increase in Hg (mainly as CH_3Hg^+, e.g., Campbell et al., 2005) from lower to upper trophic levels such that concentrations of Hg are highest in upper trophic level fishes (e.g., shark, swordfish, or tuna), aquatic mammals (e.g., seals), or land-dwelling wildlife that rely on marine biota (e.g., polar bears, seabirds) (e.g., Muir et al., 1999; Braune et al., 2005). Much of the recent focus has been on marine biota in the Arctic because of the importance of fishes and marine mammals in the diets of aboriginal peoples (e.g., Braune et al., 2005). There is a lot of evidence that human activities have increased Hg in animals in this region over the past century (e.g., Braune et al., 2005; Dietz et al., 2009).

A few studies have examined the trophic transfer of Hg through marine food webs using $\delta^{15}N$ (Atwell et al., 1998; Campbell et al., 2005; Nfon et al., 2009) and these too show that its trophic transfer varies across systems (slopes of 0.13–0.32) but is of a similar range as freshwater systems (Table 14.2). Within a particular food web, the slope of log CH_3Hg^+ versus $\delta^{15}N$ is higher (0.22) than for THg versus $\delta^{15}N$ (0.19; Campbell et al., 2003) because of the more efficient transfer and retention of CH_3Hg^+. When making comparisons across studies, it is important to note that this slope may also be affected by the type of organism included in the regression; when some of the top predators include endotherms such as polar bears or seabirds, the contaminant versus $\delta^{15}N$ slope tends to be higher than a food web containing only ectotherms (Borgå et al., 2011).

14.5.4   Biomagnification in Terrestrial Systems

Very little is known about Hg biomagnification in strictly terrestrial food webs (Gnamus et al., 2000; Rimmer et al., 2010). The Hg research community has spent little time studying and reporting on Hg in terrestrial systems, suggesting that low concentrations measured early in the period of Hg concern (i.e., post Minamata), coupled with high concentrations in aquatic top predators, shifted the focus of Hg study away from terrestrial systems. It is useful to make comparisons between terrestrial and aquatic systems by examining the three possible explanations for high concentrations in higher order consumers (Fig. 14.2).

Concentrations reported in the literature suggest that terrestrial Hg baseline levels are low. Agricultural systems give some clues as to the low likelihood of potential Hg contamination in natural terrestrial habitats. Beef cattle and domestic pigs, as primary consumers, have extremely low Hg concentrations in flesh (e.g., 5–11 ng/g, Sell et al., 1975; 1 ng/g, Celechovska et al., 2008). Terrestrial herbivores in natural ecosystems also have low concentrations. For example, THg in lichens across the Arctic was low (37–47 ng/g) and hair from reindeer that feed on the lichens had correspondingly low concentrations (15–80 ng/g) (Lokken et al., 2009), while roe deer far from industrial point sources (smelters) also had low concentrations (3 ng/g ww) (Gnamus et al., 2000). Herbivorous birds and mammals from central Europe (drakes, pheasants, fallow deer, roe deer, hares) also had low concentrations in muscle, ranging from 1 to 89 ng/g ww (Celechovska et al., 2008). Earthworms, considered to be primary consumers in soil ecosystems, actually had concentrations that were quite high for a low trophic level organism, with concentrations as high as several micrograms per gram (Ernst et al., 2008). However, CH_3Hg^+ concentrations in that study were not reported, so the high concentrations may be due to absorption of Hg^{2+} from the surrounding soil matrix.

Biomagnification of Hg in terrestrial systems has rarely been measured, never so with $\delta^{15}N$. As such, it is difficult to quantitatively compare biomagnification rates between aquatic and terrestrial systems. However, rates can be estimated using data from recently published studies. From Rimmer et al. (2010), if we assume that fir needles are at TL 1, all insects sit at TL 2, salamanders and bicknell's thrush are TL 3, and sharp-shinned hawks occupy TL 4, we can roughly estimate Hg biomagnification in a montane forest. The value for this system is an increase of ~2.4 times with each trophic level, lower than all published estimates for aquatic systems (see Section 14.5.3). Alternatively, concentrations in a plant–roe deer–lynx food chain at an uncontaminated site increased from 0.1 to 2.8 to 27.1 ng/g (Gnamus et al., 2000), suggesting average biomagnification of 18 times per trophic level, which would approach the highest values recorded. However, because baseline concentrations were so low, concentrations in the top predator (lynx) were low. Similarly, top predator brown bears also had low concentrations in central Europe (0.01 µg/g, Celechovska et al., 2006).

Food chains leading to human consumers in terrestrial systems are shorter than those in aquatic systems. While large pelagic fish that sit atop long food chains have provided protein for humans for hundreds, if not thousands of years, very rarely are terrestrial top predators (e.g., lions, hawks) consumed, likely due in part to their rarity. Instead, herbivorous mammals form the basis of meat-eating agrarian societies. By default, these species that are low on the food chain will have lower concentrations than food sourced from the ocean, lakes, or rivers.

While Hg concentrations are low in both wild and domesticated terrestrial mammals, concentrations can be high in organs such as the kidney that are often eaten by indigenous peoples (Poissant et al., 2008). This also creates difficulties in accurately measuring Hg biomagnification because these tissues may not be representative of whole body concentrations. However, in general, we can conclude that Hg originating from terrestrial production will be low in concentration and, as such, a limited threat to wildlife that feeds in these food chains.

There is reasonable evidence that aquatic Hg can enter riparian zones, particularly those sites that suffer from point source contamination (Cristol et al., 2008). Export of organic matter and associated contaminants from water to the surrounding riparian zone is a well-documented phenomenon (Walters et al., 2008). Recent evidence suggests that CH_3Hg^+ may in fact be available in some terrestrial habitats but this may also come from a partially aquatic diet by insectivores (Rimmer et al., 2005). For those species that cross boundaries between water and land, land-associated species and life stages tend to have lower Hg concentrations (e.g., amphibians, Bergeron et al., 2010), adding further evidence that Hg is less of an issue for terrestrial consumers compared to aquatic consumers.

14.6 MERCURY STABLE ISOTOPES IN BIOACCUMULATION STUDIES

Recent analytical advances have led to our ability to detect variations in the relative abundance of different isotopes of Hg in minerals and biological tissues (see Chapter 2). For most chemical elements, the fractionation of stable isotopes is caused by mass-dependent fractionation (MDF) processes. However, some isotopes of Hg, along with those of sulfur and oxygen, also undergo mass-independent fractionation (MIF). MIF is calculated based on the degree to which fractionation deviates from the predicted MDF. For more detailed discussions of the theory behind MIF, see Thiemens and Heidenreich (1983), Bigeleisen (1996), Thiemens (2006), and Zheng and Hintelmann (2010).

As in other stable isotope data, MDF of Hg uses "delta notation" and is expressed as $\delta^{XXX}Hg$. Although there are seven stable isotopes of Hg, $\delta^{202}Hg$ has been suggested as a standard measure of MDF (Bergquist and Blum, 2007). These authors report that $\delta^{202}Hg$ is positively correlated to total Hg concentrations in fish. Since THg also correlates to the size, age, and trophic position of fish, the increase in $\delta^{202}Hg$ with THg suggests that the lighter isotope of Hg is preferentially excreted from fish as they age, similar to the excretion of ^{14}N, the lighter isotope of nitrogen. Thus, so far, research indicates that $\delta^{202}Hg$ may be interpreted as an indication of the relative trophic position of an organism, although it appears that diet and habitat use by organisms of similar trophic levels also affect their Hg isotope signatures (Jackson et al., 2008).

Although this field of research is in its infancy, it seems that the complementary nature of MDF and MIF will make Hg isotopes particularly useful in elucidating the complex biogeochemical cycling of Hg. Interestingly, it has been found that only the odd-numbered isotopes of Hg undergo MIF (Bergquist and Blum, 2007). While MDF and $\delta^{202}Hg$ follow a more typical positive correlation with increasing trophic level, MIF of ^{199}Hg and ^{201}Hg occur through non-mass dependent processes such as photochemical reduction and photodemethylation of Hg. To distinguish it from MDF, Bergquist and Blum (2007) report MIF in "capital delta notation," typically as $\Delta^{199}Hg$ or $\Delta^{201}Hg$. Current values in the literature suggest that MIF in fish and other food web components varies across regions and habitats by up to 4‰ (Bergquist and Blum, 2007; Jackson et al., 2008).

Research to date indicates that the $\Delta^{199}Hg/\Delta^{201}Hg$ ratio may be a useful tracer that is specific to certain reaction pathways, and thus may serve as a means of comparison across systems. For instance, Bergquist and Blum (2007) found that the slope of the regression between $\Delta^{199}Hg$ and $\Delta^{201}Hg$ is similar for CH_3Hg^+ in fish and for the MIF signature of CH_3Hg^+ in the water column resulting from photoreduction. This also indicates that the relative proportion of ^{199}Hg to ^{201}Hg remains relatively constant once Hg has been incorporated into the food web. Therefore, the $\Delta^{199}Hg/\Delta^{201}Hg$ ratio may serve as a signature that is indicative of the degree of MIF in CH_3Hg^+ before it enters the food web.

The logical next step in Hg isotope research is to trace natural and anthropogenic sources of Hg into food webs. A few studies have examined the isotope signatures of geogenic Hg (Smith et al., 2005, 2007; Bergquist and Blum, 2007), while others have examined coal deposits, sediments, peat, and soils (Evans et al., 2001; Jackson et al., 2004; Biswas et al., 2007, 2008). As this field of research expands, Hg isotope signatures will likely serve as a means of linking Hg in contaminated ecosystems to its ultimate anthropogenic or geogenic sources.

To date, one of the most significant applications of Hg isotopes has been in tracer studies, where spikes containing mixtures of Hg of known isotopic composition have been used to characterize different sources of Hg to ecosystems. Mesocosm studies (Paterson et al., 2006; Orihel et al., 2008) and a whole lake experiment (Harris et al., 2007) used Hg isotopes to trace its uptake into organisms and the relative contribution of Hg from direct deposition, wetlands, and the terrestrial catchment. They found that Hg applied directly to the mesocosm or lake water was rapidly taken up from the water into zooplankton and macroinvertebrates, and then transferred to fish. Thus, Hg introduced to the lake surface, which under natural conditions would be mostly through precipitation, can be taken up into freshwater food webs and biomagnified into fish within short timeframes. This also implies that reductions in the output of atmospheric Hg might lead to relatively rapid declines in Hg bioaccumulation in freshwater systems. However, the whole ecosystem study also highlighted the fact that equilibrium was not reached within the three years of experimentation. This suggests that although declines in Hg bioaccumulation through the food web may occur in the short term in response to decreased inputs of Hg, it will likely take much longer for the concentrations of Hg in most lake ecosystems to reach equilibrium.

14.7   CASE STUDY—KEJIMKUJIK NATIONAL PARK AND HISTORIC SITE, NOVA SCOTIA, CANADA

Case studies of Hg biogeochemistry and food web biomagnification conducted at a particular geographic location can provide key insights into links between physical and biological processes that regulate Hg cycling. One such case study has been conducted in Kejimkujik National Park and National Historic Site (KNPNHS), located in southwestern Nova Scotia, Canada. The park encompasses 381 km^2 of mixed coniferous and hardwood forest, interspersed with ~50 lakes and ponds (Drysdale, 2005). Granite and slate bedrock underlie most of the park and provide poor buffering capacity to the park's waters (Cumming, 1985). Furthermore, peat bogs abound and acidify water flowing from the catchments; consequently, the lakes in KNPNHS are naturally acidic. Despite the park's pristine nature and remoteness from point sources of pollution, the pH in KNPNHS lakes has decreased further since industrialization because of the deposition of acidifying pollutants (Ginn et al., 2007), and has not recovered despite the stricter industrial emission standards established in recent decades (Wyn et al., 2010). Along with these acidifying pollutants, KNPNHS also receives Hg from precipitation (Banic et al., 2005). This deposition can be attributed to sources of Hg within Atlantic Canada, of which electric power generation and municipal waste incineration are the largest contributors, and to the convergence of westerly wind patterns over Nova Scotia, which transport atmospheric Hg eastward from large North American industrial centers (Rutherford, 1998).

During the mid-1990s, increased concern over Hg contamination in pristine areas led to a study of Hg concentrations in the common loon (*Gavia immer*) in five different regions of North America, including KNPNHS (Evers et al., 1998). This research found that Hg in loon blood increased across a west-to-east gradient and that Hg concentrations in individuals from KNPNHS were twice as high as levels in loons elsewhere. Thus, concern over the levels of Hg in loons prompted further investigation into the problem of Hg contamination in the park, and efforts shifted to the loon's primary prey species, the yellow perch.

In 1996–1997, Carter et al. (2001) collected yellow perch from 24 lakes in KNPNHS representing a range of chemical and physical characteristics. They reported an overall average whole body THg concentration of 0.25 ± 0.14 µg/g (ww) in yellow perch, with a total range of $0.05-0.77$ µg/g and, therefore, wide variation across lakes. Bioaccumulation rates, as measured by THg versus fork length and THg versus weight relationships, also differed significantly among lakes. To allow for comparisons across lakes in the study, a size-standardized perch Hg concentration was calculated based on the average fork length of all individuals (12 cm). This showed that THg in 12-cm perch was positively correlated to aluminum, iron, and total organic carbon concentrations in lake water, and negatively related to pH and alkalinity. These correlations have been documented in a number of other studies elsewhere in North America (Spry and Wiener, 1991; Driscoll et al., 1995; Kamman et al., 2005; Gabriel et al., 2009). Thus, it seems that there is significant variation in yellow perch Hg concentrations across lakes in KNPNHS, and that this variation depends on differences in the physicochemical characteristics of each lake, likely affecting the bioavailability of Hg at the base of the food web. The data of Carter et al. (2001) and Evers et al. (2007) suggests that yellow perch Hg in KNPNHS is within the range of concentrations reported for other areas of eastern North America.

A decade later, in 2006–2007, a follow-up study was conducted in KNPNHS to determine whether the levels of Hg in yellow perch had changed over this 10-year period. Wyn et al. (2010) returned to 16 of the 24 lakes studied by Carter et al. (2001) and found that THg concentrations in yellow perch had increased by an average of 29% in 10 of these lakes. The increase was greatest in fish from lakes with higher pH and lower DOC. This was accompanied by a second study, which investigated Hg concentrations in fish and lower trophic level organisms within the food webs of four lakes with especially high Hg in yellow perch (Wyn et al., 2009). Here, the goal was to determine whether biomagnification was greater in acidic lakes when compared to near neutral systems, perhaps explaining the higher Hg in perch from these low pH lakes. Wyn et al. (2009) measured Hg concentrations (CH_3Hg^+ in invertebrates, THg in fishes) and carbon and nitrogen stable isotopes in pelagic, profundal, and littoral invertebrates, along with yellow perch, brown bullhead (*Ameiurus nebulosus*), golden shiner (*Notemigonus crysoleucas*), and banded killifish (*Fundulus diaphanus*). To compare trophic transfer of Hg across lakes, they examined the biomagnification rate (the slope of log Hg versus $\delta^{15}N$ regression) for each lake. Despite the prediction that biomagnification rates might be higher in KNPNHS because of its acidic lakes and higher THg concentrations in top predators, the rates of Hg biomagnification in these lakes were within the range observed for systems with more neutral pH. However, CH_3Hg^+ concentrations in lower trophic levels were higher than in other systems, particularly in zooplankton, amphipods, and the dragonfly nymph *Aeshna* spp. Thus, this study concluded that differences in the extent of biomagnification could not account for the anomalously high levels of Hg observed in top predators such as loons and perch (Fig. 14.2b). Rather, the concentration of CH_3Hg^+ in lower trophic level organisms was the strongest predictor of THg in fish (Fig. 14.2a).

Ongoing research in KNPNHS is focusing on additional lakes with a range of DOC, pH, and dissolved iron concentrations, as these appear to be the strongest chemical correlates of THg in yellow perch (M. Clayden, unpublished data). In addition to more traditional carbon and nitrogen stable isotope analyses, sulfur isotopes are being used to further investigate the relationships between Hg in food webs, lake sediments, and nutrients in the water column. This case study at KNPNHS and others (e.g., Clear Lake, Suchanek et al., 2008; Everglades, Gilmour et al., 1998) have consolidated research efforts from a variety of disciplines (e.g., biogeochemistry, ecology) in a single location to better understand the complexities of Hg cycling.

14.8 CONCLUSIONS

The behavior of Hg upon entry into food webs is governed by a complex series of biochemical reactions. It is clear that contemporary Hg concentrations in fish and other wildlife remain elevated and threaten the health of the organisms themselves and their consumers. To manage the risks associated with consumption of food items with high Hg (e.g., fish), further research is needed to understand the processes that regulate and enhance Hg uptake into and movement through food webs.

Modern technology (e.g., stable isotope analysis) will continue to aid in investigations of the sources and fate of Hg in natural systems and those modified by human disturbance. Ecological tracers that link consumers to their diets and habitats will help identify prey items and hotspots that lead to high exposure levels for consumers in aquatic systems. These investigations are best carried out in conjunction with other biogeochemical measurements to better understand links between physical and biological factors that govern Hg uptake and accumulation in food webs.

REFERENCES

Adams DH. Consistently low mercury concentrations in dolphinfish, *Coryphaena hippurus*, an oceanic pelagic predator. Environ Res 2009;109(6):697–701.

Allard B, Arsenie I. Abiotic reduction of mercury by humic substances in aquatic system—an important process for the mercury cycle. Water Air Soil Pollut 1991;56:457–464.

Al-Reasi HA, Ababneh FA, Lean DR. Evaluating mercury biomagnification in fish from a tropical marine environment using stable isotopes (delta C-13 and delta N-15). Environ Toxicol Chem 2007;26(8):1572–1581.

Amyot M, Mierle G, Lean DRS, McQueen DJ. Sunlight-induced formation of dissolved gaseous mercury in lake waters. Environ Sci Technol 1994;28(13):2366–2371.

Amyot M, Mierle G, Lean D, McQueen DJ. Effect of solar radiation on the formation of dissolved gaseous mercury in temperate lakes. Geochim Cosmochim Acta 1997;61(5):975–987.

Anderson DW, Suchanek TH, Eagles-Smith CA, Cahill TM. Mercury residues and productivity in osprey and grebes from a mine-dominated ecosystem. Ecol Appl 2008;18:A227–A238.

Ariya PA, Dastoor AP, Amyot M, Schroeder WH, Barrie L, Anlauf K, Raofie F, Ryzhkov A, Davignon D, Lalonde J, Steffen A. The Arctic: a sink for mercury. Tellus B 2004;56(5):397–403.

Atwell L, Hobson KA, Welch HE. Biomagnification and bioaccumulation of mercury in an Arctic marine food web: insights from stable nitrogen isotope analysis. Can J Fish Aquat Sci 1998;55(5):1114–1121.

Babiarz CL, Hurley JP, Hoffmann SR, Andren AW, Shafer MM, Armstrong DE. Partitioning of total mercury and methylmercury to the colloidal phase in freshwaters. Environ Sci Technol 2001;35(24):4773–4782.

Banic C, Blanchard P, Dastoor A, Hung H, Steffen A, Tordon R, Poissant L, Wiens, B. Atmospheric distribution and long-range transport of mercury. In: Parsons MP, Percival JB, editors. Mercury, sources, measurements, cycles and effects. Ottawa (ON): Mineralogical Association of Canada; 2005. p 157–178.

Benoit JM, Mason RP, Gilmour CC, Aiken GR. Constants for mercury binding by dissolved organic matter isolates from the Florida Everglades. Geochim Cosmochim Acta 2001;65(24):4445–4451.

Bergeron CM, Bodinof CM, Unrine JM, Hopkins WA. Mercury accumulation along a contamination gradient and nondestructive indices of bioaccumulation in amphibians. Environ Toxicol Chem 2010;29(4):980–988.

Bergeron CM, Husak JF, Unrine JM, Romanek CS, Hopkins WA. Influence of feeding ecology on blood mercury concentrations in four species of turtles. Environ Toxicol Chem 2007;26(8):1733–1741.

Bergquist BA, Blum JD. Mass-dependent and -independent fractionation of Hg isotopes by photoreduction in aquatic systems. Science 2007;318(5849):417–420.

Bigeleisen J. Nuclear size and shape effects in chemical reactions. Isotope chemistry of the heavy elements. J Am Chem Soc 1996;118(15):3676–3680.

Bisogni JJ, Lawrence AW. Kinetics of mercury methylation in aerobic and anaerobic aquatic environments. J Water Pollut Control Fed 1975;47(1):135–152.

Biswas A, Blum JD, Bergquist BA. Variation in natural mercury isotopic ratios of coal formations. Geochim Cosmochim Acta 2007;71(15): A94–A94.

Biswas A, Blum JD, Bergquist BA, Keeler GJ, Xie ZQ. Natural mercury isotope variation in coal deposits and organic soils. Environ Sci Technol 2008;42(22):8303–8309.

Blais JM, Kimpe LE, McMahon D, Keatley BE, Mattory ML, Douglas MSV, Smol JP. Arctic seabirds transport marine-derived contaminants. Science 2005;309(5733):445–445.

Block M, Part P, Glynn AW. Influence of water quality on the accumulation of methyl (203) mercury in gill tissue of minnow (*Phoxinus phoxinus*). Comp Biochem Phys C 1997;118(2):191–197.

Bloom NS. On the chemical form of mercury in edible fish and marine invertebrate tissue. Can J Fish Aquat Sci 1992;49(5):1010–1017.

Blum JD, Bergquist BA. Reporting of variations in the natural isotopic composition of mercury. Anal Bioanal Chem 2007;388(2):353–359.

Bodaly R, Louis VS, Paterson M, Fudge R, Hall B, Rosenberg D, Rudd J. Bioaccumulation of mercury in the aquatic food chain in newly flooded areas. In: Sigel A, Sigel H, Sigel RKO, editors. Biogeochemistry, availability, and transport of metals in the environment. Boca Raton (FL): Taylor & Francis; 1997. p 259–287.

Bodaly RA, Rudd JWM, Fudge RJP, Kelly CA. Mercury concentrations in fish related to size of remote Canadian Shield lakes. Can J Fish Aquat Sci 1993;50(5):980–987.

Borgå K, Kidd KA, Muir DCG, Berglund O, Conder JM, Gobas FAPC, Kucklick J, Malm O, Powell DE. Muir DCG. Trophic magnification factors: impact of ecology, ecosystem and study design. Environ Assess Manag, 2011; In press.

Borgmann U, Whittle DM. Bioenergetics and PCB, DDE, and mercury dynamics in Lake-Ontario lake trout (*Salvelinus namaycush*) - a model based on surveillance data. Can J Fish Aquat Sci 1992;49(6):1086–1096.

Bowles KC, Apte SC, Maher WA, Kawei M, Smith R. Bioaccumulation and biomagnification of mercury in Lake Murray, Papua New Guinea. Can J Fish Aquat Sci 2001;58(5):888–897.

Bowles KC, Apte SC, Maher WA, McNamara J. Mercury speciation in waters and sediments of Lake Murray, Papua New Guinea. Mar Freshwater Res 2002;53(4):825–833.

Braune BM, Gaskin DE. Mercury levels in Bonapartes gulls (*Larus philadelphia*) during autumn molt in the Quoddy Region, New Brunswick, Canada. Arch Environ Contam Toxicol 1987;16:539–549.

Braune BM, Outridge PM, Fisk AT, Muir DCG, Helm PA, Hobbs K, Hoekstra PF, Kuzyk ZA, Kwan M, Letcher RJ, Lockhart WL, Norstrom RJ, Stern GA, Stirling I. Persistent organic pollutants and mercury in marine biota of the Canadian Arctic: an overview of spatial and temporal trends. Sci Total Environ 2005;351:4–56.

Broman D, Naf C, Rolff C, Zebuhr Y, Fry B, Hobbie J. Using ratios of stable nitrogen isotopes to estimate bioaccumulation and flux of polychlorinated dibenzo-p-dioxins (PCDDs) and dibenzofurans (PCDFs) in 2 food-chains from the Northern Baltic. Environ Toxicol Chem 1992;11(3):331–345.

Burgess NM. Mercury in biota and its effects. In: Parsons MD, Percival JW, editors. Mercury: sources, measurements, cycles and effects. Ottawa (ON): Mineralogical Association of Canada; 2005. p 235–258.

Burgess NM, Evers DC, Kaplan JD. Mercury and other contaminants in common loons breeding in Atlantic Canada. Ecotoxicology 2005;14(1,2):241–252.

Burgess NM, Meyer MW. Methylmercury exposure associated with reduced productivity in common loons. Ecotoxicology 2008;17(2):83–91.

Cabana G, Rasmussen JB. Modeling food-chain structure and contaminant bioaccumulation using stable nitrogen isotopes. Nature 1994;372(6503):255–257.

Cabana G, Tremblay A, Kalff J, Rasmussen JB. Pelagic food-chain structure in Ontario Lakes - a determinant of mercury levels in lake trout (*Salvelinus-namaycush*). Can J Fish Aquat Sci 1994;51(2):381–389.

Campbell LM, Norstrom RJ, Hobson KA, Muir DCG, Backus S, Fisk AT. Mercury and other trace elements in a pelagic Arctic marine food web (Northwater Polynya, Baffin Bay). Sci Total Environ 2005;351:247–263.

Campbell LM, Osano O, Hecky RE, Dixon DG. Mercury in fish from three rift valley lakes (Turkana, Naivasha and Baringo), Kenya, East Africa. Environ Pollut 2003;125(2):281–286.

Cardona-Marek T, Knott KK, Meyer BE, O'Hara TM. Mercury concentrations in Southern Beauport sea polar bears: variation based on stable isotopes of carbon and nitrogen. Environ Toxicol Chem 2009;28(7):1416–1424.

Carter J, Drysdale C, Burgess N, Beauchamp S, Brun G, d'Entremont A. Mercury Concentrations in Yellow Perch (*Perca flavescens*) from 24 Lakes at Kejimkujik National Park, Nova Scotia. Parks Canada—Technical Reports in Ecosystem Science; [Halifax, NS] 2001, 31.

Celechovska O, Literak I, Ondrus S, Pospisil Z. Heavy metals in brown bears from the central European Carpathians. Acta Vet Brno 2006;75(4):501–506.

Celechovska O, Malota L, Zima S. Entry of heavy metals into food chains: a 20-year comparison study in Northern Moravia (Czech Republic). Acta Vet Brno 2008;77(4):645–652.

Chadwick SP, Babiarz CL, Hurley JP, Armstrong DE. Influences of iron, manganese, and dissolved organic carbon on the hypolimnetic cycling of amended mercury. Sci Total Environ 2006;368:177–188.

Chasar LC, Scudder BC, Stewart AR, Bell AH, Aiken GR. Mercury cycling in stream ecosystems. 3. Trophic dynamics and methylmercury bioaccumulation. Environ Sci Technol 2009;43(8):2733–2739.

Chen CY, Stemberger RS, Kamman NC, Mayes BM, Folt CL. Patterns of Hg bioaccumulation and transfer in aquatic food webs across multi-lake studies in the northeast US. Ecotoxicology 2005;14(1,2):135–147.

Chételat J, Amyot M. Elevated methylmercury in high Arctic Daphnia and the role of productivity in controlling their distribution. Glob Change Biol 2009;15(3):706–718.

Chételat J, Amyot M, Cloutier L, Poulain A. Metamorphosis in chironomids, more than mercury supply, controls methylmercury transfer to fish in high Arctic lakes. Environ Sci Technol 2008;42(24):9110–9115.

Chételat J, Amyot M, Garcia E. Habitat-specific bioaccumulation of methylmercury in invertebrates of small mid-latitude lakes in North America. Environ Pollut 2011;159(1):10–17.

Chumchal MM, Hambright KD. Ecological factors regulating mercury contamination of fish from Caddo Lake, Texas, USA. Environ Toxicol Chem 2009;28(5):962–972.

Ciardullo S, Aureli F, Coni E, Guandalini E, Lost F, Raggi A, Rufo G, Cubadda F. Bioaccumulation potential of dietary arsenic, cadmium, lead, mercury, and selenium in organs and tissues of rainbow trout (*Oncorhyncus mykiss*) as a function of fish growth. J Agric Food Chem 2008;56(7):2442–2451.

Compeau GC, Bartha R. Sulfate-reducing bacteria - principal methylators of mercury in anoxic estuarine sediment. Appl Environ Microbiol 1985;50(2):498–502.

Costa M, Liss P. Photoreduction and evolution of mercury from seawater. Sci Total Environ 2000;261(1–3):125–135.

Cremona F, Hamelin S, Planas D, Lucotte M. Sources of organic matter and methylmercury in littoral macroinvertebrates: a stable isotope approach. Biogeochemistry 2009;94(1):81–94.

Cristol DA, Brasso RL, Condon AM, Fovargue RE, Friedman SL, Hallinger KK, Monroe AP, White AE. The movement of aquatic mercury through terrestrial food webs. Science 2008;320(5874):335.

Croisetière L, Hare L, Tessier A, Cabana G. Sulphur stable isotopes can distinguish trophic dependence on sediments and plankton in boreal lakes. Freshw Biol 2009;54(5):1006–1015.

Crump KL, Trudeau VL. Mercury-induced reproductive impairment in fish. Environ Toxicol Chem 2009;28(5):895–907.

Cumming LM. A Halifax slate graptolite locality, Nova Scotia. Current research, Part A. 85-1A. Geological Survey of Canada; Ottawa (ON) 1985. p 215–221.

DesGranges JL, Rodrigue J, Tardif B, Laperle M. Mercury accumulation and biomagnification in ospreys (*Pandion haliaetus*) in the James Bay and Hudson Bay regions of Quebec. Arch Environ Contam Toxicol 1998;35(2):330–341.

Desrosiers M, Planas D, Mucci A. Short-term responses to watershed logging on biomass mercury and methylmercury accumulation by periphyton in boreal lakes. Can J Fish Aquat Sci 2006;63(8):1734–1745.

Desta Z, Borgstrom R, Rosseland BO, Dadebo E. Lower than expected mercury concentration in piscivorous African sharptooth catfish *Clarias gariepinus* (Burchell). Sci Total Environ 2007;376(1–3):134–142.

Dietz R, Outridge PM, Hobson KA. Anthropogenic contributions to mercury levels in present-day Arctic animals - a review. Sci Total Environ 2009;407(24):6120–6131.

Dittman JA, Driscoll CT. Factors influencing changes in mercury concentrations in lake water and yellow perch (*Perca flavescens*) in Adirondack lakes. Biogeochemistry 2009;93(3):179–196.

Dominique Y, Muresan B, Duran R, Richard S, Boudou A. Simulation of the chemical fate and bioavailability of liquid elemental mercury drops from gold mining in Amazonian freshwater systems. Environ Sci Technol 2007;41(21):7322–7329.

Donkor AK, Bonzongo JC, Nartey VK, Adotey DK. Mercury in different environmental compartments of the Pra River basin, Ghana. Sci Total Environ 2006;368(1):164–176.

Drevnick PE, Canfield DE, Gorski PR, Shinneman ALC, Engstrom DC, Muir DCG, Smith GR, Garrison PJ, Cleckner LB, Hurley JP, Noble RB, Otter RR, Oris JT. Deposition and cycling of sulfur controls mercury accumulation in Isle Royale fish. Environ Sci Technol 2007;41(21):7266–7272.

Driscoll CT, Blette V, Yan C, Schofield CL, Munson R, Holsapple J. The role of dissolved organic-carbon in the chemistry and bioavailability of mercury in remote Adirondack lakes. Water Air Soil Pollut 1995;80(1–4):499–508.

Driscoll CT, Holsapple J, Schofield CL, Munson R. The chemistry and transport of mercury in a small wetland in the Adirondack region of New York, USA. Biogeochemistry 1998;40(2,3):137–146.

Driscoll CT, Yan C, Schofield CL, Munson R, Holsapple J. The mercury cycle and fish in the Adirondack lakes. Environ Sci Technol 1994;28(3): A136–A143.

Drysdale C. Kejimkujik National Park and National Historic Site. In: O'Driscoll NJ, Rencz AN, Lean DRS, editors. Mercury cycling in a wetland-dominated ecosystem: a multidisciplinary study. Pensacola (FL): SETAC Press; 2005.

Eagles-Smith CA, Ackerman JT, Yee J, Adelsbach TL. Mercury demethylation in waterbird livers: dose-response thresholds and differences among species. Environ Toxicol Chem 2009;28(3):568–577.

Eagles-Smith CA, Suchanek TH, Colwell AE, Anderson NL. Mercury trophic transfer in a eutrophic lake: the importance of habitat-specific foraging. Ecol Appl 2008;18(8): A196–A212.

Ernst G, Zimmermann S, Christie P, Frey B. Mercury, cadmium and lead concentrations in different ecophysiological groups of earthworms in forest soils. Environ Pollut 2008;156(3):1304–1313.

Essington TE, Houser JN. The effect of whole-lake nutrient enrichment on mercury concentration in age-1 yellow perch. Trans Amer Fish Soc 2003;132(1):57–68.

Ethier ALM, Scheuhammer AM, Bond DE. Correlates of mercury in fish from lakes near Clyde Forks, Ontario, Canada. Environ Pollut 2008;154(1):89–97.

Evans RD, Hintelmann H, Dillon PJ. Measurement of high precision isotope ratios for mercury from coals using transient signals. J Anal At Spectrom 2001;16(9):1064–1069.

Evans MS, Lockhart WL, Doetzel L, Low G, Muir D, Kidd K, Stephens G, Delaronde J. Elevated mercury concentrations in fish in lakes in the Mackenzie River basin: the role of physical, chemical, and biological factors. Sci Total Environ 2005;351:479–500.

Evers DC, Burgess NM, Champoux L, Hoskins B, Major A, Goodale WM, Taylor RJ, Poppenga R, Daigle T. Patterns and interpretation of mercury exposure in freshwater avian communities in northeastern North America. Ecotoxicology 2005;14(1,2):193–221.

Evers DC, Han YJ, Driscoll CT, Kamman NC, Goodale MW, Lambert KF, Holsen TM, Chen CY, Clair TA, Butler T. Biological mercury hotspots in the northeastern United States and southeastern Canada. Bioscience 2007;57(1):29–43.

Evers DC, Kaplan JD, Meyer MW, Reaman PS, Braselton WE, Major A, Burgess N, Scheuhammer AM. Geographic trend in mercury measured in common loon feathers and blood. Environ Toxicol Chem 1998;17(2):173–183.

Fisk AT, Moisey J, Hobson KA, Karnovsky NJ, Norstrom RJ. Chlordane components and metabolites in seven species of Arctic seabirds from the Northwater Polynya: relationships with stable isotopes of nitrogen and enantiomeric fractions of chiral components. Environ Pollut 2001;113:225–238.

Fitzgerald WF, Engstrom DR, Mason RP, Nater EA. The case for atmospheric mercury contamination in remote areas. Environ Sci Technol 1998;32(1):1–7.

Fleming EJ, Mack EE, Green PG, Nelson DC. Mercury methylation from unexpected sources: molybdate-inhibited freshwater sediments and an iron-reducing bacterium. Appl Environ Microbiol 2006;72(1):457–464.

Freije A, Awadh M. Total and methylmercury intake associated with fish consumption in Bahrain. Water Environ J 2009;23(2):155–164.

Furness RW, Muirhead SJ, Woodburn M. Using bird feathers to measure mercury in the environment-relationships between mercury content and molt. Mar Pollut Bull 1986;17:27–30.

Gabriel MC, Kolka R, Wickman T, Nater E, Woodruff L. Evaluating the spatial variation of total mercury in young-of-year yellow perch (*Perca flavescens*), surface water and upland soil for watershed-lake systems within the southern Boreal Shield. Sci Total Environ 2009;407(13):4117–4126.

Gantner N, Power M, Iqaluk D, Meili M, Borg H, Sundbom M, Solomon KR, Lawson G, Muir DC. Mercury concentrations in landlocked Arctic char (*Salvelinus alpinus*) from the Canadian Arctic. Part I: insights from trophic relationships in 18 lakes. Environ Toxicol Chem 2010;29(3):621–632.

Garcia E, Carignan R. Impact of wildfire and clear-cutting in the boreal forest on methyl mercury in zooplankton. Can J Fish Aquat Sci 1999;56(2):339–345.

Garcia E, Carignan R. Mercury concentrations in northern pike (*Esox lucius*) from boreal lakes with logged, burned, or undisturbed catchments. Can J Fish Aquat Sci 2000;57:129–135.

Garcia E, Carignan R. Mercury concentrations in fish from forest harvesting and fire-impacted Canadian boreal lakes compared using stable isotopes of nitrogen. Environ Toxicol Chem 2005;24(3):685–693.

Gilmour CC, Henry EA, Mitchell R. Sulfate stimulation of mercury methylation in freshwater sediments. Environ Sci Technol 1992;26(11):2281–2287.

Gilmour CC, Riedel GS, Ederington MC, Bell JT, Benoit JM, Gill GA, Stordal MC. Methylmercury concentrations and production rates across a trophic gradient in the northern Everglades. Biogeochemistry 1998;40(2,3):327–345.

Ginn BK, Cumming BF, Smol JP. Assessing pH changes since pre-industrial times in 51 low-alkalinity lakes in Nova Scotia, Canada. Can J Fish Aquat Sci 2007;64(8):1043–1054.

Gnamus A, Byrne AR, Horvat M. Mercury in the soil-plant-deer-predator food chain of a temperate forest in Slovenia. Environ Sci Technol 2000;34(16):3337–3345.

Gochfeld M. Cases of mercury exposure, bioavailability, and absorption. Ecotoxicol Environ Saf 2003;56(1):174–179.

Gonzalez P, Dominique Y, Massabuau JC, Boudou A, Bourdineaud JP. Comparative effects of dietary methylmercury on gene expression in liver, skeletal muscle, and brain of the Zebrafish (*Danio rerio*). Environ Sci Technol 2005;39:3972–3980.

Gorski PR, Armstrong DE, Hurley JP, Shafer MM. Speciation of aqueous methylmercury influences uptake by a freshwater alga (*Selenastrum capricornutum*). Environ Toxicol Chem 2006;25(2):534–540.

Grandjean P, Budtz-Jorgensen E, White RF, Jorgensen PJ, Weihe P, Debes F, Keiding N. Methylmercury exposure biomarkers as indicators of neurotoxicity in children aged 7 years. Am J Epidemiol 1999;150(3):301–305.

Greenfield BK, Hrabik TR, Harvey CJ, Carpenter SR. Predicting mercury levels in yellow perch: use of water chemistry, trophic ecology, and spatial traits. Can J Fish Aquat Sci 2001;58(7):1419–1429.

Gutknecht J. Inorganic mercury (Hg^{2+}) transport through lipid bilayer-membranes. J Membr Biol 1981;61:61–66.

Habicht KS, Canfield DE. Sulfur isotope fractionation during bacterial sulfate reduction in organic-rich sediments. Geochim Cosmochim Acta 1997;61(24):5351–5361.

Hall BD, Aiken GR, Krabbenhoft DP, Marvin-DiPasquale M, Swarzenski CM. Wetlands as principal zones of methylmercury production in southern Louisiana and the Gulf of Mexico region. Environ Pollut 2008;154(1):124–134.

Hall BD, Bodaly RA, Fudge RJP, Rudd JWM, Rosenberg DM. Food as the dominant pathway of methylmercury uptake by fish. Water Air Soil Pollut 1997;100(1,2):13–24.

Harris RC, Bodaly RA. Temperature, growth and dietary effects on fish mercury dynamics in two Ontario lakes. Biogeochemistry 1998;40(2,3):175–187.

Harris HH, Pickering IJ, George GN. The chemical form of mercury in fish. Science 2003;301(5637):1203–1203.

Harris RC, Rudd JWM, Amyot M, Babiarz CL, Beaty KG, Blanchfield PJ, Bodaly RA, Branfireun BA, Gilmour CC, Graydon JA, Heyes A, Hintelmann H, Hurley JP, Kelly CA, Krabbenhoft DP, Lindberg SE, Mason RP, Paterson MJ, Podemski CL, Robinson A, Sandilands KA, Southworth GR, Louis VLS, Tate MT. Whole-ecosystem study shows rapid fish-mercury response to changes in mercury deposition. Proc Natl Acad Sci U S A 2007;104(42):16586–16591.

Harris RC, Snodgrass WJ. Bioenergetic simulations of mercury uptake and retention in walleye (*Stizostedion vitreum*) and yellow perch (*Perca flavescens*). Water Pollut Res J Canada 1993;28:217–236.

Hecky RE, Ramsey DJ, Bodaly RA, Strange NE. Increased methylmercury contamination in fish in newly formed freshwater reservoirs. In: Suzuki T, Imura N, Clarkson TW, editors. Advances in mercury toxicology. New York (NY): Plenum Press; 1991. p 33–52.

Hill WR, Larsen IL. Growth dilution of metals in microalgal biofilms. Environ Sci Technol 2005;39(6):1513–1518.

Hill WR, Stewart AJ, Napolitano GE. Mercury speciation and bioaccumulation in lotic primary producers and primary consumers. Can J Fish Aquat Sci 1996;53(4):812–819.

Hines ME, Horvat M, Faganeli J, Bonzongo JCJ, Barkay T, Major EB, Scott KJ, Bailey EA, Warwick JJ, Lyons WB. Mercury biogeochemistry in the Idrija River, Slovenia, from above the mine into the Gulf of Trieste. Environ Res 2000;83(2):129–139.

Horton TW, Blum JD, Xie Z, Hren M, Chamberlain CP. Stable isotope food-web analysis and mercury biomagnification in polar bears (*Ursus maritimus*). Polar Res 2009;28(3):443–454.

Hurley JP, Benoit JM, Babiarz CL, Shafer MM, Andren AW, Sullivan JR, Hammond R, Webb DA. Influences of watershed characteristics on mercury levels in Wisconsin rivers. Environ Sci Technol 1995;29(7):1867–1875.

Jackson TA. Biological and environmental-control of mercury accumulation by fish in lakes and reservoirs of northern Manitoba, Canada. Can J Fish Aquat Sci 1991;48(12):2449–2470.

Jackson TA, Muir DCG, Vincent WF. Historical variations in the stable isotope composition of mercury in Arctic lake sediments. Environ Sci Technol 2004;38(10):2813–2821.

Jackson TA, Whittle DM, Evans MS, Muir DCG. Evidence for mass-independent and mass-dependent fractionation of the stable isotopes of mercury by natural processes in aquatic ecosystems. Appl Geochem 2008;23(3):547–571.

Jardine TD, Al TA, MacQuarrie KTB, Ritchie CD, Arp PA, Maprani A, Cunjak RA. Water striders (Family Gerridae): mercury sentinels in small freshwater ecosystems. Environ Pollut 2005;134(1):165–171.

Jardine LB, Burt MDB, Arp PA, Diamond AW. Mercury comparisons between farmed and wild Atlantic salmon (*Salmo salar* L.) and Atlantic cod (*Gadus morhua* L.). Aquac Res 2009a;40(10):1148–1159.

Jardine TD, Kidd KA, Cunjak RA, Arp PA. Factors affecting water strider (*Hemiptera: Gerridae*) mercury concentrations in lotic systems. Environ Toxicol Chem 2009b;28(7):1480–1492.

Jardine TD, Kidd KA, Fisk AT. Applications, considerations, and sources of uncertainty when using stable isotope analysis in ecotoxicology. Environ Sci Technol 2006;40(24):7501–7511.

Jarman WM, Hobson KA, Sydeman WJ, Bacon CE, McLaren EB. Influence of trophic position and feeding location on contaminant levels in the Gulf of the Farallones food web revealed by stable isotope analysis. Environ Sci Technol 1996;30(2):654–660.

Jeremiason JD, Engstrom DR, Swain EB, Nater EA, Johnson BM, Almendinger JE, Monson BA, Kolka RK. Sulfate addition increases methylmercury production in an experimental wetland. Environ Sci Technol 2006;40(12):3800–3806.

Johnson BE, Esser BK, Whyte DC, Ganguli PM, Austin CM, Hunt JR. Mercury accumulation and attenuation at a rapidly forming delta with a point source of mining waste. Sci Total Environ 2009;407(18):5056–5070.

Kamman NC, Burgess NM, Driscoll CT, Simonin HA, Goodale W, Linehan J, Estabrook R, Hutcheson M, Major A, Scheuhammer AM, Scruton DA. Mercury in freshwater fish of northeast North America - A geographic perspective based on fish tissue monitoring databases. Ecotoxicology 2005;14(1,2):163–180.

Kannan K, Smith RG, Lee RF, Windom HL, Heitmuller PT, Macauley JM, Summers JK. Distribution of total mercury and methyl mercury in water, sediment, and fish from south Florida estuaries. Arch Environ Contam Toxicol 1998;34(2):109–118.

Karimi R, Chen CY, Pickhardt PC, Fisher NS, Folt CL. Stoichiometric controls of mercury dilution by growth. Proc Natl Acad Sci U S A 2007;104(18):7477–7482.

Kelly CA, Rudd JWM, Bodaly RA, Roulet NP, St. Louis VL, Heyes A, Moore TR, Schiff S, Aravena R, Scott KJ, Dyck B, Harris R, Warner B, Edwards G. Increases in fluxes of greenhouse gases and methyl mercury following flooding of an experimental reservoir. Environ Sci Technol 1997;31(5):1334–1344.

Kidd KA, Bootsma HA, Hesslein RH, Lockhart WL, Hecky RE. Mercury concentrations in the food web of Lake Malawi, East Africa. J Great Lakes Res 2003;29:258–266.

Kidd KA, Paterson MJ, Hesslein RH, Muir DCG, Hecky RE. Effects of northern pike (*Esox lucius*) additions on pollutant accumulation and food web structure, as determined by delta C-13 and delta N-15, in a eutrophic and an oligotrophic lake. Can J Fish Aquat Sci 1999;56(11):2193–2202.

Klinck J, Dunbar M, Brown S, Nichols J, Winter A, Hughes C, Playle RC. Influence of water chemistry and natural organic matter on active and passive uptake of inorganic mercury by gills of rainbow trout (*Oncorhynchus mykiss*). Aquat Toxicol 2005;72(1,2):161–175.

Kurland LT, Faro SN, Siedler H. The outbreak of a neurologic disorder in Minamata, Japan, and its relationship to the ingestion of seafood contaminated by mercuric compounds. J Occup Med 1962;4(6):341.

Lalonde JD, Poulain AJ, Amyot M. The role of mercury redox reactions in snow on snow-to-air mercury transfer. Environ Sci Technol 2002;36(2):174–178.

Lamontagne S, Carignan R, D'Arcy P, Prairie YT, Pare D. Element export in runoff from eastern Canadian Boreal Shield drainage basins following forest harvesting and wildfires. Can J Fish Aquat Sci 2000;57:118–128.

Larsson P, Collvin L, Okla L, Meyer G. Lake productivity and water chemistry as governors of the uptake of persistent pollutants in fish. Environ Sci Technol 1992;26(2):346–352.

Larsson P, Holmqvist N, Stenroth P, Berglund O, Nystrom P, Graneli W. Heavy metals and stable isotopes in a benthic omnivore in a trophic gradient of lakes. Environ Sci Technol 2007;41(17):5973–5979.

Lasut MT, Yasuda Y, Edinger EN, Pangemanan JM. Distribution and accumulation of mercury derived from gold mining in marine environment and its impact on residents of Buyat Bay, North Sulawesi, Indonesia. Water Air Soil Pollut 2010;208(1–4):153–164.

Lebel J, Roulet M, Mergler D, Lucotte M, Larribe F. Fish diet and mercury exposure in a riparian Amazonian population. Water Air Soil Pollut 1997;97(1,2):31–44.

Lepak JM, Robinson JM, Kraft CE, Josephson DC. Changes in mercury bioaccumulation in an apex predator in response to removal of an introduced competitor. Ecotoxicology 2009;18(5):488–498.

Lokken JA, Finstad GL, Dunlap KL, Duffy LK. Mercury in lichens and reindeer hair from Alaska: 2005–2007 pilot survey. Polar Rec 2009;45(235):368–374.

Mailman M, Stepnuk L, Cicek N, Bodaly RA. Strategies to lower methyl mercury concentrations in hydroelectric reservoirs and lakes: a review. Sci Total Environ 2006;368(1):224–235.

Mason RP, Laporte JM, Andres S. Factors controlling the bioaccumulation of mercury, methylmercury, arsenic, selenium, and cadmium by freshwater invertebrates and fish. Arch Environ Contam Toxicol 2000;38(3):283–297.

Mason RP, Reinfelder JR, Morel FMM. Uptake, toxicity, and trophic transfer of mercury in a coastal diatom. Environ Sci Technol 1996;30(6):1835–1845.

Mason RP, Sullivan KA. Mercury in Lake Michigan. Environ Sci Technol 1997;31(3):942–947.

McClain WC, Chumchal MM, Drenner RW, Newland LW. Mercury concentrations in fish from Lake Meredith, Texas: implications for the issuance of fish consumption advisories. Environ Monit Assess 2006;123(1–3):249–258.

McGeer JC, Brix KV, Skeaff JM, DeForest DK, Brigham SI, Adams WJ, Green A. Inverse relationship between bioconcentration factor and exposure concentration for metals: implications for hazard assessment of metals in the aquatic environment. Environ Toxicol Chem 2003;22(5):1017–1037.

McIntyre JK, Beauchamp DA. Age and trophic position dominate bioaccumulation of mercury and organochlorines in the food web of Lake Washington. Sci Total Environ 2007;372:571–584.

Mikac N, Niessen S, Ouddane B, Wartel M. Speciation of mercury in sediments of the Seine estuary (France). Appl Organomet Chem 1999;13(10):715–725.

Morel FMM, Kraepiel AML, Amyot M. The chemical cycle and bioaccumulation of mercury. Annu Rev Ecol Syst 1998;29:543–566.

Morrissey CA, Elliott JE, Ormerod SJ. Diet shifts during egg laying: implications for measuring contaminants in bird eggs. Environ Pollut 2010;158(2):447–454.

Muir D, Braune B, DeMarch B, Norstrom R, Wagemann R, Lockhart L, Hargrave B, Bright D, Addison R, Payne J, Reimer K. Spatial and temporal trends and effects of contaminants in the Canadian Arctic marine ecosystem: a review. Sci Total Environ 1999;230(1–3):83–144.

Mzoughi N, Stoichev T, Dachraoui M, El Abed A, Amouroux D, Donard O. Inorganic mercury and methylmercury in surface sediments and mussel tissues from a microtidal lagoon (Bizerte, Tunisia). J Coast Conserv 2002;8:141–145.

Nfon E, Cousins IT, Jarvinen O, Mukherjee AB, Verta M, Broman D. Trophodynamics of mercury and other trace elements in a pelagic food chain from the Baltic Sea. Sci Total Environ 2009;407(24):6267–6274.

O'Driscoll NJ, Rencz AN, Lean DRS. Review of factors affecting mercury fate in Kejimkujik Park, Nova Scotia. In: O'Driscoll NJ, Rencz AN, Lean DRS, editors. Mercury cycling in a wetland-dominated ecosystem: a multidisciplinary study. Pensacola (FL): SETAC Press; 2005.

Olson KR, Fromm PO. Mercury uptake and ion distribution in gills of rainbow-trout (*Salmo gairdneri*)-tissue scans with an electron-microprobe. J Fish Res Board Can 1973;30(10):1575–1576.

Orihel DM, Paterson MJ, Blanchfield PJ, Bodaly RA, Gilmour CC, Hintelmann H. Temporal changes in the distribution, methylation, and bioaccumulation of newly deposited mercury in an aquatic ecosystem. Environ Pollut 2008;154(1):77–88.

Pacyna EG, Pacyna JM, Fudala J, Strzelecka-Jastrzab E, Hlawiczka S, Panasiuk D. Mercury emissions to the atmosphere from anthropogenic sources in Europe in 2000 and their scenarios until 2020. Sci Total Environ 2006;370(1):147–156.

Part P, Lock RAC. Diffusion of calcium, cadmium and mercury in a mucous solution from rainbow trout. Comp Biochem Physiol C 1983;76:259–263.

Pastershank G. Unifying ecosystem concepts and mercury biomagnification in an estuarine environment using stable isotopes (13C and 15N) [dissertation]. Ottawa (ON): University of Ottawa; 2001.

Paterson MJ, Blanchfield PJ, Podemski C, Hintelmann HH, Gilmour CC, Harris R, Ogrinc N, Rudd JWM, Sandilands KA. Bioaccumulation of newly deposited mercury by fish and invertebrates: an enclosure study using stable mercury isotopes. Can J Fish Aquat Sci 2006;63(10):2213–2224.

Peterson SA, Van Sickle J, Herlihy AT, Hughes RM. Mercury concentration in fish from streams and rivers throughout the western United States. Environ Sci Technol 2007;41(1):58–65.

Pickhardt PC, Fisher NS. Accumulation of inorganic and methylmercury by freshwater phytoplankton in two contrasting water bodies. Environ Sci Technol 2007;41:125–131.

Pickhardt PC, Folt CL, Chen CY, Klaue B, Blum JD. Algal blooms reduce the uptake of toxic methylmercury in freshwater food webs. Proc Natl Acad Sci U S A 2002;99(7):4419–4423.

Pickhardt PC, Folt CL, Chen CY, Klaue B, Blum JD. Impacts of zooplankton composition and algal enrichment on the accumulation of mercury in an experimental freshwater food web. Sci Total Environ 2005;339(1–3):89–101.

Pickhardt PC, Stepanova M, Fisher NS. Contrasting uptake routes and tissue distributions of inorganic and methylmercury in mosquitofish (*Gambusia affinis*) and redear sunfish (*Lepomis microlophus*). Environ Toxicol Chem 2006;25(8):2132–2142.

Pinkney AE, Logan DT, Wilson HT. Mercury concentrations in pond fish in relation to a coal-fired power plant. Arch Environ Contam Toxicol 1997;33(2):222–229.

Playle RC. Modelling metal interactions at fish gills. Sci Total Environ 1998;219(2,3):147–163.

Poissant L, Zhang HH, Canario J, Constant P. Critical review of mercury fates and contamination in the Arctic tundra ecosystem. Sci Total Environ 2008;400(1–3):173–211.

Porvari P, Verta M, Munthe J, Haapanen M. Forestry practices increase mercury and methyl mercury output from boreal forest catchments. Environ Sci Technol 2003;37(11):2389–2393.

Post DM. Using stable isotopes to estimate trophic position: models, methods, and assumptions. Ecology 2002;83(3):703–718.

Power M, Klein GM, Guiguer K, Kwan MKH. Mercury accumulation in the fish community of a sub-Arctic lake in relation to trophic position and carbon sources. J Appl Ecol 2002;39(5):819–830.

Ravichandran M. Interactions between mercury and dissolved organic matter - a review. Chemosphere 2004;55(3):319–331.

Regine MB, Gilles D, Yannick D, Alain B. Mercury distribution in fish organs and food regimes: significant relationships from twelve species collected in French Guiana (Amazonian basin). Sci Total Environ 2006;368(1):262–270.

Rencz AN, O'Driscoll NJ, Hall GEM, Peron T, Telmer K, Burgess NM. Spatial variation and correlations of mercury levels in the terrestrial and aquatic components of a wetland dominated ecosystem: Kejimkujik Park, Nova Scotia, Canada. Water Air Soil Pollut 2003;143(1–4):271–288.

Rimmer CC, McFarland KP, Evers DC, Miller EK, Aubry Y, Busby D, Taylor RJ. Mercury concentrations in Bicknell's thrush and other insectivorous passerines in Montane forests of northeastern North America. Ecotoxicology 2005;14(1,2):223–240.

Rimmer CC, Miller EK, McFarland KP, Taylor RJ, Faccio SD. Mercury bioaccumulation and trophic transfer in the terrestrial food web of a montane forest. Ecotoxicology 2010;19(4):697–709.

Rodgers DW. You are what you eat and a little bit more: bioenergetics-based models of methylmercury accumulation in fish revisited. In: Watras CJ, Huckabee JW, editors. Mercury pollution: integration and synthesis. Boca Raton (FL): CRC Press, Inc.; 1994. p 427.

Rolfhus KR, Sandheinrich MB, Wiener JG, Bailey SW, Thoreson KA, Hammerschmidt CR. Analysis of fin clips as a nonlethal method for monitoring mercury in fish. Environ Sci Technol 2008;42(3):871–877.

Roulet M, Lucotte M, Canuel R, Farella N, Courcelles M, Guimaraes JRD, Mergler D, Amorim M. Increase in mercury contamination recorded in lacustrine sediments following deforestation in the Central Amazon. Chem Geol 2000;165(3,4):243–266.

Roy V, Amyot M, Carignan R. Beaver ponds increase methylmercury concentrations in Canadian Shield streams along vegetation and pond-age gradients. Environ Sci Technol 2009;43(15):5605–5611.

Rudd JWM. Sources of methyl mercury to fresh-water ecosystems - a review. Water Air Soil Pollut 1995;80(1–4):697–713.

Rutherford LA. Mercury sources. In: Burgess N, Beauchamp S, Brun G, Clair T, Roberts C, Rutherford L, Tordon R, Vaidya O, editors. Mercury in Atlantic Canada: a progress report. Environment Canada-Atlantic Region; Ottawa (ON) 1998.

Rytuba JJ. Geogenic and mining sources of mercury to the environment. In: Parsons MB, JB Percival, editors. Mercury: sources, measurements, cycles and effects. Halifax,Mineralogical Association of Canada; 2005. p 21–36.

Sandheinrich MB, Wiener JG. Methylmercury in freshwater fish: recent advances in assessing toxicity of environmentally relevant exposures. In: Beyer WN, Meador JP, editors. Environmental contaminants in biota: interpreting tissue concentrations. 2nd ed. Boca Raton (FL): Taylor and Francis Publishers; 2010. p 169–192.

Sarica J, Amyot M, Hare L, Doyon MR, Stanfield LW. Salmon-derived mercury and nutrients in a Lake Ontario spawning stream. Limnol Oceanogr 2004;49(4):891–899.

Schaefer JK, Morel FMM. High methylation rates of mercury bound to cysteine by *Geobacter sulfurreducens*. Nat Geosci 2009;2(2):123–126.

Schaefer JK, Yagi J, Reinfelder JR, Cardona T, Ellickson KM, Tel-Or S, Barkay T. Role of the bacterial organomercury lyase (MerB) in controlling methylmercury accumulation in mercury-contaminated natural waters. Environ Sci Technol 2004;38(16):4304–4311.

Scheuhammer AM. Effects of acidification on the availability of toxic metals and calcium to wild birds and mammals. Environ Pollut 1991;71(2–4):329–375.

Scheuhammer AM, Meyer MW, Sandheinrich MB, Murray MW. Effects of environmental methylmercury on the health of wild birds, mammals, and fish. Ambio 2007;36(1):12–18.

Schindler DW, Kidd KA, Muir DCG, Lockhart WL. The effects of ecosystem characteristics on contaminant distribution in northern fresh-water lakes. Sci Total Environ 1995;160,161:1–17.

Schuster PF, Krabbenhoft DP, Naftz DL, Cecil LD, Olson ML, Dewild JF, Susong DD, Green JR, Abbott ML. Atmospheric mercury deposition during the last 270 years: a glacial ice core record of natural and anthropogenic sources. Environ Sci Technol 2002;36(11):2303–2310.

Sell JL, Deitz FD, Buchanan ML. Concentration of mercury in animal products and soils of North Dakota. Arch Environ Contam Toxicol 1975;3:278–288.

Sellers P, Kelly CA, Rudd JWM, MacHutchon AR. Photodegradation of methylmercury in lakes. Nature 1996;380(6576):694–697.

Senn DB, Chesney EJ, Blum JD, Bank MS, Maage A, Shine JP. Stable isotope (N, C, Hg) study of methylmercury sources and trophic transfer in the Northern Gulf of Mexico. Environ Sci Technol 2010;44(5):1630–1637.

da Silva DS, Lucotte M, Paquet S, Davidson R. Influence of ecological factors and of land use on mercury levels in fish in the Tapajos River basin, Amazon. Environ Res 2009;109(4):432–446.

da Silva DS, Lucotte M, Roulet M, Poirier H, Mergler D, Santos EO, Crossa M. Trophic structure and bioaccumulation of mercury in fish of three natural lakes of the Brazilian Amazon. Water Air Soil Pollut 2005;165:77–94.

Simoneau M, Lucotte M, Garceau S, Laliberte D. Fish growth rates modulate mercury concentrations in walleye (*Sander vitreus*) from eastern Canadian lakes. Environ Res 2005;98(1):73–82.

Smith CN, Kesler SE, Blum JD, Rytuba JJ. Isotope geochemistry of mercury in source rocks, mineral deposits and spring deposits of the California Coast Ranges, USA. Earth Planet Sci Lett 2008;269(3,4):398–406.

Smith CN, Kesler SE, Klaue B, Blum JD. Mercury isotope fractionation in fossil hydrothermal systems. Geology 2005;33(10):825–828.

Snodgrass JW, Jagoe CH, Bryan AL, Brant HA, Burger J. Effects of trophic status and wetland morphology, hydroperiod, and water chemistry on mercury concentrations in fish. Can J Fish Aquat Sci 2000;57(1):171–180.

Spry DJ, Wiener JG. Metal bioavailability and toxicity to fish in low-alkalinity lakes-a critical-review. Environ Pollut 1991;71(2–4):243–304.

Srikumar TS, Johansson GK, Ockerman PA, Gustafsson JA, Akesson B. Trace-element status in healthy-subjects switching from a mixed to a lactovegetarian diet for 12 Mo. Am J Clin Nutr 1992;55(4):885–890.

Stafford CP, Haines TA. Mercury concentrations in Maine sport fishes. Trans Amer Fish Soc 1997;126(1):144–152.

Stewart AR, Saiki MK, Kuwabara JS, Alpers CN, Marvin-DiPasquale M, Krabbenhoft DP. Influence of plankton mercury dynamics and trophic pathways on mercury concentrations of top predator fish of a mining-impacted reservoir. Can J Fish Aquat Sci 2008;65(11):2351–2366.

Stewart R, Grosell M, Buchwalter D, Fisher N, Luoma S, Mathews T, Orr P, Wang W-X. Bioaccumulation and trophic transfer of selenium. In: Chapman PM, Adams WJ, Brooks ML, Delos CG, Luoma SN, Maher WA, Ohlendorf HM, Presser TS, Shaw DP, editors. Ecological assessment of selenium in the aquatic environment. Boca Raton (FL): CRC Press; 2010. p 93–140.

St. Louis VL, Rudd JWM, Kelly CA, Beaty KG, Bloom NS, Flett RJ. Importance of wetlands as sources of methyl mercury to boreal forest ecosystems. Can J Fish Aquat Sci 1994;51(5):1065–1076.

St. Louis VL, Rudd JWM, Kelly CA, Bodaly RA, Paterson MJ, Beaty KG, Hesslein RH, Heyes A, Majewski AR. The rise and fall of mercury methylation in an experimental reservoir. Environ Sci Technol 2004;38(5):1348–1358.

Suchanek TH, Eagles-Smith CA, Slotton DG, Harner EJ, Adam DP. Mercury in abiotic matrices of Clear Lake, California: human health and ecotoxicological implications. Ecol Appl 2008;18(8): A128–A157.

Surma-Aho K, Paasivirta J, Rekolainen S, Verta M. Organic and inorganic mercury in the food-chain of some lakes and reservoirs in Finland. Chemosphere 1986;15(3):353–372.

Swanson HK, Kidd KA. Mercury concentrations in Arctic food fishes reflect the presence of anadromous Arctic charr (*Salvelinus alpinus*), species, and life history. Environ Sci Technol 2010;44(9):3286–3292.

Swanson HK, Kidd KA, Reist JD. Effects of partially anadromous Arctic charr (*Salvelinus alpinus*) populations on ecology of coastal Arctic lakes. Ecosystems 2010;13(2):261–274.

Swanson HK, Johnston TA, Schindler DW, Bodaly RA, Whittle DM. Mercury bioaccumulation in forage fish communities invaded by rainbow smelt (*Osmerus mordax*). Environ Sci Technol 2006;40(5):1439–1446.

Therien N, Surette C, Fortin R, Lucotte M, Garceau S, Schetagne R, Tremblay A. Reduction of mercury concentration in fish through intensive fishing of lakes: a preliminary testing of assumptions. In: Brebbia CA, editor. River basin management II. Southampton: Wit Press; 2003. p 365–376.

Thiemens MH. History and applications of mass-independent isotope effects. Annu Rev Earth Planet Sci 2006;34:217–262.

Thiemens MH, Heidenreich JE. The mass-independent fractionation of oxygen- a novel isotope effect and its possible cosmochemical implications. Science 1983;219(4588):1073–1075.

Tom KR, Newman MC, Schmerfeld J. Modeling mercury biomagnification (South River, Virginia, USA) to inform river management decision making. Environ Toxicol Chem 2010;29(4):1013–1020.

Tremblay A, Lucotte M, Rheault I. Methylmercury in a benthic food web of two hydroelectric reservoirs and a natural lake of Northern Quebec (Canada). Water Air Soil Pollut 1996;91(3,4):255–269.

Trudel M, Rasmussen JB. Modeling the elimination of mercury by fish. Environ Sci Technol 1997;31(6):1716–1722.

Trudel M, Rasmussen JB. Bioenergetics and mercury dynamics in fish: a modelling perspective. Can J Fish Aquat Sci 2006;63(8):1890–1902.

Tsui MTK, Finlay JC, Nater EA. Mercury bioaccumulation in a stream network. Environ Sci Technol 2009;43(18):7016–7022.

Tsui MTK, Wang WX. Uptake and elimination routes of inorganic mercury and methylmercury in *Daphnia magna*. Environ Sci Technol 2004;38(3):808–816.

Ullrich SM, Tanton TW, Abdrashitova SA. Mercury in the aquatic environment: a review of factors affecting methylation. Crit Rev Environ Sci Technol 2001;31(3):241–293.

Van Oostdam J, Gilman A, Dewailly E, Usher P, Wheatley B, Kuhnlein H, Neve S, Walker J, Tracy B, Feeley M, Jerome V, Kwavnick B. Human health implications of environmental contaminants in Arctic Canada: a review. Sci Total Environ 1999;230(1–3):1–82.

Verta M. Changes in fish mercury concentrations in an intensively fished lake. Can J Fish Aquat Sci 1990;47(10):1888–1897.

Wagemann R, Trebacz E, Hunt R, Boila G. Percent methylmercury and organic mercury in tissues of marine mammals and fish using different experimental and calculation methods. Environ Toxicol Chem 1997;16(9):1859–1866.

Walters DM, Fritz KM, Johnson BR, Lazorchak JM, McCormico FH. Influence of trophic position and spatial location on polychlorinated biphenyl (PCB) bioaccumulation in a stream food web. Environ Sci Technol 2008;42(7):2316–2322.

Watras CJ, Back RC, Halvorsen S, Hudson RJM, Morrison KA, Wente SP. Bioaccumulation of mercury in pelagic freshwater food webs. Sci Total Environ 1998;219(2,3):183–208.

Watras CJ, Bloom NS. Mercury and methylmercury in individual zooplankton-Implications for bioaccumulation. Limnol Oceanogr 1992;37(6):1313–1318.

Weech SA, Scheuhammer AM, Elliott JE, Cheng KM. Mercury in fish from the Pinchi Lake Region, British Columbia, Canada. Environ Pollut 2004;131(2):275–286.

Weir SM, Halbrook RS, Sparling DW. Mercury concentrations in wetlands associated with coal-fired power plants. Ecotoxicology 2010;19(2):306–316.

Weis JS. Reproductive, developmental, and neurobehavioral effects of methylmercury in fishes. J Environ Sci Health C 2009;27(4):212–225.

Westcott K, Kalff J. Environmental factors affecting methyl mercury accumulation in zooplankton. Can J Fish Aquat Sci 1996;53(10):2221–2228.

Wiener JG, Krabbenhoft DP, Heinz GH, Scheuhammer AM. Ecotoxicology of mercury. In: Hoffman DJ, Rattner BA, Burton GA Jr, J Cairns, editors. Handbook of ecotoxicology, 2nd ed. Boca Raton (FL): CRC Press, Inc; 2003. p 409–464.

Wolfe M, Norman D. Effects of waterborne mercury on terrestrial wildlife at Clear Lake: evaluation and testing of a predictive model. Environ Toxicol Chem 1998;17(2):214–227.

Wren CD, Scheider WA, Wales DL, Muncaster BW, Gray IM. Relation between mercury concentrations in walleye (*Stizostedion vitreum*) and northern pike (*Esox lucius*) in Ontario lakes and influence of environmental factors. Can J Fish Aquat Sci 1991;48(1):132–139.

Wright DR, Hamilton RD. Release of methyl mercury from sediments-effects of mercury concentration, low-temperature, and nutrient addition. Can J Fish Aquat Sci 1982;39(11):1459–1466.

Wyn B, Kidd KA, Burgess NM, Curry RA. Mercury biomagnification in the food webs of acidic lakes in Kejimkujik National Park and National Historic Site, Nova Scotia. Can J Fish Aquat Sci 2009;66(9):1532–1545.

Wyn B, Kidd KA, Burgess NM, Curry RA, Munkittrick KR. Increasing mercury in yellow perch at a hotspot in Atlantic Canada, Kejimkujik National Park. Environ Sci Technol 2010;44(23):9176–9181.

Zhang H, Lindberg SE. Sunlight and iron(III)-induced photochemical production of dissolved gaseous mercury in freshwater. Environ Sci Technol 2001;35(5):928–935.

Zhang JZ, Wang FY, House JD, Page B. Thiols in wetland interstitial waters and their role in mercury and methylmercury speciation. Limnol Oceanogr 2004;49(6):2276–2286.

Zheng W, Hintelmann H. Nuclear field shift effect in isotope fractionation of mercury during abiotic reduction in the absence of light. J Phys Chem A 2010;114(12):4238–4245.

Zizek S, Horvat M, Gibicar D, Fajon V, Toman MJ. Bioaccumulation of mercury in benthic communities of a river ecosystem affected by mercury mining. Sci Total Environ 2007;377(2,3):407–415.

CHAPTER 15

A REVIEW OF MERCURY TOXICITY WITH SPECIAL REFERENCE TO METHYLMERCURY

MINESHI SAKAMOTO, KATSUYUKI MURATA, AKIYOSHI KAKITA, and MASANORI SASAKI

15.1 INTRODUCTION

The epidemic known as *Minamata disease* was the first instance on record of severe methylmercury poisoning caused by man-made environmental pollution in Minamata City, Japan. It was caused by the consumption of large amounts of fish and shellfish heavily contaminated with methylmercury discharged from a chemical plant (Irukayama and Kondo, 1966). Residents living around the small Minamata Bay, who were dependent on the fish and shellfish caught in the Bay, were poisoned first. The poisoning spread to the people living around the surrounding Shiranui Sea after the company changed to release the wastewater to the mouth of the Minamata River. The first case was reported in 1956, and the discharge of methylmercury continued through 1968. The pollution level was extraordinarily high and the average hair Hg concentration in patients was an astonishing 338.4 ppm (range: 96.8-705 ppm). The principal symptoms were neurological disorders (Takeuchi et al., 1962) . After the first case, the number of patients rapidly increased. To date, more than 2200 people in the Minamata districts (1780 in Kumamoto Prefecture and 491 in Kagoshima Prefecture as of June 2011) have been certified to have Minamata disease. In 1968, patients with Minamata disease were also recognized in the Agano River basin in Niigata Prefecture (699 as of March 2011). In Minamata district, many fetuses exposed to methylmercury through the placenta displayed severe cerebral palsy-like symptoms, while their mothers had mild or no manifestation of the poisoning (Harada, 1978). Outbreaks of typical fetal-type Minamata disease occurred between 1955 and 1959, when the mercury pollution appears to have been worst

Environmental Chemistry and Toxicology of Mercury, First Edition.
Edited by Guangliang Liu, Yong Cai, and Nelson O'Driscoll.
© 2012 John Wiley & Sons, Inc. Published 2012 by John Wiley & Sons, Inc.

judging from the incidence of cases (Harada, 1978) and the methylmercury concentration in the preserved umbilical cords of inhabitants in the area (Nishigaki and Harada, 1975; Sakamoto et al., 2010). This landmark event was the first to bring to worldwide attention the risk of fetal methylmercury exposure. The epidemic showed that fetuses comprise a high risk group because of the high susceptibility of the developing brain to methylmercury exposure (Choi, 1989; WHO, 1990; Sakamoto et al., 1993). Moreover, methylmercury easily crosses the blood–placenta barrier, accumulating more in the fetus than in the mother (Choi, 1989; WHO, 1990; Sakamoto et al., 2002b, 2004b; Stern and Smith, 2003).

Mercury is released mainly as Hg(0) into the atmosphere from natural and anthropogenic sources. Recent studies indicated that human activity contributes ~50-70% of total emission into the environment, making it a large contribution to the global mercury cycle (UNEP, 2002). The effects of methylmercury exposure on fetuses is a matter of great concern, especially among populations of humans who consume large quantities of fish and sea mammals (WHO, 1990; Myers et al., 1995; Grandjean et al., 1997, 2005; NRC, 2000; Myers et al., 2003b).

15.2 GLOBAL MERCURY EMISSION INTO THE ATMOSPHERE

Fossil fuel combustion and volcanoes emit large amounts of Hg(0) and particle-bound mercury. Most mercury in the air is gaseous Hg(0) because it has a much longer retention time in the atmosphere than the other forms (UNEP, 2002). Global atmospheric releases of mercury from human activity were estimated at ~1930 t (range, 1230-2890 t) in 2005 (UNEP, 2008), which included fossil fuel combustion (878 t), artisanal and small-scale gold production (350 t), metal production excluding gold (200 t), cement production (189 t), waste incineration, waste and other (125 t), large-scale gold production (111 t), chlor-alkali industry (47 t), and dental amalgam cremation (26 t). This number is in the same range as estimates of natural emission from oceans (400–1300 t per year) plus emissions from land (500-1000 t per year). The estimated anthropogenic Hg(0) emissions from Asia are particularly high, followed by those in North America and Europe (UNEP, 2002). Further, the atmospheric mercury concentration in the Northern Hemisphere is double that in the Southern Hemisphere (UNEP, 2002). Figures indicate that global mercury emissions have increased since the industrial revolution started. The United Nations Environment Programme Global Mercury Assessment project was initiated to investigate the possibility of setting international limits on mercury emissions, deemed necessary because mercury concentrations in superficial ice in the Arctic have increased (UNEP, 2002).

Hg(0) emitted into the atmosphere is oxidized and transformed into Hg^{2+}, a portion of which is methylated (mainly by aquatic bacteria) and enters the aquatic food chain. Species high in the trophic web tend to have higher concentrations of mercury (e.g., >10 μg/g in whales (toothed) and >1 μg/g in sharks, pike, swordfish, and tuna). Although regional pollution caused by high concentrations of methylmercury such as that in Minamata, is very rare nowadays, the Hg concentrations in fish and other seafood may be increasing because of other mercury emissions of anthropogenic origin (UNEP, 2002). Recently, there have been active research programs focusing on the global mercury cycle, particularly in Western countries where emissions of Hg(0) and sulfur have polluted the environment (e.g., the American Great Lakes and Scandinavian inland waters). The pollution of these waters has raised concerns over a possible future increase in human exposure to methylmercury.

15.3   METABOLISM AND TOXICITY OF CHEMICAL FORMS OF MERCURY

Human absorption of liquid Hg(0) is minimal, and acute toxicity does not occur even when the liquid mercury used in thermometers is accidentally ingested. The problem arises when liquid mercury is heated and goes into the gaseous phase, which causes acute interstitial pneumonia when inhaled at a high concentration. Approximately 80% of inhaled gaseous Hg(0) is absorbed into the blood and easily passes through the blood-brain barrier in its unoxidized form, thereby reaching the brain and damaging the central nervous system. With time, gaseous Hg(0) in the body is oxidized to Hg^{2+}, which accumulates in the kidneys and causes damage there (WHO, 1991). The biological half-life of Hg absorbed from vapor into the blood is approximately two to four days when 90% is excreted through urine and feces. Absorption of Hg^{2+} through the digestive tract is comparatively low. However, a large intake of Hg^{2+}, such as in accidental or suicidal ingestion, causes digestive tract and kidney disorders resulting in death (WHO, 1991). Methylmercury is readily absorbed by the digestive tract and enters the central nervous system after passing the blood-brain barrier, thereby causing degeneration and dysfunction of nerve cells (Takeuchi, 1982; WHO, 1991).

Methylmercury transport into tissues appears to be mediated by the formation of a methylmercury-cysteine conjugate, which is transported into cells via a neutral amino acid carrier protein (WHO, 1990; NRC, 2000). The brain of the developing fetus is very sensitive to methylmercury. In addition, the methylmercury concentration in fetal blood reaches ~1.6-fold higher (range: 1.03-2.23) than that of the mother, as summarized in Table 15.1, because of active methylmercury transport across the placenta (WHO, 1990; NRC, 2000). Thus, fetuses are recognized as the highest risk group for methylmercury.

15.3.1   Exposure Evaluation

For determining the effects of methylmercury on the human body, the preferred biomarker is one that occurs in the body and reflects the methylmercury concentration in the brain, since the brain is the major target organ. In humans, methylmercury has an average biological half-life of ~70 days (whole body) (WHO, 1990). Generally, the amount retained in the body becomes stable

TABLE 15.1 Total Mercury (T-Hg) and Methylmercury (MeHg) Concentrations in Maternal and Cord Blood in Study Populations

Study Site	Measure	No. of Samples	Mean Maternal Blood	Mean cord	Cord/ Maternal blood Ratio	References
Seville, Spain	T-Hg μg/L	24	6.23	6.43	1.03	Soria et al. (1992)
China	T-Hg μg/L	9	6.77	10.4	1.54	Yang et al. (1997)
Greenland	T-Hg μg/L	178	16.8	35.6	2.12	Bjerregaard and Hansen (2000)
Quebec, Canada	T-Hg μg/L	92	0.48	0.52	1.08	Morrissette et al. (2004)
Tehran, Iran	T-Hg μg/L	365	1.34	1.7	1.27	Vigeh et al. (2006)
Arctic Canada	T-Hg μg/L	402	2.96	5.8	1.96	Butler Walker et al. (2006)
Fukuoka, Japan	T-Hg ng/g	115	5.18	9.81	1.89	Sakamoto et al. (2007b)
Istanbul, Turkey	T-Hg μg/L	143	0.38	0.5	1.32	Unuvar et al. (2007)
Taipei, Taiwan	T-Hg ng/g	65	9.1	10	1.1	Hsu et al. (2007)
Slovakia	T-Hg μg/L	99	0.63	0.8	1.27	Palkovicova et al. (2008)
Seville, Spain	MeHg μg/L	17	4.97	5.25	1.06	Soria et al. (1992)
China	MeHg μg/L	9	2.5	4.18	1.67	Yang et al. (1997)
Solna, Sweden	MeHg μg/L	98	0.73	1.4	1.92	Vahter et al. (2000)
Quebec, Canada	MeHg μg/L	92	0.23	0.39	1.7	Morrissette et al. (2004)
Arctic Canada	MeHg μg/L	402	2.2	4.9	2.23	Butler Walker et al. (2006)
Fukuoka, Japan	MeHg ng/g	115	4.77	9.32	1.95	Sakamoto et al. (2007b)

under constant methylmercury exposure, and depends on dietary intake. Animal experiments indicate that the ratio of the Hg concentration in the blood to that in the brain becomes fixed under steady-state conditions. Therefore, the mercury concentration in the blood is a good biomarker of the concentration in the brain (WHO, 1990). The mercury concentration in the hair also reflects blood methylmercury concentration during hair formation and is frequently used as a biomarker for evaluating methylmercury exposure (WHO, 1990). Generally, the Hg concentration in the hair is 250-fold higher than that in the blood, because sulfur-containing proteins in the hair bind to methylmercury.

The major form of mercury in the urine is inorganic mercury, and the total mercury concentration in the urine reflects the amount of inorganic mercury accumulated in the kidney, which is a good biomarker for evaluating inorganic mercury exposure (WHO, 1995). On the other hand, elevated exposure to gaseous elemental mercury at high concentration causes acute toxicity, (e.g., respiratory distress, breathing difficulty, bronchitis, and renal tubular damage) (WHO, 1995). Consequently, the lungs are another target organ for acute exposure.

15.3.1.1 Exposure Evaluation for the Fetus and Breast-Fed Offspring.
The National Research Council (NRC, 2000) has recommended umbilical cord

blood mercury as the best biomarker for fetal exposure to methylmercury. In addition, cord tissue mercury concentration was used as a predictor of the effects of fetal methylmercury exposure (Grandjean et al., 2005). We have reported that the cord tissue total mercury and methylmercury have strong correlations with cord blood mercury (Sakamoto et al., 2007b). Thanks to the traditional Japanese custom of preserving umbilical cord tissue at the time of birth, this preserved cord tissue is useful to estimate past methylmercury exposure. Practically, methylmercury concentration in preserved umbilical cords has been used as a biomarker for the exposure in Minamata district (Nishigaki and Harada, 1975; Akagi et al., 1998; Sakamoto 2010).

The risk of fetal exposure to methylmercury is very high. However, the mercury levels in the blood of infants decreased drastically during breast feeding in both animal and human studies. The brain Hg concentration also dramatically decreased during breast-feeding (Sandborgh-Englund et al., 2001; Sakamoto et al., 2002a,b) because the contribution of breast milk to methylmercury transfer to infants seems limited. However, based on multiple studies, the rate of methylmercury excretion is thought to be low, and the biological half-time of methylmercury in lactating women is shorter than that in nonlactating women (WHO, 1990). Suckling mice are incapable of excreting methylmercury (WHO, 1990). In Iraq, human milk was the suspected source of methylmercury exposure in poisoned infants (Amin-Zaki et al., 1981). These phenomena may suggest that breast-fed infants also seem to be at high risk for methylmercury poisoning. However, as demonstrated by our animal and human studies, after neonates are separated from the active intrauterine amino acid transport system, methylmercury transfer depends on the milk in which the methylmercury concentration is low. Offspring grow rapidly after birth, and the growth may dilute methylmercury concentrations in the body and brain (Sakamoto et al., 2002a).

15.3.1.2 *Methylmercury Intoxication in Adults.* The symptoms of the typical cases of Minamata disease were sensory disturbance, constriction of visual fields, hearing loss, tremors, and cerebellar ataxia (Tokuomi et al., 1961; Okajima et al., 1976). Large-scale Iraqi poisoning incidents in 1972-1973 were caused by wheat seed disinfected with methylmercury. These incidents afflicted more than 6000 people and resulted in 400 deaths; the main symptoms were similar to those in Minamata disease (Bakir et al., 1973). The study in Iraq showed that thresholds of methylmercury body burden at case diagnosis were as follows: abnormal sensory perception, $\sim$25 mg (equivalent to a mercury concentration in blood of 250 μg/L); ataxia, $\sim$50 mg; articulation disorders, $\sim$90 mg; hearing loss, $\sim$180 mg; and death, $>$200 mg (Bakir et al., 1973).

15.3.1.3 *Methylmercury Intoxication in Fetus.* Patients with typical fetal-type Minamata disease born during the severe methylmercury pollution in 1955-1959 in the Minamata area exhibited mental retardation, primitive reflexes, cerebellar ataxia, disturbances in physical growth, dysarthria, and limb deformities

(a)

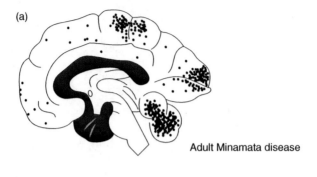

Adult Minamata disease

(b)

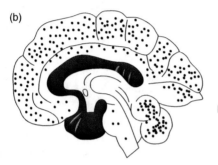

Fetal-type Minamata disease

Figure 15.1 Comparisons of the distribution of lesions in (a) adult Minamata disease and (b) fetal-type Minamata disease.

similar to the symptoms of cerebral palsy (Harada, 1978). Most severely affected children in Iraq manifested severe sensory impairments, general paralysis, hyperactive reflexes, and impaired mental development (Amin-Zaki et al., 1974).

15.3.2 Distinct Pattern of Neuronal Degeneration in the Developing Brain

15.3.2.1 Human Study. In the tragic methylmercury pollution cases in Japan, many infants were congenitally affected by methylmercury (Harada, 1978). Different from patients with adult-type Minamata disease, patients with typical fetal-type Minamata disease revealed widespread severe neuronal degeneration in the central nervous system, as shown in Fig. 15.1 (Takeuchi et al., 1962), and showed cerebral palsy-like symptoms. In the adult cases, neuronal degeneration was observed mainly in the cerebral cortex (parietal, occipital, and temporal lobes), cerebellum, and peripheral nerves; and showed the main symptoms of sensory disturbance, cerebellar sensory ataxia, constriction of visual fields, and hearing impairment, reflecting the place where the nerves were damaged.

15.3.2.2 Rat Studies. In the rat brain, the postnatal development stage corresponds to the third trimester in humans (Dobbing and Sands, 1979; Choi,

1989), when many histogenetic events such as gliogenesis, elaboration of neuronal dendritic arbors, synaptic connection, and rapid growth of blood vessels occur. Therefore, determining effects of methylmercury on the postnatal developing rat nervous system will help understand neurotoxicity in the human fetal brain. There are distinct patterns of neuronal degeneration in the developing brain exposed to methylmercury at various phases of brain development (Wakabayashi et al., 1995). Moreover, prolonged exposure of neonatal rats to methylmercury for >30 days revealed widespread neuronal degeneration in the cerebral neocortex and spinal sensory ganglia (Sakamoto et al., 1998). The widespread distribution resembled that in patients with fetal-type Minamata disease in Minamata, Japan. These series of rat experiments indicated that the pattern of damage in the brain clearly changes with the timing of methylmercury exposure at various stages of brain development, and the widespread neuronal degeneration in fetal-type human Minamata disease could be caused by prolonged methylmercury exposure during brain growth, but not short-term exposure.

15.3.3   Cohort Study on the Effect of Prenatal Exposure to Low Level of Methylmercury

Three cohort studies were done in New Zealand (Kjellström et al., 1989), Faroe Islands (Grandjean et al., 1992), and Seychelles (Marsh et al., 1995; Shamlaye et al., 1995), for risk assessment of prenatal exposure to methylmercury in the 1980s, and the results have been published since 1989 (Kjellstrom et al., 1989; Grandjean et al., 1992, 1997; Marsh et al., 1995; Shamlaye et al., 1995; Davidson et al., 1998; Murata et al., 1999; Sørensen et al., 1999). Thereafter, a workshop on the scientific issues relevant to assessment of health effects of methylmercury exposure was organized at the request of the White House in November 1998 (NRC, 2000). At that time, most discussions focused on two of the three epidemiologic studies; the Faroese Birth Cohort Study and the Seychelles Child Development Study, associating methylmercury exposure with an array of developmental measures in children. The maternal hair mercury levels at parturition were between 0.2 and 39.1 µg/g (median 4.5 µg/g) among the Faroese cohort (1023 mother-infant pairs) and between 0.5 and 26.7 µg/g (mean 6.8 µg/g) among the Seychellois cohort (779 pairs).

The Faroese population has eaten whale meat and blubber at least since the early eighteenth century. For this reason, most of the Faroese have been exposed to methylmercury and/or polychlorinated biphenyls (PCBs) and the children would also be exposed to these substances *in utero*. When the birth cohort was 7 and 14 years old, neuropsychological, neurobehavioral, and neurophysiological tests were carried out. The Faroese Birth Cohort Study consistently demonstrated adverse effects of methylmercury on child neurodevelopment including finger tapping speed, reaction time on a continued performance task, cued naming, systolic blood pressure, brainstem auditory evoked potential latencies, and heart rate variability (HRV) (Grandjean et al., 1997, 2004; Murata et al., 1999, 2004; Sørensen et al., 1999; Debes et al., 2006). On the other hand, the cord PCB concentration was associated with deficits on the Boston naming test, the continuous performance test reaction time, and the California verbal learning test at age seven years, but such adverse effects of PCBs disappeared in the process of data analysis after the adjustment for mercury (Grandjean et al., 2001; Budtz-Jørgensen et al., 2002).

Seychellois consume a high quantity and a wide variety of ocean fish on a regular basis (Shamlaye et al., 1995). Fish is the main source of methylmercury, protein, and n-3 polyunsaturated fatty acids. Neurodevelopmental outcomes in the Seychellois at 66 and 107 months of age were examined (Davidson et al., 1998; Myers et al., 2003b). According to the studies' reports, methylmercury had both an adverse and a beneficial association with some of 34 endpoints; for instance, increased exposure to methylmercury was associated with decreased performance in the grooved pegboard using the nondominant hand in males and improved scores in the hyperactivity index of the Conner's teacher rating scale. Consequently, the Seychelles child development study noted no consistent pattern suggesting an adverse association at the level of prenatal exposure (Myers et al., 2003a), whereas the Iraqi data analyzed by the same research group demonstrated a dose-response relationship that suggested the fetal lowest effect level was indicated by a maximum maternal hair mercury level during pregnancy in the range of 10-15 µg/g (Marsh et al., 1987; Cox et al., 1989). After this, the Seychelles child development nutrition study with 229 mother-infant pairs observed not only a significant correlation coefficient ($r = 0.31$) between maternal hair mercury and n-3 polyunsaturated fatty acids but also a significant adverse association between prenatal methylmercury and 30-month psychomotor developmental index of the Bayley Scales of Infant Development when the n-3 polyunsaturated fatty acid measures were included in the regression analysis (Strain et al., 2008). Davidson et al. (2008) also suggested a possible confounding role of maternal nutrition in studies examining associations between prenatal methylmercury exposures and developmental outcomes in children. There seemed to be subtle but adverse effects of methylmercury on child development in Seychelles, unless the researchers overlooked crucial confounders.

15.3.4 Reproductive Outcomes

Itai et al. (2004) reported increased fetal death (i.e., stillbirth and spontaneous abortion) in the period from 1956 to 1968 in Minamata City, Japan. Sakamoto et al. (2001) also reported a decreased male sex ratio in offspring among fishing families in the overall city population, and in mothers who were recognized as having Minamata disease in the city in 1955-1959, when methylmercury pollution was most severe. An increase in the proportion of male stillborn fetuses in the city was also observed at the time. It is possible that male fetuses were more susceptible to the pollution than female, and this could be a cause for the lower number of male offspring at birth.

15.3.5 Cardiovascular Effects

Since 1995, there has been much debate over the cardiovascular effects of low level exposure to methylmercury. The first evidence was that fish consumption and mercury levels in hair were associated with an increased risk of myocardial infarction (MI) among residents of Eastern Finland (Salonen et al., 1995). A research group then observed an association between the risk of MI and total mercury exposure (Guallar et al., 2002), but data from another group did not exactly support it (Yoshizawa et al., 2008). This debate has been dampened by many studies stressing the beneficial effects of fish oil such as n-3 polyunsaturated fatty acids on MI and child development except for a few reports (Sørensen et al., 1999; Choi et al., 2009), and whether low level exposure to methylmercury affects the cardiovascular system remains unclear.

By using HRV, Oka et al. (2002) reported that methylmercury exposure at parturition was associated with decreased vagal modulation in patients with fetal Minamata disease. Thereafter, two reports observed similar results; cord blood mercury was negatively correlated with autonomic activities of HRV in 14-year-old Faroese children (Grandjean et al., 2004) and cord tissue methylmercury was negatively correlated with parasympathetic components in 7-year-old Japanese children (Murata et al., 2006). In addition, an intervention study using subjects exposed to methylmercury at the provisional tolerable weekly intake (TWI) level (3.4 µg/kg body weight/week) through consumption of bigeye tuna and swordfish for 14 weeks, confirmed that the sympathovagal balance index of HRV was significantly elevated after the exposure (mean hair mercury, 2.30 µg/g before exposure vs 8.76 µg/g after exposure), and decreased to baseline levels after a 15-week washout period following the cessation of exposure (Yaginuma-Sakurai et al., 2009). Such changes in HRV parameters were not found in the control group with a mean hair mercury level of around 2.1 µg/g. These data indicate that long-term exposure to methylmercury may pose a potential risk for cardiac events involving sympathovagal imbalance among fish-consuming populations.

15.4 RISK ASSESSMENT OF PRENATAL EXPOSURE TO METHYLMERCURY

Tolerable intake levels of methylmercury for pregnant women are decided by relevant authorities in each country, taking into account fetal safety factors. The Joint Food and Agriculture Organization of the United Nations/World Health Organization Expert Committee on Food Additives (JECFA, 2003) established a provisional tolerable intake for methylmercury at 1.6 µg Hg/kg body weight/week (equivalent to a hair mercury concentration of approximately 2.3 µg/g), with an uncertainty factor of 6.4. The United States Environmental Protection Agency (USEPA, 2001) set 0.1 µg Hg/kg body weight/day (equivalent to a hair mercury concentration of 1.0 µg/g) as the reference dose, using an uncertainty factor of 10. The amount of fish and other seafood consumed by people in Japan and other Asian countries bordering the sea is higher than by Europeans and Americans. The average mercury concentration in the hair of women of childbearing age (15-49 years) in Japan is 1.4 µg/g (Yasutake et al., 2003). In June 2003, the Japanese

Ministry of Health, Labour, and Welfare issued advice to limit the consumption of toothed whales, red snapper, swordfish, bluefin tuna, and other fish by pregnant women. The standards were issued because these high trophic marine species have high methylmercury concentrations as a result of biomagnification through the food chain. In August 2005, the Food Safety Commission, which had been requested by the Japanese Ministry of Health, Labour, and Welfare to evaluate TWI, established a methylmercury TWI of 2.0 μg Hg/kg body weight/week (Japan Food Safety Commission, 2005) using an uncertainty factor of 4. This TWI corresponds to a hair mercury concentration of ~2.8 μg/g.

15.5 RISKS AND BENEFITS OF FISH CONSUMPTION FOR BRAIN DEVELOPMENT

Methylmercury is one of the substances most risky to fetal brain development, and most of the exposure to methylmercury is through maternal fish consumption. On the other hand, docosahexaenoic acid (DHA), which is important for the fetal brain and its growth, is also derived from maternal fish consumption. If human exposure to methylmercury were independent of nutrition from fish, we would aim at zero exposure. However, fish plays an important role among fish-eating populations and contains n-3 polyunsaturated fatty acids, such as DHA.

Maternal and fetal blood DHA concentrations are significantly correlated, indicating that fetal exposure to methylmercury and DHA strongly reflected each maternal exposure level. Sakamoto et al. (2004a) reported that methylmercury was directly correlated with DHA in the fetal circulation. These results suggest that fish consumption may have been the source of both methylmercury and DHA in maternal circulation that was subsequently transferred to the fetus. If fish consumed are low in methylmercury but rich in DHA, the health of the children will likely improve, but if the fish methylmercury concentrations are sufficiently elevated to cause deleterious outcomes the beneficial aspects of DHA intake may be negated. Accordingly, fish consumption would then have an adverse effect on child development. This salient issue makes the placental transfer of methylmercury and DHA and their relationship to fetal and maternal blood circulation important factors for determining the risks and benefits of maternal fish consumption during gestation. In light of low exposure levels to methylmercury, further research will be necessary to clarify the combined effects of methylmercury and other potential risks, and benefits originating from fish consumption on child development.

15.6 EXCEPTIONAL METHYLMERCURY EXPOSURE THROUGH RICE

Fish consumption is the primary pathway for methylmercury exposure. However, Horvat et al. (2003) reported elevated levels of methylmercury in rice grain in some regions near mercury mines in China. The maximum methylmercury value in the grain was 144 ng/g. Therefore, methylmercury exposure to the people also occurs through rice ingestion as an exceptional case (Sakamoto et al., 2007a; Li et al., 2009).

15.7 SUMMARY

Most human exposure to methylmercury is through fish/shellfish consumption. Methylmercury exposure levels depend on the amount and species of fish/shellfish consumed daily. The developing brain in the late gestation period is known to be most vulnerable. Further, more methylmercury accumulates in fetuses than in mothers. Therefore, efforts must be made to protect fetuses from the risk of methylmercury, especially in populations that consume a lot of fish/shellfish containing high methylmercury, such as pilot whale, shark, and sword fish. However, fish is an important protein source for many people around the world and contains n-3 polyunsaturated fatty acids. Pregnant women must consider the risks and benefits of fish consumption during the gestation period.

REFERENCES

Akagi H, Grandjean P, Takizawa Y, Weihe P. Methylmercury dose estimation from umbilical cord concentrations in patients with Minamata disease. Environ Res 1998;77:98–103.

Amin-Zaki L, Elhassani S, Majeed MA, Clarkson TW, Doherty RA, Greenwood M. Intra-uterine methylmercury poisoning in Iraq. Pediatrics 1974;54:587–595.

Amin-Zaki L, Majeed MA, Greenwood MR, Elhassani SB, Clarkson TW, Doherty RA. Methylmercury poisoning in the Iraqi suckling infant: a longitudinal study over five years. J Appl Toxicol 1981;1:210–214.

Bakir F, Damluji SF, Amin-Zaki L, Murtadha M, Khalidi A, al-Rawi NY, Tikriti S, Dahahir HI, Clarkson TW, Smith JC, Doherty RA. Methylmercury poisoning in Iraq. Science 1973;181:230–241.

Bjerregaard P, Hansen JC. Organochlorines and heavy metals in pregnant women from the Disko Bay area in Greenland. Sci Total Environ 2000;245:195–202.

Budtz-Jørgensen E, Keiding N, Grandjean P, Weihe P. Estimation of health effects of prenatal methylmercury exposure using structural equation models. Environ Health 2002;1:2.

Butler Walker J, Houseman J, Seddon L, McMullen E, Tofflemire K, Mills C, Corriveau A, Weber JP, LeBlanc A, Walker M, Donaldson SG, Van Oostdam J. Maternal and umbilical cord blood levels of mercury, lead, cadmium, and essential trace elements in Arctic Canada. Environ Res 2006;100:295–318.

Choi BH. The effects of methylmercury on the developing brain. Prog Neurobiol 1989;32:447–470.

Choi AL, Weihe P, Budtz-Jørgensen E, Jørgensen PJ, Salonen JT, Tuomainen TP, Murata K, Nielsen HP, Petersen MS, Askham J, Grandjean P. Methylmercury exposure and adverse cardiovascular effects in Faroese whaling men. Environ Health Perspect 2009;117 367–372.

Cox C, Clarkson TW, Marsh DO, Amin-Zaki L, Tikriti S, Myers GG. Dose-response analysis of infants prenatally exposed to methyl mercury: an application of a single compartment model to single-strand hair analysis. Environ Res 1989;49:318–332.

Davidson PW, Myers GJ, Cox C, Axtell C, Shamlaye C, Sloane-Reeves J, Cernichiari E, Needham L, Choi A, Wang Y, Berlin M, Clarkson TW. Effects of prenatal and postnatal methylmercury exposure from fish consumption on neurodevelopment: outcomes at 66 months of age in the Seychelles Child Development Study. JAMA 1998;280:701–707.

Davidson PW, Strain JJ, Myers GJ, Thurston SW, Bonham MP, Shamlaye CF, Stokes-Riner A, Wallace JM, Robson PJ, Duffy EM, Georger LA, Sloane-Reeves J, Cernichiari E, Canfield RL, Cox C, Huang LS, Jaciuras J, Clarkson TW. Neurodevelopmental effects of maternal nutritional status and exposure to methylmercury from eating fish during pregnancy. Neurotoxicology 2008;29:767–775.

Debes F, Budtz-Jorgensen E, Weihe P, White RF, Grandjean P. Impact of prenatal methylmercury exposure on neurobehavioral function at age 14 years. Neurotoxicol Teratol 2006;28:536–547.

Dobbing J, Sands J. Comparative aspects of the brain growth spurt. Early Hum Dev 1979;3:79–83.

Grandjean P, Weihe P, Jorgensen PJ, Clarkson T, Cernichiari E, Videro T. Impact of maternal seafood diet on fetal exposure to mercury, selenium, and lead. Arch Environ Health 1992;47:185–195.

Grandjean P, Weihe P, White RF, Debes F, Araki S, Yokoyama K, Murata K, Sorensen N, Dahl R, Jørgensen PJ. Cognitive deficit in 7-year-old children with prenatal exposure to methylmercury. Neurotoxicol Teratol 1997;19:417–428.

Grandjean P, Weihe P, Burse VW, Needham LL, Storr-Hansen E, Heinzow B, Debes F, Murata K, Simonsen H, Ellefsen P, Budtz-Jørgensen E, Keiding N, White RF. Neurobehavioral deficits associated with PCB in 7-year-old children prenatally exposed to seafood neurotoxicants. Neurotoxicol Teratol 2001;23:305–317.

Grandjean P, Murata K, Budtz-Jørgensen E, Weihe P. Cardiac autonomic activity in methylmercury neurotoxicity: 14-year follow-up of a Faroese birth cohort. J Pediatr 2004;144:169–176.

Grandjean P, Budtz-Jørgensen E, Jørgensen PJ, Weihe P. Umbilical cord mercury concentration as biomarker of prenatal exposure to methylmercury. Environ Health Perspect 2005;113:905–908.

Guallar E, Sanz-Gallardo MI, van't Veer P, Bode P, Aro A, Gomez-Aracena J, Kark JD, Riemersma RA, Martin-Moreno JM, Kok FJ. Mercury, fish oils, and the risk of myocardial infarction. N Engl J Med 2002;347:1747–1754.

Harada M. Congenital Minamata disease: intrauterine methylmercury poisoning. Teratology 1978;18:285–288.

Horvat M, Nolde N, Fajon V, Jereb V, Logar M, Lojen S, Jacimovic R, Falnoga I, Liya Q, Faganeli J, Drobne D. Total mercury, methylmercury and selenium in mercury polluted areas in the province Guizhou, China. Sci Total Environ 2003;304:231–256.

Hsu CS, Liu PL, Chien LC, Chou SY, Han BC. Mercury concentration and fish consumption in Taiwanese pregnant women. BJOG 2007;114:81–85.

Irukayama K, Kondo T. Studies on the organomercury compound in the fish and shellfish from Minamata Bay and its origin. VII. Synthesis of methylmercury sulfate and its chemical properties. Nippon Eiseigaku Zasshi 1966;21:342–343.

Itai Y, Fujino T, Ueno K, Motomatsu Y. An epidemiological study of the incidence of abnormal pregnancy in areas heavily contaminated with methylmercury. Environ Sci 2004;11:83–97.

Japan Food Safety Commission. Safety Risk Assessment Related to Methylmercury in Seafood. 2005 Available on http://www.fsc.go.jp/english/topics/methylmercury_risk_assessment.pdf.

Joint Food and Agriculture Organization/World Health Organization Expert Committee on Food Additives (JECFA). Summary Report of the Sixty-first JECFA Meeting. Geneva: WHO, 2003.

Kjellström T, Kennedy P, Wallis S. Physical and Mental Development of Children with Prenatal Exposure to Mercury from Fish. Stage 2: Interviews and Psychological Test at Age 6. Report. Stockholm: National Swedish Environmental Protection Board; 1989. 3642.

Li P, Feng X, Qiu G, Li Z, Fu X, Sakamoto M, Liu X, Wang D. Mercury exposures and symptoms in smelting workers of artisanal mercury mines in Wuchuan, Guizhou, China. Environ Res 2008;107:108–114.

Marsh DO, Clarkson TW, Cox C, Myers GJ, Amin-Zaki L, Al-Tikriti S. Fetal methylmercury poisoning. Relationship between concentration in single strands of maternal hair and child effects. Arch Neurol 1987;44:1017–1022.

Marsh DO, Clarkson TW, Myers GJ, Davidson PW, Cox C, Cernichiari E, Tanner MA, Lednar W, Shamlaye C, Choisy O, et al. The Seychelles study of fetal methylmercury exposure and child development: introduction. Neurotoxicology 1995;16:583–596.

Morrissette J, Takser L, St-Amour G, Smargiassi A, Lafond J, Mergler D. Temporal variation of blood and hair mercury levels in pregnancy in relation to fish consumption history in a population living along the St. Lawrence River. Environ Res 2004;95:363–374.

Murata K, Weihe P, Araki S, Budtz-Jorgensen E, Grandjean P. Evoked potentials in Faroese children prenatally exposed to methylmercury. Neurotoxicol Teratol 1999;21:471–472.

Murata K, Weihe P, Budtz-Jorgensen E, Jorgensen PJ, Grandjean P. Delayed brainstem auditory evoked potential latencies in 14-year-old children exposed to methylmercury. J Pediatr 2004;144:177–183.

Murata K, Sakamoto M, Nakai K, Dakeishi M, Iwata T, Liu XJ, Satoh H. Subclinical effects of prenatal methylmercury exposure on cardiac autonomic function in Japanese children. Int Arch Occup Environ Health 2006;79:379–386.

Myers GJ, Marsh DO, Davidson PW, Cox C, Shamlaye CF, Tanner M, Choi A, Cernichiari E, Choisy O, Clarkson TW. Main neurodevelopmental study of Seychellois children following in utero exposure to methylmercury from a maternal fish diet: outcome at six months. Neurotoxicology 1995;16:653–664.

Myers G, Cox C, Davidson PW, Huang LS, Clarkson T. Authors' reply. Lancet 2003a;362:665.

Myers GJ, Davidson PW, Cox C, Shamlaye CF, Palumbo D, Cernichiari E, Sloane-Reeves J, Wilding GE, Kost J, Huang LS, Clarkson TW. Prenatal methylmercury exposure from ocean fish consumption in the Seychelles child development study. Lancet 2003b;361:1686–1692.

National Research Council (NRC). Toxicological effects of methylmercury. Washington (DC): Academic Press; 2000.

Nishigaki S, Harada M. Methylmercury and selenium in umbilical cords of inhabitants the Minamata area. Nature (London) 1975;258:324–325.

Oka T, Matsukura M, Okamoto M, Harada N, Kitano T, Miike T, Futatsuka M. Autonomic nervous functions in fetal type Minamata disease patients: assessment of heart rate variability. Tohoku J Exp Med 2002;198:215–221.

Okajima T, Mishima I, Tokuomi H. Minamata disease with a long-term follow-up. Int J Neurol 1976;11:62–72.

Palkovicova L, Ursinyova M, Masanova V, Yu Z, Hertz-Picciotto I. Maternal amalgam dental fillings as the source of mercury exposure in developing fetus and newborn. J Expo Sci Environ Epidemiol 2008;18:326–331.

Sakamoto M, Nakano A, Kajiwara Y, Naruse I, Fujisaki T. Effects of methyl mercury in postnatal developing rats. Environ Res 1993;61:43–50.

Sakamoto M, Wakabayashi K, Kakita A, Hitoshi T, Adachi T, Nakano A. Widespread neuronal degeneration in rats following oral administration of methylmercury during the postnatal developing phase: a model of fetal-type Minamata disease. Brain Res 1998;784:351–354.

Sakamoto M, Nakano A, Akagi H. Declining Minamata male birth ratio associated with increased male fetal death due to heavy methylmercury pollution. Environ Res 2001;87:92–98.

Sakamoto M, Kakita A, Wakabayashi K, Takahashi H, Nakano A, Akagi H. Evaluation of changes in methylmercury accumulation in the developing rat brain and its effects: a study with consecutive and moderate dose exposure throughout gestation and lactation periods. Brain Res 2002a;949:51–59.

Sakamoto M, Kubota M, Matsumoto S, Nakano A, Akagi H. Declining risk of methylmercury exposure to infants during lactation. Environ Res 2002b;90:185–189.

Sakamoto M, Kubota M, Liu XH, Murata K, Nakai K, Satoh H. Maternal and fetal mercury and n-3 polyunsaturated fatty acids as a risk and benefit of fish consumption to fetus. Environ Sci Technol 2004a;38:3860–3863.

Sakamoto M, Kubota M, Liu XJ, Murata K, Nakai K, Satoh H. Maternal and fetal mercury and n−3 polyunsaturated fatty acids as a risk and benefit of fish consumption to fetus. Environ Sci Technol 2004b;38:3860–3863.

Sakamoto M, Feng X, Li P, Qiu G, Jiang H, Yoshida M, Iwaia T, Liu XJ, Murata K. High exposure of Chinese mercury mine workers to elemental mercury vapor and increased methylmercury levels in their hair. Environ Health Prev Med 2007a;12:66–70.

Sakamoto M, Kaneoka T, Murata K, Nakai K, Satoh H, Akagi H. Correlations between mercury concentrations in umbilical cord tissue and other biomarkers of fetal exposure to methylmercury in the Japanese population. Environ Res 2007b;103:106–111.

Sakamoto M, Murata K, Tsuruta K, Miyamoto K, Akagi H Retrospective study on temporal and regional variations of methylmercury concentrations in preserved umbilical cords collected from inhabitants of the Minamata area, Japan. Ecotoxicol Environ Saf 2010; 73:1144–1149.

Salonen JT, Seppänen K, Nyyssönen K, Korpela H, Kauhanen J, Kantola M, Tuomilehto J, Esterbauer H, Tatzber F, Salonen R. Intake of mercury from fish, lipid peroxidation, and the risk of myocardial infarction and coronary, cardiovascular, and any death in eastern Finnish men. Circulation 1995;91:645–655.

Sandborgh-Englund G, Ask K, Belfrage E, Ekstrand J. Mercury exposure in utero and during infancy. J Toxicol Environ Health A 2001;63:317–320.

Shamlaye CF, Marsh DO, Myers GJ, Cox C, Davidson PW, Choisy O, Cernichiari E, Choi A, Tanner MA, Clarkson TW. The Seychelles child development study on neurodevelopmental outcomes in children following in utero exposure to methylmercury from a maternal fish diet: background and demographics. Neurotoxicology 1995;16:597–612.

Sørensen N, Murata K, Budtz-Jorgensen E, Weihe P, Grandjean P. Prenatal methylmercury exposure as a cardiovascular risk factor at seven years of age. Epidemiology 1999;10:370–375.

Soria ML, Sanz P, Martinez D, Lopez-Artiguez M, Garrido R, Grilo A, Repetto M. Total mercury and methylmercury in hair, maternal and umbilical blood, and placenta from women in the Seville area. Bull Environ Contam Toxicol 1992;48:494–501.

Stern AH, Smith AE. An assessment of the cord blood: maternal blood methylmercury ratio: implications for risk assessment. Environ Health Perspect 2003;111:1465–1470.

Strain JJ, Davidson PW, Bonham MP, Duffy EM, Stokes-Riner A, Thurston SW, Wallace J, Robson PJ, Shamlaye CF, Georger LA, Sloane-Reeves J, Cernichiari E, Canfield RI, Cox C, Huang LS, Janciuras J, Myers GJ, Clarkson TW. Associations of maternal long-chain polyunsaturated fatty acids, methyl mercury, and infant development in the Seychelles child development nutrition study. Neurotoxicology 2008;29:776–782.

Takeuchi T. Pathology of Minamata disease. With special reference to its pathogenesis. Acta Pathol Jpn 1982;32(1 Suppl): 73–99.

Takeuchi T, Morikawa N, Matsumoto H, Shiraishi Y. A pathological study on Minamata disease in Japan. Acta Neuropathol 1962;2:40–57.

Tokuomi H, Okajima T, Kanai J, Tsunoda M, Ichiyasu Y, Misumi H, Shimomura K, Takaba M. Minamata disease. World Neurol 1961;2:536–545.

UNEP. Global mercury assessment. Geneva, UNEP Chemicals Mercury Programme: 2002.

UNEP. The global atmospheric mercury assessment: sources, emission, transport. Geneva: UNEP Chemicals Branch; 2008.

US Environmental Protection Agency (EPA). Water Quality Criterion for the Protection of Human Health: Methylmercury, Final. EPA-823-R-01-001. Washington, DC: EPA, 2001.

Unuvar E, Ahmadov H, Kiziler AR, Aydemir B, Toprak S, Ulker V, Ark C. Mercury levels in cord blood and meconium of healthy newborns and venous blood of their mothers: clinical, prospective cohort study. Sci Total Environ 2007;374:60–70.

Vahter M, Akesson A, Lind B, Bjors U, Schutz A, Berglund M. Longitudinal study of methylmercury and inorganic mercury in blood and urine of pregnant and lactating women, as well as in umbilical cord blood. Environ Res 2000;84:186–194.

Vigeh M, Yokoyama K, Ramezanzadeh F, Dahaghin M, Sakai T, Morita Y, Kitamura F, Sato H, Kobayashi Y. Lead and other trace metals in preeclampsia: a case-control study in Tehran, Iran. Environ Res 2006;100:268–275.

Wakabayashi K, Kakita A, Sakamoto M, Su M, Iwanaga K, Ikuta F. Variability of brain lesions in rats administered methylmercury at various postnatal development phases. Brain Res 1995;705:267–272.

WHO. Methylmercury. Environmental Health Criteria 101. Geneva: World Health Organization; 1990.

WHO. Inorganic mercury. Environmental Health Criteria 118. Geneva: World Health Organization; 1991.

World Health Organization (WHO). Environmental Health Criteria 165: Inorganic Lead. Geneva: WHO, 1995.

Yaginuma-Sakurai K, Murata K, Shimada M, Nakai K, Kurokawa N, Kameo S, Satoh H. Intervention study on cardiac autonomic nervous effects of methylmercury from seafood. Neurotoxicol Teratol. 32:240–245; 2009.

Yang J, Jiang Z, Wang Y, Qureshi IA, Wu XD. Maternal-fetal transfer of metallic mercury via the placenta and milk. Ann Clin Lab Sci 1997;27:135–141.

Yasutake A, Matsumoto M, Yamaguchi M, Hachiya N. Current hair mercury levels in Japanese: survey in five districts. Tohoku J Exp Med 2003;199:161–169.

Yoshizawa K, Rimm EB, Morris JS, Spate VL, Hsieh CC, Spiegelman D, Stampfer MJ, Willett WC. Mercury and the risk of coronary heart disease in men. N Engl J Med 2002;347:1755–1760.

CHAPTER 16

METALLOMICS OF MERCURY: ROLE OF THIOL- AND SELENOL-CONTAINING BIOMOLECULES

FEIYUE WANG, MARCOS LEMES, and MOHAMMAD A.K. KHAN

16.1 INTRODUCTION

As shown in the previous chapters, extensive studies in the past 50 years have greatly advanced our understanding of mercury (Hg) as a global contaminant and as a toxic substance to biota including humans. It is now well established that the mobility, chemical reactivity, and bioavailability of Hg in the environment are determined not by its total concentration but by its speciation, that is, the distribution of Hg among its specific forms defined as to isotopic composition (e.g., ^{200}Hg, ^{202}Hg), electronic or oxidation states (e. g., Hg(0), Hg(I), Hg(II)), and/or molecular structure (e.g., Hg(OH)$^+$, HgCl$_2$, CH$_3$Hg$^+$) (Templeton et al., 2000). Although the same holds true when it comes to the toxicity of Hg inside a biological system (hereafter defined as the whole body, a specific organ, or a cell), the molecular-level processes governing the uptake and metabolism of Hg in biological systems are less well known.

Following a recently emerged metallomics approach, molecular-level inter-actions of Hg species in biological systems, their implications on Hg uptake, toxicity, and detoxification, and analytical and modeling approaches for such studies are discussed in this chapter.

16.2 METALLOMICS OF MERCURY

The term *metallomics* was first coined by Hiroki Haraguchi in 2004 to highlight the growing recognition of the roles metal ions (including metalloids) have in

Environmental Chemistry and Toxicology of Mercury, First Edition.
Edited by Guangliang Liu, Yong Cai, and Nelson O'Driscoll.
© 2012 John Wiley & Sons, Inc. Published 2012 by John Wiley & Sons, Inc.

the functions of genes and proteins, and to facilitate the integration of various fields related to the biometal science (Haraguchi, 2004). Similar to the genome in genomics and the proteome in proteomics, the metallome can be thought of as the entirety of metal species present in a biological system, including free metal ions (i.e., aquo complexes), their complexes with inorganic ligands (e.g., Cl^-), and metal-containing biomolecules (e.g., metal-complexed amino acids, metalloproteins, and metalloenzymes) (Lobinski et al., 2010). Metallomics thus refers to the study of the metallome, interactions, and functional connections of metal species with genes, proteins, metabolites, and other biomolecules in a biological system (Lobinski et al., 2010).

Different from the essential metals such as Cu and Zn, Hg is not required for any known essential biochemical functions of genes or proteins for any life form. Therefore, the metallomics of Hg focuses on how the presence of Hg adversely affects the normal functions of genes and proteins in the cell or whole body ("toxic effects"), and how such adverse effects can be alleviated ("detoxification") by the self-defense machinery of the cell or by remediation strategies.

Figure 16.1 is a schematic representation of the domains of Hg geochemistry in the environment and Hg metallomics in a biological system. In the environment, Hg cycling is mainly controlled by redox reactions between elemental Hg (Hg(0)) and divalent Hg(II) and complexation reactions of Hg^{2+}. Monovalent Hg(I) can also be found in the atmosphere, but it tends to disproportionate rapidly in aqueous solution (Hepler and Olofsson, 1975). Of particular importance is the complexation of Hg^{2+} by methyl anions (CH_3^-) to form monomethylmercury (CH_3Hg^+ and its complexes; hereafter MeHg), a process known as *Hg methylation*. Other alkyl mercuric species (e.g., ethylmercury or EtHg) also appear in the environment, but their concentrations are usually much lower and thus will not be included in the discussion in this chapter.

Hg(0), inorganic Hg(II), and MeHg can all be taken up by biota, and the chemical processes governing their uptake and subsequent *in vivo* transformation and transport are the domain of Hg metallomics (Fig. 16.1). Similar to that found in the environment, the metallome of Hg in a biological system is also composed of Hg(0) and complexes of inorganic Hg(II) and MeHg (Fig. 16.2). However, there is one major difference: while inorganic sulfides (DeVries and Wang, 2003), polysulfides (Wang and Tessier, 2009), and small molecular weight thiols (Zhang et al., 2004) can be present at considerable concentrations in certain environmental compartments (e.g., sediment porewaters, deeper layers of lakes and oceans), thiol- and selenol-containing amino acids, proteins, and enzymes are abundant in all the biological systems on Earth. The strong binding affinity (Sections 16.3 and 16.4) and lability (Section 16.5) of Hg^{2+} and CH_3Hg^+ ions for thiol and selenol groups dictate that the Hg metallomics in biological systems is dominated by their interactions with thiol- and selenol-containing biomolecules.

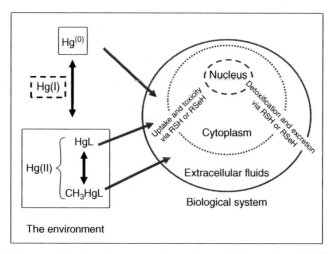

Figure 16.1 The metallomics of mercury: interactions of Hg species with biomolecules in and across a biological system (the whole body or its component). The metallomics of Hg is controlled primarily by thiol- and selenol-containing biomolecules (RSH and RSeH, respectively, where R denotes functional groups ranging from amino acids to proteins), whereas Hg geochemistry in the environment is dominated by redox (Hg(0), Hg(I), and Hg(II)) and complexation (by CH_3^- or other ligands L).

16.3 MERCURY AND METHYLMERCURY COMPLEXES WITH THIOL-CONTAINING BIOMOLECULES

Both inorganic Hg^{2+} and CH_3Hg^+ ions are soft Lewis acids, and therefore have strong thermodynamic affinities for thiolic groups that are soft Lewis bases (Pearson, 1963). Thiolic groups in a biological system are present mainly in cysteine, tripeptide glutathione, and cysteine residues of proteins and enzymes. These thiolic groups are known to play fundamentally important structural and functional roles in protein chemistry, being located within the active sites of many enzymes and directly involved in catalysis (Fasman, 1989). With their Hg and MeHg complexes typically having a formation constant in the range of $10^{15}-10^{30}$ (Zhang et al., 2004), these thiolic groups are the primary sites of Hg binding in biological systems.

16.3.1 Cysteine Complexes

Cysteine ($HSCH_2CH(NH_3^+)COO^-$ or CysSH) is an essential amino acid. Although the intracellular concentration of "free" CysSH is usually low, CysSH is the most abundant peptide- or protein-bound thiol (cysteine moieties) in biological systems. As such, CysSH is often used as a model thiol for the study of Hg and MeHg binding with thiol-containing peptides and proteins.

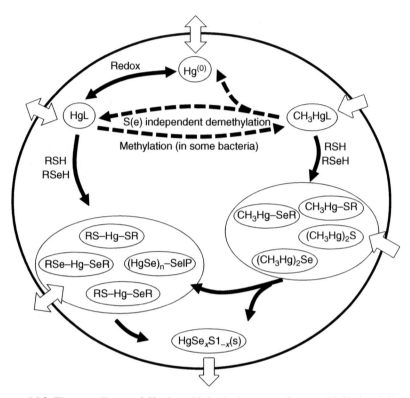

Figure 16.2 The metallome of Hg in a biological system. L, non-thiol/selenol ligands (e.g., Cl^-); R, functional groups (small amino acids to proteins); SelP, selenoprotein P; n, an integer number; and $0 \leq x \leq 1$.

16.3.1.1 Hg Cysteinates. The most stable and abundant Hg cysteinate is the near-linear (S–Hg–S bond angle: $\sim 170°$; Taylor and Carty, 1977), two-coordinated $Hg(SCys)_2$ (for simplicity, no charge will be shown for this and other complexes because of the complication due to the potential protonation of the NH_2 group and/or ion-pair formation; Jalilehvand et al., 2006). Higher coordinated $Hg(SCys)_3$ and $Hg(SCys)_4$ have also been reported in aqueous solutions (Jalilehvand et al., 2006). The Hg–S bond length in these complexes ranges from 2.3 to 2.5 Å, increasing with an increasing Hg coordination number (Taylor and Carty, 1977; Jalilehvand et al., 2006). The formation of multinuclear species is also possible (Taylor and Carty, 1977), but they are of negligible significance in Hg metallomics since the intracellular concentration of Hg is usually much lower than that of CysSH.

16.3.1.2 MeHg Cysteinates. $CH_3HgSCys$ is the simplest and probably the most important MeHg-cysteinate because of its capability of crossing the blood–brain barrier (BBB) (Section 16.6). When compared with $Hg(SCys)_2$,

$CH_3HgSCys$ is less polar and has a more linear $C-Hg-S$ bond ($\sim179°$; Taylor and Carty, 1977; Lemes, 2010). The $Hg-S$ and $Hg-C$ bond lengths are ~2.35 and 2.10 Å, respectively (Taylor et al., 1975; Hoffmeyer et al., 2006; Lemes, 2010). Higher coordination number complexes such as $CH_3Hg(SCys)_2$ and $CH_3Hg(SCys)_3$ and multinuclear complexes such as $(CH_3Hg)_2SCys$ (where one Hg is bond to the sulfur site and the other to the carboxylic group) have also been reported (Canty et al., 1994; Hoffmeyer et al., 2006).

16.3.2   Glutathione Complexes

Glutathione (γ-glutamyl-cysteinyl-glycine, GSH) is the most abundant cellular "free" thiol in animal tissues, plants, and microorganisms. Millimolar levels (up to 10 mM) of GSH can be found in mammalian cells with micromolar levels typically present in the blood plasma, accounting for more than 90% of the total non-protein sulfur in many cells (Meister, 1988). GSH serves as a storage and transport form of CysSH moieties, and performs diverse functions in catalysis, metabolism, and transport (Meister, 1988). It participates in reactions involving the synthesis of proteins and nucleic acids and in those that detoxify free radicals and peroxides. GSH is a cofactor for various enzymes, and forms complexes with a variety of toxic substances including Hg and MeHg.

16.3.2.1   Hg Glutathionates. Hg binding to GSH occurs primarily with the -SH group on its CysSH moiety. $Hg(SG)_2$ is the dominant complex between Hg^{2+} and GSH under physiological pH; however, $Hg(SG)_3$ and $Hg(SG)_4$ have been reported and can be present at considerable concentrations (Cheesman et al., 1988; Mah and Jalilehvand, 2008). No crystal structures have been reported for these complexes, but X-ray absorption measurements of their aqueous solutions showed similar $Hg-S$ bond lengths to those in the corresponding $Hg-CysSH$ complexes (Mah and Jalilehvand, 2008).

16.3.2.2   MeHg Glutathionates. No crystal structure data are available for CH_3HgSG, probably because of the amorphous nature of the compound (Lemes, 2010).

16.3.3   Homocysteine Complexes

Homocysteine ($HSCH_2CH_2CH(NH_3^+)COO^-$ or HcySH) is a nonessential, non-protein-forming thiolic amino acid. Produced from the intracellular metabolism of methionine, it can undergo transsulfuration to CysSH, or remethylation back to methionine (Selhub, 1999). Similar to its CysSH counterparts, experimental studies have shown that HcySH complexes of Hg^{2+} and CH_3Hg^+ can be transported across biological membranes via certain amino acid transporters and organic anion transporters (Bridges and Zalups, 2004, 2010; Zalups et al., 2007). Although no structural or thermodynamic data are available for these complexes, they are expected to be similar to the corresponding Hg^{2+} or CH_3Hg^+ complexes with CysSH.

16.3.4   Cysteine-Containing Proteins

CysSH is present as a common moiety in many important proteins such as met-allothioneins (MTs), the metalloregulatory protein MerR (in some bacteria), and serum albumins and hemoglobin (in mammals). The binding of Hg^{2+} to these proteins, despite their large sizes and potential steric hindrance, can be very strong because of the presence of multiple CysSH residues and thus possible formation of polydentate complexes. Of particular interest are MTs, which are low molecular mass proteins (6000–7000 Da) that typically consist of 20 CysSH residues (Stillman, 1995). MTs occur in all animals, and some plants, fungi, and bacteria, and serve important functions in transporting and detoxifying metals ions including Hg. The formation of Hg_m-MT with m up to 18 has been reported, where Hg^{2+} binding can be via various $Hg(SCys)_n$ ($n = 2$–4) environments (Stillman, 1995). CH_3Hg^+ binding with MTs is, however, less well known, but the affinity of MTs for CH_3Hg^+ seems to be much weaker than for Hg^{2+}, and the binding is most probably via a diagonal $CH_3HgSCys$ environment (Leiva-Presa et al., 2004).

16.4   MERCURY AND METHYLMERCURY BINDING TO SELENOL-CONTAINING BIOMOLECULES

Selenium is an essential micronutrient for many organisms. Since selenols chemically resemble thiols and can readily replace thiols in amino acids, Hg and MeHg complexes with selenol-containing biomolecules widely occur in biological systems. There is, however, one major difference—selenols are in general more powerful nucleophiles than thiols. For instance, the -SeH group of seleno-cysteine has a pK_a of 5.7 (at $25°C$ and $I = 0\,M$; NIST, 2004) and is thus mostly deprotonated (i.e., as $-Se^-$) at the physiological pH, whereas the -SH group of CysSH has a pK_a of 8.4 (see Table 16.2) and is thus predominantly protonated (i.e., as -SH) at the physiological pH. Therefore, thermodynamically, Hg and MeHg complexes with selenols tend to be even more stable than their thiol analogs, a property that is particularly important in the Hg–Se antagonism (Section 16.7).

16.4.1   Selenoamino Acid Complexes

Selenocysteine ($HSeCH_2CH(NH_3^+)COO^-$ or CysSeH) is the twenty-first amino acid present in biological systems. While free, unbound CysSeH may be present *in vivo* as a degradation product from selenoproteins and selenomethionine, the majority of CysSeH is bound in selenoproteins as CysSeH residues. Human blood typically contains 0.5–2.5 μM Se and it is assumed that most of it is present as CysSeH (Reilly, 2006). Selenoglutathione (GSeH) is a physiological source of CysSeH. Another selenoamino acid is selenomethionine (SeMet), which is the major Se species naturally occurring in most foods and is generally thought as the most bioavailable and bioactive form of Se (Reilly, 2006).

Despite major interest in inorganic Hg complexes with CysSH and GSH, no structural or thermodynamic data have been reported for their CysSeH and GSeH analogs. Data are however available for a few MeHg complexes with selenoamino acids, including $CH_3HgSeCys$ (Canty et al., 1983), CH_3HgSeG (Khan et al., 2009), and two CH_3Hg^+ –SeMet complexes (one via a Hg–Se bonding and the other a Hg–N bonding; Khan et al., 2009). Different from CysSeH and GSeH, SeMet is not a selenol as the Se is bound with two carbon atoms. As such the binding affinity of SeMet for CH_3Hg^+ is much weaker. In all these complexes, the Hg–Se bond length is longer than in their sulfur analogs, but the complexes are thermodynamically more stable (Carty et al., 1979; Asaduzzaman et al., 2010) because of the higher nucleophilicity of selenols, as mentioned earlier.

16.4.2 Selenoproteins

So far, about 25 selenoprotein families are known in bacteria, single-celled eukaryotes, or vertebrates (including humans), with another $\sim$20 selenoproteins being discovered through bioinformatics approaches. In all these proteins, Se is present predominately as CysSeH residues (Gladyshev, 2006). Among the most important and well-studied selenoproteins are GSH peroxidases (GPx), which are highly efficient antioxidant enzymes that catalyze GSH-dependent hydroperoxide reduction, and selenoprotein P (SelP) which is the only selenoprotein that contains multiple CysSeH residues (10 in humans and 17 in zebrafish) (Gladyshev, 2006). SelP is the major plasma selenoprotein; it is synthesized in the liver and delivers Se to other organs and tissues, although the brain appears to have the ability to synthesize its own pool of SelP (Gladyshev, 2006).

16.4.2.1 Hg Binding to Selenoproteins. Despite the presence of many nucleophilic SeH groups, as well as SH groups, SelP surprisingly does not show high affinity for inorganic Hg^{2+} ions (Suzuki et al., 1998). One possible reason for the weak affinity is thought to be the formation of ionic bonds in SelP between the cationic centers composed of imidazolyl groups of histidinyl residues and anionic centers composed of carboxyl functional groups; this ionic interaction may have masked the Hg–Se or Hg–S interactions (Suzuki et al., 1998). However, what is remarkable is that SelP was found to be able to bind and solubilize HgSe, which is otherwise essentially insoluble, following administration of high doses of $HgCl_2$ and selenite to rats or to plasma added with GSH (Yoneda and Suzuki, 1997a). The binding is attributed to the formation of a $(HgSe)_n$ polymer that is held onto SelP by the intramolecular ionic interaction (Yoneda and Suzuki, 1997a). Suzuki et al. (1998) further suggested that the complex is in the form of $([HgSe]_n)_m$-SelP, where n is the number of Hg–Se complexes ($\sim$100) and m the number of binding sites ($\leq$35) in SelP. The nature of this unusual bonding and its relevance in biological systems remains to be further investigated (Burk and Hill, 2005).

A different mechanism was proposed by Gailer et al. (2000), in which selenide binds with albumin-bound Hg to form a $(HgSe)_n$ core. At the surface of the core, GSH (or other thiols) molecules are attached via either Se or Hg atoms to make the $(HgSe)_n$ core water soluble. The interaction with SelP is then suggested to proceed with the replacement of two units of GSH with SelP.

16.4.2.2 MeHg Binding to Selenoproteins. Although the activity of several selenoproteins including GPx (Watanabe et al., 1999) and selenoprotein W (SelW) (Kim et al., 2005) has been shown to be affected by MeHg, no structural or thermodynamic data are available for the interactions between CH_3Hg^+ and selenoproteins. If the weak affinity of SelP for Hg^{2+} could be used as an indicator, CH_3Hg^+ would not be expected to bind strongly on selenoproteins.

16.5 LABILITY OF MERCURY OR METHYLMERCURY COMPLEXES WITH THIOLS OR SELENOLS

Despite very high thermodynamic formation constants, Hg^{2+} or CH_3Hg^+ complexes with thiols or selenols are kinetically labile and undergo rapidly ligand exchange in the presence of free thiols or selenols. This was first demonstrated by nuclear magnetic resonance (NMR) studies (Rabenstein et al., 1982; Rabenstein and Reid, 1984; Cheesman et al., 1988). The ligand exchange occurs via an associative mechanism involving a three-coordinated Hg intermediate (Rabenstein and Reid, 1984; Cheesman et al., 1988):

$$RS(e)–Hg–S(e)R + R'S(e)^- \rightleftharpoons RS(e)–Hg \genfrac{}{}{0pt}{}{-S(e)R}{\diagdown S(e)R'} \rightleftharpoons RS(e)–Hg–S(e)R' + RS(e)^-$$

$$H_3C–Hg–S(e)R + R'S(e)^- \rightleftharpoons H_3C–Hg \genfrac{}{}{0pt}{}{-S(e)R}{\diagdown S(e)R'} \rightleftharpoons H_3C–Hg–S(e)R' + RS(e)^-$$

where $RS(e)^-$ and $R'S(e)^-$ refer to two identical (when $R = R'$) or different thiols or selenols. The equilibrium composition favors the complex with a higher formation constant (Rabenstein and Reid, 1984).

The recent development of a new high performance liquid chromatography-inductively coupled plasma-mass spectrometry (HPLC-ICP-MS) analytical technique (Lemes and Wang, 2009) allows us to directly examine such ligand exchange in aqueous solutions. The addition of free CysSH into a 30-nM solution of CH_3HgSG (Fig. 16.3a) resulted in a decrease in the peak height of CH_3HgSG and a corresponding increase in $CH_3HgSCys$, suggesting the conversion of CH_3HgSG into $CH_3HgSCys$. Similarly, the addition of free GSH into a 75-nM solution of $CH_3HgSCys$ (Fig. 16.3b) resulted in a decrease in $CH_3HgSCys$ and a corresponding increase in CH_3HgSG, though the decrease in $CH_3HgSCys$ was less extensive. The results confirm that CH_3Hg^+ exchanges ligand between CysSH and GSH, and that the formation constant of $CH_3HgSCys$ is higher than that of CH_3HgSG.

This rapid thiolic/selenolic ligand exchange may have played several key roles in the Hg metallomics as follows:

1. *Enhanced Mobility*: The exchange between the free and complexed forms of a thiol (when $R = R'$), particularly GSH which is the most abundant

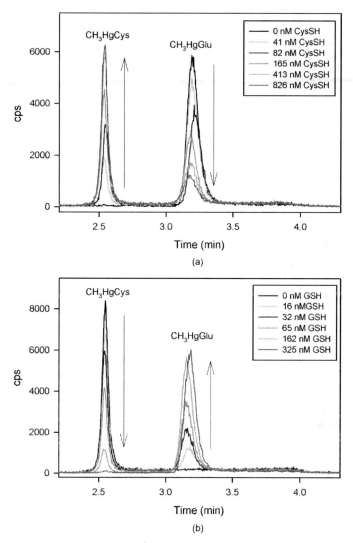

Figure 16.3 HPLC-ICP-MS chromatograms of (a) titration of a 30-nM CH₃HgSG with various concentrations of free CysSH and (b) titration of a 75-nM CH₃HgSCys with various concentrations of free GSH. The arrows show the direction of increasing concentration of CysSH (a) or GSH (b).

intracellular thiol, likely facilitates the transport of Hg or MeHg in the biological system (Rabenstein and Reid, 1984; Cheesman et al., 1988).

2. *Reduced Selectivity*: The capability of exchanging Hg^{2+} or CH_3Hg^+ between different thiols or selenols (when $R \neq R'$) makes every thiol- or selenol-containing protein a potential target for Hg or MeHg binding, which may have contributed to its wide-spectrum toxicity.

3. *Possibility for Detoxification*: Rapid ligand exchange also makes it possible for detoxifying Hg or MeHg by the *in vivo* presence of selenols, or by therapeutic application of other thiols (e.g., 2,3-dimercapto-propanol; 2,3-dimercaptopropanesulfonic acid; penicillamine; Cheesman et al., 1988) to "extract" Hg or MeHg from their thiol complexes in the body fluids and tissues.

16.6 THIOL-CONTAINING BIOMOLECULES IN THE UPTAKE AND METABOLISM OF MERCURY

Several recent reviews are available on the uptake, transport, metabolism, and toxic effects of Hg(0), Hg(I), inorganic Hg(II), MeHg, and EtHg in humans (Clarkson, 2002; Clarkson and Magos, 2006; Mutter et al., 2007; Bridges and Zalups, 2010), which will not be repeated here. Instead, we provide a brief overview of the general processes governing the uptake and metabolism in biological systems (not limited to humans) of three environmentally significant Hg species: Hg(0), inorganic Hg(II), and MeHg. The emphasis will be on the roles of thiol-containing biomolecules in these processes.

16.6.1 Hg(0)

When taken up by biota, Hg(0) can readily cross cellular membranes and be carried out to all tissues in the body (Table 16.1). This is not necessarily exclusively because of the lipid solubility and diffusivity of Hg(0); uptake through a protein-lined transport channel is also possible (Clarkson and Magos, 2006). Hg(0) can also be formed *in vivo* as a result of Hg(II) reduction (Section 16.6.2) or MeHg demethylation (Section 16.6.3). Once into a cell, Hg(0) can be rapidly oxidized to inorganic Hg(II) by the catalase—H_2O_2 pathway (Clarkson and Magos, 2006); the remaining unoxidized Hg(0) is exhaled out of the body. The capability of Hg(0) transporting across the BBB (Clarkson, 2002; Clarkson and Magos, 2006) and its subsequent oxidation to Hg(II) give rise to the neurotoxicity of inorganic Hg, though this is usually of negligible concern when compared with MeHg (Section 16.6.3) because of the generally low concentrations of Hg(0) in the environment.

There is no evidence that thiol-containing biomolecules are involved in the uptake, transport, or excretion of Hg(0). However, since the *in vivo* oxidation of Hg(0) to Hg(II) is the primary mode of activation for its toxicity (Clarkson and Magos, 2006), GSH and anti-oxidative selenoenzymes or selenoproteins (e.g., GPx) may alleviate the toxicity of Hg(0) by controlling the level of H_2O_2 in the cell. Furthermore, as shown in Table 16.1, once oxidized to Hg(II), thiol-containing biomolecules become its major binding targets.

16.6.2 Inorganic Hg(II)

Greater uncertainties exist in how inorganic Hg(II) is taken up through cellular membranes. Both passive and facilitated uptake pathways have been suggested

TABLE 16.1 Known and Postulated Hg Species Involved in the Uptake and Transport of Hg in Mammalian Organs

Organ	Direction of Transport	Hg(0)	Inorganic Hg(II)	MeHg
Brain	Uptake	Hg(0)		$CH_3HgSCys$; $CH_3HgSHcy$
	Export	Hg(0)		
Erythrocytes	Uptake	Hg(0)		CH_3HgSG; $CH_3HgSCys$
	Export	Hg(0)		
Intestine	Absorption	Hg(0)	HgL; $Hg(SR)_2$	CH_3HgSG; $CH_3HgSCys$
	Secretion	Hg(0)	$Hg(SR)_2$	CH_3HgSG; $CH_3HgSCys$
Kidney	Uptake	Hg(0)	$Hg(SR)_2$	$CH_3HgSCys$
	Export	Hg(0)	$Hg(SR)_2$	CH_3HgSR
Liver	Uptake	Hg(0)	$Hg(SR)_2$	CH_3HgSR
	Export	Hg(0)	$Hg(SR)_2$	CH_3HgSR
Placenta	Uptake	Hg(0)	$Hg(SR)_2$	CH_3HgSR
	Export	Hg(0)	$Hg(SR)_2$	CH_3HgSR

HgL, inorganic Hg(II) complexes with non-thiol-containing molecules (e.g., Cl^-); R, thiol-containing molecules.
Source: Based on Clarkson and Magos (2006); Bridges and Zalups (2010).

in the literature. The passive pathway would favor the uptake of nonpolar or neutral complexes such as $HgCl_2$ (Mason et al., 1996) and HgS(0) (Benoit et al., 1999) which diffuse more readily across cellular membranes. The facilitated pathway, however, suggests that cellular uptake of all the Hg(II) species is possible (Golding et al., 2002, 2007).

Of particular importance is the recent finding that the uptake of inorganic Hg(II) from aqueous solution by a sulfate-reducing bacterium (SRB) *Geobacter sulfurreducens*, a known Hg methylator, is promoted by the presence of L-CysSH (Schaefer and Morel, 2009). This was attributed to the formation of a Hg–CysSH complex, presumably $Hg(SCys)_2$. Since $Hg(SCys)_2$ is highly polar, its uptake across membranes is likely via a mechanism different from passive diffusion. Similar enhanced uptake of inorganic Hg(II) was also observed in a facultative anaerobic bacteria *Vibrio anguillarum* in the presence of histidine under anaerobic conditions (Golding et al., 2007), suggesting that the enhanced uptake may be ubiquitous to essential amino acids and not necessarily involving the S–Hg interaction. It is interesting to note that in both cases, the enhanced uptake occurred under anaerobic conditions; under aerobic conditions, the presence of histidine did not result in enhanced uptake of Hg(II) by *V. anguillarum* (Golding et al., 2007).

As shown in Table 16.1, once in the biological system, the transport of inorganic Hg(II) is almost exclusively via Hg^{2+} complexes with thiolic complexes $Hg(SR)_2$. The kidneys are the primary organ where inorganic Hg(II) accumulates, resulting in nephrotoxicity. One postulated mechanism for inorganic Hg(II) to transport across the plasma membranes in renal proximal tubular epithelial cells involves $Hg(SCys)_2$ and $Hg(SHcy)_2$ complexes, which may be transported by system $b^{0,+}$ amino acid transporter because of the molecular mimicry between these complexes and cystine (Bridges and Zalups, 2004, 2010; Bridges et al., 2004). There is no evidence, however, that $Hg(SCys)_2$, $Hg(SG)_2$, or inorganic Hg(II) in general can cross the BBB; therefore, inorganic Hg(II) in brain must be formed *in vivo* from the oxidation of Hg(0) or demethylation of MeHg (Section 16.6.3).

16.6.3 MeHg

Although abiotic methylation of inorganic Hg(II) to MeHg can and do occur in the environment, the majority of MeHg is thought to be formed microbially. Several species of SRB and Fe(III)-reducing bacteria are known to be able to methylate Hg(II) (Compeau and Bartha, 1985; Fleming et al., 2006; Kerin et al., 2006). There is no conclusive evidence that Hg methylation occurs *in vivo* in animals; instead, animals, including humans, take up MeHg primarily from their diets. To most human populations, for example, this is via consumption of fish and seafood (Clarkson, 2002; Sunderland, 2007) in which MeHg concentrations are elevated because of biomagnification. Indigenous people in the circumpolar Arctic may take up a significant amount of MeHg via consumption of marine mammal tissues that have been shown to contain high levels of MeHg (Lockhart et al., 2005; Gaden et al., 2009). Elevated concentrations of MeHg have also been reported recently in rice grown from mining impacted areas (Horvat et al., 2003; Feng et al., 2008; Li et al., 2010).

As shown in Table 16.1, the transport of MeHg between various organs is exclusively via CH_3Hg^+ complexes with thiols, presumably in the form of CH_3HgSR. However, one important difference from that of inorganic Hg(II) is that MeHg can also cross the BBB, and thus cause neurotoxicity. The BBB transfer of MeHg is generally thought to be due to the formation of the CH_3Hg^+ complex with L-CysSH, $CH_3HgSCys$ (Aschner and Clarkson, 1989), and possibly with DL-HcySH, $CH_3HgSHcy$ (Mokrzan et al., 1995). These complexes are transported into the brain capillary endothelial cells through the L-type large neutral amino acid transporters (LAT 1 and 2) (Kerper et al., 1992; Mokrzan et al., 1995; Bridges and Zalups, 2010). The observations that CH_3Hg^+ complexes with D-CysSH and GSH do not transport across the BBB suggest that molecular mimicry between $CH_3HgSCys$ (or $CH_3HgSHcy$) and the essential amino acid methionine, which is known to be transported by LAT, might be at play (Kerper et al., 1992; Clarkson, 1993; Mokrzan et al., 1995; Simmons-Willis et al., 2002). However, recent studies suggest that such mimicry occurs only in the $L\alpha$ region of the molecules (Hoffmeyer et al., 2006).

MeHg is known to gradually demethylate to inorganic Hg (Hg(II) and Hg(0)) *in vivo* (Norseth and Clarkson, 1970; Mehra and Choi, 1981). In fact, inorganic Hg(II) present in the brain, liver, and kidneys is mainly because of demethylation of MeHg (Lind et al., 1988; Hansen et al., 1989). Since Hg^{2+} binds to thiol-containing biomolecules stronger than CH_3Hg^+, the *in vivo* demethylation of MeHg to inorganic Hg(II) could enhance the toxicity unless the resulted Hg(II) is immobilized to HgS(s) or HgSe(s) (Section 16.7). There is reason to believe that the neurotoxicity of MeHg is due to its transportability across the BBB and subsequent demethylation to Hg^{2+} in the brain.

MeHg is excreted mainly through the bile and through urine to some extent (Norseth and Clarkson, 1971; Refsvik and Norseth, 1975; Hirata and Takahashi, 1981). MeHg complexes excreted in bile are mostly associated with small molecular weight thiols that can be reabsorbed from the intestine. This circulation is one of the major reasons responsible for the long half-life of MeHg in animals (Hirata and Takahashi, 1981).

16.7 SELENIUM AIDED BIOMINERALIZATION OF MERCURY AND METHYLMERCURY

Since Parízek and Oštádalová's (1967) discovery of the protective effect of Se on kidney intoxication by Hg in laboratory rats, extensive studies have demonstrated that Se can modify the toxicity of both inorganic Hg and MeHg in the laboratory and in nature. While the majority of the studies reported antagonistic interactions between Se and Hg, synergistic interactions have also been documented (Khan and Wang, 2009a).

In a recent review (Khan and Wang, 2009a), we have summarized several potential molecular-level mechanisms for the Hg–Se antagonism. The presence or addition of Se-containing biomolecules could decrease the toxicity of inorganic Hg(II) or MeHg by (i) the formation of Hg–selenol or MeHg–selenol compounds, which prevents the binding of Hg^{2+} or CH_3Hg^+ to thiolic sites; (ii) demethylation of MeHg to form biologically "inert" HgSe(s); (iii) redistribution of Hg among various organs; (iv) inhibition of methyl radicals from MeHg; and/or (v) prevention of Hg-induced Se deficiency. It is possible that all of these processes may have contributed to the well-documented Hg–Se antagonism, though their relative importance may differ in different biological systems under different physiological conditions.

Mechanisms (i) and (ii) are of particular interest in the metallomics of Hg. As discussed earlier, selenol groups on Se-containing biomolecules tend to form thermodynamically more stable complexes with Hg^{2+} or CH_3Hg^+; therefore, their presence in the biological system would tend to "extract" Hg^{2+} or CH_3Hg^+ from thiolic sites and thus decrease their toxicity effects. What is even more important is that Se compounds also provide effective and efficient pathways for converting both inorganic Hg(II) and MeHg to chemically and biologically inert HgSe(s). HgSe(s) granules or nanoparticles have indeed been reported in the liver and kidneys of marine mammals and sea birds (Martoja and Viale, 1977; Martoja and Berry, 1980; Nigro, 1994; Rawson et al., 1995; Nigro and Leonzio, 1996; Arai et al., 2004), and most recently in human brain (Korbas et al., 2010).

16.7.1 Se-Aided Biomineralization of Inorganic Hg(II)

Suzuki and colleagues were the first to report the occurrence of a soluble $(HgSe)_n$ polymer (n is an integer) on SelP upon addition of Hg(II) and selenite *in vivo* or *in vitro* (Yoneda and Suzuki, 1997a,b; Suzuki et al., 1998). Gailer et al. (2000) later showed that the solubilization of $(HgSe)_n$ does not necessarily involve SelP; GSH alone could solubilize HgSe formed from the interaction between Hg(II) and selenite. We have recently showed that the GSH-aided solubilization is a pH reversible reaction (Khan and Wang, 2009b) (Fig. 16.4, left panel): in the presence of excess amount of GSH, selenide produced from the reduction of selenite reacts with Hg(II) to produce HgSe, which is held soluble by forming $GS_m-(HgSe)_n$ species ("black solution") at neutral to slightly alkaline pH. Upon acidification, however, hydrogen bonding results in the formation of $\{(GS)_m - HgSe)_n\}_p$ nanoclusters that precipitate out from the solution ("black precipitation") and eventually age to HgSe(s). This precipitation–dissolution process is reversible simply by changing the pH of the solution (Khan and Wang, 2009b), which could potentially explain the lack of HgSe(s) in the blood plasma in marine mammals. At the physiological pH of the blood ($\sim$7.4), HgSe nanoparticles are present as water-soluble $GS_m-(HgSe)_n$ and thus do not form HgSe(s) granules. In the gastric fluid, where pH is much lower (2.0), $GS_m-(HgSe)_n$ would aggregate into insoluble HgSe nanoclusters and eventually result in HgSe(s). We further showed that the similar process could happen with HgS(s) resulting in the biomineralization of a mixed solid in the form of $HgSe_xS_{1-x}$ ($0 \leq x \leq 1$) (Khan and Wang, 2009b).

16.7.2 Se-Aided Biomineralization of MeHg

Owing to the kinetic stability of the C–Hg bond (Stumm and Morgan, 1996), MeHg demethylation in nature is thought to occur primarily via photolysis or microbial processes (Fitzgerald et al., 2007). The first established mechanism for chemical demethylation of MeHg in nature is the reaction between MeHg and H_2S via a bis(methylmercuric)sulfide (($CH_3Hg)_2S$) intermediate, ultimately forming HgS(s) (Rowland et al., 1977; Craig and Bartlett, 1978).

As mentioned earlier, demethylation of MeHg is known to occur readily in the biological systems, and Se has long been postulated to be involved in this demethylation process (Khan and Wang, 2009a). Indirect evidence has suggested that the Se-aided demethylation may have involved the formation of bis(methylmercuric) selenide (($CH_3Hg)_2Se$) (Naganuma et al., 1980; Masukawa et al., 1982), similar to $(CH_3Hg)_2S$ in the H_2S case. We have recently confirmed this pathway when synthesizing MeHg complexes with various selenoamino acids, including CysSeH, GSeH, selenopenicillamine, and selenomethionine (Khan and Wang, 2010). Black precipitates were observed from aqueous solutions of all these complexes, which were characterized to be HgSe(s) by X-ray powder diffraction (XRD). The presence of $(CH_3Hg)_2Se$ and $(CH_3)_2Hg$ were confirmed by NMR and gas chromatography (GC)-MS, respectively. The proposed mechanism is shown also in Fig. 16.4 (right panel). A similar demethylation process may also occur for MeHg complexes with thiol-containing amino acids such as CysSH and GSH (Lemes, 2010), but binding to selenoamino acids seems to have enhanced the demethylation process.

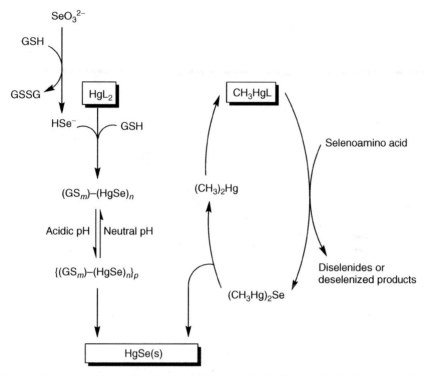

Figure 16.4 Se-aided biomineralization of inorganic Hg(II) and MeHg based on Khan and Wang (2009b, 2010). *m, n, p*: integer numbers.

Although Se-aided biomineralization occurs with both inorganic Hg(II) and MeHg, the later is likely the main pathway for HgSe(s) granules found in the liver of marine mammals where exposure to Hg is almost exclusively via dietary uptake of MeHg (Khan and Wang, 2010). This is further supported by the recent X-ray absorption spectroscopic evidence of the presence of HgSe nanoparticles in frozen tissues of human brain following acute poisoning of MeHg or fish consumption (Korbas et al., 2010). The occurrence of the nonpolar $(CH_3Hg)_2Se$ as an intermediate during the demethylation also provides a new mechanism for the transfer of MeHg across the BBB. Furthermore, it is possible that selenoamino acid-aided MeHg demethylation may occur in the aquatic environment where MeHg is primarily formed. Although there has been no report on the concentrations of selenoamino acids in natural waters, nanomolar to micromolar levels of their sulfur counterparts have been reported in surface and sediment pore waters (Zhang et al., 2004).

16.8 ANALYTICAL AND MODELING APPROACHES

At the center of metallomics study is the identification and quantification of various chemical species making up the metallome in a biological system (Haraguchi,

2004; Lobinski et al., 2010). Since different chemical species of a metal exhibit different degrees of mobility, transportability, chemical reactivity, and thus toxicity, the measurement of the total concentration of the metal of interest in the whole body or among various tissues is rarely sufficient. Instead, chemical speciation information on spatially or temporally resolved scales is needed.

In the case of Hg, while it has become a routine analysis in many laboratories for the differentiation of MeHg from Hg(0), inorganic Hg(II) and other organic Hg (e.g., EtHg), the identification and quantification of molecular forms of inorganic Hg(II) or MeHg in environmental or biological samples have only recently become possible, thanks to the technological breakthroughs in high resolution and highly sensitive molecular speciation techniques. However, given the complexity and thermodynamic nature of metal speciation in biological systems, it is unlikely that an analytical technique will ever become available which is capable of analyzing all possible species of a metal in a biological system. Therefore, in addition to the continuous development and refinement of analytical techniques, computational approaches and thermodynamic modeling provide important alternatives that will help shed new insights into molecular-level processes underlying the Hg metallomics.

16.8.1 HPLC-MS

HPLC is a versatile group of separation techniques for molecular species. When coupled with atomic (e.g., by ICP) or molecular (e.g., by electrospray ionization, ESI) MS, HPLC-MS provides a powerful means for the separation and quantification of Hg and MeHg species. For example, the presence of $Hg(SeCys)_2$ and/or $Hg(SCys)_2$ in salmon egg cell cytoplasm (Hasegawa et al., 2005) and the *in vitro* and *in vivo* formation of SelP-bound $(HgSe)_n$ (Suzuki et al., 1998) were all reported on the basis of HPLC-ICP-MS evidence.

Hintelmann and Simmons (2003) were the first to use ESI-MS to study MeHg speciation in aqueous solutions. The method was able to differentiate polynuclear complexes such as $[(CH_3Hg)_2OH]^+$ and $[(CH_3Hg)_3O]^+$, but had limited applicability in environmental or biological samples because of insufficient detection limits (Krupp et al., 2008). By interfacing HPLC with ICP-MS and ESI-MS, Krupp et al. (2008) were successful in determining $CH_3HgSCys$ and CH_3HgSG in aqueous solutions spiked with laboratory standards, but were not able to determine MeHg speciation in real-world plant samples because of the difficulty in extracting these compounds from the samples.

Lemes and Wang (2009) were the first to develop a HPLC-ICP/ESI-MS method for quantitative measurement of MeHg–thiol complexes in biological tissues, and reported the first direct analytical evidence for the presence and dominance of $CH_3HgSCys$, the MeHg species that is thought to be able to cross the BBB, in dogfish muscle (*Squalus acanthius*). The method was subsequently applied for the speciation analysis of MeHg in rice (*Oryza sativa L.*) grains grown from a Hg-mining area (Li et al., 2010). Similar to fish muscle, MeHg in the uncooked rice is found to be dominated by $CH_3HgSCys$. Interestingly, although cooking does not change the total Hg or total MeHg concentration in rice, no $CH_3HgSCys$ was measurable after cooking, suggesting that most, if not all, of the $CH_3HgSCys$ is converted to other forms of MeHg, the identity and toxicity of which remain elusive (Li et al., 2010). Most recently, the HPLC-ICP-MS method was used to determined MeHg and Se speciation in the muscle, brain, liver, and kidneys of beluga whales from the western Canadian Arctic (Lemes et al. 2011). MeHg in all the tissues analyzed was found to be dominated by $CH_3HgSCys$, with CH_3HgSG also detected in the muscle, and to a much lesser extent in the liver, and brain tissues. Furthermore, a profound inorganic Hg peak was detected in the liver and brain tissues, which showed the same retention time as a Se peak, suggesting the presence of a Hg-Se complex, most likely an inorganic Hg complex with a selenoamino acid (Lemes et al. 2011).

As an isotope-specific detector after HPLC separation, ICP-MS offers superior sensitivity and isotopic capability, but itself does not differentiate molecular forms of Hg; molecular identities of the species measured by ICP-MS have to be deduced on the basis of HPLC separation. In contrast, ESI-MS (and other soft-ionization MS) retains molecular information of parent or daughter species, but its application is often complicated by the presence of concomitant ions generated by matrix components that can suppress the ionization of the species of interest and thus compromise the detection limit, as well as introduce interference ions (Lobinski et al., 2010). As a result, many laboratories including ours have been actively pursuing simultaneous ICP-MS and ESI-MS determinations after HPLC separation. Instrumental development in tandem (in space or in time) ICP/ESI-MS would make this technique particularly useful for metallomics studies.

16.8.2 Capillary Electrophoresis (CE)

CE is another versatile technique that can offer such advantages as high resolution, low surface-to-volume ratio, short analysis time, low sample size requirement, and low cost. Through careful selection of background electrolyte, the electrophoretic separation can be operated under physiological or near-physiological buffer conditions (Li et al., 2006). Moreover, unlike HPLC, there is no interaction between the analytes and the stationary phase in CE, making CE an excellent tool to study the interaction between Hg species and biomolecules with minor disturbance of the existing Hg–biomolecule equilibria (Silva da Rocha et al., 2000, 2001; Li et al., 2005, 2006, 2007; Li, 2011). For instance, a CE technique coupled with flame-heated furnace atomic absorption spectrometry (FHF-AAS) has been developed, which is capable of speciating MeHg and inorganic Hg in fish muscle samples (Li et al., 2005). Subsequently, the method has been successfully used in probing the interactions of Hg(II), MeHg, EtHg, and phenylmercury (PhHg) with DNA, and provided direct evidence for the formation of Hg–DNA adducts, revealing the fastest binding of MeHg to DNA (Li et al., 2006). A similar Hg speciation technique has been developed for CE-ICP-MS (Silva da Rocha et al., 2001; Li, 2011).

16.8.3 Synchrotron-Based X-ray Absorption Spectroscopy (XAS)

Another powerful technique for Hg speciation in biological samples is synchrotron-based X-ray absorption spectroscopy (XAS). X-ray absorption near-edge spectroscopy (XANES) provides information about oxidation states of the Hg atoms to be probed, whereas extended X-ray absorption fine structure (EXAFS) can elucidate structural information about the atomic neighborhood of the Hg metal atom of interest (e.g., coordination number, the identity of the ligand atoms, and the bond length). When combined, XANES and EXAFS can probe both atomic and molecular information of Hg species in a biological sample; in particular, they can be readily used to "map" the spatial distribution of Hg species in a sample.

By comparing the Hg L_{III} XANES of swordfish muscle (*Xiphias gladiu*) spectrum with the spectra of several MeHg standards, Harris et al. (2003) provided the first analytical evidence for the dominance of MeHg–thiol complexes in the fish muscle. However, since XAS can only probe the bonding environment immediately to the Hg atom, it cannot deduce to which thiol (CysSH or GSH or other thiols) the Hg atom is bonded. The complex was later identified to be $CH_3HgSCys$ by the aforementioned HPLC-ICP/ESI-MS technique (Lemes and Wang, 2009). XAS has also been successfully used in identifying the bonding environment of Hg^{2+} and CH_3Hg^+ with sulfur-containing proteins such as MTs (Stillman, 1995; Leiva-Presa et al., 2004). Most recently, XAS analysis of human brain samples following MeHg poisoning or environmental exposure has confirmed the presence of inorganic and methyl Hg complexes with thiols and selenols, as well as HgSe nanoparticles (Korbas et al., 2010).

16.8.4 Computational Chemistry Approaches

Where analytical techniques are not available or incapable of deducing Hg speciation information in biological systems, computational chemistry approaches can be used to model structural, electronic, and thermodynamic properties of all possible Hg complexes. They can also be used as secondary evidence to support or critique analytical or experimental data.

A variety of computational approaches have been used in the study of the metallomics of Hg, including the Hartree–Fock theory, many-body perturbation theory, configuration interactions, coupled cluster theory, and the density functional theory (Koch and Holthausen, 2000), and by several software packages such as Gaussian 03 (Frisch et al., 2004), HONDO (Dupuis et al., 1988), and GAMESS (Schmidt et al., 1993). To account for the relativistic effect of Hg, relativistic effective core potential-type basis sets such as Stuttgart–Dresden basis set (SDD) (Figgen et al., 2005) and 6-31+G, 6-31+G(d) (Krishnan et al., 1980) are commonly used along with functionals such as B3LYP (Lee et al., 1988; Becke, 1993) and B3-PW91 (Perdew et al., 1996). These basis sets neglect core electrons but properly describe their effects upon the valence electrons, with relativistic effects incorporated. Additional basis functions of d type (polarization functions) are added to each of the non-H atoms to better account for the polarization of the electron density during bond formation. To account for the solvent effect or to optimize compounds in solution, the Conductor Polarizable Continuum Model (CPCM) (Cossi et al., 2003) or Isodensity Polarized Continuum Method (IPCM) (Wiberg et al., 1996) may be used.

For instance, Tai and Lim (2006) carried out computational calculations to study the coordination stereochemistry, bonding, and metal selectivity of Hg and reported the differences between inorganic Hg^{2+} and CH_3Hg^+ in their interactions with different ligands of biological interest. Their results reveal that, relative to Hg^{2+}, the lower positive charge on CH_3Hg^+ results in a longer and weaker bond with a given ligand, in accord with the observed kinetic lability of CH_3Hg^+ complexes. They also found that Hg^{2+} is a far better electron acceptor than Zn^{2+}, enabling Hg^{2+} to displace the native cofactor from essential Zn-containing enzymes and proteins which may have contributed to the Hg toxicity. In another example, our recent computational calculations (Asaduzzaman et al., 2010) show that, although the Hg–S bond strength in MeHg complexes with sulfur-containing amino acids is greater than the Hg–Se bond strength in their corresponding selenoamino acid complexes, MeHg–selenoamino acid complexes are thermodynamically more favorable than those of the corresponding amino acid complexes. This can be attributed to the lower stability of the reactant selenoamino acids. Such different stability and favorability of formation might have contributed to the Hg–Se antagonism.

16.8.5   Thermodynamic Modeling

The lability of Hg^{2+} and CH_3Hg^+ complexes with thiols and selenols (Section 16.5) makes thermodynamic modeling of Hg and MeHg speciation in the presence of thiols or selenols a promising alternative to direct analytical measurements. A prerequisite for such modeling is, however, the availability of accurate information on the stoichiometries and formation constants of all possible complexes under the conditions relevant to the biological systems. This is unfortunately not the case: only limited data are available for Hg and MeHg complexes with thiol- or selenol-containing amino acids; and most notably almost no such thermodynamic data are available for thiol- or selenol-containing proteins or enzymes. Even for those whose formation data have been reported, large uncertainties exist and it is not unusual to see the formation constant for the same species reported by different studies differ by several orders of magnitude (Berthon, 1995). Furthermore, much of the available data were determined under laboratory conditions that may bear no relevance to the concentration ranges, temperature, ionic strength, and matrix conditions found in biological systems. There is a clear need for the determination and evaluation of high quality and self-consistent dataset of thermodynamic constants for such systems.

Nevertheless, MeHg complexes with small thiol- and seleno-containing amino acids have been better studied than the corresponding Hg complexes (Berthon, 1995; NIST, 2004). Table 16.2 summarizes the best available thermodynamic constants for MeHg complexes with CysSH, GSH, and CysSeH, along with

TABLE 16.2 Thermodynamic Constants for MeHg Complexes with Small Molecular Weight Biogenic Thiols and Selenols, as well as with Inorganic Ligands (OH^-, Cl^-, and Sulfide) ($t = 25°C$; $I = 0$)

Reaction	log K	References
$MeHg^+ + H_2O = MeHgOH + H^+$	-4.53	NIST (2004)
$MeHg^+ + Cl^- = MeHgCl$	5.45^a	NIST (2004)
$H_2S = H^+ + HS^-$	-7.02	NIST (2004)
$MeHg^+ + HS^- = MeHgS^- + H^+$	$7.0^{a,b}$	NIST (2004)
$2MeHg^+ + HS^- = (MeHg)_2S + H^+$	$23.52^{a,b}$	NIST (2004)
$3MeHg^+ + HS^- = (MeHg)_3S^+ + H^+$	$30.52^{a,b}$	NIST (2004)
$CysS^{2-} + H^+ = HCysS^-$	10.74	NIST (2004)
$CysS^{2-} + 2H^+ = H_2CysS$	19.10	NIST (2004)
$CysS^{2-} + 3H^+ = H_3CysS^+$	20.80	NIST (2004)
$CH_3Hg^+ + CysS^{2-} = CH_3HgSCys^-$	16.90^a	NIST (2004)
$CH_3Hg^+ + CysS^{2-} + H^+ = CH_3HgSCysH$	26.07^a	NIST (2004)
$GS^{3-} + H^+ = HGS^{2-}$	10.17^a	NIST (2004)
$GS^{3-} + 2H^+ = H_2GS^-$	19.25^a	NIST (2004)
$GS^{3-} + 3H^+ = H_3GS$	22.96^a	NIST (2004)
$GS^{3-} + 4H^+ = H_4GS^+$	25.04^a	NIST (2004)
$CH_3Hg^+ + GS^{3-} = CH_3HgSG^{2-}$	16.66^a	NIST (2004)
$CH_3Hg^+ + GS^{3-} + H^+ = CH_3HgSGH^-$	26.35^a	NIST (2004)
$CH_3Hg^+ + GS^{3-} + 2H^+ = CH_3HgSGH_2$	30.01^a	NIST (2004)
$CysSe^{2-} + H^+ = HCysSe^-$	11.24^c	Arnold et al. (1986)
$CysSe^{2-} + 2H^+ = H_2CysSe$	16.95^c	Arnold et al. (1986)
$CysSe^{2-} + 3H^+ = H_3CysSe^+$	19.15^c	Arnold et al. (1986)
$CH_3Hg^+ + CysSe^{2-} = CH_3HgSeCys^-$	17.94^c	Arnold et al. (1986)

[a]Recalculated from $I = 0.1$ M to $I = 0$ M using the Davis equation.
[b]Data for 20°C.
[c]Recalculated from $I = 0.3$ M to $I = 0$ M using the Davis equation.

OH^-, Cl^-, and inorganic sulfide (HS^-), all corrected to $I = 0$ M and $t = 25°C$. On the basis of these constants, MeHg speciation modeling for two different scenarios was performed (Fig. 16.5). Scenario 1 is a hypothetic freshwater system with the following composition: $[MeHg] = 1$ pM, $[Cl^-] = 1$ mM, $[HS^-]_T = 1$ µM, and $[CysSH]_T = [GSH]_T = [CysSeH]_T = 0.1$ µM, $I = 0.1$ M, and $t = 25°C$. Except for CysSeH for which no field data are available, such conditions typically exist in uncontaminated freshwater lakes (Zhang et al., 2004; Wang and Tessier, 2009). As shown in Fig. 16.5a, the model predicts that in such a freshwater system, MeHg speciation would be dominated by thiol complexes when pH<6 and by inorganic sulfide complexes when pH>6. The dominance of MeHg–thiol complexes under acidic conditions are potentially of major importance as SRB-mediated Hg methylation is known to be favored under acidic conditions (Compeau and Bartha, 1985).

Figure 16.5b shows the competition between CysSH and GSH for MeHg under Scenario 2, a hypothetic solution similar to human blood ($[MeHg] = 10$ nM,

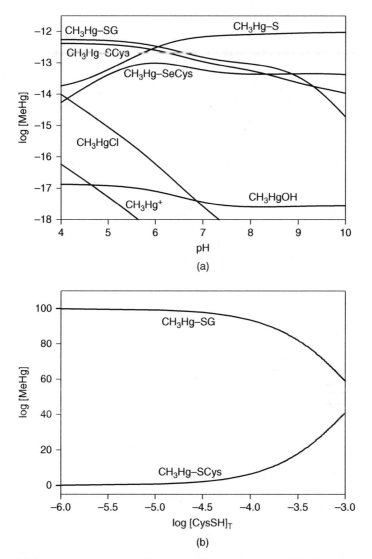

Figure 16.5 Thermodynamic modeling of MeHg speciation in (a) a hypothetic natural water as a function of pH ([MeHg] $= 1 \times 10^{-12}$ M, [Cl$^-$] $= 1 \times 10^{-3}$ M, [HS$^-$]$_T$ $= 1 \times 10^{-6}$ M, [CysSH]$_T$ $=$ [GSH]$_T$ $=$ [CysSeH]$_T$ $= 1 \times 10^{-7}$ M, $I = 0.1$ M, $t = 25°$C) and (b) a hypothetical biological fluid as a function of total CysSH concentration ([MeHg] $= 1 \times 10^{-8}$ M, [Cl$^-$] $= 1 \times 10^{-3}$ M, [GSH]$_T$ $= 1 \times 10^{-3}$ M, pH $= 7.4$, $I = 0.1$ M, $t = 25°$C). The formation constants for Hg and MeHg complexes were taken from Table 16.2. The calculation was done with the computer software MINEQL+ Version 4.5 (Schecher and McAvoy, 2003).

[GSH]$_T$ = 1 mM, pH = 7.4, I = 0.1 M). Note that since temperature correction to 37°C is not available for most of these constants, t = 25°C is used in the calculation. Free CysSH concentration in human blood is in the micromolar level (Mills and Lang, 1996), about three orders of magnitude lower than GSH. Under such conditions, MeHg speciation is almost exclusively present as MeHg-SG, which is expected to facilitate the transport of MeHg around various organs but does not cross the BBB (Table 16.1). However, as shown in Fig. 16.5b, an increase in the concentration of CysSH would result in an increase in the concentration MeHg–SCys that can cross the BBB; when the CysSH concentration equals to that of GSH, ~40% of MeHg would be present as CH$_3$HgCys. Such a high concentration of CysSH is unlikely to occur in human blood, but the example shows how a change in the *in vivo* thiol concentration could result in major changes in MeHg speciation and thus its potential neurotoxicity.

16.9 CONCLUSION

Several factors make thiol- and seleno-containing biomolecules of major interest in the Hg metallomics: (i) thiols and, to a lesser extent, selenols are abundant in all biological systems; (ii) thiols and selenols have very high thermodynamic affinity for Hg^{2+} or CH$_3$Hg$^+$, and thus are primary sites where Hg and MeHg are bound in biological systems; (iii) since thiols and selenols are involved in many essential and critical biological functions, the binding of Hg^{2+} and CH$_3$Hg$^+$ may alter these essential functions giving rise to their wide-spectrum toxicity; (iv) the Hg or MeHg complexes with thiols or selenols are highly labile which facilitates the transformation and transport of Hg and MeHg among various organs in a biological system; and (v) selenols are also effectively involved in detoxifying Hg or MeHg by ultimately transforming Hg or MeHg to the chemically inert HgSe(s). In addition to their *in vivo* roles in Hg and MeHg toxicity, evidence is emerging that biogenic thiols (and potentially selenols) in the environment may also affect the bioavailability and biological uptake of Hg and MeHg. Therefore, molecular-level understanding of the roles of thiols and selenols will greatly advance our understanding of the metallomics of Hg in the biological system, the interactions at the biointerfaces, as well as the development of bioremediation techniques.

ACKNOWLEDGMENT

This work was financially supported by the Natural Science and Engineering Research Council (NSERC) of Canada.

REFERENCES

Arai T, Ikemoto T, Hokura A, Terada Y, Kunito T, Tanabe S, et al. Chemical forms of mercury and cadmium accumulated in marine mammals and seabirds as determined by XAFS analysis. Environ Sci Technol 2004;38:6468–6474.

Arnold AP, Tan KS, Rabenstein DL. Nuclear magnetic resonance studies of the solution chemistry of metal complexes. 23. Complexation of methylmercury by selenohydryl-containing amino acids and related molecules. Inorg Chem 1986;25:2433–2437.

Asaduzzaman AM, Khan MAK, Schreckenbach G, Wang F. Computational studies of structural, electronic, spectroscopic, and thermodynamic properties of methylmercury amino acid complexes and their Se analogues. Inorg Chem 2010;49:870–878.

Aschner M, Clarkson TW. Methyl mercury uptake across bovine brain capillary endothelial cells in vitro: the role of amino acids. Pharmacol Toxicol 1989;64:293–297.

Becke AD. Density-functional thermochemistry. 3. The role of exact exchange. J Chem Phys 1993;98:5648–5652.

Benoit JM, Gilmour CC, Mason RP, Heyes A. Sulfide controls on mercury speciation and bioavailability to methylating bacteria in sediment pore waters. Environ Sci Technol 1999;33:951–957.

Berthon G. The stability constants of metal complexes of amino acids with polar side chains. Pure Appl Chem 1995;67:1117–1240.

Bridges CC, Bauch C, Verrey F, Zalups RK. Mercuric conjugates of cysteine are transported by the amino acid transporter system $b^{0,+}$: Implications of molecular mimicry. J Am Soc Nephrol 2004;15:663–673.

Bridges CC, Zalups RK. Homocysteine, system $b^{0,+}$ and the renal epithelial transport and toxicity of inorganic mercury. Am J Pathol 2004;165:1385–1394.

Bridges CC, Zalups RK. Transport of inorganic mercury and methylmercury in target tissues and organs. J Toxicol Environ Health B 2010;13:385–410.

Burk RF, Hill KE. Selenoprotein P: an extracellular protein with unique physical characteristics and a role in selenium homeostasis. Annu Rev Nutr 2005;25:215–235.

Canty AJ, Carty AJ, Malone SF. Methylmercury(II) selenolates. Synthesis and characterization of MeHgSeMe and MeHgSePh and ^{1}H and [199]Hg NMR studies of ligand exchange in methylmercury(II) thiolates and selenolates, including amino acid complexes. J Inorg Biochem 1983;19:133–142.

Canty AJ, Colton R, D'Agostino A, Traeger JC. Positive and negative ion electrospray mass spectrometry studies of some amino acids and glutathione, and their interactions with alkali metal ions and methylmercury. Inorg Chim Acta 1994;223:103–107.

Carty AJ, Malone SF, Taylor NJ. The selenium-mercury interaction: synthesis, spectroscopic and x-ray structural studies of methylmercury-selenourea complexes. J Organomet Chem 1979;172:201–211.

Cheesman BV, Amold AP, Rabenstein DL. Nuclear magnetic resonance studies of the solution chemistry of metal complexes. 25. Hg(thiol)$_3$ complexes and Hg(II)-thiol ligand exchange kinetics. J Am Chem Soc 1988;110:6359–6364.

Clarkson TW. Molecular and ionic mimicry of toxic metals. Annu Rev Pharmacol Toxicol 1993;33:545–571.

Clarkson TW. The three modern faces of mercury. Environ Health Perspect 2002;110:11–23.

Clarkson TW, Magos L. The toxicology of mercury and its chemical compounds. Crit Rev Toxicol 2006;36:609–662.

Compeau GC, Bartha R. Sulfate-reducing bacteria: principal methylators of mercury in anoxic estuarine sediment. Appl Environ Microbiol 1985;50:498–502.

Cossi M, Rega N, Giovanni S, Barone V. Energies, structures, and electronic properties of molecules in solution with the C-PCM solvation model. J Comp Chem 2003;24:669–681.

Craig PJ, Bartlett PD. The role of hydrogen sulphide in environmental transport of mercury. Nature 1978;275:635–637.

DeVries CR, Wang F. In situ two-dimensional high-resolution profiling of sulfide in sediment interstitial waters. Environ Sci Technol 2003;37:792–797.

Dupuis M, Watts JD, Villar HO, Hurst GJB. HONDO 7.0. QCPE Program No. 544. QCPE Bull 1988;8:79.

Fasman GD. Prediction of protein structure and the principles of protein conformation. New York: Penum Press; 1989.

Feng X, Li P, Qiu G, Wang S, Li G, Shang L, et al. Human exposure to methylmercury through rice intake in mercury mining areas, Guizhou Province. China Environ Sci Technol 2008;42:326–332.

Figgen D, Rauhat G, Dolg M, Stoll H. Energy-consistent pseudopotentials for group 11 and 12 atoms: adjustment to multi-configuration Dirac-Hartree-Fock data. Chem Phys 2005;311:227–244.

Fitzgerald WF, Lamborg CH, Hammerschmidt CR. Marine biogeochemical cycling of mercury. Chem Rev 2007;107:641–662.

Fleming EJ, Mack EE, Green PG, Nelson DC. Mercury methylation from unexpected sources: molybdate inhibited freshwater sediments and iron-reducing bacterium. Appl Environ Microbiol 2006;72:457–464.

Frisch MJ, Trucks GW, Schlegel HB, Scuseria GE, Robb MA, Cheeseman JR, et al. GAUSSIAN-03. Wallingford (CT): Gaussian, Inc; 2004.

Gaden A, Ferguson SH, Harwood L, Melling H, Stern GA. Mercury trends in ringed seals (*Phoca hispida*) from the western Canadian Arctic since 1973: Associations with length of ice-free season. Environ Sci Technol 2009;43:3646–3651.

Gailer J, George GN, Pickering IJ, Madden S, Prince RC, Yu EY, et al. Structure basis of the antagonism between inorganic mercury and selenium in mammals. Chem Res Toxicol 2000;13:1135–1142.

Gladyshev VN. Selenoproteins and selenoproteomes. In Hatfield DL, Berry MJ, Gladyshev VN, editors. Selenium. Its molecular biology and role in human health. 2nd ed. New York (NY): Springer; 2006. p 99–110.

Golding GR, Kelly CA, Sparling R, Loewen PC, Barkay T. Evaluation of mercury toxicity as a predictor of mercury bioavailability. Environ Sci Technol 2007;41:5685–5692.

Golding GR, Kelly CA, Sparling R, Loewen PC, Rudd JWM, Barkay T. Evidence for facilitated uptake of Hg(II) by *vibrio anguillarum* and *escherichia coli* under anaerobic and aerobic conditions. Limnol Oceanogr 2002;47:967–975.

Hansen JC, Reske-Nielsen E, Thorlacius-Ussing O, Rungby J, Dansher G. Distribution of dietary mercury in a dog: quantification and localization of total mercury in organs and central nervous system. Sci Total Environ 1989;78:23–43.

Haraguchi H. Metallomics as integrated biometal science. J Anal At Spectrom 2004;19:5–14.

Harris HH, Pickering IJ, George GN. The chemical from of mercury in fish. Science 2003;201:1203.

Hasegawa T, Asano M, Takatani K, Matsuura H, Umemura T, Haraguchi H. Speciation of mercury in salmon egg cell cytoplasm in relation with metallomics research. Talanta 2005;68:465–469.

Hepler LG, Olofsson G. Mercury. Thermodynamic properties, chemical equilibriums, and standard potentials. Chem Rev 1975;75:585–602:

Hintelmann H, Simmons DA. Determination of aqueous methylmercury species using electrospray mass spectrometry. Can J Anal Sci Spectrosc 2003;48:244–249.

Hirata E, Takahashi H. Degradation of methyl mercury glutathione by pancreatic enzymes in bile. Toxicol Appl Pharmacol 1981;58:483–491.

Hoffmeyer RE, Singh SP, Doonan CJ, Ross ARS, Hughes RJ, Pickering IJ, et al. Molecular mimicry in mercury toxicology. Chem Res Toxicol 2006;19:753–759.

Horvat M, Nolde N, Fajon V, Jereb V, Logar M, Lojen S, et al. Total mercury, methylmercury and selenium in mercury polluted areas in the province Guizhou, China. Sci Total Environ 2003;304:231–256.

Jalilehvand F, Leung BO, Izadifard M, Damian E. Mercury(II) cysteine complexes in alkaline aqueous solution. Inorg Chem 2006;45:66–73.

Kerin EJ, Gilmour CC, Roden E, Suzuki MT, Coates JD, Mason RP. Mercury methylation by dissimilatory iron-reducing bacteria. Appl Environ Microbiol 2006;72:7919–7921.

Kerper LE, Ballatori N, Clarkson TW. Methylmercury transport across the blood-brain barrier by an amino acid carrier. Am J Physiol 1992;262: R761–R765.

Khan MAK, Asaduzzaman AM, Schreckenbach G, Wang F. Synthesis, characterization and structures of methylmercury complexes with selenoamino acids. Dalton Trans 2009;29:5766–5772.

Khan MAK, Wang F. Mercury-selenium compounds and their toxicological significance: toward a molecular understanding of the mercury-selenium antagonism. Environ Toxicol Chem 2009a;28:1567–1577.

Khan MAK, Wang F. Reversible dissolution of glutathione-mediated $HgSe_xS_{1-x}$ nanoparticles and possible significance in Hg-Se antagonism. Chem Res Toxicol 2009b;22:1827–1832.

Khan MAK, Wang F. Chemical demethylation of methylmercury by selenoamino acids. Chem Res Toxicol 2010;23:1202–1206.

Kim YJ, Chai YG, Ryu JC. Selenoprotein W as molecular target of methylmercury in human neuronal cells is down-regulated by GSH depletion. Biochem Biophys Res Commun 2005;330:1095–1102.

Koch W, Holthausen MC. A chemist's guide to density functional theory. New York (NY): Wiley Verlag Chemie; 2000.

Korbas M, O'Donoghue JL, Watson GE, Pickering IJ, Singh SP, Myers GJ, et al. The chemical nature of mercury in human brain following poisoning or environmental exposure. ACS Chem Neurosci 2010;1:810–818.

Krishnan R, Binkley JS, Seeger R, Pople JA. Self-consistent molecular orbital methods. XX. A basis set for correlated wave functions. J Chem Phys 1980;72:650–654.

Krupp EM, Milne BF, Mestrot A, Meharg AA, Feldmann J. Investigation into mercury bound to biothiols: structural identification using ESI–ion-trap MS and introduction of a method for their HPLC separation with simultaneous detection by ICP–MS and ESI–MS. Anal Bioanal Chem 2008;390:1753–1764.

Lee C, Yong W, Parr RG. Development of the colle-salvetti correlation-energy formula into a functional of the electron density. Phys Rev B 1988;37:785–789.

Leiva-Presa A, Capdevila M, Cols N, Atrian S, Gonzalez-Duarte P. Chemical foundation of the attenuation of methylmercury(II) cytotoxicity by metallothioneins. Eur J Biochem 2004;271:1323–1328.

Lemes M. A new analytical method for methylmercury speciation and its application for the study of methylmercury-thiol complexes Ph.D. [dissertation]. Winnipeg: Department of Chemistry, University of Manitoba; 2010. p 122.

Lemes M, Wang F. Methylmercury speciation in fish muscle by HPLC-ICP-MS following enzymatic hydrolysis. J Anal At Spectrom 2009;24:663–668.

Lemes M, Wang F, Stern GA, Ostertag S, Chan HM. Methylmercury and selenium speciation in different tissues of beluga whales (*Delphinapterus leucas*) from the Western Canadian Arctic. Environ Toxicol Chem 2011 (in press).

Li BH. Rapid speciation analysis of mercury by short column capillary electrophoresis on-line coupled with inductively coupled plasma mass spectrometry. Anal Methods 2011;3:116–121.

Li L, Wang F, Meng B, Lemes M, Feng XB, Jiang GB. Speciation of methylmercury in rice grown from a mercury mining area. Environ Pollut 2010;158:3103–3107.

Li Y, Jiang Y, Yan XP. On-line hyphenation of capillary electrophoresis with flame-heated furnace atomic absorption spectrometry for trace mercury speciation. Electrophoresis 2005;26:661–667.

Li Y, Jiang Y, Yan XP. Probing mercury species-DNA interactions by capillary electrophoresis with on-line electrothermal atomic absorption spectrometric detection. Anal Chem 2006;78:6115–6120.

Li Y, Yan XP, Chen C, Xia YL, Jiang Y. Human serum albumin-mercurial species interactions. J Proteome Res 2007;6:2277–2286.

Lind B, Friberg L, Nylander M. Primary studies on methylmercury biotransformation and clearance in the brain of primates. II Demethylation of mercury in brain. J Trace Elem Exp Med 1988;1:49–56.

Lobinski R, Becker JS, Haraguchi H, Sarkar B. Metallomics: guidelines for terminology and critical evaluation of analytical chemistry approaches (IUPAC Technical Report). Pure Appl Chem 2010;82:493–504.

Lockhart WL, Stern GA, Wagemann R, Hunt RV, Metner DA, DeLaronde J, et al. Concentrations of mercury in tissues of beluga whales (*Delphinapterus leucas*) from several communities in the Canadian Arctic from 1981 to 2002. Sci Total Environ 2005;351–352:391–412.

Mah V, Jalilehvand F. Mercury(II) complex formation with glutathione in alkaline aqueous solution. J Biol Inorg Chem 2008;13:541–553.

Martoja R, Berry JP. Identification of tiemannite as a probable product of demethylation of mercury by selenium in cetaceans. A complement to the scheme of the biological cycle of mercury. Vie Milieu 1980;30:7–10.

Martoja R, Viale D. Accumulation de granules de seleniure mercurique dans le foie d'odontocetes (Mammiferes, Cetaces): Un mecanisme possible de detoxication du methylmercure par le selenium. C R Hebd Seances Acad Sci Paris D 1977;285:109–112.

Mason RP, Reinfelder JR, Morel FMM. Uptake, toxicity, and trophic transfer of mercury in a coastal diatom. Environ Sci Technol 1996;30:1835–1845.

Masukawa T, Kito H, Hayashi M, Iwata H. Formation and possible role of bis(methylmercury) selenide in rats treated with methylmercury and selenite. Biochem Pharmacol 1982;31:75–78.

Mehra M, Choi BH. Distribution and biotransformation of methyl mercuric chloride in different tissues of mice. Acta Pharmacol Toxicol 1981;49:28–37.

Meister A. Glutathione metabolism and its selective modification. J Biol Chem 1988;263:17205–17208.

Mills BJ, Lang CA. Differential distribution of free and bound glutathione and cyst(e)ine in human blood. Biochem Pharmacol 1996;52:401–406.

Mokrzan EM, Kerper LE, Ballatori N, Clarkson TW. Methylmercury thiol uptake into cultured brain capillary endothelial cells on amino acid system L. J Pharmacol Exp Ther 1995;272:1277–1284.

Mutter J, Naumann J, Guethlin C. Comments on the article "The toxicology of mercury and its chemical compounds" by Clarkson and Magos (2006). Crit Rev Toxicol 2007;37:537–549.

Naganuma A, Kojima Y, Imura N. Interaction of methylmercury and selenium in mouse: formation and decomposition of bis(methylmercuric)selenide. Res Commun Chem Pathol Pharmacol 1980;30:301–316.

Nigro M. Mercury and selenium localization in macrophages of the striped dolphin, *Stenella coeruleoalba*. J Mar Biol Assoc UK 1994;74:975–978.

Nigro M, Leonzio C. Intracellular storage of mercury and selenium in different marine vertebrates. Mar Ecol Prog Ser 1996;135:137–143.

NIST. Database 46: NIST Critically selected stability constants of metal complexes database, Version 8. Gaitherburg (MD): National Institute of Standards and Technology; 2004.

Norseth T, Clarkson TW. Studies on the biotransformation of [203]Hg-labelled methyl mercury chloride in rats. Arch Environ Health 1970;21:717–727.

Norseth T, Clarkson TW. Intestinal transport of [203]Hg-labelled methylmercury cysteine. Arch Environ Health 1971;22:568–577.

Parízek J, Oštádalová I. The protective effect of small amounts of selenite in sublimate intoxication. Experientia 1967;23:142–143.

Pearson RG. Hard and soft acids and bases. J Am Chem Soc 1963;85:3533–3539.

Perdew JP, Burke K, Ernzerhof M. Generalized gradient approximation made simple. Phys Rev Lett 1996;77:3865–3868.

Rabenstein DL, Isab AA, Reid RS. A proton nuclear magnetic resonance study of the binding of methylmercury in human erythrocytes. Biochim Biophys Acta 1982;720:53–64.

Rabenstein DL, Reid RS. Nuclear magnetic resonance studies of the solution chemistry of metal complexes. 20. Ligand-exchange kinetics of methylmercury(II)-thiol complexes. Inorg Chem 1984;23:1246–1250.

Rawson AJ, Bradley JP, Teetsov A, Rice SB, Haller EM, Patton GW. A role for airborne particulates in high mercury levels of some cetaceans. Ecotoxicol Environ Saf 1995;30:309–314.

Refsvik T, Norseth T. Methylmercuric compounds in the bile. Acta Pharmacol Toxicol 1975;36:67–78.

Reilly C. Selenium in food and health. New York (NY): Springer; 2006.

Rowland IR, Davies MJ, Grasso P. Volatilisation of methylmercuric chloride by hydrogen sulphide. Nature 1977;265:718–719.

Schaefer JK, Morel FMM. High methylation rates of mercury bound to cysteine by *Geobacter sulfurreducens*. Nat Geosci 2009;2:123–126.

Schecher WD, McAvoy DC. MINEQL+: A chemical equilibrium program for personal computers-User's manual. Hallowell, (ME): Environmental Research Software; 2003.

Schmidt MW, Baldridge KK, Boatz JA, Elbert ST, Gordon MS, Jensen JH, et al. General atomic and molecular electronic structure system. J Comput Chem 1993;14:1347–1363.

Selhub J. Homocysteine metabolism. Annu Rev Nutr 1999;19:217–246.

Silva da Rocha M, Soldado AB, Blanco-Gonzalez E, Sanz-Medel A. Speciation of mercury by capillary electrophoresis-inductively coupled plasma mass spectrometry. Biomed Chromatogr 2000;14:6–7.

Silva da Rocha M, Soldado AB, Blanco E, Sanz-Medel A. Speciation of mercury using capillary electrophoresis coupled to volatile species generation-inductively coupled plasma mass spectrometry. J Anal At Spectrom 2001;16:951–956.

Simmons-Willis TA, Koh AS, Clarkson TW, Ballatori N. Transport of a neurotoxicant by molecular mimicry: the methylmercury-$_L$-cysteine complex is a substrate for human L-type large neutral amino acid transporter (LAT) 1 and LAT2. Biochem J 2002;367:239–246.

Stillman MJ. Metallothioneins. Coord Chem Rev 1995;144:461–511.

Stumm W, Morgan JJ. Aquatic chemistry. New York (NY): John Wiley & Sons; 1996.

Sunderland EM. Mercury exposure from domestic and imported estuarine and marine fish in the U.S. seafood market. Environ Health Perspect 2007;115:235–242.

Suzuki KT, Sasakura C, Yoneda S. Binding sites for the (Hg-Se) complex on selenoprotein P. Biochim Biophys Acta 1998;1429:102–112.

Tai HC, Lim C. Computational studies of the coordination stereochemistry, bonding, and setal selectivity of mercury. J Phys Chem A 2006;2006:452–462.

Taylor NJ, Carty AJ. Nature of Hg^{2+}-L-cysteine complexes implicated in mercury biochemistry. J Am Chem Soc 1977;99:6143–6145.

Taylor NJ, Wong YS, Chieh PC, Carty AJ. Syntheses, X-ray crystal structure, and vibrational spectra of L-cysteinatomethylmercury(II) monohydrate. J Chem Soc Dalton Trans Inorg Chem 1975;5:438–442.

Templeton DM, Ariese F, Cornelis R, Danielsson LG, Muntau H, Van Leeuwen HP, et al. Guidelines for terms related to chemical speciation and fractionation of elements. Definitions, structural aspects and methodological approaches. Pure Appl Chem 2000;72:1453–1470.

Wang F, Tessier A. Zero-valent sulfur and metal speciation in sediment porewaters of freshwater lakes. Environ Sci Technol 2009;43:7252–7257.

Watanabe C, Yin KYK, Satoh H. In utero exposure to methylmercury and Se deficiency converge on the neurobehavioral outcome in mice. Neurotoxicol Teratol 1999;21:83–88.

Wiberg KB, Castejon H, Keith TA. Solvent effects: 6. A comparison between gas phase and solution acidities. J Comput Chem 1996;17:185–190.

Yoneda S, Suzuki KT. Detoxification of mercury by selenium by binding of equimolar Hg-Se complex to a specific plasma protein. Toxicol Appl Pharmacol 1997a;143:274–280.

Yoneda S, Suzuki KT. Equimolar Hg-Se complex binds to selenoprotein P. Biochem Biophys Res Commun 1997b;231:7–11.

Zalups RK, Koropatnick J, Joshee L. Mouse monocytes (RAW CELLS) and the handling of cysteine and homocysteine S-conjugates of inorganic mercury and methylmercury. J Toxicol Environ Health A 2007;70:799–809.

Zhang J, Wang F, House JD, Page B. Thiols in wetland interstitial waters and their role in mercury and methylmercury speciation. Limnol Oceanogr 2004;49:2276–2286.

CHAPTER 17

HUMAN HEALTH SIGNIFICANCE OF DIETARY EXPOSURES TO METHYLMERCURY

ANNA L. CHOI and PHILIPPE GRANDJEAN

17.1 INTRODUCTION

Dietary intake of fish and seafood is the dominant source of human exposure to methylmercury, a toxicant that can have serious adverse effects on the developing nervous system and may promote heart diseases. Methylmercury is an organic form of mercury that is formed from inorganic mercury primarily in microorganisms in the aquatic environment. The microorganisms in turn are consumed by fish, and methylmercury is biomagnified in the aquatic food chains so that the highest concentrations occur in large and long-lived predatory fish and marine mammals at the top tropic levels (NRC, 2000). Releases of and increased exposures to inorganic mercury may occur from volcanos and from industrial processes, such as mercury mining, mercury catalysts at chlor-alkali plants, fluorescent lamp factories, and artisanal and small-scale gold mining operations (IPCS, 1990; Mergler et al., 2007). Current concerns related to human exposures particularly emphasize dietary intakes of fish and other seafood products as the dominant source of human exposure to methylmercury.

Evidence from methylmercury poisoning outbreaks in Japan and Iraq has clearly demonstrated the severe and widespread damage that may occur to the brain when exposed to methylmercury during development. The poisoning in Minamata, Japan, occurred because of long-term exposure through the ingestion of methylmercury-contaminated fish (Harada, 1995). The infants were born with serious neurological damage, even when their exposed mothers were virtually unaffected. However, serious delays affected the recognition of methylmercury as a cause of the serious human poisonings, and the vulnerability of the developing nervous system was not taken into account in risk assessment

Environmental Chemistry and Toxicology of Mercury, First Edition.
Edited by Guangliang Liu, Yong Cai, and Nelson O'Driscoll.
© 2012 John Wiley & Sons, Inc. Published 2012 by John Wiley & Sons, Inc.

internationally until ~50 years later (Grandjean et al., 2010). In Iraq, exposure was a result of the consumption of homemade bread that was made with grain treated with methylmercury as a fungicide (Bakir et al., 1973). Neurologic signs caused by methylmercury poisoning include paresthesias, ataxia, sensory disturbances, tremors, impairment of hearing, and walking difficulties. The effect in offspring who were exposed to methylmercury in utero were more serious, as the severe and widespread damage that may occur to the brain when exposed to methylmercury during development were clearly demonstrated in the poisoning outbreaks. Recent epidemiological studies have found more subtle adverse effects on brain functions at lower levels of methylmercury (Grandjean et al., 1997; Debes et al., 2006). A recent case-control study found that an increased blood mercury concentration was associated with attention-deficit hyperactivity disorder (Cheuk and Wong, 2006), although the premorbid exposure level was unknown. Recent studies suggest that methylmercury may promote or predispose to heart attacks and other clinical events associated with cardiovascular disease (Salonen et al., 1995; Yoshizawa et al., 2002; Virtanen et al., 2005). The intima media thickness of the carotid arteries was apparently associated with mercury exposure from fish (Salonen et al., 2000). A recent study also found significant associations between mercury exposure and increased blood pressure and intima media thickness in whaling men aged 30–70 years (Choi et al., 2009). However, fish and seafood also contain important nutrients, such as ω-3 fatty acids that may provide beneficial effects, thereby possibly counteracting or obscuring the adverse effects of methylmercury.

This chapter reviews the existing evidence on methylmercury developmental neurotoxicity and the emerging evidence that methylmercury may promote the development of heart diseases. Methylmercury risks may have been underestimated in the past, in part because of the confounding effects of nutrients from seafood and fish. Risk assessment, nutrients, and co-contaminants are also discussed.

17.2 METHYLMERCURY EXPOSURE

Mercury is a widespread contaminant found in the environment in both its metallic form and in various inorganic and organic complexes (NRC, 2000). The natural global biogeochemical cycling of mercury includes a conversion of mercury from inorganic into an organic form—methylmercury primarily in microorganisms in the aquatic environment, which are consumed by fish. Methylmercury bioaccumulates up the aquatic food chain so that the highest concentrations occur in large, long-lived predatory fish and marine mammals at the top trophic levels (NRC, 2000). Fish and seafood therefore provide an important pathway for human exposure to methylmercury in freshwater and marine food chains, and methylmercury contamination is the main reason for fishing advisories in the United States (US EPA, 2004). Moreover, different types of fish do not contain similar proportions of mercury contamination and nutrients, as methylmercury bioaccumulates through multiple levels of the aquatic food web. Total mercury concentrations vary widely across fish and shellfish, and mean values differ by as much as 100-fold (Keating et al., 1997). Farmed fish is not free of methylmercury because of the presence of the contaminant in the feed (Choi and Cech, 1998). The European Food Safety Authority, in assessing the differences between wild and farmed fish, concluded that there is no general difference in safety between the two kinds of fish when the same species and the same locations are compared (EFSA, 2006). Options, however, are available to produce farmed fish with lower methylmercury by controlling the feed. Other possible sources of methylmercury in the human diet include rice cultivated in mercury-contaminated areas (Zhang et al., 2010), organ meats of terrestrial animals (Ysart et al., 2000), and chicken and pork, probably as a result of using fish meal as livestock feed (Lindberg et al., 2004).

High levels of mercury exposure have been documented in fish-eating populations. The median mercury concentration of maternal hair in the Faroe Islands was 4.5 μg/g, with 27% above 10 μg/g (Grandjean et al., 1992), and in the Seychelles an average of 5.8 μg/g (Cernichiari et al., 1995). Populations in the Amazon communities who rely on freshwater fish have median hair-mercury levels ranging from 5 to 15 μg/g (Cordier et al., 1998; Dorea et al., 2003).

The exposure depends not only on the frequency of fish intake and the size of each meal, but also on the species consumed. High concentrations of methylmercury can be found in predatory fish and marine mammals at the top trophic levels, as methylmercury biomagnifies in the aquatic food chains. Sharks, king mackerel, swordfish, and tilefish are among the predatory fish with high methylmercury concentrations and are on the national advisories list of fish to avoid for women of childbearing age and young children (US EPA, 2004). Results of recent studies found elevated blood and hair-mercury levels in Chinese adults and children (Choy et al., 2002; Ip et al., 2004). Shark fin soup, a Chinese delicacy, is an important dietary source of methylmercury exposure in this population (Choy et al., 2002). The European Union has to comply with a high contamination limit of 1 μg/g due to a large number of fish species that are known to accumulate high mercury concentrations.

In prospective studies, biomarkers of exposure include maternal hair, cord blood, and cord tissue. Maternal dietary questionnaires have also been used to obtain information on the frequency of fish and seafood consumption. Blood gives an estimate of most recent exposure, with the half-life of methylmercury in blood being 50–70 days, while hair may provide a calendar of mercury exposure (Cernichiari et al., 1995). Although hair growth rates are known to vary, a 9-cm hair sample obtained at parturition or shortly thereafter would be thought to represent the average mercury exposure during the whole pregnancy (Grandjean et al., 2005a,b). Hair mercury is predominantly in the form of methylmercury, constituting 80–98% of hair total mercury. Generally, hair is 250–300 times higher in mercury than blood (IPCS, 1990). However, because of the binding to fetal hemoglobin, cord blood contains higher concentrations, thus making the difference from hair only about 180-fold (Grandjean et al., 1992).

Studies of the cardiovascular effect of mercury have used mercury levels in toenails and fingernails as biomarkers of mercury exposure (Guallar et al., 2002; Yoshizawa et al., 2002), although the extent to which these reflect organic or inorganic mercury exposure is unclear. The fact that dentists have increased toenail-mercury concentrations (Yoshizawa et al., 2002) would suggest that this biomarker reflects the methylmercury exposure as well as others. Urinary mercury excretion levels have been used in some studies (Berglund et al., 2005; Ohno et al., 2007), but the concentrations mainly reflect inorganic mercury and is not considered a useful biomarker of methylmercury exposure (Berglund et al., 2005).

17.3   NUTRIENTS IN FISH AND SEAFOOD

17.3.1   Long-Chain n-3 Polyunsaturated Fatty Acids

Certain essential nutrients in fish and seafood may provide beneficial effects on brain development and may protect against the development of heart disease. Fish and seafood are rich in long-chain n-3 polyunsaturated fatty acids (LCP-UFAs), which are particularly important in human nutrition (NAS/NRC, 2005). Two mainly important LCPUFAs are docosahexaenoic acid (DHA, 22:6n-3) and eicosapantaenoic acid (EPA, 20:5n-3) (Hearn et al., 1987; Raper et al., 1992). Fatty acids have specific functions in cell membranes that are important to normal metabolism, including the binding between molecules and receptors, the cellular interactions, and the transport of nutrients (Bourre et al., 1989). DHA and EPA are formed in animal, fish, and shellfish tissues, but not plant tissues. DHA is a component of membrane structural lipids that are enriched in non-myelin membranes of the nervous system and certain phospholipid components of the retina. EPA is a precursor of the n-3 eicosanoids, which have beneficial effects in the prevention of ventricular arrhythmias, thrombosis, and atherosclerosis (Kinsella et al., 1990; Connor, 2000; Mahaffey, 2004). Although fish and seafood are a primary source of EPA and DHA (IOM/NAS, 2007), eggs and chickens may contribute to the EPA and DHA content if frequently consumed. However, they are not particularly rich sources. Plant sources, such as walnuts and flaxseed oil, contain α-linolenic acid (ALA, 18:3n-3) that can be converted to EPA and DHA, but humans do not convert EPA or DHA from ALA at rates high enough to reach recommended intake levels (Pawlosky et al., 2001).

17.3.2   Selenium

Selenium is a trace mineral that is essential to health. Fish and seafood, eggs, meats, and vegetables are good sources of selenium. Selenium is a constituent of selenoproteins, which are important antioxidant enzymes and catalysts for the production of thyroid hormone (Rayman, 2000). Although the physiologic functions of selenium in the brain are not well understood, studies have found that selenium and certain selenoproteins are particularly well maintained despite prolonged selenium deficiency, suggesting the important role of selenium in this organ (Whanger, 2001; Chen and Berry, 2003). Low selenium levels have been reported to associate with accelerated progression of carotid atherosclerosis (Salonen et al., 1991), but other studies have not shown a clear relationship (Rayman, 2000).

17.3.3   Vitamin E

Vitamin E may interact with selenium additively because of their similar antioxidant roles (Maberly et al., 1994). Fish is a source of vitamin E, although vegetable oils are the most abundant sources. Selenium and vitamin E in a diet may alter methylmercury reproductive and developmental toxicity in some animal studies (Beyrouty and Chan, 2006). Although experimental studies have suggested that selenium may decrease methylmercury toxicity under certain exposure regimens (Ganther et al., 1972), little epidemiological evidence has been found to support the animal findings (Steuerwald et al., 2000; Watanabe, 2002; Choi et al., 2008).

17.3.4   Iron

Iron is an essential component of proteins involved in oxygen transport and for the regulation of cell growth and differentiation (Andrews, 2000). Deficiency in iron may impact brain growth, neurotransmitter levels, as well as toxicity or intracellular deficiency in the central nervous system (Pollitt, 1993). Adverse effects of iron deficiency on the cognitive and psychomotor development of children have been found in some studies (Lozoff et al., 1987; Akman et al., 2004). However, associations between iron status and coronary heart disease have been inconsistent. High iron stores have been linked with increased risk of coronary heart disease in some studies (Salonen et al., 1992, Sempos et al., 1994), but not others (Danesh and Appleby, 1999; Ma and Stampfer, 2002).

17.3.5   Iodine

Iodine, a trace element, is an essential component of thyroid hormones. Development of the central nervous system depends on an adequate supply of thyroid hormone, which requires iodine for biosynthesis (Maberly, 1994). Fish and seafood are rich sources of iodine. Children with iodine deficiency are at risk for poor mental and psychomotor development (Morreale de Escobar et al., 1989; Bleichrodt and Born, 1994). The disorders increase with the extent of deficiency, with overt endemic cretinism as the severest consequence, resulting in irreversible mental retardation, neurological damage, and thyroid failure (Delange, 2000).

17.4   MAJOR PROSPECTIVE COHORT STUDIES

Major prospective cohort studies of methylmercury-exposed children have been conducted in New Zealand, the Faroe Islands, and the Seychelles. Table 17.1

TABLE 17.1 Main Characteristics of Three Major Prospective Studies of Methylmercury-Exposed Children

Attribute	New Zealand	Faroes	Seychelles
Sources of exposure	Shark and ocean fish	Whale, ocean fish, and shellfish	Ocean fish
Mercury exposure assessment	Maternal hair	Cord blood, cord tissue, and maternal hair	Maternal hair, adjusted for child's hair-mercury
Mercury effect	Significant	Significant	Not significant
Effect of maternal fish intake	Mothers were matched for high fish intake	Adjustment for maternal fish intake increased mercury effect	Maternal fish intake not included in first study
Other toxicant exposures	Lead in house paint and air	PCBs (whale blubber)	Tropical pesticide use
Language	English (and Pacific languages)	Faroese (and Danish)	Creole (English and French)
Socioeconomic setting	Industrialized Western	Industrialized Scandinavian	Middle-income developing
Family-setting	Urban, mixed cultures	Traditional	Mainly matriarchal
Outcome tests	Omnibus	Domain-related and neurophysiological	Omnibus and domain-related
Clinical examiners	Clinical specialists	Clinical specialists	Nurse/student

outlines the major differences between these three prospective studies. Several published smaller cohorts and cross-sectional studies support the notion of developmental neurotoxicity associated with methylmercury in contaminated fish and seafood (NRC, 2000), although the main evidence comes from the three largest cohorts.

17.4.1 New Zealand

A cohort of 11,000 mothers, who gave birth to children in 1978, was initially screened (Kjellström et al., 1986). Hair-mercury concentrations were determined for 1000 mothers, who had consumed three fish meals per week during pregnancy. The high exposure group consisted of 73 mothers who had a hair-mercury level above 6 μg/g. At the first follow-up at age four years, 31 high exposure children and 31 reference children with lower exposure were matched for potential confounders (i.e., mother's ethnic group, age, child's birthplace, and birth date). The high exposure group showed significantly lower scores on childhood mental and motor development. A follow-up of the original cohort was carried out at age six years with three control groups with lower prenatal mercury exposure. During pregnancy, mothers in two of these control groups had high fish consumption and average hair-mercury concentrations of 3–6 μg/g and 0–3 μg/g, respectively. At this time, 61 of the high exposure children were available for examinations. A three-point decrement in intelligence quotient (IQ) was noted in children born to women with mercury concentrations in hair greater than 6 μg/g (Kjellström et al., 1989).

17.4.2 Faroe Islands

The Faroe Islands are located in the North Atlantic between Norway, Shetland, and Iceland. Excess exposure to methylmercury is mainly due to the traditional habit of eating meat from the pilot whale in this fishing community. Fish intake varied but shows a positive association with whale intake. Ingestion of whale blubber causes exposure to lipophilic contaminants, notably polychlorinated biphenyls (PCBs). The first birth cohort consisted of 1022 children born during a 21-month period in 1986–1987 (Grandjean et al., 1997). Prenatal methylmercury exposure was determined from mercury concentrations in cord blood and maternal hair, both spanning a range of about 1000-fold. A total of 917 eligible children (90.3%) participated in the detailed examination at school age (seven years). The geometric mean for maternal hair-mercury concentration collected at delivery was 4.3 μg/g. The physical examination included a sensory function assessment and a functional neurological examination with emphasis on motor coordination and perceptual-motor performance. The main emphasis was placed on detailed neurophysiological and neuropsychological function tests that had been selected as sensitive indicators of abnormalities thought to be caused by methylmercury. A repeat examination was carried out at age 14 years, again with a high participation rate. The clinical test battery was similar to the one at seven years. At the 7-year and 14-year follow-up examinations, decrements in attention, language, verbal memory, and, to a lesser extent, motor speed and visuospatial function were associated with prenatal methylmercury exposure (controlled for age, sex, and confounders). Delayed latencies of the brainstem auditory evoked potentials (BAEPs) and decreased heart rate variability were also associated with mercury exposure (Grandjean et al., 1997; Murata et al., 2004; Debes et al., 2006).

Another prospective study (cohort 2) of 182 singleton term births were examined by the neurological optimality score (NOS) at age two weeks. Detailed information was obtained on exposures both to methylmercury and to lipophilic pollutants. The NOS showed significant decreases at higher cord blood mercury concentrations, but neither with PCB nor with LCPUFAs (Steuerwald et al., 2000).

In both cohorts, no evidence was found that selenium was an important protective factor against methylmercury neurotoxicity (Steuerwald et al., 2000; Choi et al., 2008).

17.4.3 Seychelles

A pilot cohort study and a main study, each with approximately 800 mother–child pairs, were conducted in the Seychelles, an archipelago in the Indian Ocean

(Shamlaye et al., 1995). A hair sample was obtained from the mother six months after parturition. The hair segment that represented the pregnancy period was identified from the assumption that hair grows 1.1 cm per month. A subset of 217 children from the pilot cohort was evaluated at 66 months (Myers et al., 1995). After outliers were excluded, maternal hair mercury remained significantly associated with auditory comprehension, but not with the neurodevelopmental outcomes. The main study included evaluation of the children at 6.5, 19, 29, and 66 months of age, and again at 8 years. No clear association with maternal hair mercury was found for most end points in these children (Myers et al., 1995; Myers et al., 2003). The results were adjusted for the child's postnatal methylmercury exposure, but not for maternal fish intake.

A new longitudinal study of 300 Seychellois mother–child pairs was undertaken to assess the relationship between maternal mercury exposure and measures of LCPUFA with neurodevelopment of the children (Myers et al., 2007; Strain et al., 2008). Psychomotor development at nine months of age was positively associated with maternal serum LCPUFA concentration and decreased with increasing maternal hair methylmercury concentration at 30 months of age. The adverse associations with methylmercury appeared only when nutrient status was added as a covariate, whereas the positive associations of developmental tests with LCPUFA likewise became much stronger after adjustment for methylmercury.

17.5 HEALTH EFFECTS

17.5.1 Neurodevelopmental Outcomes

Tools used for outcome measurement need to be sensitive, specific, and as independent as possible from study-specific administration procedures and cultural environment. Many studies employed a battery of neurobehavioral tests, some of which appeared to be more sensitive to mercury neurotoxicity than others, possibly due to superior psychometric properties, but not necessarily greater sensitivity to mercury. A simple comparison of regression coefficients may provide suggestions for the most sensitive parameter, at least within the confines of a particular study. To facilitate such a comparison, the regression coefficient may be expressed as a proportion of the standard deviation of the test result or as a delay in mental development calculated from the regression coefficient for age (Grandjean et al., 1997, 1999). Benchmark dose levels may also be used as a basis for comparison. Thus, the most sensitive neurological, neuropsychological, and neurophysiological effect parameters all exhibit benchmark dose levels of 5–10 µg/g in hair (NRC, 2000; Murata et al., 2004). Despite the great variability of the study settings and the outcome variables, a substantial degree of concordance exists, and the combined evidence is quite convincing in regard to the dose–response relationship.

17.5.2 Neurological Tests

Neurological examination has been included in prospective studies (Steuerwald et al., 2000) and cross-sectional studies (Marsh et al., 1995; Cordier et al., 2002). The clinical tests, however, provide only suggestive evidence linking low dose methylmercury exposures to detectable abnormalities. The absence of clear, positive findings most probably reflects the lack of sensitivity of this type of examination within this range of exposures and the potential imprecision in assessment due to the subjectivity of the evaluation.

17.5.3 Neuropsychological Tests

Neuropsychological tests are likely to be more sensitive in revealing early neurotoxic changes. However, they require standardized administration and may show examiner dependence. In addition, they may be sensitive to details in the test situation, such as the use of an interpreter, differences in temperature, and other aspects that may be important when a test is used for the first time in a particular culture. In New Zealand, two psychologists tested the same children with shortened version of the test battery and documented a high level of agreement (Kjellström et al., 1989). In the Faroes and several other studies, each test was administered to all children by the same examiner, thus limiting the possible impact of examiner-related differences.

Traditionally, studies in this field have included standard intelligence batteries. For example, the Wechsler Intelligence Scale for Children (WISC) and the McCarthy Scale of Children's Abilities were included in the New Zealand (Kjellström et al., 1989) as well as the Seychelles examinations (Davidson et al., 2001; Myers et al., 2003). These intelligence tests may not be the most sensitive for methylmercury toxicity, although significant results were found on WISC and McCarthy in the New Zealand study. Some WISC subtests were used under different circumstances in the cross-sectional studies administered by an interpreter, for example, in Madeira (Murata et al., 1999a,b), thereby making the test results less reliable. The Faroe Islands study emphasized neurobehavioral tests that reflected functional domains (e.g., attention, motor speed, verbal memory) that are mostly likely to be affected by developmental methylmercury exposure, as determined from the location of neuropathological lesions in poisoning cases and as illustrated by studies on other developmental neurotoxicants, especially lead. The Boston Naming test (language) showed a wide range of responses and appeared to be the most sensitive and reliable outcome (NRC, 2000).

Similar outcomes have been used in studies of dietary long-chained n-3 polyunsaturated fatty acids (LCPUFAs), which are transferred via the placenta or supplied in human milk as necessary nutrients for normal brain growth and development in infancy and also likely to play an important role in the development of infant cognition (Willatts and Forsyth, 2000; Lucas et al., 1992).

17.5.4 Neurophysiological Tests

As an objective evaluation of brain dysfunction that is probably less sensitive to motivation of socioeconomic confounding, neurophysiological tests have been applied in several studies. Their applicability requires advanced instrumentation and depends on skilled examiners. BAEPs is an outcome that has been previously found to be sensitive to lead exposure. They are recorded using surface electrodes placed on the skull while the child listens to a stimulus in one ear. The transmission of the electrical signals within the brain is then recorded as peaks that represent the acoustic nerve, an intermediate connection in the pons, and the midbrain. Patients from Minamata, Japan, with congenital methylmercury poisoning exhibited delays in auditory brainstem evoked potential latencies (Hamada et al., 1982). The latency of peak III was significantly increased at higher intrauterine exposure to mercury. Parallel associations were found in seven-year-old children in the Faroes (Murata et al., 1999a) and in Madeira (Murata et al., 1999b). This observation was replicated in the Faroese cohort when examined at 14 years (Murata et al., 2004). This study showed that delays in peak V were associated with the adolescents' current exposure and that early effects occurred at very low exposure levels (Fig. 17.1) (Murata et al., 2004). As a parameter primarily affected by postnatal exposure, peak V delays may provide unique insight in

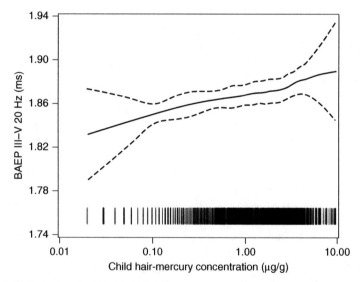

Figure 17.1 Latency of peak V of the brainstem auditory evoked potentials recorded in 859 Faroese children at 14 years and adjusted for sex and age. The association is estimated in a generalized additive model analysis, using the current hair-mercury concentration as an indicator of current exposure. The broken lines indicate the point-wise 95% confidence interval for the dose–response relationship. Each vertical line above the horizontal axis represents one observation at the exposure level indicated. *Source*: Redrawn from Murata et al. (2004).

comparison with majority of functions that are mainly sensitive to methylmercury during fetal development.

17.6 CARDIOVASCULAR OUTCOMES

Although the developing brain is considered the critical target organ in regard to methylmercury, recent evidence has suggested that mercury from fish and seafood may promote or predispose one's development of heart disease. Several cohort studies have found an inverse relationship between fish consumption and LCPUFA and mortality from coronary heart disease, although not all studies were supportive of a cardioprotective effect of LCPUFA (Hallgren et al., 2001; Mozaffarian and Rimm, 2006; IOM/NAS, 2007). While this evidence is not yet conclusive, it deserves attention because it suggests that a narrow definition of subpopulations of interest, that is, pregnant women, might leave out other vulnerable groups.

The first studies of methylmercury-associated cardiovascular disease were carried out in Finland (Salonen et al., 1995). One important study showed that the intima–media thickness of the carotid arteries was in apparent association with the degree of mercury exposure from fish (Salonen et al., 2000). More recent information tends to support these findings. A later study of Finnish men reported that an increased mercury exposure was associated with increased risk of acute coronary events and cardiovascular mortality and that mercury also seemed to attenuate the protective effects of fish on cardiovascular health (Virtanen et al., 2005). A large multicenter study from Europe showed an increased risk of cardiovascular disease associated with toenail-mercury concentrations and that high mercury content may diminish the cardioprotective effect of fish intake (Guallar et al., 2002). In a US study of health care workers, only a minimal risk was seen even with the adjustment of n-3 fatty acid intake from fish in the multivariate models. However, after the exclusion of dentists with high toenail-mercury concentrations most likely a result of amalgam exposures, the mercury-associated risk in other health professionals was similar to the one observed in the European study, although not statistically significant (Yoshizawa et al., 2002).

A possible mechanism may be the induction of lipid peroxidation. In this regard, it is interesting to note that while essential fatty acids from fish may reduce the risk of acute coronary events, a high mercury content in fish could attenuate this beneficial effect (Rissanen et al., 2000). The increased risk seems to occur at hair-mercury concentrations above 2 µg/g, that is, only twice the level corresponding to the US Environmental Protection Agency (US EPA) Reference Dose, RfD (a daily intake level designed to be without a significant risk of adverse effects over a lifetime).

Regular consumption of fish oil supplements appears to reduce the risk of coronary artery disease in some observational studies (Von Schacky et al., 1999; Saldeen et al., 2002), but not others (Sacks et al., 1995). Randomized controlled trials have shown that LCPUFA in fish oil or fish can play a role in secondary prevention of coronary heart disease (Kris-Etherton et al., 2002; Harper and Jacobson, 2005). For example, the Diet And Reinfarction Trial (DART) reported a reduction in all-cause mortality in male myocardial infarction survivors advised to increase their intake of oily fish (Burr et al., 1989). However, a Norwegian study reported no benefit in patients with myocardial infarction who were given fish oil capsules compared with placebo, possibly due to the high habitual fish consumption among the general population in the area, with fish oil supplementation conferring no additional benefit (Nilsen et al., 2001). Results of the GISSI trial, the largest prevention study, found that polyunsaturated fatty acid (PUFA) supplements, but not Vitamin E, significantly reduced the risk of total mortality, nonfatal myocardial infarction, and stroke (GISSI-Prevenzione Investigators, 1999). The relative risks of cardiovascular death and of sudden death were also significantly reduced. These benefits were apparent within four months of randomization. The available studies point to an antiarrhythmic effect as a beneficial mechanism of LCPUFA on coronary heart disease (Kris-Etherton et al., 2002). However, a recent study found that low dose supplementation with EPA-DHA or ALA in margarine did not significantly reduce the rate of major cardiovascular events among patients who had had a myocardial infarction (Kromhout et al., 2010).

17.7 NUTRIENT AND METHYLMERCURY EXPOSURE AS PREDICTORS OF DEVELOPMENTAL OUTCOMES

Only a small number of studies have aimed at examining the effects of both nutrient and contaminant intakes at the same time as predictors of developmental outcomes. A beneficial association on developmental score with fish intake by the mother during pregnancy and by the infant postnatally was reported, but no effect of low mercury concentrations in umbilical cord tissue (wet weight) was found (Daniels et al., 2004). However, the validity of the latter finding is uncertain because of the imprecision of the mercury exposure biomarker. In the Faroes, adverse neonatal neurological function was associated with increased prenatal methylmercury exposure, but neither LCPUFA nor selenium provided any detectable beneficial or protective effect on this outcome (Steuerwald et al., 2000). No evidence was found that selenium provided any important protection against methylmercury-associated deficits on neuropsychological tests in two separate Faroese birth cohorts (Choi et al., 2008). In a Polish cohort, maternal fish intake during pregnancy was positively related to both maternal and cord blood mercury concentrations, which were associated with delayed psychomotor development of infants in the first year of life (Jedrychowski et al., 2006). Three studies, in particular, showed that the effects of both nutrient and contaminant intakes were strengthened when both maternal fish intake and prenatal methylmercury exposure were adjusted in modeling the same neurodevelopmental outcomes (Oken et al., 2005; Budtz-Jørgensen et al., 2007; Strain et al., 2008). Thus, both the beneficial and the adverse effects of fish and seafood intake should be assessed at the same time to separate opposite impacts on the outcomes. Only then will the full impact of methylmercury toxicity (and the beneficial effects of the nutrients) be apparent. As a corollary, optimizing the benefits of fish and seafood consumption requires a prudent choice of species high in nutrients and as low as possible in methylmercury contamination.

17.8 CONFOUNDING VARIABLES

One major reason a mercury effect might have been overestimated may be due to possible association of mercury intake with exposure to other neurotoxic pollutant(s) and other types of residual confounding (NIEHS, 1998). The best protection against confounding problems is to select a study setting where such concerns are unlikely and, if relevant, may be adjusted for appropriately. Thus, a homogenous society with limited difference in socioeconomic and cultural factors should be preferred. Although the existence of residual confounding can never be fully excluded, careful attention should be paid in the inclusion of relevant covariates such that biologically plausible associations between methylmercury exposure and adverse effects would not be explained away. Disproportionate attention is usually concentrated on confounders that affect the outcomes in the same direction as the exposure under study. However, the control for negative confounding (opposite effect of the exposure) can be crucial in epidemiological studies. The absence of proper adjustment will lead to underestimation of the toxicity of the exposure on the outcome and the benefits of the confounder (Choi et al., 2009). In the case of methylmercury and fish, the toxicity of mercury and the benefits of the nutrients in fish and seafood will both be underestimated.

Socioeconomic conditions vary substantially between the three major prospective studies on the neurotoxicity of methylmercury—New Zealand (Kjellström et al., 1986, 1989), the Faroe Islands (Grandjean et al., 1997; Debes et al., 2006), the Seychelles (Myers et al., 2003; Davidson et al., 2006)—as well as other cross-sectional studies. Within each study, socioeconomic differences may be important and dependent on mercury exposures and should then be included in the confounder adjustment. For example, high intakes of methylmercury have been reported in certain ethnic groups (Innis et al., 2006; Sweeney et al.,; 2006) and in social strata with a high sushi intake (Hightower and Moore, 2003). Furthermore, vulnerability to contaminant effects may differ between socioeconomic groups.

Potential confounding was taken into account in previous studies of methylmercury neurotoxicity. For example, in the follow-up of the New Zealand birth cohort at ages four and six years, children whose mother had high hair-mercury concentrations and reference children with lower exposure were matched for potential confounders, including mother's ethnic group, age, child's birthplace, and birth date. In addition, study and control children were stratified according to fish consumption of mothers during pregnancy (Kjellström et al., 1986; Kjellström et al., 1989). Significant decrements in test performance in the children prenatally exposed to increased doses of methylmercury were found.

Other potential confounders include the family and home environment, which are documented as important determinants of childhood development. In the New

Zealand study, low social class and non-English home language reduced the score on some tests, and more than six months of breast-feeding increased the score on some tests (Kjellström et al., 1989). These variables were accounted for in the analysis.

Exposure to other toxicants should also be considered. The Faroese, for example, people are exposed to PCBs from eating whale blubber (Grandjean et al., 1997). However, no important impact of PCB exposure on the neurotoxicity outcomes were shown from detailed analyses of the Faroes data (Steuerwald et al., 2000; Budtz-Jørgensen et al., 2010). The relative importance of PCB and mercury was assessed in structural equation analysis taking into account the imprecision in both variables. The inclusion of PCB exposure attenuated the mercury effect, but mercury remained statistically significant, while PCB was far from that (Budtz-Jørgensen et al., 2010). In New Zealand and Seychelles, the ocean fish consumed is unlikely to be contaminated by PCB, and the same would be the case with freshwater fish in the Amazon Basin (Grandjean et al., 1999).

17.9 RISK ASSESSMENT AND EXPOSURE IMPRECISION

The purpose of an exposure assessment is to provide a correct measure of exposure in terms of the amount that has reached the toxicological target during the relevant time period. Because the validity depends on the degree to which the exposure biomarkers reflect the "true" exposure, they can be considered only proxy variables, which are always imprecise to some extent (Grandjean et al., 2005b). In addition, the degree of imprecision of the exposure data is usually unknown. This issue is important since exposure misclassification (i.e., errors in matching the exposure-based biomarker of dose to the observed effect) is likely to cause underestimation of the true effect of the exposure.

In prospective studies, samples for mercury analysis have included maternal hair, cord blood, and cord tissue. Scalp hair is the most frequently used sample for methylmercury exposure assessment (Grandjean et al., 2002). However, hair-mercury concentration is subject to variability such as hair type, hair color, external contamination, and leaching due to permanent hair treatments (Yamamoto and Suzuki, 1978; Grandjean et al., 2002; Yasutake et al., 2003). These factors might well account for the greater overall imprecision of this biomarker. The blood concentration of methylmercury is often considered the appropriate indicator of the absorbed dose and the amount systemically available, but this biomarker may also be subject to possible variation (Grandjean and Budtz-Jørgensen, 2007). The dry-weight-based mercury concentration of the cord tissue seems to be a more precise parameter than the level expressed on a wet-weight basis (Grandjean et al., 2005b).

In assessing exposure biomarker imprecision and providing proper adjustment for its consequences, cord blood has been documented to be the best available indicator of prenatal methylmercury exposure (Grandjean and Budtz-Jørgensen, 2007). However, the results also suggested that even the best exposure biomarker may be much more imprecise than suggested by laboratory quality data. Exposure imprecision and thus misclassification will generally be nondirectional, leading to an underestimation of dose–effect relationships (Grandjean et al., 2003). This problem may be exaggerated by potential confounders that are correlated with the exposure. Inclusion of these variables in a regression may further add to the bias toward the null hypothesis, even in the cases where the potential confounder has no independent effect on the outcome (Budtz-Jørgensen et al., 2003).

Maternal dietary questionnaires have also been used to obtain information on the frequency of fish and seafood consumption. If detailed data on nutrient absorption levels are absent in the dietary questionnaire, the crude dietary variable will have substantial imprecision, thereby limiting the power to identify the effect of fish intake, the confounder. This imprecision also causes an underestimation of the fish-adjusted mercury effect (Budtz-Jørgensen et al., 2007). The distribution of mercury (and other chemicals) and LCPUFA (and other nutrients) are not homogenous in species of fish and seafood. There is a potential problem when established categories of fish consumption do not reflect well on mercury exposure. A recent observational study found no support for the advice that women of childbearing age should avoid high mercury fish and eat up to 340 g of fish and shellfish per week (Hibbeln et al., 2007). This conclusion might have been obscured by the use of an exposure variable reflecting LCPUFA contents rather than methylmercury (Mahaffey and Schoeny, 2007).

The RfD for methylmercury derived by the US EPA was 0.1 µg/kg/day based on the conclusion of the National Research Council (NRC, 2000). This was based on a series of end points associated with a median cord blood mercury level of 58.0 µg/L. In calculating the RfD, EPA assumed that the cord blood and maternal blood mercury levels were equivalent. It should be noted that because the RfD is a dose on a $\mu g/kg_{bw}$/day basis, the total methylmercury intake depends on the individual's body weight. The quantity of fish that can be safely consumed reflects the concentration of mercury in the fish and the frequency of fish consumption (Mahaffey et al., 2008). Imprecision of the exposure assessment will bias the methylmercury neurotoxicity toward the null, and adjustment for imprecision in the Faroes study resulted in a calculated RfD that was about 50% below the level used by the US EPA (Grandjean and Budtz-Jørgensen, 2010).

17.10 CONCLUSIONS

This review outlines the substantial scientific evidence on the developmental neurotoxicity and the emerging evidence of possible promotion or predisposition to the development of heart diseases of methylmercury, a worldwide contaminant found in seafood and freshwater fish. The relationship between the benefits and risks associated with fish and seafood consumption is an important public health issue. On one hand, fish and seafood provide an important pathway for human exposures because of the biomagnifications of methylmercury in freshwater and marine food chains. On the other, fish contains essential nutrients that may provide beneficial effects on brain development and prevent cardio-vascular disease, thereby counteracting the adverse effects of methylmercury (Anonymous, 2007).

With regard to existing research studies, these effects in opposite directions have served to bias the observed methylmercury toxicity toward lower and less apparent levels (Budtz-Jørgensen et al., 2007). These adverse effects are likely to occur even at exposures thought to be fairly low. The developing human brain is inherently more susceptible to injury caused by toxic agents such as methylmer-cury than is the brain of the adult, and neurodevelopmental disorders can cause lifelong disability (Grandjean and Landrigan, 2006). In terms of public health relevance, even a subtle delay in mental development may be important, espe-cially because vast populations may be affected. The Faroes study showed that each doubling in prenatal methylmercury exposure corresponded to a delay of one or two months in mental development at age seven years (Grandjean et al., 1997), which may correspond to an approximate deficit of about 1.5 IQ points, had an IQ scale been used. A similar result was seen in the New Zealand study (Kjellström et al., 1989), while comparable adjusted data are not available from the Seychelles. Small shifts in a measure of the central tendency of the IQ dis-tribution may be associated with large changes in the tails of the distribution. The lesson from lead neurotoxicity suggests that such effects are likely to be permanent and that they may even become more apparent over time (Grandjean et al., 2005b). Although the evidence on cardiovascular effects of methylmercury is less certain, it suggests that avoidance of increased methylmercury exposure would be a safe and prudent strategy for the population at large. Occupational exposure to elemental mercury has been found to alter certain immune parame-ters (NRC, 2000). A recent study found an inverse association between prenatal methylmercury exposure and grass-specific IgE levels (an indicator of allergic sensitization) and a positive but weak association with total IgE concentrations (Grandjean et al., 2010).

Most observational studies in this field have focused either on the risk of methylmercury or on nutrient benefits. Future studies should assess both beneficial and adverse effects of fish and seafood intake, taking into account the species consumed and the consumption frequency at the same time to separate opposite impacts of the outcome. Two key messages should be clarified—first, fish and seafood provide beneficial nutrients, and the fish that are high in LCPUFA should be favored; second, advisories against methylmercury exposure should emphasize that the contamination is the greatest in larger and older fish, especially in species high in the food chain and in those originating from contaminated waters. The ratio of LCPUFA and methylmercury concentration in individual fish and seafood species varies considerably (Mahaffey, 2004; NAS/NRC, 2006). Fortunately, certain types of fish and seafood have a high content of beneficial nutrients but do not necessarily contain much methylmercury (Table 17.2). Consumption of fish with low levels of methylmercury and organic contaminants and high levels of ω-3 fatty acids constitute a "win win" situation and should be encouraged regardless of the

TABLE 17.2 Concentrations of the Long-Chain ω-3 fatty acids (Eicosapentaenoic and Docosahexaenoic Acid) in Fish and Shellfish Commonly Consumed in the United States and their Corresponding Mean Hg Concentrations

Species	EPA + DHA mg/100 g Fish	Mercury mg/1000 g Fish
Mackerel (except King)	1790	0.09–0.22
Salmon	1590	0.04–0.13
Sardines	980	0.02–0.03
Bass (freshwater)	640	0.38
Tuna (all, average)	630	0.24–0.48
Canned light (skipjack)	270	0.11–0.12
Canned white (albacore)	862	0.35–0.37
Trout	580	0.14–0.15
Swordfish	580	0.98–1.03
Walleye	530	0.52
Seabass	490	0.14–0.22
Mackerel, King	401	0.73–1.06
Shrimp	390	0.03–0.04
Crayfish	380	0.03
Lobster	360	0.10–0.28
Oysters	350	0.01–0.07
Mussels	350	0.03–0.08
Other shellfish	310	Not applicable
Perch	300	0.09–0.11
Catfish	280	0.16
Scallops	270	0.05
Pollock	260	0.02–0.06
Clams	240	0.01–0.06
Cod	240	0.06–0.11
Shark	220	0.75–0.99
Haddock	180	0.03–0.06
Pike	140	0.31

Ranges in Hg concentrations shown represent variability in sample means across different harvesting regions (Mahaffey et al., 2011).

underlying nature of the ω-3-methylmercury interaction (Mergler et al., 2007). Regulatory agencies therefore need to develop risk communication strategies for balanced messages regarding nutrients and mercury to assist the consumers in making this choice (Grandjean et al., 2005b).

REFERENCES

Akman M, Cebeci D, Okur V, Angin H, Abali O, Akman AC. The effects of iron deficiency on infants' developmental test performance. Acta Paediatr 2004;93:1391–1396.

Andrews NC. Disorders of iron metabolism. N Engl J Med 2000;341:1986–1995.

[Anonymous]. The Madison declaration on mercury pollution. Ambio 2007;36:62.

Bakir F, Damluji SF, Amin-Zaki L, Murtadha M, Khalidi A, Al-Rawi NY, Tikritia S, Dahahir HI, Clarkson TW, Smith JC, Doherty RA. Methylmercury poisoning in Iraq. Science 1973;181:230–241.

Berglund M, Lind B, Bjornberg KA, Palm B, Einarsson O, Vahter M. Inter-individual variations of human mercury exposure biomarkers: a cross-sectional assessment. Environ Health 2005;4:20.

Beyrouty P, Chan HM. Co-consumption of selenium and vitamin E altered the reproductive and developmental toxicity of methylmercury in rats. Neurotoxicol Teratol 2006;28:49–58.

Bleichrodt N, Born MP. A metaanalysis of research on iodine and its relationship to cognitive development. In: Stanbury JB, editor. The damaged brain of iodine deficiency. New York (NY): Cognizant Communication; 1994. p 195–200.

Bourre JM, Dumont O, Piciotti M, Pascal G, Durand G. Polyunsaturated fatty acids of the n-3 series and nervous system development. In: Galli C and Simopoulos AP, editors. Dietary ω3 and ω6 fatty acids, biological effects and nutritional essentiality. New York (NY): Plenum Press; 1989. p 159–175.

Budtz-Jørgensen E, Debes F, Weihe P, Grandjean P. Structural equation models for meta-analysis in environmental risk assessment. Environmetrics 2010;21:510–527.

Budtz-Jørgensen E, Grandjean P, Weihe P. Separation of risks and benefits of seafood intake. Environ Health Perspect 2007;115:323–327.

Budtz-Jørgensen E, Keiding N, Grandjean P, Weihe P, White RF. Consequences of exposure measurement error for confounder identification in environmental epidemiology. Stat Med 2003;22:3089–3100.

Burr ML, Fehily AM, Gilbert JF, Rogers S, Holliday RM, Sweetnam PM, Elwood PC, Deadman NM. Effects of changes in fat, fish, and fibre intakes on death and myocardial reinfarction: diet and reinfarction trial (DART). Lancet 1989;2:757–761.

Cernichiari E, Brewer R, Myers GJ, Marsh DO, Lapham LW, Cox C, Shamlaye CF, Berlin M, Davidson PW, Clarkson TW. Monitoring methylmercury during pregnancy: maternal hair predicts fetal brain exposure. Neurotoxicol 1995;16:711–716.

Chen J, Berry MJ. Selenium and selenoproteins in the brain and brain diseases. J Neurochem 2003;86:12.

Cheuk DK, Wong V. Attention-deficit hyperactivity disorder and blood mercury level: a case-control study in Chinese children. Neuropediatrics 2006;37:234–240.

Choi AL, Budtz-Jørgensen E, Jørgensen PJ, Steuerwald U, Debes F, Weihe P, Grandjean P. Selenium as a potential protective factor against mercury developmental neurotoxicity. Environ Res 2008;107:45–52.

Choi MH, Cech JJ. Unexpectedly high mercury level in pelleted commercial fish feed. Environ Toxicol Chem 1998;17:1979–1981.

Choi AL, Cordier S, Weihe P, Grandjean P. Negative confounding in the evaluation of toxicity: the case of methylmercury in fish and seafood. Crit Rev Toxicol 2008;38:877–893.

Choi AL, Weihe P, Budtz-Jørgensen E, Jørgensen PJ, Salonen JT, Tuomainen TP, Murata K, Nielsen HP, Petersen MS, Askham J, Grandjean P. Methylmercury exposure and adverse cardiovascular effects in Faroese whaling men. Environ Health Perspect 2009;117:367–372.

Choy CMY, Lam WK, Cheung LTF, Briton-Jones CM, Cheung LP, Haines CJ. haines, infertility, blood mercury concentrations and dietary seafood consumption: A case-control study. Br J Obstet Gynaecol 2002;109:1121–1125.

Connor WE. Importance of n-3 fatty acids in health and disease. Am J Clin Nutr 2000;71(Suppl): 171S–175S.

Cordier S, Garel M, Mandereau L, Morcel H, Doineau P, Gosme-Seguret S, Josse D, White R, Amiel-Tison C. Neurodevelopmental investigations among methylmercury-exposed children in French Guiana. Environ Res 2002;89:1–11.

Cordier S, Grasmick C, Passelaigue MP, Mandereau L, Weber JP, Jouan M. Mercury exposure in French Guiana: levels and determinants. Arch Environ Health 1998;53:209–303.

Danesh J, Appleby P. Coronary heart disease and iron status: meta-analyses of prospective studies. Circulation 1999;99:852–854.

Daniels JL, Longnecker MP, Rowland AS, Golding J, ALSPAC Study Team. Fish intake during pregnancy and early cognitive development of offspring. Epidemiology 2004;15:394–402.

Davidson PW, Kost J, Myers GJ, Cox C, Clarkson TW. Methylmercury and neurodevelopment: reanalysis of the Seychelles Child Development Study outcomes at 66 Months of age. JAMA 2001;285:1291–1293.

Davidson PW, Myers GJ, Cox C, Wilding GE, Shamlaye CF, Huang LS, Cernichiari E, Sloane-Reeves J, Palumbo D, Clarkson TW. Methylmercury and neurodevelopment: longitudinal analysis of the Seychelles child development cohort. Neurotoxicol Teratol 2006;28:529–535.

Debes F, Budtz-Jørgensen, Weihe P, White RF, Grandjean P. Impact of prenatal methylmercury exposure on neurobehavioral function at 14 years. Neurotoxicol Teratol 2006;28:363–375.

Delange F. The role of iodine in brain development. Proc Nutr Soc 2000;59:75–79.

Dorea J, Barbosa AC, Ferrari I, de Souza JR. Mercury in hair and in fish consumed by Riparian women of the Rio Negro, Amazon, Brazil. Int J Environ Health Res 2003;13:239–248.

EFSA (European Food Safety Authority). 2006. Opinion of the scientific panel on contaminants in the food chain [CONTAM] related to the safety assessment of wild and farmed fish. Available at http://www.efsa.europa.eu/EFSA/efsa_locale-1178620753812_1178620762697.htm. Accessed 2007 Apr 17.

Ganther HE, Goudie C, Kopecky MJ, Wagner P, Oh SH, Hoekstra WG. Selenium, relation to decreased toxicity of methylmercury added to diets containing tuna. Science 1972;175:1122–1124.

GISSI-Prevenzione Investigators. Dietary supplementation with n-3 polyunsaturated fatty acids and vitamin E after myocardial infarction: results of the GISSI-Prevenzione trial. Lancet 1999;354:447–455.

Grandjean P, Budtz-Jørgensen E. Total imprecision of exposure biomarkers: implications for calculating exposure limits. Am J Ind Med 2007;50:712–719.

Grandjean P, Budtz-Jørgensen E. An ignored risk factor in toxicology: the total imprecision of exposure assessment. Pure Appl Chem 2010;82(2):383–391.

Grandjean P, Budtz-Jørgensen E, Jørgensen PJ, Weihe P. Umbilicial cord mercury concentration as biomarker of prenatal exposure to methylmercury. Environ Health Perspect 2005a;113:905–908.

Grandjean P, Landrigan P. Developmental neurotoxicity of industrial chemicals. Lanet 2006;368:2167–2178.

Grandjean P, Cordier S, Kjellström T, Weihe P, Budtz-Jørgensen E. Health effects and risk assessments. In: Pirrone N, Mahaffey KR, editors. Dynamics of mercury pollution on regional and global scales: atmospheric processes and human exposures around the world. Norwell (MA): Springer; 2005b. p 499–523.

Grandjean P, Budtz-Jørgensen E, Keiding N, Weihe P. Underestimation of risk due to exposure misclassification. Eur J Oncol Suppl 2003;2:165–172.

Grandjean P, Budtz-Jørgensen E, White RF, Jørgensen PJ, Weihe P, Debes F, Keiding N. Methylmercury exposure biomarkers as indicators of neurotoxicity in children aged 7 Years. Am J Epidemiol 1999;14:301–305.

Grandjean P, Jørgensen PJ, Weihe P. Validity of mercury exposure biomarkers. In: Wilson SH, Suk WA, editors. Biomarkers of environmentally associated disease. Boca Raton (FL): CRC Press/Lewis Publishers; 2002. p 235–247.

Grandjean P, Poulsen LK, Heilmann C, Steuerwald U, Weihe P. Allergy and sensitization during childhood associated with prenatal and lactational exposure to marine pollutants. Environ Health Perspect 2010;118:1429–1433.

Grandjean P, Satoh H, Murata K, Eto K. Adverse effects of methylmercury: environmental health research implications. Environ Health Perspect 2010;118:1137–1145.

Grandjean P, Weihe P, Jorgensen PJ, Clarkson T, Cernichiari E, Videro T. Impact of maternal seafood diet on fetal exposure to mercury, selenium and lead. Arch Environ Health 1992;47:185–195.

Grandjean P, Weihe P, White RF, Debes F, Araki S, Yokoyama K, Murata K, Sorensen N, Dahl R, Jorgensen PJ. Cognitive deficit in 7-year-old children with prenatal exposure to methylmercury. Neurotoxicol Teratol 1997;19:417–428.

Grandjean P, White R, Nielsen A, Cleary D, de Oliveira Santos E. Methylmercury neuro-toxicity in Amazonian children downstream from gold mining. Environ Health Perspect 1999;107:587–591.

Guallar E, Sanz-Gallardo I, van't Veer P, Bode P, Aro A, Gomez-Aracena J, Kark JD, Riemersma RA, Marint-Mereno JM, Kok FJ. Mercury, fish oils, and the risk of myocar-dial infarction. N Engl J Med 2002;347:1747–1754.

Hallegren CG, Hallmans G, Jansson JH, Marklund SL, Huhtasaari F, Schutz A, Stromberg U, Vessby B, Skerfving S. Markers of high fish intake are associated with decreased risk of a first myocardial infarction. Br J Nutr 2001;86:397–404.

Hamada R, Yoshida Y, Kuwano A, Mishima I, Igata A. Auditory brainstem responses in fetal organic mercury poisoning (in Japanese). Shinkei-Naika 1982;16:282–285.

Harada M. Minamata disease: methylmercury poisoning in Japan caused by environmental pollution. Crit Rev Toxicol 1995;25:1–24.

Harper CR, Jacobson TA. Usefulness of omega-3 fatty acids and the prevention of coro-nary heart disease. Am J Cardiol 2005;96:1521–1529.

Hearn TL, Sgoutas SA, Hearn JA, Sgoutas DS. Polyunsaturated fatty acids and fat in fish flesh for selecting species for health benefits. J Food Sci 1987;52:1209–1211.

Hibbeln JR, Davis JM, Steer C, Emmett P, Rogers I, Williams C, Golding J. Maternal seafood consumption in pregnancy and neurodevelopmental outcomes in childhood (ALSPAC study): an observational cohort study. Lancet 2007;369:578–585.

Hightower J, Moore D. Mercury levels in high-end consumers of fish. Environ Health Perspect 2003;111:604–608.

Innis SM, Palaty J, Vaghri Z, Lockitch G. Increased levels of mercury associated with high fish intakes among children from Vancouver, Canada. J Pediatr 2006;148:759–763.

IOM/NAS (Institute of Medicine/National Academy of Sciences) Food and Nutrition Board. Seafood choices: balancing benefits and risks. Washington (DC): The National Academies Press; 2007.

Ip P, Wong V, Ho M, Lee J, Wong W. Environmental mercury exposure in children: south china's experience. Pediatr Int 2004;46:715–721.

IPCS (International Programme on Chemical Safety). Environmental Health Criteria 101: Methylmercury. Geneva: World Health Organization; 1990.

Jedrychowski W, Jankowski J, Flak E, Skarupa A, Mroz E, Sochacka-Tatara E, Lisowska-Miszczyk I, Szpanowska-Wohn A, Rauh V, Skolicki Z, Kaim I, Perera F. Effects of prenatal exposure to mercury on cognitive and psychomotor function in one-year-old infants: epidemiologic cohort study in Poland. Ann Epidemiol 2006;16:439–447.

Keating MH, Mahaffey KR, Schoeny R, Rice GE, Bullock OR, Ambrose RB, Swartout J, Nocolas JW. Mercury Study Report to Congress, Vol. III: fate and transport of mercury in the environment. Office of Air Quality Planning and Standards and Office of Research and Development, US Environmental Protection Agency, Washington, DC: Environmental Protection Agency; 1997. EPA-452/R-97-005.

Kinsella JE, Lokesh B, Stone RA. Dietary ω-3 polyunsaturated fatty acids and amelioration of cardiovascular disease: possible mechanisms. Am J Clin Nutr 1990;52:1–28.

Kjellström T, Kennedy TP, Wallis S. Physical and mental development of children with prenatal exposure to mercury from fish. Stage 2, interviews and psychological tests at age 6. Stockholm: National Swedish Environmental Protection Board; 1989. 3642.

Kjellström T, Kennedy TP, Wallis S, Mantell C. Physical and mental development of children with prenatal exposure to mercury from fish. State 1: preliminary tests at age 4. Stockholm: National Swedish Environmental Protection Board; 1986. 3080.

Kris-Etherton PM, Harris WS, Appel LJ. Fish consumption, fish oil, omega-3 fatty acids, and cardiovascular disease. Circulation 2002;106:2747–2757.

Kromhout D, Giltay EJ, Geleijnse JM, Alpha Omega Trial Group. n-3 fatty acids and cardiovascular events. N Engl J Med 2010;363(21):2015–2026.

Lindberg A, Bjornberg KA, Berglund M. Exposure to methylmercury in non-fish-eating people in Sweden. Environ Res 2004;96:28–33.

Lozoff B, Brittenham GM, Wolf AW, McClish DK, Kuhnert PM, Jimenez E, Jimenez R, Mora LA, Gomes I, Krauskoph D. Iron deficiency anemia and iron therapy effects on infant developmental test performance. Pediatr 1987;79:981–995.

Lucas A, Morley R, Cole TJ, Lister G, Leeson-Payne C. Breast milk and subsequent intelligence quotient in children born preterm. Lancet 1992;339:261–264.

Ma J, Stampfer MJ. Body iron stores and coronary heart disease. Clin Chem 2002;48:601–603.

Maberly GF. Iodine deficiency disorders: contemporary scientific issues. J Nutr 1994;124: 1473S–1478S.

Mahaffey KR. Fish and shellfish as dietary sources of methylmercury and the ω-3 fatty acids, eicosahexaenoic acid and docosahexaenoic acid: risks and benefits. Environ Res 2004;95:414–428.

Mahaffey KR, Choeny R. Maternal seafood consumption and children's development. Lancet 2007;370:216–217.

Mahaffey KR, Clickner RP, Jeffries RA. Methylmercury and omega-3 fatty acids: co-occurrence of dietary sources with emphasis on fish and shellfish. Environ Res 2008;107:20–29.

Mahaffey KR, Sunderland EM, Chan HM, Choi AL, Grandjean P, Mariën K, Oken E, Sakamoto M, Schoeny R, Weihe P, Yan CH, Yautake A. Balancing the benefits of n-3 polyunsaturated fatty acids and the risks of methylmercury exposure from fish consumption. Nutr Rev 2011;69:493-5-8.

Marsh DO, Turner MD, Smith JC, Perez VMH, Allen P, Richdale N. Fetal Methylmercury study in a Peruvian fish eating population. Neurotoxicity 1995;16:717–726.

Mergler D, Anderson HA, Chan LHM, Mahaffey KR, Murray M, Sakamoto M, Stern AH. Methylmercury exposure and health effects in humans: a worldwide concern. Ambio 2007;36:3.

Morreale de Escobar G, Ruiz de Oña C, Obregón MJ, Escobar del Rey F. Models of fetal iodine deficiency. In: Delong GR, Robbins J, Condliffe PG, editors. Iodine and the brain. New York (NY): Plenum Press; 1989. p 187–201.

Mozaffarian D, Rimm EB. Fish intake, contaminants, and human health. JAMA 2006;296:1885–1899.

Murata K, Weihe P, Araki S, Budtz-Jørgensen E, Grandjean P. Evoked potentials in Faroese children prenatally exposed to methylmercury. Neurotoxicol Teratol 1999a;2:471–472.

Murata K, Weihe P, Renzoni A, Debes F, Vasconcelos R, Zino F, Araki S, Jørgensen PJ, White RF, Grandjean P. Delayed evoked potentials in children exposed to methylmercury from seafood. Neurotoxicol Teratol 1999b;21:343–348.

Murata K, Weihe P, Budtz-Jørgensen E, Jørgensen PJ, Grandjean P. Delayed brainstem auditory evoked potential latencies in 14-year-old children exposed to methylmercury. J Pediatr 2004;144:177–183.

Myers GJ, Davidson PW, Cox C, Shamlaye CF, Palumbo D, Cernichiari E, Sloane-Reeves J, Wilding GE, Kost J, Huang LS, Clarkson TW. Prenatal methylmercury exposure from ocean fish consumption in the Seychelles Child Development Study. Lancet 2003;361:1686–1692.

Myers GJ, Davidson PW, Cox C, Shamlaye CF, Tanner MA, Marsh DO, Cernichiari E, Lapham LW, Berlin M, Clarkson TW. Summary of the Seychelles child development study on the relationship of fetal methylmercury exposure to neurodevelopment. Neurotoxicology 1995;16:711–716.

Myers GJ, Davidson PW, Strain JJ. Nutrient and methyl mercury exposure from consuming fish. J Nutr 2007;137:2805–2808.

NAS/NRC. Dietary reference intakes for energy, carbohydrate, fiber, fat, fatty acids, cholesterol, protein, and amino acids (macronutrients). Washington (DC): National Academy of Sciences/National Research Council; 2005.

NAS/NRC. Seafood choices: balancing benefits and risks. Washington (DC): National Academy of Sciences/National Research Council; 2006.

NIEHS. 1998. Workshop organized by the Committee on Environmental and Natural Resources (CENR), Office of Science and Technology Policy (OSTP), The White House: scientific issues relevant to assessment of health effects from exposure to methylmercury. Available at http://ntp.niehs.nih.gov/index.cfm?objectid = 03614B65-BC68-D231 4E915F93AF9A6872#execsumm. Accessed 2007 Apr 16.

Nilsen DW, Albrekten G, Landmark K, Moen S, Aarsland T, Woie L. Effects of a high-dose concentrate of n-3 fatty acids or corn oil introduced early after an acute myocardial infarction on serum triacylglycerol and HDL cholesterol. Am J Clin Nutr 2001;74:50–56.

NRC (National Research Council). Toxicological effects of methylmercury. Washington (DC): National Academy Press; 2000.

Ohno T, Sakamoto M, Kurosawa T, Dakeishi M, Iwata T, Murata K. Total mercury levels in hair, toenail and urine among women free from occupational exposure and their relations to tubular renal functions. Environ Res 2007;103:191–197.

Oken E, Wright RO, Kleinman KP, Bellinger D, Amarasiriwardena CJ, Hu H, Rich-Edwards JW, Gillman MW. Maternal fish consumption, hair mercury, and infant cognition in a U.S. cohort. Environ Health Perspect 2005;113:376–1380.

Pawlosky RJ, Hibbeln JR, Novotny JA, Salem Jr N. Physiological compartmental analysis of alpha-linolenic acid metabolism in adult humans. J Lipid Res 2001;42:1257–1265.

Pollitt E. Iron deficiency and cognitive function. Annu Rev Nutr 1993;13:521–537.

Raper NR, Cronin FJ, Exler J. Omega-3 fatty acid content of the US food supply. J Am Coll Nutr 1992;11:304–308.

Rayman MP. The importance of selenium to human health. Lancet 2000;356:233–241.

Rissanen T, Voutilainen S, Nyyssonen K, Lakka TA, Salonen JT. Fish oil-derived fatty acids, docosahexaeonoic acid and docosapentaeonoic acid, and the risk of acute coronary events: the Kuopio ischaemic heart disease risk factor study. Circulation 2000;102:2677–2679.

Sacks FM, Stone PH, Gibson CM, Siverman DI, Rosner B, Pasternak RC. Controlled trial of fish oil for regression of human coronary atherosclerosis. HARP Research Group. J Am Coll Cardiol 1995;25:1492–1498.

Saldeen TG, Mehta JL. Dietary modulations in the prevention of coronary artery disease: a special emphasis on vitamins and fish oil. Curr Opin Cardiol 2002;17:559–567.

Salonen JT, Nyyssönen K, Korpela H, Tuomilehto J, Seppänen R, Salonen R. High stored iron levels are associated with excess risk of myocardial infarction in eastern Finnish men. Circulation 1992;86:803–811.

Salonen JT, Salonen R, Seppänen K, Kantola M, Suntioinen S, Korpela H. Interactions of serum copper, selenium, and low density lipoprotein cholesterol in atherogenesis. Br Med J 1991;302:756–760.

Salonen JT, Seppänen K, Lakka TA, Salonen R, Kaplan G. Mercury accumulation and accelerated progression of carotid atherosclerosis: a population-based prospective 4-year follow-up study in men in eastern Finland. Atherosclerosis 2000;148:265–273.

Salonen JT, Seppänen K, Nyyssönen K, Korpela H, Kauhanen J, Kantola M, Tuomilehto J, Esterbauer H, Tatzber F, Salonen R. Intake of mercury from fish, lipid, peroxidation, and the risk of myocardial infarction and coronary, cardiovascular, and any deaths in eastern Finnish men. Circulation 1995;91:645–655.

Sempos CT, Looker AC, Gillum RF, Makuc DM. Body iron stores and the risk of coronary heart disease. N Engl J Med 1994;330:1119–1124.

Shamlaye CF, Marsh DO, Myers GJ, Cox C, Davidson PW, Choisy O, Cernichiari E, Choi A, Tanner MA, Clarkson TW. The Seychelles child development study on neurodevelopmental outcomes in children following in utero exposure to methylmercury from a maternal fish diet: background and demographics. Neurotoxicol 1995;16:597–612.

Sweeney M, Peck K, Schantz L, Gardiner C, Gasior M, Batizy H, Fitzpatrick D, Kostyniak J. Contaminant profiles in southeast Asian immigrants consuming fish from Northeastern Wisconsin waters. Epidemiol 2006;17(Suppl):S340.

Steuerwald U, Weihe P, Jørgensen PJ, Bjerve K, Brock J, Heinzow B, Budtz-Jørgensen, Grandjean P 2000. Maternal seafood diet, methylmercury exposure, and neonatal neurologic function. J Pediatr 136:599–605.

Strain JJ, Davidson PW, Bonham MP, Duffy EM, Stokes-Riner A, Thurston SW, Wallace JMW, Robson PJ, Shamlaye CF, Georger LA, Sloan-Reeves J, Cernichiari E, Canfield RL, Cox C, Huang LS, Janciuras J, Myers GJ, Clarkson TW. Associations of maternal long-chain polyunsaturated fatty acids, methyl mercury, and infant development in the Seychelles Child Development Nutrition Study. Neurotoxicol 2008;29:776–782.

US Environmental Protection Agency (US EPA). 2004. National listing of fish advisories. Available at http://www.epa.gov/waterscience/fish/advisories/fs2004.pdf. Accessed 2007 Mar 2.

Virtanen JK, Voutilainen S, Rissanen TH, Mursu J, Tuomainen TP, Korhonen MJ, Volkonen VP, Seppänen K, Laukkanen JA, Salonen JT. Mercury, fish oils, and risk of acute coronary events and cardiovascular disease, coronary heart disease, and all-cause mortality in men in eastern Finland. Arterioscler Thromb Vasc Biol 2005;25:228–233.

Von Schacky C, Angerer P, Kothny W, Theisen K, Mudra H. The effect of dietary ω-3 fatty acids on coronary atherosclerosis: a randomized, double-blind, placebo-controlled trial. Ann Intern Med 1999;130:554–562.

Watanabe C. Modification of mercury toxicity by selenium: practical importance? Tohoku J Exp Med 2002;80:71–77.

Whanger PD. Selenium and the brain: a review. Nutr Neurosci 2001;4:81–97.

Willatts P, Forsyth JS. The role of long-chain polyunsaturated fatty acids in infant cognitive development. Prostaglandins Leukot Essent Fatty Acids 2000;63:95–100.

Yamamoto R, Suzuki T. Effects of artificial hair-waving on hair mercury values. Int Arch Occup Environ Health 1978;42:1–9.

Yasutake A, Matsumoto M, Yamaguchi M, Hachiya N. Current hair mercury levels in the Japanese: survey in five districts. Tohoku J Exp Med 2003;199:161–169.

Yoshizawa K, Rimm EB, Morris JS, Spate VL, Hsieh CC, Spiegelman D, Stampfer MJ, Willet WC. Mercury and the risk of coronary heart disease in men. New Engl J Med 2002;347:1755–1760.

Ysart G, Miller P, Croasdale M, Crews H, Robb P, Baxter M, de L'Argy C, Harrison N. 1997 UK Total Diet Study–dietary exposures to aluminium, arsenic, cadmium, chromium, copper, lead, mercury, nickel, selenium, tin, and zinc. Food Addit Contam 2000;17:775–786.

Zhang H, Feng X, Larssen T, Qui G, Vogt RD. In inland China, rice, rather than fish, is the major pathway for methylmercury exposure. Environ Health Perspect 2010;118:1183–1188.

INDEX

Environmental Chemistry and Toxicology of Mercury, First Edition.
Edited by Guangliang Liu, Yong Cai, and Nelson O'Driscoll.
© 2012 John Wiley & Sons, Inc. Published 2012 by John Wiley & Sons, Inc.

569

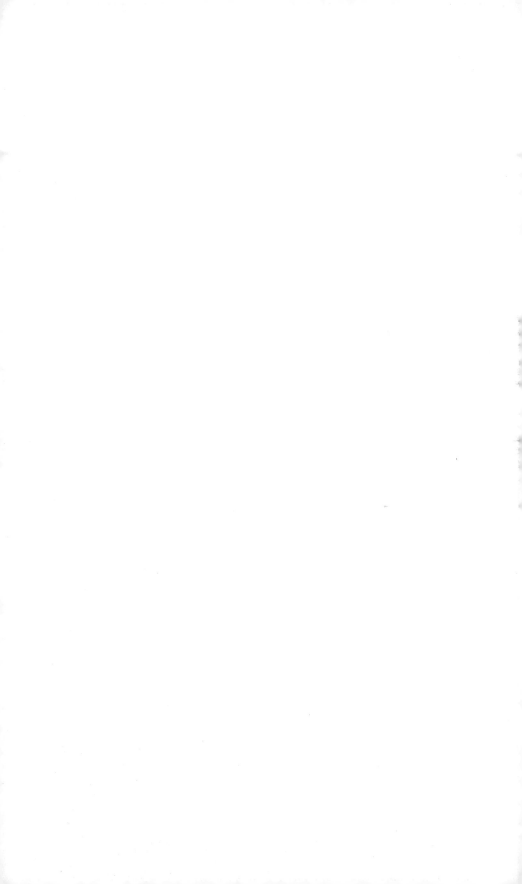